Instructor's Manual and Testbank to Accompany Brunner and Suddarth's Textbook of Medical-Surgical Nursing

Ninth Edition

INSTRUCTOR'S MANUAL
Mary Jo Boyer, RN, D.N.Sc.
Dean
Allied Health and Nursing
Delaware County Community College
Media, Pennsylvania

TESTBANK
Karen L. Cobb, RN, EdD
Associate Professor of Nursing
Indiana University School of Nursing
Indianapolis, Indiana

GUIDELINES FOR CRITICAL THINKING AND TESTBANK
Katherine H. Dimmock, RN, MSN, EdD, JD
Former Associate Professor of Nursing
University of Indianapolis
Indianapolis, Indiana

Visit Lippincott's Nursing Center Website at:
http://www.nursingcenter.com/booklink

Visit the Lippincott Williams & Wilkins Website at:
http://www.lww.com

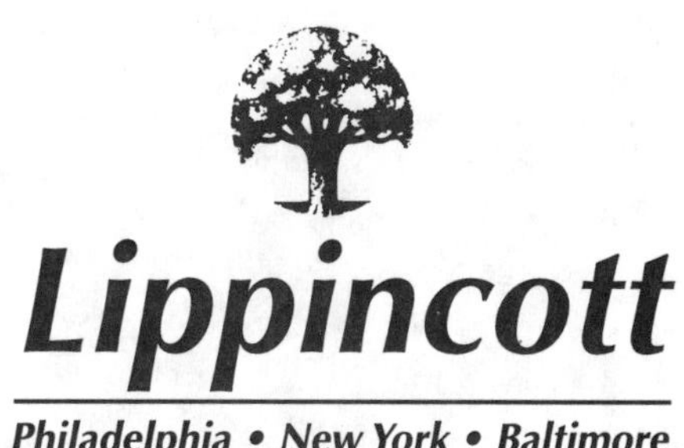

Ancillary Editor: *Doris S. Wray*
Production Service: *Pine Tree Composition, Inc.*
Printer/Binder: *Victor Graphics*

9th Edition

ISBN: 0–7817–2306–X

9 8 7 6 5 4 3 2 1

Introduction

This Instructor's Manual has been developed to accompany *Brunner and Suddarth's Textbook of Medical-Surgical Nursing, Ninth Edition.* As in previous editions of the Textbook, the ninth edition emphasizes the use of the nursing process as a framework for nursing practice. This Manual provides many suggestions for learning activities and experiences that assist students in understanding and applying the nursing process in caring for patients.

This Manual is organized to support the content of the Textbook. However, the replication of the Textbook's learning objectives and a content outline have purposely been omitted. The Learning Objectives Section has been designed to provide space for the faculty member to supplement each chapter with personal learning objectives that may be unique to a particular program of study. The section on Collaborative Learning Activities was designed to support the role of faculty as "learning facilitators" who engage students in collaborative learning activities both inside and outside the formal structure of a classroom setting. Team Discussion Questions/Seminar Topics encourage active, participatory student learning, a process that faculty are being challenged to measure under the title "classroom assessment."

An analytical approach to problem solving forms the basis for the section on Critical Thinking Exercises. Analysis, assimilation, and date-driven decision making are weaved throughout case studies and nursing care plans. This focus supports the National League of Nursing's mandate to assess and encourage critical thinking skills among students.

This Manual is designed to be used as a workbook for faculty to help supplement instructional delivery. Therefore, an Instructional Improvement Tool is provided for faculty at the end of every unit.

This Manual was written to be "user friendly," to help faculty create analytical and experiential learning activities for students. It was also designed to be a "time-saver" for faculty who are being challenged to do more with less, to do it better and to be more efficient in the process. I have brought a professional and personal perspective to this new format based on 14 years of teaching nursing students. I hope you find it useful and I hope it makes your teaching preparation time a little easier. Please let me know how you like it or how it could be improved.

Mary Jo Boyer, DNSc, RN

Contents

Unit 5: Gas Exchange and Respiratory Function 262

Unit 6: Cardiovascular, Circulatory, and Hematologic Function 265

Unit 7: Digestive and Gastrointestinal Function 270

Unit 8: Metabolic and Endocrine Function 272

Unit 9: Urinary and Renal Function 275

Unit 10: Reproductive Function 277

Unit 11: Immunologic Function 280

Unit 12: Integumentary Function 283

Unit 13: Sensorineural Function 284

SECTION 1

INSTRUCTOR'S MANUAL

UNIT I

BASIC CONCEPTS IN NURSING PRACTICE

1

Health Care Delivery and Nursing Practice

I. LEARNING OBJECTIVES

In addition to the learning objectives on page 3, I want my students to be able to:

1. ______________________________

2. ______________________________

3. ______________________________

II. TOP TERMS

1. Advanced Nursing Practice
2. Case Management
3. Clinical Pathways
4. Continuous Quality Improvement
5. Diagnosis Related Groups (DRGs)
6. Health Maintenance Organizations (HMOs)
7. Managed Health Care
8. Preferred Provider Organizations (PPOs)
9. Professional Standards Review Organizations (PSROs)
10. Wellness-Illness Continuum

III. COLLABORATIVE LEARNING ACTIVITIES

Team Discussion Questions/Seminar Topics

1. Have students discuss how current changes in managed care are affecting the delivery of nursing care in acute care, long-term care, and community-based health settings (reference pages 9–14).

Activities

Assign students to:

- choose a current journal or newpaper article and present a topical summary.
- interview a nursing administrator in each of three settings and present a summary of his or her perspective of the impact of HMOs and PPOs.
- create a vision of how managed care will influence nursing practice in the years 2000–2005.

2. Health care reform may increase the number of nurse-managed centers in the United States. Choose several teams of students to develop three arguments to counteract the American Medical Association's position that this movement will not be beneficial for patient care. Each team must use some form of documented data (statistics, research article, government document) to support one of their three arguments (reference pages 9–14).

IV. CRITICAL THINKING ACTIVITIES

In-Class Team Exercises

1. Assign students to work in groups of four or five per team. Each team should list every category of Maslow's needs and choose an example of patient behavior that reflects an unmet need for each category. Use the chart below and direct teams to share their results (reference pages 4–7 and Figure 1–1).

Physiologic (sample)	Talks incessantly about food (sample)

2. Choose one statement in the AHA's Patient's Bill of Rights and have a team of students argue in support and in opposition to the statement (reference pages 7–9, Chart 1–1).

Send-Home Assignments

Gathering data is the easiest way to begin problem solving in a continuous quality improvement cycle. Expose the students to this process by asking them to construct a check sheet similar to the following. Data should be recorded using the outline below (reference pages 7–11).

What to Observe: The frequency of nursing care events that you observe that can be improved.

Time Period: Eight clinical days

Categories: Individually chosen based on judgment and experiences.

SAMPLE CHECK SHEET
CQI

Giving Patient Information	1	2	3	4	5	6	7	8	Total
Total									

2

Community-Based Nursing Practice

I. LEARNING OBJECTIVES

In addition to the learning objectives on page 15, I want my students to be able to:

1. ______________________________

2. ______________________________

3. ______________________________

II. TOP TERMS

1. Community-Based Health Care
2. Community/Public Health Care
3. Diagnosis Related Groups (DRGs)
4. Health Maintenance Organizations (HMOs)
5. Home Health Care
6. Managed Health Care Systems
7. Nurse Managed Center
8. Nurse Practitioner
9. OSHA
10. Preferred Provider Organizations (PPOs)

III. COLLABORATIVE LEARNING ACTIVITIES

Team Discussion Questions/Seminar Topics

1. Require that students distinguish between the role, responsibilities, and scope of practice for community-based health care nurses and community/public health care nurses (reference pages 16–17).
2. Direct students to explain why accurate documentation is so important for reimbursement for home care services (reference page 17).
3. Ask students to compare the educational preparation, job responsibilities, and expanded role of a nurse practitioner and school nurse (reference page 20).

IV. CRITICAL THINKING ACTIVITIES

In-Class Team Exercises

1. Divide the class into teams of four. Each team should develop a home situation that reflects a safety problem that the community-based home care nurse might encounter during a visit—e.g., a family member is usually intoxicated when the nurse arrives. Each team should also present this situation and challenge the other students to develop creative ways to handle safety concerns (reference pages 16–20 and Chart 2–1).

Send-Home Assignments

1. Tell students to complete the following assessment outline by drafting four specific questions for each heading (reference pages 18–20).

Assessment Guide

Assessment of the need for continued home care visits for an 80-year-old who lives alone and is recovering from a prostectomy secondary to cancer. This is the second week of home care.

1. The patient's current health status:

   a. ______________________ c. ______________________

   b. ______________________ d. ______________________

2. The level of self-care abilities:

   a. ______________________ c. ______________________

   b. ______________________ d. ______________________

3. The level of nursing care needed:

   a. ______________________ c. ______________________

   b. ______________________ d. ______________________

4. Prognosis:

   a. ______________________ c. ______________________

   b. ______________________ d. ______________________

5. Patient education needs:

   a. ______________________ c. ______________________

   b. ______________________ d. ______________________

6. Mental status:

   a. ______________________ c. ______________________

   b. ______________________ d. ______________________

7. The home environment:

   a. ______________________ c. ______________________

   b. ______________________ d. ______________________

8. The level of adherence:

   a. ______________________ c. ______________________

   b. ______________________ d. ______________________

2. Assign the following case study. Direct students to choose one of the three options and prepare an argument to support their decision. Recommend that the "Guidelines" be used in their clinical practice.

Case Study: An Unsafe Discharge

A 72-year-old male patient was admitted to your institution with chest pain. He had a long history of untreated hypertension and alcohol abuse. Laboratory studies and serial ECGs reveal that the patient had suffered a myocardial infarction. A myocardial catheterization subsequently showed that he had severe three-vessel coronary artery disease, and he underwent a seven-vessel coronary artery bypass graft surgery seven days ago. Despite some persistent problems with an oozing saphenous vein graft wound and a mild pulmonary infiltrate, the patient is now ready for discharge.

Your problem is that this patient is homeless. It is midwinter, there are three inches of ice and slush on the ground, and the patient thinks that the shelter in which he usually stays is probably full because of the cold weather. The patient seems unconcerned about the weather; with prescriptions and a clinic appointment card in hand, he appears eager to leave. There is a prediction of a snowstorm within the next 48 hours, and the emergency department is full of patients waiting for a bed on your unit. What do you do?

Dilemma: The obligation to protect the patient from harm conflicts with the obligation to respect the patient's freedom (beneficence versus autonomy). The obligation to protect the patient from harm conflicts with the obligation to care for other patients (beneficence versus justice).

Option 1: Refuse to discharge the patient, or convince the physician to delay the discharge until the weather is better.

Rationale: The obligation to protect the patient from harm is more important than respecting the patient's autonomy or attending to the needs of other potential patients.

Implications of Choosing This Position: In these days of decreasing hospital reimbursement for underinsured patients, you may not be able to obtain a delay of this patient's discharge if the patient is medically ready for discharge. If you are able to postpone the discharge, however, remember that a delay does not remedy the underlying problem of the patient's homelessness. Additionally, this action serves the needs of this patient but ignores the needs of other patients needing medical care (the patients in the ER who require admission).

Option 2: Discharge the patient.

Rationale: Nurses do not have the resources to or the power to address complex social problems such as homelessness. The needs of the patients in the ER outweigh the needs of this one patient who is medically ready for discharge.

Implications of Choosing This Position: The patient will be at risk for hypothermia, fatigue, injury, and pneumonia. That patient's hospital bed will be available for another patient. The nurse feels powerless to intervene with such difficult problems.

Option 3, Potential Compromise: Discharge the patient with as much preparation as possible to help to ensure his well-being (e.g., a guaranteed spot in the shelter, appointment with a visiting nurse who will see him in the shelter, arrangements for food stamps or meals, a social contact, a cab ride to the shelter, sufficient clothing, prescriptions filled, etc.).

Rationale: The respect for the autonomy of the patient, the obligation to protect this patient from harm, and the obligation to care for future patients are the basis for this position.

Implications of Choosing This Position: This position tries to meet the needs of this patient as well as other patients in the ER who require hospital admission. The patient is still at risk for exposure and other medical problems; however, he is less at risk due to better planning and attention to detail.

Guidelines for the Nurse Preparing a Patient for a Risky Discharge

1. Assess every patient on admission for the ability to perform the activities of daily living, home situations and social (family, friends) support. Identify patients who are at-risk for an unsafe discharge (e.g., the patient who lives alone and is unable to care for himself; the patient who is confused and lives without supervision; the patient whose home environment is unsafe (abusive family, home is a fire hazard, or the patient has no home)) and make early referrals to the social worker.
2. Advance planning is essential for the patient with a potentially risky discharge. Initiate consultations with the social worker, physician, risk manager, and adult protective services as needed to assess the home situation and begin a discharge plan. A person who is aware of the resources available in the community, for example, a social worker, is invaluable. Be creative in pulling together available resources to meet the needs of the patient.
3. Consult with the physician to plan a discharge date that maximizes the benefits to the patient but also takes into consideration the needs of other patients (for needed hospital care).

Bibliography

Abramson, M. (1983, Fall). Model for Organizing an Ethical Analysis of the Discharge Planning Process. *Social Work in Health Care,* 9(1): 45–52.

Case Presentation 2: The Unsafe Hospital Discharge. (1990). HEC (Hospital Ethics Committee) Forum, 2(4): 279–284.

Cookfair, J. M. (1996). *Nursing Care in the Community* (2nd ed.). St. Louis: Mosby-Year Book.

Dubler, NN. (1988, June). Improving the Discharge Planning Process. Distinguishing Between Coercion and Choice. *The Gerontologist,* Supplement, 28(3): 76–81.

Johnson, J. Y., Smith-Temple, A. J., & Carr, P. (1998). *Nurses' Guide to Home Health Procedures.* Philadelphia: Lippincott, Williams, & Wilkens.

McNeal, G. J. (1996). High-Tech Home Care: An Expanding Critical Care Frontier. *Critical Care Nurse,* 16(5), 51–58.

Zotti, M. E., Brown, P., & Storts, R. C. (1996). Community-Based Nursing Versus Community Health Nursing, What Does It All Mean? *Nursing Outlook,* 44(5), 211–217.

3

Critical Thinking, Ethical Decision Making, and the Nursing Process

I. LEARNING OBJECTIVES

In addition to the learning objectives on page 22, I want my students to be able to:

1. ______________________________

2. ______________________________

3. ______________________________

II. TOP TERMS

1. Advanced Directives
2. Assessment
3. Collaborative Problems
4. Critical Thinking
5. Ethical Theories
6. Evaluation
7. Expected Outcomes
8. Implementation
9. Morality
10. Nursing Diagnosis
11. Nursing Goals
12. Preventive Ethics

III. COLLABORATIVE LEARNING ACTIVITIES

Team Discussion Questions/Seminar Topics

For each of the following nursing diagnoses, assign teams to choose goals and expected outcomes for each nursing action (reference pages 28–37 and Chart 3–5).

1. Activity intolerance related to leg pain associated with prolonged bed rest.

Goals: ______________________________

____

____

Expected Outcomes: ______________________________

____

____

2. Ineffective breathing patterns related to altered ventilatory capacity subsequent to recent chest trauma.

Goals: ______________________________

____

____

Expected Outcomes: ______________________________

____

____

3. Sleep pattern disturbances related to anxiety associated with a diagnosis of cancer.

Goals: ______________________________

____

____

Expected Outcomes: ______________________________

____

____

IV. CRITICAL THINKING ACTIVITIES

In-Class Team Exercises

Use Linda Carpenito's schematic that illustrates a decision-making tree for distinguishing nursing diagnoses from collaborative problems (page 34, Figure 3–2). Assign groups to fill in the appropriate blanks and compare their answers.

A Possible Problem with Circulation

The nurse can legally order the primary interventions.

Nursing Diagnoses:

1. ______________
2. ______________
3. ______________

Nursing Interventions for Prevention, Treatment, and Promotion:

1. ______________
2. ______________
3. ______________

Medical and Nursing Interventions Needed to Achieve Goals Such as:

1. ______________
2. ______________
3. ______________
4. ______________
5. ______________

Collaborative Problems That Prescribe, Monitor, Implement, and Evaluate:

1. ______________
2. ______________
3. ______________

Send-Home Assignments

Planning nursing care involves setting priorities and distinguishing problems that need urgent attention from those that can be deferred to a later time or referred to a physician. For each of the following patient care problems, ask each student to circle the **initial priority of nursing care** and write a rationale for that choice. Ask each student to be prepared to discuss collaborative problems that require physician consultation (pages 33–34).

1. Activity intolerance related to inadequate oxygenation.

   Problems: a. Dyspnea

   b. Fatigue

   c. Hypotension

   Rationale for choice: ______________________________

   ____

   ____

   ____

2. Alterations in bowel elimination: constipation, related to prolonged bed rest.

   Problems: a. Abdominal pressure and bloating

   b. Palpable impaction

   c. Straining at stool

   Rationale for choice: ______________________________

   ____

3. Altered oral mucous membrane related to stomatitis.

   Problems: a. Erythema of oral mucous

   b. Intolerance to hot foods

   c. Oral pain

   Rationale for choice: ______________________________

   ____

4

Health Education and Promotion

I. LEARNING OBJECTIVES

In addition to the learning objectives on page 40, I want my student to be able to:

1. ______________________________

2. ______________________________

3. ______________________________

II. TOP TERMS

1. Adherence
2. Experiential Readiness
3. Health Promotion
4. Learner Readiness
5. Learning Environment
6. Teaching–Learning Process

III. COLLABORATIVE LEARNING ACTIVITIES

Team Discussion Questions/Seminar Topics

1. Ask a team of students to elaborate on the statement that health education is "directed toward promotion, maintenance, and restoration of health, and the adaptation to prevention of illness" (reference page 41).
2. Ask students to compile a list of health promotion activities that each of them can do, while healthy, to maintain health (reference pages 47–48).

IV. CRITICAL THINKING EXERCISES

In-Class Team Exercises

1. Ask students to give specific examples, from their personal clinical experiences, of how patient education can:

   a. reduce costs of hospitalization

   ____

   ____

   ____

   b. decrease hospital lengths of stay

   ____

   ____

   ____

   c. avert malpractice suits

   ____

   ____

   ____

2. Ask students to identify specific criteria that they can evaluate to determine if non-adherence to a therapeutic regimen among the elderly leads to:

   a. increased morbidity

   ____

   ____

   b. increased mortality

   ____

   ____

   c. increased cost of treatment

   ____

   ____

Send-Home Assignments

1. Multiple factors influence a patient's adherence to a therapeutic regime for health promotion and maintenance. Ask each student to consider a recent clinical experience and identify variables for each category that influenced patient adherence (reference pages 41–43).

   a. Demographic variables:

   ____

   ____

   b. Illness variables:

   ____

   ____

c. Therapeutic regimen variables:

____

____

d. Psychosocial variables:

____

____

2. Ask students to identify realistic goals for each of the following nursing diagnoses. For each goal, students should write a relevant nursing action with supporting rationales and expected patient care outcomes. The following format should be used as a guide (reference pages 44–46).

Nursing Diagnosis: ______________________

Goals	Nursing Actions	Rationale	Expected Outcomes

a. Constipation related to an inadequate intake of fiber and water.
b. Decreased cardiac output related to enlargement of the heart compensatory to congestive failure.
c. Impairment of skin integrity related to full-thickness burns of the right hand.
d. Sleep pattern disturbances related to excess intake of caffeine in the early evening hours.

3. Assign the following case study. Direct students to choose one of the two options and prepare an argument to support their position. Recommend that the "Guidelines" be used in their clinical picture.

Case Study: Patient Competency

An 82-year-old patient is admitted to the hospital from home with a diagnosis of weakness and dehydration after a neighbor found her on the floor unable to get up. The patient has been living alone. On admission she is found to be slightly malnourished, unsteady on her feet, and occasionally confused and incontinent. The patient is treated with IV fluids and electrolytes and physical therapy. When she is unable to eat more that 800 calories per day, a feeding tube is inserted.

The patient is pleasant but has some short-term memory loss and is occasionally confused about time and place. She sometimes believes she is at home, and she tried to get out of bed once to go to the kitchen to get herself some dinner. She is unable to perform the activities of daily living without assistance and has pulled out the feeding tube three times despite wrist restraints. After several consultations with the patient's son, arrangements are made to admit the patient to a local nursing home. Her nutritional status remains a problem since she does not consume enough calories. The feeding tube was discontinued after she pulled it out a third time. The patient's son gives permission to the physician to insert a gastrostomy tube for feeding purposes so that his mother will be able to be admitted to a nursing home.

When the patient is taken to the operating room to have the gastrostomy tube inserted, the surgeon approaches her and asks her if she's ready for surgery. "I'm having surgery?" she asks. "What for?" The surgeon tells her that he is going to insert a feeding tube. "I don't want any tube in my stomach," the woman insists, "besides, I'm too old for surgery." When the surgeon insists and explains that she needs the feeding tube so that she will get enough food, the patient interrupts him. "I eat as much as I want to. No tube for me, thank you."

Should the feeding tube be inserted into this patient or not?

Dilemma: The obligation to respect the individual's autonomy conflicts with the obligation to do what is best for the patient (autonomy versus beneficence). The ability of the patient to be autonomous is at issue here: Is she able to understand the pertinent information about the issue and weigh the risks and the benefits of surgery? Competency is the legal term for the patient's ability to make decisions. Patients are legally assumed to be competent until in a court of law they are proved (with evidence such as physician testimony, psychiatric evidence, and observation) to be incompetent and a guardian is appointed.

Option 1: The surgery should proceed as planned.

Rationale: The patient is unable to make a rational decision. Her history of confusion and the fact that she has pulled out three feeding tubes despite restraints indicates that she may not be able to make rational decisions. The patient needs the gastrostomy tube in order to be admitted to the nursing home, and nursing home placement is necessary because she cannot safely live alone in her apartment. Beneficence outweighs autonomy here because the patient's autonomy is in question.

Implications of Choosing This Position: The evaluation of the patient's ability to make a decision does not meet accepted criteria for patient competency. A history of confusion and self-extubation are not in themselves proof that the patient is unable to make a rational decision. Therefore, if this position is chosen, it may tend to erode patient rights in this institution. The patient may be angry and uncooperative after the gastrostomy tube is inserted. The patient may pull out the gastrostomy tube and harm herself. The patient may experience side effects from the surgery, anesthesia, or tube insertion.

Option 2: The surgery should be delayed until the patient's ability to make an autonomous decision is evaluated further.

Rationale: The patient's comments indicate that she is able to comprehend some of the pertinent information about the issue at hand and that she is able—at least to some degree—to weigh the risks and the benefits of surgery. The patient is showing that she can make a rational decision, albeit one that conflicts with the decisions of her physician and her son. Procedures should not be performed on competent patients without their permission; therefore, the surgery should be postponed until the patient's ability to make a decision can be evaluated further (such as consultation with a psychiatrist). Postponing the surgery will pose no risk to the patient.

Implications of Choosing This Position: The patient's discharge planning may be made more difficult if a feeding tube is not inserted. Without a feeding tube, she may experience problems with malnutrition. This position tends to reinforce the primacy of autonomy and the protective legal standards for competency.

Guidelines for the Nurse Caring for a Patient Whose Ability to Make Rational Decisions Is in Question:

1. Assess the patient carefully. Determine the presence and degree of confusion, if any. Observe the patient's behavior. Is the patient cooperative and able to follow directions? Is the patient able to comprehend and manipulate information in a rational manner? Are there patterns of confusion? For example, is the confusion worse or present only at night?
2. Read the chart carefully and scrutinize the patient's course of treatment and past history. Is the patient's behavior consistent with her history? Is there a reason that the patient is confused or has memory problems, such as drug effect, hypoxia, or an electrolyte imbalance? Are advance directives present, and if so, what do they say?
3. Consider if the patient is being assumed to be unable to make rational decisions because she falls into a category of persons who are often subjected to discrimination. For example, is there evidence of ageism, sexism, racism, prejudice against a cultural practice, or a psychiatric problem? In the above case, for example, was the patient discriminated against because she is an elderly female with periods of mild confusion?

4. Consult with the physician to establish a plan of care that enables the patient to be as alert and conversive as possible. Collaborate with the physician to correct fluid and electrolyte imbalances and eliminate medications that may adversely affect the patient's cognitive abilities.
5. From a nursing perspective, ensure that communication with the patient is not a barrier to preserving the patient's rights. Utilize hearing aids, dentures, and interpreters if needed to maintain optimum communication with the patient. Consider a speech therapy evaluation, if appropriate. Try to ensure that evaluations of the patient's ability to make decisions are conducted at the best time of day for the patient, that is, a time when the patient is awake, alert, and not under the influence of sedatives or other medications that can cause drowsiness.
6. If the patient is clearly unable to comprehend information about a procedure and make a rational decision, make sure that the information is documented, for example, "Several attempts were made to explain to the patient that she requires surgery for a feed tube insertion; however, the patient was unable to repeat back to me either that she needed surgery or why. Her comments kept focusing on a friend she had as a child." When it is documented that the patient is clearly unable to make a decision, decision making then falls to the next of kin or the person named on the advance directive. No court proceeding is required.
7. If you find that your patient has been labeled as incompetent but in fact appears to you to be able to make rational decisions, document your observations. For example, "The patient was able to tell me that the doctor wants her to have a feeding tube because he thinks she does not eat enough, but that she thinks she eats enough for an old person and does not think she needs a tube for food." Notify the physician of your observations.
8. When a patient's competency is in question, a psychiatric consultation is invaluable to help evaluate the patient's abilities.
9. If there is a disagreement about a patient's ability to make decisions, arrange a patient care conference. If disagreement persists, consult with the Ethics Committee. Remember, the patient is legally considered competent until a court declares the patient otherwise. If disagreement persists, consult with the legal resources in your hospital about pursuing a court hearing for the patient.

Bibliography

Barry, R., & Burggraf, V. (1996). Healthy People: Objective Look at the Elderly. *Journal of Gerontological Nursing,* 22(10): 9–11.

Downie, R. S., Fyfe, C., & Tannahill, A. (1990). *Health Promotion: Models and Values.* New York: Oxford University Press.

Eliopoulos, C. (1997). *Gerontological Nursing.* Philadelphia: Lippincott, Williams, & Wilkins.

Jurchak, M. (1990, September). Competence and the Nurse-Patient Relationship. *Critical Care Nursing Clinics North America* 2(2): 453–459.

Lev, E. L., & Owen, S. V. (1996). A Measure of Self-Care Self-Efficacy: Strategies Used by People to Promote Health. *Research in Nursing & Health,* 19(5), 421–425.

Lidz, C. W., et al. (1983, October). Barriers to Informed Consent. *Annals of Internal Medicine,* 99(4): 539–543.

Perry, C. B., & Applegate, W. B. (1985, May). Medical Paternalism and Patient Self-Determination. *Journal of the American Geriatrics Society,* 33(4): 353–359.

Wheeler, L. (1991). Court Weights Fate of Woman Refusing Lifesaving Surgery. *The Washington Post,* February 8, p. C1.

5

Health Assessment

I. LEARNING OBJECTIVES

In addition to the learning objectives on page 51, I want my students to be able to:

1. ______________________________

2. ______________________________

3. ______________________________

II. TOP TERMS

1. Anthropometric
2. Body Mass Index (BMI)
3. Chief Complaint
4. Clinical Interview
5. Database
6. Food Guide Pyramid
7. Functional Status
8. Genogram
9. Ideal Body Weight
10. Midarm Circumference
11. Patient Profile
12. Systems Review
13. Triceps Skinfold Thickness

III. COLLABORATIVE LEARNING ACTIVITIES

Team Discussion Questions/Seminar Topics

1. Separate students into teams. Direct each team to develop a data sheet for obtaining a comprehensive health history that would be appropriate to use in a clinical setting. Include the components listed on pages 52–57 of the text and modify them as you feel necessary.
2. Take the nursing databases developed by each team. Assign one member from each team to interview a classmate from another team who assumes one on the following roles:
   a. An 18-year-old college student whose chief complaints are right lower quadrant pain, nausea, and a temperature of 102° F.

b. A 40-year-old mother of five whose chief complaint is tenderness and warmth in her left calf. She has calf pain with dorsiflexion and is unable to bear weight without pain.
c. An 82-year-old diabetic whose chief complaint is inability to walk because of a blackened great toe on his right foot.

3. Use the information obtained from each nursing database and conduct a complete physical assessment using pages 57–66 as a guide.

IV. CRITICAL THINKING ACTIVITIES

In-Class Team Exercises

Ask students to bring to class a completed Weekly Diary of Daily Food Intake using the Food Guide Pyramid (reference Figure 5–9, page 65—also included as an overhead transparency).

1. Encourage students to discuss their reactions to keeping the diary. What did they learn? How do they feel? Are they interested in modifying their diets?
2. Help students calculate their frame size using Chart 5–3 as a reference. Note: Several tape measures will be needed for this exercise.
3. Help students determine their Body Mass Index using Figure 5–8. This will show students whether they are at ideal body weight, overweight, or underweight.
4. Show students how to calculate their Ideal Body Weight (IBW) using Chart 5–2 as a reference.
5. Have each student estimate his or her daily caloric intake based on their IBW. Some will need to reduce calories while others will need to increase calories. Students can use these general steps for estimating daily caloric intake.
   a. Convert IBW in pounds to kilograms (÷2.2)

      ________ = ________
      IBW (lbs.) kg
      Example: 130 lbs. = 59 kg
   b. Basal energy needs = 1 Kcal/kg/hr. Therefore, multiply ___ kg × 24 hrs. = ______ calories.
      Example: 59 kg × 24 hours = 1,418 daily calories
   c. Increase by 40% for moderate activity levels (for students)

      ____________ × ____________ = ____________
      daily calories percent
      Example: 1,418 calories × 40% (moderate activity) = 1,985 calories
   d. Divide calories by percentage distribution of carbohydrate, fat, and protein
      Carbohydrate = 50% of ______ = ______ calories
      (50% of 1,985 = 992 calories)
      Fat = 30% of _____ = _______calories
      (30% of 1985 = 596 calories)
      Protein = 20% of ______ = ______calories
      (20% of 1985 = 397 calories)
   e. Estimate grams for each
      Carbohydrates ______ calories ÷ 4 gms/cal = _______ grams
      Fats ______ calories ÷ 9 gms/cal = _______ grams
      Protein ______ calories ÷ 4 gms/cal = _______ grams

Send-Home Assignments

1. Tell students to complete a weekly diary of their daily food intake, listing foods according to servings per food group. Ask students to estimate calories for each serving using a reference calorie book. Use the chart provided. The (#) refers to the number of servings per group and the (C) refers to calories.

DAY OF WEEK	M		T		W		T		F		S		S	
FOOD GROUP / Group/Servings/Calories	#	C	#	C	#	C	#	C	#	C	#	C	#	C
Bread, cereal, rice, pasta														
Fruit														
Vegetable														
Meat, poultry, fish														
Milk, yogurt, cheese														
Fats, oils, sweets														
Daily Totals														

2. Assign the following case study. Direct students to choose one of the three options and prepare an argument to support their position. Recommend that the "Guidelines" be used in their clinical practice.

Case Study: Confidentiality

A 35-year-old male patient is in your care on a medical floor of a general hospital. His diagnosis is pneumonia. Further tests reveal that the patient is HIV positive and that he has pneumocystis pneumonia, a sign of AIDS. Upon learning of his diagnosis, the patient becomes quite upset but reveals to you and the physician that he is bisexual and has been having unprotected sex with his lover and his wife. The physician urges the patient to notify his sexual partners that he is HIV positive. The patient promises that he will; but after the physician leaves the patient confides to you that he is afraid to inform his wife because of his fear that she will leave him if she learns that he is HIV positive.

Later that shift, a young woman eight months pregnant approaches you. She identifies herself as your patient's wife and demands to know more information about his illness. "I've never seen anyone so sick from pneumonia. What kind of pneumonia does he have? What's his problem anyway? How does a healthy man his age get pneumonia? Why does he have to take so much medicine?"

What information should you reveal?

Dilemma: The privacy of the patient conflicts with others' need to know about the patient's health status in order to protect their own health and prevent the spread of the HIV virus (autonomy versus justice).

Option 1: Inform the woman that the patient is HIV positive and has AIDS.

Rationale: The need of the wife to know about the patient's disease to protect herself and her unborn child is more important than the patient's right to privacy. The breach in privacy is considered to be justified by the need to stop the spread of the HIV virus.

Implications of Choosing This Option: The violation of his right to privacy and confidentiality without his knowledge or consent will undoubtedly upset the patient and will disrupt the nurse–patient relationship. HIV positive people in general might forgo necessary medical care if they believed that their confidentiality could be violated at any time and without their consent. A policy of reporting HIV status might cause people to lie about their HIV infection. The information you release about the patient may threaten his job, his housing, his marriage, and his health insurance. Furthermore, the woman to whom you are speaking may not be the patient's wife; does she have a need to know?

Option 2: Do not inform the woman that the patient is HIV positive.

Rationale: The patient's confidentiality is more important than preventing the spread of the HIV virus, and it is even more important than insuring treatment for your patient's wife, unborn child and your patient's lover. Any breach of confidentiality will disrupt the nurse–patient and physician–patient relationship. The release of devastating information about HIV status can harm the patient you are trying to help. The woman may not be the patient's wife and may not have a need to know.

Implications of Choosing This Option: The patient's lover, wife, and unborn child will suffer harm and potentially the loss of their lives without the knowledge that they are at risk of being HIV infected. AIDS and HIV infection will spread because the contacts of the patient will not know to curb their own high-risk behavior.

Option 3, Potential Compromise: Refuse to reveal confidential information to this woman at this time but take steps to strongly encourage your patient to identify those he has put at risk for HIV infection. Those people who have had sexual or needle-sharing contact with an HIV-positive person can then be notified and testing can be encouraged.

Rationale: It is important to maintain patient confidentiality because patients need to feel free to reveal personal information to their caregivers. However, it is also true that sexual and needle-sharing partners of HIV-positive patients have a right to know of their own risk for HIV so they can seek treatment and change their own high-risk behavior to stem the spread of the virus.

Implications of Choosing This Option: The breach of confidentiality will become a moot point if you obtain the patient's permission to contact those people with whom he has had sexual contact or shared needles. Confidentiality of the patient will be enhanced if the anonymity of the patient is paramount during the notification process. If the patient desires this approach, a health care professional can make the appropriate notifications and refuse to reveal the name of the patient. For example, "A patient of this clinic has tested HIV positive and has named you as a previous sexual partner. You are urged to seek confidential HIV testing at. . . ." The patient may or may not produce reliable information about his sexual and needle-sharing partners. The alternative to seeking the patient's cooperation is to rely on the unreliable guess of the health care professional as to the identity of the patient's sexual and needle-sharing partners.

Guidelines for the Nurse Receiving Request for Information about an HIV Infected Patient:

1. Never reveal confidential information (diagnosis, HIV status, current treatment) about your patient unless you have the patient's permission AND you have verified the person's identity.
2. If someone presses you for information, apologize for your inability to help, explain that as a nurse you are required to uphold the patient's confidentiality, and refer the person to the patient, if he or she wants more information.
3. Practice universal precautions. Avoid trying to "flag" the patient (ominous warning on chart, use of more infection control measures that required) that could result in public attention to the possibility that the patient has AIDS.
4. Teach the patient how the HIV virus is spread and encourage him or her to inform his or her contacts who may be at risk for HIV infection. Emphasize the importance of early identification and treatment of HIV infection. Counsel the patient about ways to reduce the risk to him- or herself and others. Refer the patient to a local AIDS information center.
5. Discuss with the patient's physician the plan to encourage the patient to notify those at risk from his or her HIV infection. Encourage the physician to strongly urge the patient to notify those at risk for HIV infection. Remember that notification does not require identification of the patient, just that the person being notified is at risk for HIV infection.
6. If the patient refuses to notify those at risk for HIV infection, encourage the physician to inform the patient that HIV infection and AIDS are conditions that health care professionals are required to report to public health authorities. This may encourage the patient to cooperate with efforts to notify at-risk partners of HIV infection.

Bibliography

Alfaro-LeFevre, R. (1997, April 7). Critical Thinking. *The Nursing Spectrum,* p. 4.

Ballinger, D. (1997). Is It Ever Acceptable to Deceive a Patient? *Nursing Times,* 93(35), 44–45.

Bosek, M. S. D., & Mixon D. K. (1993, February). Caring for Patients with AIDS: Conflicting Duties in Ethical Decision Making. *MEDSURG Nursing,* 2(1): 82–83.

Daly, B. (1997, September/October). Nursing Ethical Code Reflects Changing Times. *The American Nurse,* p. 9.

Sherman, D. W. (1996). Taking the Fear Out of AIDS Nursing: Voices from the Field. *Journal of the New York State Nurses Association,* 27(1): 4–8.

Marcus, E. (1991). AIDS Patient Sues Hospital Over Privacy; Says Therapist Violated His Privacy. *The Washington Post,* July 22, pp. D1, D2.

INSTRUCTIONAL IMPROVEMENT TOOL FOR UNIT 1

Student feedback/evaluation indicated that I need to improve my classroom presentation by:

Adding Content

1. ______________________________

2. ______________________________

3. ______________________________

Deleting Content

1. ______________________________

2. ______________________________

3. ______________________________

Emphasizing/Deemphasizing the Following Content

1. ______________________________

2. ______________________________

3. ______________________________

Questions students asked that I need to research for the future are:

1. ______________________________

2. ______________________________

3. ______________________________

UNIT 2

BIOPHYSICAL AND PSYCHOSOCIAL CONCEPTS IN NURSING PRACTICE

6

Homeostasis, Stress, and Adaptation

I. LEARNING OBJECTIVES

In addition to the learning objectives on page 71, I want my students to be able to:

1. ______________________________

2. ______________________________

3. ______________________________

II. TOP TERMS

1. Adaptation
2. Catecholamines
3. General Adaptation Syndrome
4. Hans Selye
5. Homeostasis
6. Hypothalamic-Pituitary Response
7. Inflammation
8. Local Adaptation Syndrome
9. Maladaptive Responses
10. Negative Feedback
11. Stressor
12. Sympathetic-Adrenal-Medullary Response

III. COLLABORATIVE LEARNING ACTIVITIES

Team Discussion Questions/Seminar Topics

1. For each of the situations below, ask students to compare their expected coping behavior with that of a classmate (reference pages 74–78).
   a. You arrive home from school to find that your house has been robbed.
   b. The school nurse calls and asks you to meet her at the hospital because your son needs stitches in his face.
   c. Your parents announce their divorce after thirty years of marriage.
2. Ask students to identify the physiological signals that make them aware that they are responding to stress (reference pages 74–78).

3. Have students describe patterns of coping behavior that have worked well for them in the past and would be used again during a stressful event (reference pages 84–86).
4. Require each student to name several daily stressors in their lives. Have students compare their lists with other classmates and compare their coping mechanisms (reference pages 84–86).

IV. CRITICAL THINKING ACTIVITIES

In-Class Team Exercises

Ask students to identify an expected pathophysiologic response to hypertensive heart disease. Starting with decreased renal blood flow and ending with fluid invasion of the alveolar spaces, have each student draw an illustration of the maladaptive, pathophysiological response. Use the following diagram. A physiology textbook should be used as a reference along with pages 74–78, Figure 6–2, and Table 6–1.

Flow Chart: Pathophysiologic Process: Hypertensive Heart Disease

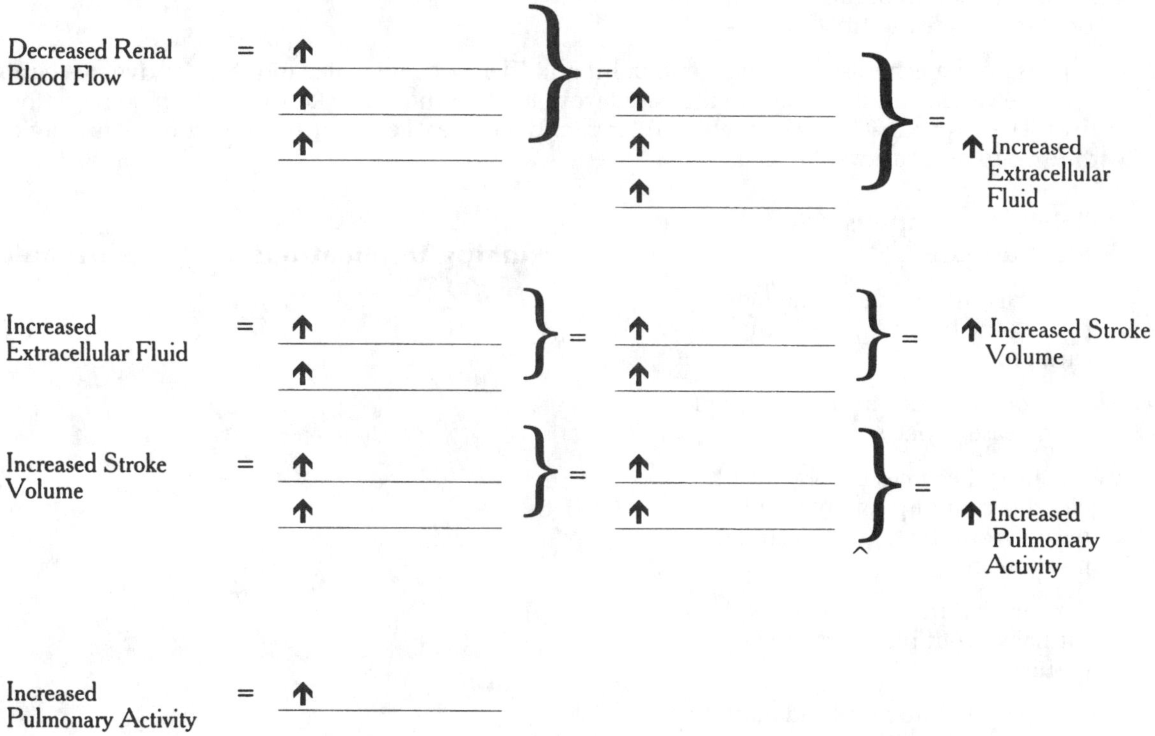

Decreased Renal Blood Flow = ↑ ______ ↑ ______ ↑ ______ } = ↑ ______ ↑ ______ ↑ ______ } = ↑ Increased Extracellular Fluid

Increased Extracellular Fluid = ↑ ______ ↑ ______ } = ↑ ______ ↑ ______ } = ↑ Increased Stroke Volume

Increased Stroke Volume = ↑ ______ ↑ ______ } = ↑ ______ ↑ ______ } = ↑ Increased Pulmonary Activity

Increased Pulmonary Activity = ↑ ______

Send Home Assignments

Ask students to reference the team exercise outlining an expected pathophysiologic response to hypertensive heart disease. Each student should construct an outline of nursing implications and supporting rationales to meet identified patient needs related to three compensatory mechanisms. The nursing process must be used as a guide for developing nursing implications.

1. Persistent arteriolar constriction results in increased cardiac output to overcome peripheral resistance. Sympathetic nervous system stimulation increases the heart rate, while selective vasoconstriction facilitates the return of more blood to the heart.

Selected Compensatory Mechanisms	Nursing Implications	Rationale
a. Arterial pressure rises in response to increased peripheral resistance.		
b. The heart rate increases to increase cardiac output.		
c. Vasoconstriction occurs in peripheral organs to increase stroke volume.		

2. Compensatory mechanisms reach an end point and then become maladaptive. Adaptive mechanisms to increase cardiac output create an increased work load on the heart. Resistance to blood ejection increases. The left ventricle hypertrophies, dilates, and enlarges. Left ventricular failure eventually occurs with forward and backward effects.

Selected Compensatory Mechanisms	Nursing Implications	Rationale
a. Coronary arteries degenerate, depleting the blood supply to the myocardium.		
b. Cardiomegaly occurs in an attempt to increase stroke volume.		
c. The heart becomes engorged with blood it cannot pump out. This results from the renin-aldosterone mechanism.		
d. Forward failure is associated with low cardiac output plus decreased tissue perfusion.		
e. Backward failure raises end diastolic pressure and is reflected in pulmonary congestion.		

3. As backward heart failure progresses, gas exchange is disrupted. Fluid shifts occur, leading to pulmonary edema. Right failure eventually occurs. The body is in total failure and close to death.

Selected Compensatory Mechanisms	Nursing Implications	Rationale
a. Fluid exudes from the capillaries into the alveolar spaces.		
b. Backward progression leads to congestion in the veins and organs drained by the venae cavae.		

7

Individual and Family Considerations Related to Illness

I. LEARNING OBJECTIVES

In addition to the learning objectives on page 89, I want my students to be able to:

1. ______________________________

2. ______________________________

3. ______________________________

II. TOP TERMS

1. "Accepted" Illness
2. Death and Dying
3. Denial
4. Depression
5. Emotional Health
6. Elizabeth Kübler-Ross
7. Posttraumatic Stress Syndrome
8. Remissions
9. Restitution Period
10. Stages of Illness

III. COLLABORATIVE LEARNING ACTIVITIES

Team Discussion Questions/Seminar Topics

1. Assign students to several teams. Ask each team to develop a definition of "posttraumatic stress disorder." What precipitates it and exaggerates it? What emotional responses are involved? What coping mechanisms can help? Ask students to share definitions and discuss responses (reference page 94).
2. Read students this exercise: Compare your emotional reaction to an acute illness with that of a classmate who has experienced an acute illness. Discuss the coping mechanisms that helped you adjust to an altered self-image. Based on your prior experience, how would you alter your behavior if you experienced another acute illness? Discuss how these learned behaviors would assist you in coping with a chronic illness. Share the similarities and differences of your team's emotional reactions with other teams reference pages 90–94).

IV. CRITICAL THINKING ACTIVITIES

In-Class Team Exercises

Divide students into teams of four. Have each team complete the following chart and share their answers. Encourage dialogue about the various stages of adjustment to illness.

A 19-year-old professional ice skater is diagnosed as having rheumatoid arthritis. She can no longer skate because of inflamed joints. She lives at home with her parents (reference pages 90–94).

Patho-physiological Change	Emotional Reaction	Specific Nursing Interventions	Evaluation Criteria

Send-Home Assignments

1. Assign students to interview a family member or friend who is experiencing an acute or chronic illness and complete the following assessment form:

ASSESSMENT FORM

Human Response to Illness

Individual: ______________________ Stage of Illness: ______________________

Illness: ______________________

Emotional Responses Exhibited: ______________________

____

Unmet Basic Needs: ______________________

____

Self-Image Changes: ______________________

____

Current Coping Strategies: ______________________

____

____

List several activities that you can do to promote more-effective coping strategies: ______________________

____

____

____

2. Assign the following case study. Direct students to choose one of the three options and prepare an argument to support their position. Recommend that the "Guidelines" be used in their clinical practice.

Case Study: A Patient's Desperate Request

You are the home care nurse for a 47-year-old male patient terminally ill with pancreatic cancer. His symptoms have proven difficult to manage: severe pain, nausea, vomiting, diarrhea, and skin breakdown. Despite these problems, he has ready outlived his original three-month prognosis and his vital signs remain stable.

On a Monday morning, you receive a report that he contacted the on-call nurse three separate times over the weekend because of his pain, and that his IV morphine was increased from 40 mg/hr to 50 mg/hr over the course of two days in an attempt to control the pain. When you visit him that afternoon, you find him anxious and in pain. He indicates that he cannot stand the pain any more. He feels his life is not worth living in this painful condition. He wants to die, and he wants you to help him. What should you do?

Dilemma: The obligation to respect the patient's autonomy conflicts with the obligation to do the patient no harm (autonomy versus nonmaleficence). Another way to frame the debate is that the patient's autonomy conflicts with the standards of the nursing profession (autonomy verus the integrity of the nursing profession).

Option 1: Agree to assist the patient with his suicide.

Rationale: The autonomy of the patient in choosing his death and the timing of his death is more important than an obligation not to harm him. Indeed, not to agree to assist him in his suicide would be to harm him by allowing him to continue to suffer.

Implication of Choosing This Position: You may face criminal charges by following this plan. Your advice or actions in assisting with the patient's suicide may injure him but not cause his death. You might assist in the suicide of a patient who may have changed his mind at another time under different circumstances.

Option 2: Refuse to participate in any way with this patient's plan.

Rationale: The duty to do no harm and prevent killing is more important than the autonomy of this patient.

Implication of Choosing This Position: The patient may continue to live and suffer in pain. The nurse-patient relationship may be disrupted.

Option 3, Potential Compromise: Talk with the patient and discuss why he wants to commit suicide. Is his pain the problem, or are there other factors—such as a family dispute or a money problem—at issue? Explore with the patient possible alternatives to his pain treatment or other problem. Obtain medical, psychiatric, pastoral care, social work, or pharmacist consultations as needed to seek resolution to these problems. Explain your reasons—legal, ethical—why you will not assist in his suicide.

Rationale: This approach respects autonomy by engaging the patient as a partner in solving problems, but also prevents harm to the patient.

Implications of Choosing This Position: The patient may continue to suffer if the cause of his suffering is not easily remedied. The nurse-patient relationship is maintained. There are no legal problems involved in this approach, and the nurse does not violate her profession's standards. The patient receives attention to his problems and emotional support.

Guidelines for the Nurse Whose Assistance Is Requested in Committing Suicide:

1. Never assist in the suicide of a patient. It is illegal.
2. Explore with your patient the reasons he is considering suicide. Frequently, depression or poor pain control is the source of suicidal thoughts for the terminally ill patient.

3. Initiate appropriate consultations, e.g. chaplain, psychiatric nurse, social worker. With these consultants and the physician, formulate a plan to treat the cause of the patient's distress, such as poor pain control.
4. Provide emotional support to the patient and family.

Bibliography

ACG Panel on Chronic Pain in Older Persons. (1998, May). Clinical Practice Guidelines: The Management of Chronic Pain in Older Patients. *Journal of the American Geriatric Society,* 46(5): 635–651.

Averill, P. M., et al. (1996, April). Correlates of Depression in Chronic Pain Patients: A Comprehensive Examination. *Pain,* 65(1): 93–100.

Cassel, C. K., & Meier D. E. (1990, September). Morals and Moralism in the Debate over Euthanasia and Assisted Suicide. *New England Journal of Medicine,* 323(11):750–752.

Cate, S. (1991, July). Death by Choice. *American Journal of Nursing,* 91(7):33–34.

Singer, P. A., & Seigler M. (1990, June 28). Euthanasia: A Critique. *New England Journal of Medicine,* 322(26):1881–1883.

Malek, C. J. (1996, May). Pain Management: Documenting the Decision Making Process. *Nursing Case Management,* 1:64–74.

Yeates, C., & Caine, E. D. (1991, October 10). Rational Suicide and the Right to Die: Reality and Myth. *New England Journal of Medicine,* 325(15):1100–1102.

8

Perspectives in Transcultural Nursing

I. LEARNING OBJECTIVES

In addition to the learning objectives on page 102, I want my students to be able to:

1. ______________________________

2. ______________________________

3. ______________________________

II. TOP TERMS

1. Acculturation
2. Acupuncture
3. Cultural Taboos
4. Eye Contact
5. Folk Healers
6. Minority
7. Spiritualist
8. Subculture
9. Transcultural Nursing
10. Yin/Yang

III. COLLABORATIVE LEARNING ACTIVITIES

Team Discussion Questions/Seminar Topics

1. Instruct students to compare and contrast Dr. Madeleine Leininger's definition of culture (1988) with Sir Edward Taylor's original definition (1871) (reference pages 103–104).
2. Ask students to explain variations in interpreting the concepts of space, distance, and time relative to communication among several cultures (reference pages 105–106).
3. Ask students to explain the naturalistic view of the cause of illness and disease (reference pages 106–107).

IV. CRITICAL THINKING ACTIVITIES

In-Class Team Exercises

Divide the class into groups of four. Have each group choose one of Leninger's terms used to describe her theory of "Cultural Care Diversity and Universality." Each group should define and explain the term relative to several culture groups: African Americans, Hispanics, Native Americans, Asians, and Indo-Chinese (reference pages 103–104).

Terms to Use:

- Cultural Care Accommodation
- Cultural Care Repatterning
- Culturally Congruent Nursing
- Acculturation
- Cultural Blindness
- Cultural Imposition
- Cultural Taboos

Send-Home Assignments

1. Assign students to interview a fellow student, friend, neighbor, or family member who represents a different culture. The content of the interview can be individually determined. What is most important in the dialogue is identification of communication barriers and methods used to overcome those barriers (reference pages 103–106, Chart 8–1).
2. Assign the following case study. Direct students to choose one argument. Recommend that the "Guidelines" be used in their clinical practice.

Case Study: What Part Does Culture Play in Deciding Whether to Tell a Patient He Has a Life-Threatening Illness?

Situation: Mr. Chavez, a 55-year-old man of Mexican descent, is on your unit for removal of a possibly cancerous thyroid growth. He is told that surgery is necessary to remove the growth, and he consents to the operation. After the operation, the surgeon informs Mrs. Chavez that the tumor could not be totally removed. At this time, Mrs. Chavez asks you (the primary nurse) and the physician not to tell Mr. Chavez. She explains that it is customary in her culture that the family assumes a protective role in keeping news that might "harm" the patient from the patient.

Dilemma: Conflict between the nurse's responsibility to act as patient advocate and truth teller and the nurse's responsibility to respect a patient's culture and customs.

Arguments for Not Telling the Patient: Some cultures may not place great importance on patients having all the information. In some cultures the family as a unit is the decision maker and the patient receives information through the family. In honoring Mrs. Chavez's request, the nurse might be protecting the family integrity and in so doing protecting the patient from information that he might be unable to handle.

Implications of Choosing Not to Tell: If the patient will not be told that he will die from the tumor, the nursing staff and the physician will have to filter any negative information concerning the patient's condition through the patient's wife. A practical issue that arises is that the health care staff does not know first hand what the patient wants. If he questions the nursing staff about his diagnosis or prognosis, the nursing staff will be unable to interact in a therapeutic relationship with him.

Arguments Against Not Telling: The patient has an autonomous right to know all information regarding his care and diagnosis so that he can make decisions that affect the rest of his life. Having a timetable and knowing his diagnosis may give him an opportunity to resolve unresolved situations if that is his desire. Additionally, he might suspect that his family and others are acting strangely around him and wonder why.

Implications of Full Disclosure (Telling): If the patient is told his diagnosis, he may appreciate knowing the information. On the other hand, withholding information may indeed be the way the family copes with bad situations. In such a case, the patient's new knowledge may impair whatever coping mechanisms might be in place.

Potential Compromise: The nurse should endeavor to find out from cultural experts, e.g. priest or clergy person, cultural leaders of the community, translators, friends, if this is the cultural pattern that is followed. Perhaps the wife is mistaken and the husband might want to know. We don't have enough information to make the assumption without further data.

Guidelines for Nursing Care:

1. Explore what the patient's cultural patterns really are.
2. Discuss with the wife and other family members the implications of abiding by their requests that differ from the dominant way of providing patient care.
3. Discuss in nursing and medical conferences how the news might affect the patient.
4. Observe how the patient interacts with the family. Does he seem willing to accept the family's leadership role?
5. Arrange for a patient care conference with the family, surgeon and nursing staff and see what compromises may be acceptable.
6. Discuss with nursing staff the issues of beneficence and harm. By not telling the patient about the nature of his condition, is the healthcare staff being beneficent (doing good) or harmful to the patient.

Bibliography

Alfaro-LeFevre, R. (1997, April 7). Critical Thinking. *The Nursing Spectrum:* 4.

Ballinger, D. (1997) Is It Ever Acceptable to Deceive a Patient? *Nursing Times,* 93(35): 44–45.

Caws P. (1978, October). On the Teaching of Ethics in a Pluralistic Society. *Hastings Center Report,* 8(5):32–39.

Daly, B. (1997, September/October). Nursing Ethical Code Reflects Changing Times. *The American Nurse:* 9.

Edwards, B. S. (1994, January). When the Family Won't Give Up. *American Journal of Nursing,* 94(1):52–56.

Engelhardt, H. T. (1989, September/October). Can Ethics Take Pluralism Seriously? *Hastings Center Report,* 19(5):33–34.

Erlen, J. A. (1997). Everyday Ethics. *Orthopaedic Nursing,* 16(4), 60–63.

International Perspectives on Biomedical Ethics. (1988, August/September) *Hastings Center Report,* Special Supplement, 18(4): 1–31.

Marty, M. E. & Vaux, K. L. (Eds) (1986). *Health/Medicine and the Faith Traditions.* Book series. Various authors. Published volumes include the Anglican, Catholic, Islamic, Jewish, Lutheran, and Reformed traditions. New York: Crossroad Publishing Co.

Mason, S. (1997). The Ethical Dilemma of the Do Not Resuscitate Order. *British Journal of Nursing,* 6(11):646–649.

9

Chronic Illness

I. LEARNING OBJECTIVES

In addition to the learning objectives on page 110, I want my students to be able to:

1. ______________________________

2. ______________________________

3. ______________________________

II. TOP TERMS

1. Adherence
2. Chronic Illness
3. Collaborative Management
4. Contextual Conditions
5. Continuum
6. Disabling
7. Health Maintenance
8. Prevalence
9. Reciprocal Impact
10. Trajectory Framework

III. COLLABORATIVE LEARNING ACTIVITIES

Team Discussion Questions/Seminar Topics

1. Divide students into two teams to support the following statement by presenting arguments and examples: "Patients with chronic health care problems may function independently and lead a full life" (reference pages 111–115).
2. Have students trace the prevalence and causes of chronic illnesses and identify specific interventions that can decrease frequency and virulence (reference pages 110–114).

IV. CRITICAL THINKING EXERCISES

In-Class Team Exercises

1. Ask students to list the variables that have caused chronic illnesses to become a major health problem in developed countries today. Each group should list how group members, as nursing professionals, can intervene to help prevent the rise of chronic illnesses, especially those common among the elderly (references pages 111–114 and Table 9–1)
2. Divide the class into two groups. Ask each group to debate opposing viewpoints to the following statement: "Advanced technology has greatly increased the survival rates of severely premature infants at the same time that it has made them vulnerable to complications, such as ventilator dependence and blindness." Students should use current articles to support their positions (reference pages 111–114).
3. Separate students into five teams, each team representing one of five age groups: (a) those under 18 years, (b) those between 18 and 44, (c) those between 45 and 64, (d) those between 65 and 74, and (e) those older than 75 years. Ask each team to present the most common chronic condition for its category and the challenges to lifestyle adjustment and self-image changes (reference pages 110–115 and Figures 9–1 and 9–2).

10

Principles and Practices of Rehabilitation

I. LEARNING OBJECTIVES

In addition to the learning objectives on page 119, I want my students to be able to:

1. ______________________________

2. ______________________________

3. ______________________________

II. TOP TERMS

1. Activities of Daily Living (ADL)
2. Barthel Index
3. Disability
4. Functional Ability
5. Independence Measure
6. Isometric Exercises
7. Orthoses
8. Physiatrist
9. PULSES
10. Range of Motion
11. Rehabilitation
12. Shearing Force

III. COLLABORATIVE LEARNING ACTIVITIES

Team Discussion Questions/Seminar Topics

1. Ask for student volunteers to discuss a personal rehabilitative experience. Direct discussion around the frustrations associated with a slow and gradual physical improvement. Students should also describe emotional responses to such an illness, from diagnosis through dependency and eventual adjustment and/or independence (reference pages 119–123).
2. Assign the following exercise: Look around your house environment and make a list of those areas you would need to change if you were suddenly confined to a wheelchair. Is a bathroom accessible without climbing stairs? Can you safely reach the stove or oven to prepare a meal? How would you reach the freezer to get ice cubes for your soda? How would you carry a hot beverage from the stove to a table?

3. Ask students to share independently designed nursing care plans that have well-defined goals and priorities to help a disabled (choose any disability) person maximize abilities and take control of his or her life (reference pages 123–129)

IV. CRITICAL THINKING ACTIVITIES

Send-Home Assignments

Tell students to read the following case studies and circle the correct answers.

Case Study: Pressure Ulcers

Quincy, age 82, was hospitalized two weeks ago for insulin shock. He is obese, has joint stiffness due to osteoarthritis, and has been in bed for the duration of his stay (reference pages 135–141).

1. During his morning care the nurse notices a reddened area about 5 cm in diameter on Quincy's coccygeal area. To diagnose the presence of a pressure sore, the nurse should:
   a. assess how long hyperemia persists after removal of pressure.
   b. palpate for increased skin temperature.
   c. press on the area to determine blanching.
   d. do all of the above.
2. The nurse knows that to relieve pressure, Quincy will have to be turned every:
   a. 30 minutes.
   b. 1 to 2 hours.
   c. 2 to 4 hours.
   d. 8 to 10 hours.
3. The nursing plan of care for Quincy should include:
   a. keeping the skin clean.
   b. removing pressure from the area.
   c. supplying adequate nutrients.
   d. all of the above.
4. Nursing interventions that would prevent extension of the pressure sore include:
   a. initiating a 2-hour turning schedule.
   b. obtaining an alternating pressure pad mattress.
   c. using pillows to position bony prominences and support the extremities.
   d. all of the above.

Case Study: Assisted Ambulation: Crutches

Rita, a 17-year-old college student, is in a full leg cast because of a compound fracture of the left femur. Rita is to be discharged from the hospital in several days. She lives with her parents in a split-level house (reference pages 131–135 and Chart 10–2).

1. The exercises that the nurse would recommend to strengthen Rita's upper extremity muscles are:
   a. isometric exercises of the biceps.
   b. push-ups performed in a sitting position.
   c. gluteal setting.
   d. quadriceps setting.
2. Rita is 5 feet 5 inches tall. Her crutches should measure:
   a. 45 inches.
   b. 49 inches.
   c. 54 inches.
   d. 59 inches.

3. Before teaching a crutch gait, the nurse directs Rita to assume the tripod position. In this basic crutch stance, the crutches are placed in front and to the side of Rita's toes, at an approximate distance of:
   a. 4 to 6 inches.
   b. 6 to 8 inches
   c. 8 to 10 inches.
   d. 10 to 12 inches.

4. Because Rita is not allowed to bear weight on her casted leg, she should be taught the:
   a. two-point gait.
   b. three-point gait.
   c. four-point gait.
   d. swing-through gait.

11

Health Care of the Older Adult

I. LEARNING OBJECTIVES

In addition to the learning objectives on page 148, I want my students to be able to:

1. ____________________

2. ____________________

3. ____________________

II. TOP TERMS

1. Ageism
2. Alzheimer's Disease
3. Benign Senescent Forgetfulness
4. Delirium
5. Dementia
6. Ego Integrity
7. Frail Elderly
8. Gerontology
9. Intrinsic vs. Extrinsic Aging
10. Multi-Infarct Dementia

III. COLLABORATIVE LEARNING ACTIVITIES

Team Discussion Questions/Seminar Topics

1. Separate students into teams. Ask each team to discuss behaviors that would be expected among the elderly who are depressed. For each behavior, have students list several nursing interventions that would assist the patient with coping (references pages 156–157).
2. Direct students to list the ways in which various drug classifications can alter a person's nutritional status. For example, antacids are known to produce thiamin deficiency; therefore, vitamin supplements should be provided for a patient who cannot alter his or her antacid intake (reference pages 164–165).

IV. CRITICAL THINKING ACTIVITIES

In-Class Team Exercises

1. For each drug classification listed, tell students to document several nursing interventions for administering these drugs to the elderly. Cite a rationale for each nursing intervention (reference pages 164–165).

MEDICATIONS FOR THE ELDERLY		
Drug Classification	**Nursing Interventions**	**Rationale**
Opiates		
Sedatives and hypnotics		
Salicylates		
Tranquilizers		
Central nervous system stimulants		
Cardiac glycosides		
Diuretics		

2. Ask students to answer the following questions about Alzheimer's disease (reference pages 159–162).
   a. The cause is believed to be affected by a decrease in the enzyme ______________________________ .
   b. List interventions a nurse can perform to
      (1) support cognitive functioning: ______________________________
      ____
      (2) promote physical safety: ______________________________
      ____
      (3) improve communication: ______________________________
      ____
   c. Provide a rationale for each of the following nursing interventions:
      (1) Be predictable in your manner and conversation.
      ____
      (2) Avoid use of constraints. ______________________________
      ____
      (3) Treat the patient as a person with feelings. ______________________________
      ____

Send-Home Assignments

1. Give students directions for completing the following interview and self-appraisal. Choose an elderly family member or friend and complete the following assessment. Bring the completed paper back to class and share your findings with your classmates (used with permission, Nursing Department, Delaware County Community College, Media, PA.).

Guidelines for the Interview

(Suggested questions to ask the older adult)

a. Describe a typical day.
b. How would you describe your health?
c. What factors in your life contribute to your health?
d. Tell me about your home and your neighborhood and what they mean to you.
e. Summarize the living situation:
   - How long have you lived here?
   - If the older adult is in a new living situation, ask what circumstances precipitated the change.
   - If the older adult has lived in the present environment for a long time, ask how he or she has managed to be so successful at home.
f. What has helped the older adult to maintain independence at home?
g. Topic: Adaptation to Aging: Defining Healthy Aging

   Place of Meeting ____________________

   Age of Older Adult ____________________

   - Discuss impressions, general reactions, and feelings regarding your first visit.
   - How did the older adult describe "health" and "old age"?
   - What factors were described by the older adult as essential for a healthy adaptive lifestyle?
   - Identify factors that enable the older adult to maintain independence at home.

2. Complete the "Self-Appraisal of Aging" activity.

   a. Current age: ____________________
   b. Projected life expectancy: ____________________
   c. Define health: ____________________
   d. What parts of you are currently healthy? ____________________

      ____
   e. Describe the environment you wish to live in when you are older:

      ____

      ____
   f. Describe the roles you expect to have: ____________________

      ____
   g. What social activities will be important to you? ____________________

      ____
   h. Make a statement of the legacy you wish to leave: ____________________

      ____

      ____

3. Assign the following case study. Direct students to choose one of the three options and prepare an argument to support their decision. Recommend that the "Guidelines" be used in their clinical practice.

Case Study: The Use of Restraints

An 89-year-old woman is admitted to your unit with a diagnosis of pneumonia and dehydration. She lives by herself in an assisted living apartment. She is malnourished, underweight, and lethargic, and IV fluids and antibiotics are prescribed. By day three of her hospital stay, her serum sodium level is 121 mEQ/l and her caloric intake (she needs to be fed) is less than 500 calories per day. The physician orders a feeding tube inserted and tube feedings started. It is now day six. She is on her third feeding tube, having pulled the other two out. The nurse who gave you report tells you that the doctor wants the patient's hands tied "at all times" so this tube will not be pulled out. "Our job is to keep that tube in," she reports. On your rounds, you find a frail elderly woman who appears to be alert and oriented. "Honey, won't you please untie me?" she says. "And take this nasty thing out of my nose! I don't want it!"

Dilemma: The obligation to respect the patient's autonomy by releasing her from her restraints at her request conflicts with the obligation to protect her from harming herself by removing or dislodging the feeding tube (autonomy versus beneficence).

Option 1: Keep the patient restrained.

Rationale: The duty to protect the patient from harm is more important than respecting the patient's autonomy. The patient's autonomy is suspect because she has tried three times to pull out her feeding tube. The physician has ordered that the patient be restrained. The patient must be restrained to prevent the feeding tube from being removed or dislodged.

Implications of Choosing This Position: The patient may be upset, humiliated, and angered at the continued use of the restraints. The patient may remove or dislodge the feeding tube despite the restraints. Nursing observation of the patient may decrease if the nurse believes the restraints are keeping the patient safe. The physician may become upset that it was not communicated to him that an alert and oriented patient requested that the feeding tube be removed. The patient may experience an injury to herself because of the restraints. The patient may be incontinent because the restraints prevent her from getting up to use the bathroom.

Option 2: Remove the restraints.

Rationale: The obligation to respect the patient's autonomy is more important than the obligation to protect the patient from harm. If the patient wants to remove the feeding tube, it is her right to make that choice.

Implications of Choosing This Position: The patient may remove or dislodge the feeding tube and cause herself harm, such as aspiration pneumonia. The patient's nutritional status may worsen. The patient may receive trauma to her nasal passages due to repeated insertions of feeding tubes. The physician may be angry that you discontinued the restraints and allowed the patient to pull out her feeding tube.

Option 3, Potential Compromise: Release the restraints while you are with the patient and take a few minutes to observe her behavior. Evaluate if the patient is able to understand the reason for the feeding and the tube and the risks and benefits of the tube and the restraints. Explain the reason for the restraints and restrain the patient again before you leave the bedside. Review the chart for the patient's current lab values, plan of care, reason for restraints, and information about the patient's psychological status. Inform the physician of your observations about the patient's mental status and her request for the feeding tube to be removed. With the physician, form a plan of care that addresses the patient's autonomy as well as her caloric and safety needs.

Rationale: The safety of the patient and the autonomy of the patient are both important, but safety wins out until the ability of the patient to give an informed consent to have the feeding tube removed is clarified.

Implications of Choosing This Position: If this patient is alert and oriented, restraining her after assessing her may be insulting, humiliating, and may anger the patient. Beneficence may not be totally upheld since the patient could still remove or dislodge the feeding tube with the restraints in place.

Guidelines for the Nurse Caring for a Patient for Whom Restraints Are Being Considered:

1. Assess the patient, paying particular attention to the patient's ability to follow directions and understand the risks and benefits of the treatments. If confusion is present, consider its possible cause. Assess the reason for the behavior the patient is exhibiting: Does the patient get out of bed often because of urinary frequency or diarrhea? Is the patient confused because he or she is hypoxic? Does the patient with an unsteady gait require a walker or physical therapy?
2. Review the patient's chart, laboratory results, and medication as possible sources of information about the problems for which restraints are being considered. Does the patient have a low serum sodium? Is he or she experiencing the side effects of a sleeping pill? Does he or she have a hearing or language problem that is being mistaken for confusion? Does he or she have a urinary tract infection? Is he or she undergoing withdrawal from alcohol? Consult with your peers, the physicians on the case, a pharmacist, and other specialists to help find the cause of____ and identify a treatment for______, the patient's underlying problem.
3. Consider alternatives to restraints, such as increasing the frequency of your observations of the patient or having the patient's family or friends to stay with him or her.
4. Weigh the risks and benefits of using restraints. Remember, restraints may aggravate the patient's condition by increasing agitation, causing injuries, and contributing to incontinence and weakness.
5. Consult with the physician before or immediately after restraints are required. Form a plan of care for removing the restraints. Explain your rationale for the restraints to the patient and family. Document your reason for the need for restraints in the patient record.
6. If restraints are required, use the least restrictive kind necessary for the least amount of time.
7. Increase your observation of the patient in restraints, paying particular attention to the nutritional, ventilatory, circulation, and elimination needs of these immobile patients.
8. Continue your nursing interventions to resolve the cause of the need for restraints.

Bibliography

Benaski, S. H. (1998). Delirium in Hospitalized Geriatric Patients. *American Journal of Nursing,* 98(4): 16D-16L.

Evans, M. L., & Strumpf, N. E. (1990 Spring). Myths About Elder Restraint. *Image: The Journal of Nursing Scholarship,* 22(2): 124–128.

Morse J. M., & McHutchion, E. (1991). Releasing Restraints: Providing Safe Care for the Elderly. *Research in Nursing and Health,* 14: 187–196.

Sullivan-Marx, E. M. (1996). Restraint-Free Care: How Does a Nurse Decide? *Journal of Gerontologic Nursing,* 22(9):7–14.

Weick M. D. (1992, November). Physical Restraints: A FDA Update. *American Journal of Nursing,* 92 (11): 74–80.

INSTRUCTIONAL IMPROVEMENT TOOL FOR UNIT 2

Student feedback/evaluation indicated that I need to improve my classroom presentation by:

Adding Content

1. ______________________________
____

2. ______________________________
____

3. ______________________________
____

Deleting Content

1. ______________________________
____

2. ______________________________
____

3. ______________________________
____

Emphasizing/Deemphasizing the Following Content

1. ______________________________
____

2. ______________________________
____

3. ______________________________
____

Questions students asked that I need to research for the future are:

1. ______________________________
____

2. ______________________________
____

3. ______________________________
____

UNIT **3**

CONCEPTS AND CHALLENGES IN PATIENT MANAGEMENT

12

Pain Management

I. LEARNING OBJECTIVES

In addition to the learning objectives on page 175, I want my students to be able to:

1. ______________________________

2. ______________________________

3. ______________________________

II. TOP TERMS

1. Antagonist
2. Endorphins
3. Enkephalins
4. "Gate Control" Theory of Pain
5. Nociceptive System
6. Opioid
7. Placebo
8. Prostaglandins
9. Referred Pain
10. Tolerance

III. COLLABORATIVE LEARNING ACTIVITIES

In-Class Team Exercises

1. Help students list several noninvasive categories of nursing activity that can be used to assist a patient with pain experience. For each category, ask students to document a rationale and an example of an associated activity. Use the following format as a guide (reference pages 195–196).

Category	Rationale	Example
Relaxation techniques (Sample)	Relaxation measures help to reduce muscle tension, thus decreasing the intensity of pain or increasing pain tolerance.	Teach the patient to use slow, rhythmic abdominal breathing at 6–9 breaths per minute and maintain a slow, constant, counting rhythm.

2. Ask students to draft a nursing care plan for a 55-year-old woman with intractable pain associated with breast cancer and bone metastasis. She was independent, worked full-time, and lived alone prior to her recent hospital admission for chemotherapy and radiation. Tell students to write a nursing care plan based on the patient's need for pain management and independence.

Nursing Diagnosis: Alteration in comfort related to breast cancer and bone metastasis.

Sample Goals: Patient will experience a decrease in the intensity of pain or relief of pain. Patient will manage episodes of pain and maintain a realistic level of independence in activities of daily living.

Nursing Actions	Rationale	Expected Outcomes

IV. CRITICAL THINKING ACTIVITIES

Send-Home Assignments

1. Recommend that students use the Pain Assessment Tool and Visual Analogue Scale (Figures 12–4 and 12–5, pages 181–183) to assess the pain of someone they know (family member, neighbor, friend) who is experiencing either acute or chronic pain. Each student should bring the completed tool back to school and share the results with classmates in a collaborative discussion group.

Pain Assessment Tool

NAME: ________________________ **DATE:** ________________________

LOCATION: Describe or point to area of pain. ________________________

QUALITY: What words best describe your pain?________________________

____

INTENSITY: Rate your pain on a scale of 0 (no pain) to 10 (worst pain possible)

At present ________________ 1 hour after medication ________________

Worst it gets ________________ Best it gets ________________

ONSET: When did pain begin? ____________ What time of day does it occur ____________

How often does it occur? ____________ How long does it last? ____________

EFFECT OF PAIN: What relieves the pain?________________________

What makes the pain worst? ________________________

What other problems/symptoms occur with the pain?________________

How does the pain affect your life and your activities?________________

PLAN: ____

____

Visual Analogue Scale

0 ____ 10

No Pain Visual Analogue Scale Worst Possible Pain

2. Assign the following case study. Direct students to choose a position, either in favor or in opposition to aggressive management of pain. Have each student defend his/her position with logical problem analysis. Recommend that the "Guidelines" be used in their clinical practice.

Case Study: How Does the Nurse Determine Whether the Patient Should Have the Prescribed Dosage of a Drug or Whether the Dosage Will Cause the Patient's Death?

Situation: Mrs. Jones, a 34-year-old woman dying of metastatic bone cancer secondary to breast cancer, is crying out for pain relief. You have a standing order to administer morphine sulfate up to 15 mg, IV, as needed for pain relief. However, in administering this dose, you are afraid that you will sedate her and cause her to stop breathing.

Dilemma: The nurse is caught between two ethical principles: beneficence (benefiting) versus nonmaleficence (doing no harm).

Arguments for Giving IV Morphine: The patient is dying of her disease, not the morphine. Rather, morphine is given to relieve pain and provide some comfort.

Implications of Giving the Morphine: The patient may not be conscious and may be heavily sedated from the bolus of medication. Her respirations may decrease as she sleeps. The nurse is giving relief to the patient.

Arguments Against Giving the Morphine: The patient may die from the bolus of morphine. The nurse doesn't want to be responsible for the death of the patient.

Implications of Choosing to Give the Morphine: The patient's pain may not be relieved. The patient may die anyway.

Potential Compromise: Instead of giving one bolus of morphine sulfate IV, the nurse could administer the medication on a timed basis, i.e., 1 to 3 mg at a time titrated to pain relief. In such a case, the patient would remain conscious and able to interact with the environment and the pain would be relieved as well.

Guidelines for the Nursing Care

1. In administering large doses of narcotic analgesics, understand what the doctrine of double effect means in the care of a terminally ill patient (see Bibliography, especially Beauchamp and Childress, 1994, pp. 206–211).
2. Understand the physiologic strain for the patient in severe pain.
3. Understand why the respiratory rate changes when pain is relieved.
4. Think about measures that are available in addition to narcotics to help the nurse relieve pain.
5. Investigate administering narcotic analgesics in other ways than IV bolus.
6. Analyze how the nurse can continually assess the patient's oxygen saturation level after administering the pain medication.
7. Understand how to give medications for pain relief in divided doses.

Bibliography

Agency for Health Care Policy and Research (AHCPR) Guidelines: Acute Pain Management: Operative or Medical Procedures and Trauma. Clinical Practice Guideline, AHCPR Publication No. 920032. Rockville, MD: Agency for Health Care Policy and Research, Public Health Service, US Department of Health and Human Services, February, 1992.

Bosek, M. S. D. (1993, June). The Ethics of Pain Management. *MEDSURG Nursing,* 2(3): 218–220.

Cleeland, C. S., et al. (1997, November). Pain and Treatment of Pain in Minority Patients with Cancer. *Annals of Internal Medicine,* 127(9): 813–816.

Connor, M., & Deane D. (1995, May). Patterns of Patient-Controlled Analgesia and Intramuscular Analgesia. *Applied Nursing Research,* 8(2): 67–92.

Gureje, O., Von Korff, M., Simon, G. E., & Gater, R. (1998, July 8). Persistent Pain and Well-Being. *Journal of American Medical Association,* 280 (2): 147–151.

Management of Cancer Pain. Clinical Practice Guideline, AHCPR Publication No. 94–0592. Rockville, MD: Agency for Health Care Policy and Research, Public Health Service, U.S. Department of Health and Human Services, March, 1994.

McCaffery, M., & Ferrell, B. R. (1997, September). Nurses' Knowledge of Pain Assessment and Management: How Much Progress Have We Made? *Journal of Pain Symptom Management,* 14(3): 175–188.

McCaffery, M., & Ferrell, B. R. (1994, July). How to Use the New AHCPR Cancer Pain Guidelines. *American Journal of Nursing,* 94(7): 42–46.

Wilson, W. C., et al. (1992, February 19). Ordering and Administration of Sedatives and Analgesics During the Withholding and Withdrawal of Life Support from Critically Ill Patients. *Journal of the American Medical Association,* 267(7): 949–953.

13

Fluid and Electrolytes: Balance and Disturbances

I. LEARNING OBJECTIVES

In addition to the learning objectives on page 201, I want my students to be able to:

1. ______________________________

2. ______________________________

3. ______________________________

II. TOP TERMS

1. Acid-Base Disturbances
2. Baroreceptors
3. Electrolytes
4. Hypervolemia
5. Hypotonic Solution
6. Insensible Fluid Loss
7. Osmolality
8. Renin-Angiotensin-Aldosterone System
9. Serum Osmolality
10. Sodium-Potassium Pump

III. COLLABORATIVE LEARNING ACTIVITIES

Team Discussion Questions

Direct students to analyze each statement and discuss its physiological rationale based on the principles of fluid and electrolyte balance.

1. Confusion can be an early sign of hyponatremia in the elderly (reference pages 213–217).
2. Administered potassium is usually retained in the elderly and can rise to dangerous levels because renal function decreases with advancing age (reference pages 218–221).
3. Bed rest for the elderly person with osteoporosis can cause impaired calcium metabolism (reference pages 221–224).
4. Alcohol and caffeine in high doses are known to inhibit calcium absorption (reference pages 221–224).
5. Local symptoms of infiltration of an intravenous solution are edema, coolness at the site of infiltration, and decreased flow rate (reference pages 240–242).

IV. CRITICAL THINKING ACTIVITIES

In-Class Team Exercises

Tell students to read the following case study and circle the correct answer.

Case Study: Postoperative Intravenous Infusion

Keith, age 16, has been admitted to the hospital for an arthroscopy of his right knee. He returns from the operating room at 12:00 noon with 750 ml remaining in a 1-liter bottle of Ringer's solution. The solution was ordered to be administered over an 8-hour period. The drop factor is 15 drops per milliliter (reference pages 234–242).

1. The nurse knows that the infusion should be absorbed by:
   a. 4:00 PM.
   b. 6:00 PM.
   c. 8:00 PM.
   d. 10:00 PM.
2. The nurse checks the intravenous flow rate to make certain that it is calculated to drip at:
   a. 21 drops per minute.
   b. 25 drops per minute.
   c. 31 drops per minute.
   d. 40 drops per minute.
3. When the nurse inspects the intravenous site, she notes the presence of inflammation. This complication is evidenced by:
   a. heat.
   b. pain.
   c. swelling.
   d. all of the above.
4. Nursing actions for discontinuing an infusion include:
   a. applying gentle counteraction to the skin while removing the needle.
   b. placing a dry, sterile sponge over the infusion site as the needle is removed.
   c. applying firm pressure to the puncture site until the bleeding has stopped.
   d. all of the above.

Send-Home Assignments

Assign this three-column matching test and review the following directions.

First, match the statement about body fluid listed in Column III with its body fluid space listed in Column II. Then match the fluid space in Column II with an associated fact in Column I. (reference pages 203–206).

Column I

__ 1. third space fluid shift
__ 2. the smallest compartment of ECF space
__ 3. space where plasma is contained
__ 4. comprises the intravascular, interstitial, and transcellular fluid
__ 5. comprises about 60% of body fluid
__ 6. comprises fluid surrounding cell

Column II

__ a. intracellular space
__ b. extracellular fluid compartment
__ c. intravascular space
__ d. transcellular space
__ e. interstitial space
__ f. intravascular fluid volume deficit

Column III

__ I. comprises the cerebrospinal and pericardial fluids
__ II. is equal to about 8 L in an adult
__ III. signs include: hypotension, edema, and tachycardia
__ IV. found mostly in skeletal muscle mass
__ V. comprises about one-third of body fluid
__ VI. comprises 50% of blood volume

14

Shock and Multisystem Failure

I. LEARNING OBJECTIVES

In addition to the learning objectives on page 244, I want my students to be able to:

1. ______________________________

2. ______________________________

3. ______________________________

II. TOP TERMS

1. Anaphylactic shock
2. Cardiogenic Shock
3. Crystalloid and Colloid Solutions
4. Distributive Shock
5. Dopamine (Intropin)
6. Hypovolemic Shock
7. Intra-Aortic Balloon Counterpulsation
8. Mean Arterial Pressure (MAP)
9. Septic Shock
10. Shock Syndrome
11. Vasoactive Drug Therapy

III. COLLABORATIVE LEARNING ACTIVITIES

Team Discussion Questions/Seminar Topics

Advise students to analyze each statement and present a supporting physiological rationale.

1. In the initial stage of shock, damage has already begun at the cellular and tissue levels when blood pressure has dropped. Explain (reference pages 245–247).
2. During the compensated stage of shock the blood pressure is normal yet the organs are showing clinical signs of decreased perfusion. Explain (reference pages 247–248).
3. A crystalloid solution such as Ringer's lactate is used to treat hypovolemic shock because it contains the lactate ion. Explain (reference pages 249–251).

IV. CRITICAL THINKING ACTIVITIES

In-Class Team Exercises

Direct students to chart the physiologic sequence of events in hypovolemic shock. (Legend: ↓ = decreased) (reference pages 252–254 and Figure 14–3).

Flow Chart: Hypovolemic Shock

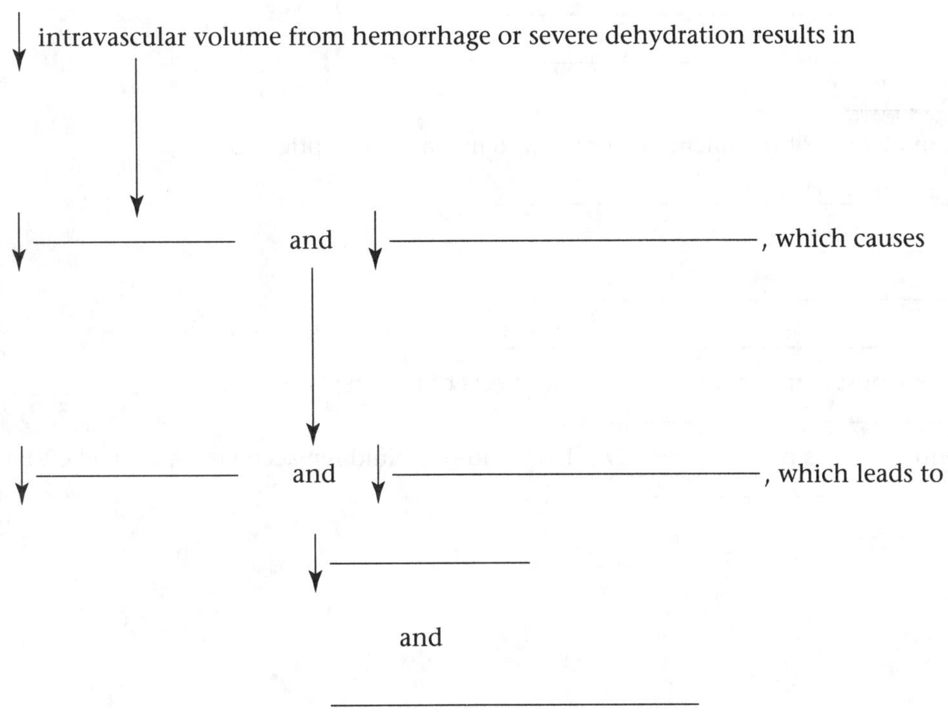

Send-Home Assignments

Tell students to read the following case study and fill in the blanks with the correct answer (reference pages 257–259).

Case Study: Septic Shock

Mr. Dressler, a 43-year-old Caucasian, was admitted to the medical-surgical unit on this third postoperative day following a vertical bonded gastroplasty for morbid obesity. He had initially transferred to the ICU from the recovery room.

Mr. Dressler had a normal postoperative recovery period until his first afternoon on the unit. The RN went into his room to assess 4:00 PM vital signs and noted that his temperature was 102°, he was shaking with chills, his skin was warm and dry, yet his extremities were cool to the touch. Vital signs were 70/50, 124, and 36, and his urinary drainage bag only had 200 ml from 7:00 AM. The nurse, assessing that Mr. Dressler was probably experiencing septicemia, immediately notified the physician.

Answer the following questions, based on your knowledge of speticemia and shock.

1. Septic shock is most commonly caused by gram-negative organisms. Give an example of a common gram-negative bacteria: ____________________
2. The nurse knows that the mortality rate associated with septic shock is between ____% and ____%.
3. The nurse expects that the physician will request body fluid specimens for culture and sensitivity tests. She prepares to collect specimens of
   a. ____
   b. ____
   c. ____
   d. ____
4. Four modalities of treatment are essential to manage the septic shock:
   a. ____
   b. ____
   c. ____
   d. ____
5. The two most common and serious side effects of fluid replacement are: ____________________________ and ____________________________.
6. A central venous pressure line (CVP) helps monitor fluid replacement. A normal CVP value is ____________________________.

15

Oncology: Nursing Management in Cancer Care

I. LEARNING OBJECTIVES

In addition to the learning objectives on page 263, I want my students to be able to:

1. ____

2. ____

3. ____

II. TOP TERMS

1. Biologic Response Modifiers
2. Carcinogenesis
3. Cytokines
4. Interferon
5. Interleukins
6. Metastases
7. Myelosuppression
8. Neoplasia
9. Palliation
10. Staging
10. Vesicant Drugs

III. COLLABORATIVE LEARNING ACTIVITIES

Team Discussion Questions/Seminar Topics

1. In 1997, five-year survival rates for cancer were 44% for African Americans and 60% for Caucasians. Ask students to explain why mortality for African Americans is higher than any other race in the United States (reference page 264).
2. Direct students to discuss the three-step cellular process that is believed to be part of the malignant transformation that occurs with carcinogenesis (reference pages 267–268).
3. Direct students to discuss the use of radiation therapy to interrupt cellular growth. Ask them to answer the following questions: What type of ionizing radiation exists? What cells are most valuable? How do radiation implants work? How is toxicity determined and treated? (reference pages 274–276)

IV. CRITICAL THINKING ACTIVITIES

In-Class Team Exercise

Have students work in two teams and identify seven cellular characteristics of malignant neoplasms (reference pages 266–267 and Table 15–2). Have each team describe the physiological processes that alter cellular growth.

Cell Characteristics	Altered Effect
1. Peripheral growth (sample)	1. infiltrate and destroy surrounding tissues
2. ________________	2. ________________
3. ________________	3. ________________
4. ________________	4. ________________
5. ________________	5. ________________
6. ________________	6. ________________
7. ________________	7. ________________

Send-Home Assignments

1. Toxicity following chemotherapy affects various body systems. For each system below, ask students to list two symptoms of toxicity and explain the rationale for each nursing intervention (reference pages 276–281).

Body System	Symptoms	Rationale for Nursing Action
1. Gastrointestinal	Nausea (sample) Vomiting (sample)	Administer serotonin blockers (Ondansetron) to decrease stimulation of the chemoreceptor trigger zone in the brain's vomiting center.
2. Hematopoietic	________________ ________________	________________ ________________ ________________
3. Renal	________________ ________________	________________ ________________ ________________
4. Cardiopulmonary	________________ ________________	________________ ________________ ________________

2. Tell students to read the following case study and fill in the blanks or circle the correct answers.

Case Study: Cancer of the Lung

Mr. Donato is a 43-year-old accountant who has been a one-pack-a-day smoker for 23 years. He has had a persistent cough for one year that is hacking and nonproductive and has had repeated unresolved upper respiratory tract infections. He went to see his physician because he was fatigued, had been anorexic, and lost 12 pounds over the last three months. Diagnostic evaluation led to a diagnosis of a localized tumor with no evidence of metastatic spread. He was scheduled for a lobectomy in three days (reference: nursing care plan, 15–1 on pages 282–290).

1. Because infection is the leading cause of mortality in the oncology population, the nurse preoperatively notes the significance a(n):
   a. basophil count of 1.3%.
   b. eosinaphil count of 4.5%.
   c. lymphocyte count of 23%.
   d. neutrophil count of 20%.
2. The nurse is concerned that the patient's nutritional status is compromised based on his recent weight loss. Impaired nutritional status contributes to:

   a. ______________________ d. ______________________

   b. ______________________ e. ______________________

   c. ______________________
3. List five factors that the nurse would assess to determine the patient's experience with pain in order to develop a plan of care for pain management.

   a. ______________________ d. ______________________

   b. ______________________ e. ______________________

   c. ______________________
4. The nurse knows that a diagnosis of cancer is accompanied by grieving. Usually the first reaction to the grieving process is:

   a. bargaining. c. denial.

   b. acceptance. d. depression.
5. List four activities the nurse can do to support the patient and family during the grieving process.

   a. ______________________ c. ______________________

   b. ______________________ d. ______________________
6. The nurse knows that postoperative care needs to be directed toward the prevention of ______________________, the leading cause of death in cancer patients.
7. Two major gram-negative bacilli that cause infection in an immunosuppressed patient are: ______________________ and ______________________.
8. The nurse will also assess for the postoperative complication of septic shock, which is not associated with:

   a. dysrhythmias. c. metabotic acidosis.

   b. hypertension. d. oliguria.

3. Assign the following ethical case study. Direct students to choose one of the two positions and prepare an argument to support their position. Recommend that the "Guidelines" be used in their clinical practice.

ETHICAL QUESTION: WHEN IS STOPPING TREATMENT THE ETHICAL ACTION?

Situation: A 65-year-old man with multisystem disease has signed a life prolongation document stating that he wants to have all treatments available to him to be kept alive. Shortly after signing the document, he was readmitted to the hospital and rapidly became comatose. When family members arrive at the hospital, they ask the staff to stop all treatments. The physician agrees that the treatments represent futile medical care and the resources could be better used elsewhere. As the nurse in charge, you know the wishes of the patient. And you seem to be the only health care provider that is paying attention to them.

Dilemma: The nurse is caught in a conflict between the prior wishes of the patient and the present wishes of others.

Arguments for Stopping Treatment: The patient is going to die anyway, and he no longer has any say in what is to be done with him. The family and physician agree that treatment will have no benefit, nor will it change the course of the disease.

Implications of Choosing to Stop Treatment: The patient's prior wishes are going to be disregarded. The patient will die. It is not clear what the patient would want if he knew that the treatments would be futile.

Arguments Against Stopping Treatment: The patient signed a life prolongation document in which he stated he wanted everything done. It is not clear if he knew what "everything" entailed. If prior documents are disregarded when the patient cannot make his wishes known, what is the purpose of signing the document in the first place?

Implications of Choosing Not to Stop Treatment: Patients may be less likely to document their wishes in advance if the wishes are to be disregarded.

Potential Compromise: Give the treatments a chance to effect a clinical remission of disease before stopping treatment. Then if the treatments do not help, stop them and let the patient die. In choosing the compromise, the patient's prior wishes are honored. Treatments are tried, but if they are unhelpful, they can be stopped. The nurse remains the patient's advocate. The family does not feel that they ignored the wishes of the patient.

Guidelines for Nursing Care:

1. When providing care for patients with advance directives, know the policies of the institution.
2. Know how to access the ethics committee if an unresolvable conflict arises.
3. Support the family, but make it known to the family and the physician what the wishes of the patient were prior to his becoming comatose.
4. Know what the nurse's ethical obligations (morally and clinically) are to the patient and the family.
5. Know the criteria for determining when a treatment is futile.

Bibliography

Cherny, N.I., Coyle, N., & Foley, K.M. (1996, February). Guidelines in the Care of the Dying Cancer Patient. *Hematology/Oncology Clinics of North America,* 10(1): 261–286.

Council on Ethical and Judicial Affairs. American Medical Association. (1991, April 10). Guidelines for the Appropriate Use of Do-Not-Resuscitate Orders. *Journal of the American Medical Association,* 265(14): 1868–1875.

Kellermann, A., et al. (1993, September 22/29). Predicting the Outcome of Unsuccessful Prehospital Advanced Cardiac Life Support. *Journal of the American Medical Association,* 270(12): 1433–1436.

Lichtman, S. M. (1995, September). Physiologic Aspects of Aging: Implications for the Treatment of Cancer. *Drugs and Aging,* 7(3): 212–225.

INSTRUCTIONAL IMPROVEMENT TOOL FOR UNIT 3

Student feedback/evaluation indicated that I need to improve my classroom presentation by:

Adding Content

1. ______________________________

____

2. ______________________________

____

3. ______________________________

____

Deleting Content

1. ______________________________

____

2. ______________________________

____

3. ______________________________

____

Emphasizing/Deemphasizing the Following Content

1. ______________________________

____

2. ______________________________

____

3. ______________________________

____

Questions students asked that I need to research for the future are:

1. ______________________________

____

2. ______________________________

____

3. ______________________________

____

UNIT 4
PERIOPERATIVE CONCEPTS AND NURSING MANAGEMENT

16

Preoperative Nursing Management

I. LEARNING OBJECTIVES

In addition to the learning objectives on page 315, I want my students to be able to:

1. ______________________________

2. ______________________________

3. ______________________________

II. TOP TERMS

1. Ambulatory Surgery
2. Anesthesia
3. Cognitive Coping Strategies
4. Diaphragmatic Breathing
5. Elective Surgery
6. Informed Consent
7. Intraoperative Phase
8. Perioperative Period
9. Pharmacokinetics
10. Preadmission Testing (PAT)

III. COLLABORATIVE LEARNING ACTIVITIES

Team Discussion Questions/Seminar Topics

Nutrients are essential for wound healing and recovery in surgery. Direct students to look at the nutrients listed in Table 16–3 on page 321 and discuss nursing interventions necessary to overcome the results of possible nutrient deficiencies.

IV. CRITICAL THINKING ACTIVITIES

In-Class Team Exercises

Divide students into two teams to complete the following table. List specific teaching guidelines that a nurse can use preoperatively to prepare a patient for postoperative rehabilitation (reference pages 322–327 and Figure 16–1).

Preoperative Teaching Guidelines

Deep Breathing, Coughing, and Relaxation Skills	Turning and Active Body Movement	Pain Control and the Use of Medications	Cognitive Control

Send-Home Assignments

Give students the following assignment. In the second column list a common function for each vitamin listed in the first column. In the third column identify symptoms of vitamin deficiency that would influence a patient's preoperative course.

Vitamin Functions and Deficiencies

Vitamin	Function	Symptoms Associated with Deficiency
Retinal (A)		
Thiamin (B1)		
Riboflavin (B2)		
Ascorbic Acid (C)		
Calciferol (D)		
Menadione (K)		

See textbook chapters on vitamins in Suitor, C.W. and Hunter, M.R. *Nutrition: Principles and Application in Health Promotion* (Philadelphia: JB Lippincott), for assistance in completing of this chart.

17

Intraoperative Nursing Management

I. LEARNING OBJECTIVES

In addition to the learning objectives on page 329, I want my students to be able to:

1. ____

2. ____

3. ____

II. TOP TERMS

1. Anesthesiologist
2. Anesthetist
3. Circulatory Nurse
4. Conscious Sedation
5. General Anesthesia
6. Malignant Hyperthermia
7. Neuromuscular Blocker
8. Regional Anesthesia
9. Scrub Nurse
10. Trendelenburg Position

III. COLLABORATIVE LEARNING ACTIVITIES

Team Discussion Questions/Seminar Topics

Divide students into five teams. Assign each to a different classification of anesthesia (general, intravenous, neuromuscular blocking, regional, and local). Ask each team to complete the following chart for its drug category. Students need to identify a minimum of four common agents for each category, action and type of administration, several advantages and disadvantages of use, implications for use, and significant related nursing actions (reference pages 334–341 and Tables 17–2 to 17–5).

Types of Anesthesia

Category	Agent	Action	Type of Administration	Advantages	Disadvantages	Implications for Use	Nursing Actions
General							
Intravenous							
Neuromuscular Blocking							
Regional							
Local							

IV. CRITICAL THINKING ACTIVITIES

Send-Home Assignments

1. Tell students to list three perioperative nursing actions and rationales for each listed phase of care for a patient undergoing a surgical intervention (reference pages 344–345).

Nursing Actions

Assessment

1. ______________________________

2. ______________________________

3. ______________________________

Planning

1. ______________________________

2. ______________________________

3. ______________________________

Intervention

1. ______________________________

2. ______________________________

3. ______________________________

Evaluation

1. ______________________________

2. ______________________________

3. ______________________________

2. Tell students to read the following case studies and circle the correct answers.

Case Study: Spinal Anesthesia

Colleen, an 18-year-old college student, is to receive a spinal anesthetic for surgery on her left leg (reference pages 338–342, Table 17–5, and Figure 17–2).

1. Preoperatively the nurse needs to make sure that Colleen knows that during surgery she will:
   a. be awake.
   b. feel paralysis initially in her toes and then in her perineum, legs, and abdomen.
   c. not feel pain.
   d. experience all of the above.

2. A major nursing intervention after administration of a spinal anesthetic is to:
   a. assess vital signs.
   b. document the time and amount of the first postoperative voiding.
   c. log-roll the patient from side to side, as needed, for the first 8 hours after surgery.
   d. record the time when sensation returns to the toes.
3. Nursing measures to alleviate a post-spinal-anesthesia headache include all of the following except:
   a. ambulating the patient.
   b. increasing body hydration.
   c. keeping the patient flat in bed.
   d. providing a quiet environment.

Case Study: Malignant Hyperthermia

Rachel, a healthy 3-year-old, is scheduled for hernia repair. During her intubation the anesthesiologist notes that her jaw is rigid and that she is developing tachypnea and tachycardia (reference pages 343–344).

1. Based on these assessment data, the circulating nurse prepares to institute emergency nursing measure to treat probable:
   a. profound cardiovascular collapse.
   b. malignant hyperthermia.
   c. respiratory obstruction.
   d. tetany.
2. Anticipating the progression of the symptoms, the circulating nurse knows that she will need to plan for:
   a. measures aimed at reducing body temperature.
   b. administration of drugs to reverse metabolic alkalosis.
   c. insertion of transvenous pacemaker.
   d. prompt and rapid transfusion of whole blood.
3. If Rachael had a family history of this pharmacogenic syndrome, it is possible that she would have received prophylactic treatment with:
   a. antitetanus serum.
   b. epinephrine.
   c. aminophylline.
   d. dantrolene sodium.

3. Assign the following ethical case studies. Direct students to choose one of the two positions in each study and prepare an argument to support their position. Recommend that the "Guidelines" for each be used in their clinical practice.

CASE STUDY: WHAT ARE THE OBLIGATIONS OF HEALTH CARE PROVIDERS TO GETTING AN INFORMED CONSENT FOR A PROCEDURE?

Situation: A 78-year-old man was admitted via the Emergency Department to your unit. His abdomen was rigid and grossly distended. A nasogastric tube was inserted and a CT scan was performed disclosing no obstruction. A Cantor tube was inserted to replace the nasogastric tube. After 3 days the patient began to improve as evidenced by formed stools. The Cantor tube was clamped overnight and the patient did not experience nausea or vomiting. The surgeon came in the next morning, briefly assessed the patient, and announced that the patient would be scheduled for an exploratory laparotomy at 9:30 am. The physician gave the patient a consent form to sign and briefly explained the risks as "usual and expected problems." There was no explanation to the patient of why the surgery was needed or what would be done if "something" was found. The physician did not refer to the patient's prognosis without surgery nor were alternatives to the procedure discussed. After the physician left, the patient gave the nurse a very puzzled look and stated, "He's the surgeon, so I guess he knows best."

Dilemma: There is no ethical conflict here between two or more ethical oughts. What the surgeon is doing is clearly wrong. The only conflict is whether the nurse should act as the patient advocate and make sure that the patient understands what the surgeon wishes to do and why.

Arguments for Making Sure the Patient's Consent Is Informed: It is the right of every patient or guardian to know what is done to or for him or her. It is the nurse's obligation—both clinically and morally—to make sure patients understand what is going to be done. The nurse's obligation is to witness the informed consent for a procedure that someone else is going to do.

Implications of Choosing to Inform the Patient: The nurse should inform the surgeon that the patient did not understand the consent. If the surgeon persists in scheduling the patient for surgery, the nurse should contact the anesthesiologist (who also has obligations, both ethically and clinically) that the patient signed a consent for surgery without knowing what the surgery was for. Clinically there appears to be no indication for the surgery, and the nurse should contact the nursing supervisor to see what can be done and to see if the surgery is justified.

Arguments Against Making Sure Patient Consent is Informed: By not acting as the patient's advocate, the nurse may avoid conflict with the surgeon. The patient would have the surgery without knowing what was done or why it was done.

Implications of Choosing Not to Inform the Patient: The patient would have the surgery. The surgeon's status would be reinforced with the concept that whatever he or she wanted to do to a patient would be supported by the nursing staff. The nurse would not learn the surgeon's reasoning—maybe there were other clinical reasons for the surgery that were not demonstrated in the patient's current clinical presentation. The patient might be undergoing an "unnecessary" surgery. The patient's rights would be violated.

Potential Compromise: The nurse can ask the surgeon to explain the clinical reasoning for the surgery. If the surgeon refuses, then call for an ethics committee consultation. Make sure the nursing supervisor is aware of the problem. In choosing to compromise, the nurse makes sure that the patient's rights are protected. Nurses on staff are perceived as professionals. The surgeon can share information that he or she has and in so doing improve the patient's postoperative care.

Guideline for Nursing Care:

1. Understand patient rights with regard to informed consent.
2. Know that the basis for informed consent includes the following standards:
   a. Disclosure—information is given to the patient about diagnosis and prognosis, a course of action is proposed, risks and benefits are explained. The disclosure is based on what a reasonable person would want to know.
   b. Cognition—information is absorbed and understood by the patient.
   c. Consent, refusal, choice—the patient makes the choice based on his or her values and life plan and the nurse understands that the patient needs to have the conditions of informed consent followed.
   d. Freedom—the patient has the ability and chance to choose either to accept or refuse the treatment proposal.
   e. Competence—the patient has the requisite capacity for making an informed choice.

Bibliography

Lidz, C. W., Appelbaum, P. S., & Meisel, A. (1988). Two models of implementing informed consent. *Archives of Internal Medicine 148,* 1385–1389.

Drane, J. F. (1984). Competency to give informed consent. *Journal of the American Medical Association 252,* 925–927.

Faden, R. R., & Beauchamp, T. L. (1986). *A history and theory of informed consent.* New York: Oxford University Press.

President's Commission for the Study of Ethical Problems in Medicine and Biomedical and Behavioral Research, Making Health Care Decisions. Government Printing Office, 1982.

CASE STUDY: IS IT POSSIBLE FOR A PATIENT TO HAVE A DO-NOT-RESUSCITATE DIRECTIVE IN THE OPERATING ROOM?

Situation: Your hospital has developed a policy, authorized through the medical staff, that allows for patients to have a do not resuscitate (DNR) order in place during a surgical procedure. This policy follows the guidelines of the American Society of Anesthesiologists for DNR in the Operating Room (OR). You are getting a patient ready for surgery and the anesthesiologist who will administer the anesthetic writes an order for the DNR to be rescinded during surgery. The physician is refusing to talk to the patient concerning the DNR.

Dilemma: Conflict between the directive of the patient and the authorized policy and the directive of the physician.

Arguments for Honoring the DNR: The patient's wishes will be followed.

Implications of Choosing to Honor the DNR: It is imperative that the patient understand that he or she will be intubated and ventilated during the surgery irrespective of having or not having a DNR directive. The patient and the physician both need to know each other's understanding of the DNR directive.

Arguments Against Honoring the DNR: The patient's wishes will not be followed. The anesthesiologist goes against the hospital policy. Perhaps he or she did not understand the patient's request for the DNR directive.

Implications of Choosing Not to Honor the DNR:. There is no communication between the patient and the physician.

Potential Compromise: A patient, family, nurse, physician conference on the DNR directive and its implications in the OR can be scheduled so that the patient's wishes and the physician's understanding of clinical management of a patient in the OR are communicated and understood.

Guidelines for Nursing Care:

1. When providing care for a patient undergoing surgery, understand the hospital and staff policies regarding DNR in the OR.
2. Help the patient understand what he or she is requesting.
3. Contact the ethics committee if there is a conflict between physician and patient.

Bibliography

Keffer, M. J., & Keffer, H. L. (1992). Do-not-resuscitate in the operating room: Moral Obligations of anesthesiologists. *Anesthesia & Analgesia 74,* 901–905.

Keffer, M. J., & Keffer, H. L. (1994). The do-not-resuscitate order: Moral responsibilities of the perioperative nurse. *AORN Journal 59*(3), 641–650.

Margolis, J. O., McGrath, B. J., Kussin, P. S., & Schwinn, D. A. (1995). Do not resuscitate (DNR) orders during surgery: Ethical foundations for institutional policies in the United States. *Anesthesia & Analgesia 80,* 806–9.1.2.

18

Postoperative Nursing Management

I. LEARNING OBJECTIVES

In addition to the learning objectives on page 347, I want my students to be able to:

1. ______________________________

2. ______________________________

3. ______________________________

II. TOP TERMS

1. Aspiration
2. Atelectasis
3. Deep Vein Thrombosis
4. Dehiscence
5. Epidural Infusion
6. Evisceration
7. First Intention Healing
8. Hypoxemia
9. Paralytic Ileus
10. Post-Anesthesia Care Unit (PACU)
11. Proliferative Phase of Wound Healing
12. Serosanguineous

III. COLLABORATIVE LEARNING ACTIVITIES

Team Discussion Questions/Seminar Topics

1. Ask students to outline collaborative nursing interventions for the nursing diagnosis, "Impaired skin integrity related to incision and drainage site." Tell students to list supporting rationales for each nursing action (reference pages 362–367 and Tables 18–2 to 18–4).
2. Direct students to discuss the gerontologic considerations related to the postoperative management of a patient with deep vein thrombosis (reference pages 361–362 and Figure 18–6).

IV. CRITICAL THINKING ACTIVITIES

In-Class Team Exercises

For each of the nursing diagnoses listed below, direct students to list one patient goal and two nursing interventions for assisting the patient toward goal achievement.

1. Nursing Diagnosis: Ineffective airway clearance related to the depressant effects of medications and anesthetic agents

   Goal: ______________________________

   Nursing Interventions: ______________________________

   ____

2. Nursing Diagnosis: Pain and other postoperative discomforts

   Goal: ______________________________

   Nursing Interventions: ______________________________

   ____

3. Nursing Diagnosis: Alteration in tissue perfusion, systemic, secondary to hypovolemia, peripheral blood pooling, and possible vasoconstriction

   Goal: ______________________________

   Nursing Interventions: ______________________________

   ____

4. Nursing Diagnosis: Potential fluid volume deficit

   Goal: ______________________________

   Nursing Interventions: ______________________________

   ____

Send-Home Assignments

1. Most surgical patients have a nursing diagnosis of impaired skin integrity related to the surgical incision. Patient goals for this nursing diagnosis are evidenced by participation in self-care and the ability to identify initial symptoms of hematoma and infection. Ask students to describe four areas of patient education for care of a wound before suture removal (reference pages 362–367).

   a. ______________________________

   b. ______________________________

   c. ______________________________

   d. ______________________________

2. Tell students to read the following case study and circle the correct answers.

Case Study: Hypovolemic Shock

Mario is admitted to the emergency department with a diagnosis of hypovolemic shock secondary to a 30% blood volume loss resulting from a motorcycle accident (reference pages 350–351 and Table 18–1).

1. A primary nursing objective is to:
   a. administer vasopressors.
   b. ensure a patent airway.
   c. minimize energy expenditure.
   d. provide external warmth.
2. With a diagnosis of hypovolemic shock, the nurse expects to assess all of the following except:
   a. a decreased and concentrated urinary output.
   b. an elevated central venous pressure reading.
   c. hypotension with a small pulse pressure.
   d. tachycardia and a thready pulse.
3. The nurse takes blood pressure readings every 5 minutes. She knows that shock is well advanced when the systolic reading drops below:
   a. 90 mm Hg.
   b. 100 mm Hg.
   c. 110 mm Hg.
   d. 120 mm Hg.
4. A urinary catheter is inserted to measure hourly output. The nurse knows that inadequate volume replacement is reflected by an output less than:
   a. 30 ml/hr.
   b. 50 ml/hr.
   c. 80 ml/hr.
   d. 100 ml/hr.
5. The physician prescribes crystalloid solution to be administered to restore blood volume. The nurse knows that a crystalloid solution is:
   a. a blood transfusion.
   b. lactated Ringer's solution.
   c. plasma or a plasma substitute.
   d. serum albumia.

INSTRUCTIONAL IMPROVEMENT TOOL FOR UNIT 4

Student feedback/evaluation indicated that I need to improve my classroom presentation by:

Adding Content

1. ______________________________
____

2. ______________________________
____

3. ______________________________
____

Deleting Content

1. ______________________________
____

2. ______________________________
____

3. ______________________________
____

Emphasizing/Deemphasizing the Following Content

1. ______________________________
____

2. ______________________________
____

3. ______________________________
____

Questions students asked that I need to research for the future are:

1. ______________________________
____

2. ______________________________
____

3. ______________________________
____

UNIT 5
GAS EXCHANGE AND RESPIRATORY FUNCTION

19

Assessment of Respiratory Function

I. LEARNING OBJECTIVES

In addition to the learning objectives on page 373, I want my students to be able to:

1. ____

2. ____

3. ____

II. TOP TERMS

1. Alveoli
2. Apneustic Center
3. Crackles
4. Cyanosis
5. Dyspnea
6. Hematemesis
7. Hering-Breuer Reflex
8. Hypoxia
9. Partial Pressure
10. Pulmonary Perfusion
11. Rales
12. Rhonchi
13. Sibilant Wheezes
14. Surfactant
15. Tachypnea
16. Tactile Fremitus

III. COLLABORATIVE LEARNING ACTIVITIES

Team Discussion Questions/Seminar Topics

1. Ask students to compare and contrast the various respiratory processes: ventilation, perfusion, diffusion, and shunting. Have students explain the relationship of the pulmonary circulation to these processes (reference pages 378–380 and Chart 19–2).
2. Ask students to explain the differences and clinical significance between adventitious breath sounds: (crackles, rales, rhonchi, wheezes and pleural friction rub) (reference pages 390–392 and Table 19–4).

IV. CRITICAL THINKING ACTIVITIES

In-Class Team Exercises

Assign students to teams of four. Have each student assess the breath sounds of three of his or her classmates. Complete the following chart, identifying as many characteristics as possible (reference pages 390–392 and Table 19–4).

Breath Sounds Assessment

	Description of Sound in Your Words	Sound Duration	Location of Various Intensities	Expiratory Sound Intensity	Expiratory Sound Pitch
Vesicular					
Broncho-Vesicular					
Bronchial					
Tracheal					

20

Management of Patients with Upper Respiratory Tract Disorders

I. LEARNING OBJECTIVES

In addition to the learning objectives on page 401, I want my students to be able to:

1. ______________________________

2. ______________________________

3. ______________________________

II. TOP TERMS

1. Dysphasia
2. Epistaxis
3. Heimlich Maneuver
4. Herpes Simplex Virus
5. Laryngectomy
6. Nasal Polyps
7. Pharyngitis
8. Rhinitis

III. COLLABORATIVE LEARNING ACTIVITIES

Team Discussion Questions/Seminar Topics

1. Ask students to describe what an individual should do to help someone who has a nosebleed. Students should list criteria to use to determine when a person should go to the emergency room (reference pages 411–412).
2. Direct students to answer the following: Describe the appearance of a herpes simplex canker sore. Why does it appear? What are common preventive measures and treatment modalities? How can its spread be contained? (reference page 402 and Chart 20–1)
3. Encourage several members of the class to describe their personal experiences with acute or chronic sinusitis. What were their symptoms? How do they manage to control and treat the disorder and carry on with their home and school responsibilities? Ask if anyone who has had surgery for this condition would share his or her experiences (reference pages 403–406).

III. CRITICAL THINKING ACTIVITIES

In-Class Team Exercises

1. Assign students to a partner and ask each student to demonstrate the Heimlich maneuver on his or her partner (reference pages 413–414 and Guidelines 20–1).
2. Assign students to two teams. Have each team design a poster for a college/school bulletin board. The first poster should include information for students about recognizing and preventing upper respiratory tract infections. The second poster should include information about the symptoms of the common cold, recognizable symptoms, and measures to prevent its spread (reference pages 402–403 and 409–410).

Send-Home Assignments

Tell students to read the following case study and fill in the blanks or circle the correct answers.

Case Study: The Common Cold

Carol, a 28-year-old bank teller, felt very lethargic when she went to work on Monday. Her symptoms of fatigue were vague, but her muscles ached and she had a headache. By the afternoon, she had nasal congestion, a sore throat, and chills. Two of her co-workers, feeling the same way, had gone home earlier. Carol decided to stay at work because she felt she "just had a cold" (reference pages 402–403).

1. Based on your knowledge about the common cold, list eight characteristic symptoms that Carol might experience.

   a. ______________________________

   b. ______________________________

   c. ______________________________

   d. ______________________________

   e. ______________________________

   f. ______________________________

   g. ______________________________

   h. ______________________________

2. Carol's virus is highly contagious because the virus is shed for _____(hours/days) before symptoms appear.
   a. 48 hours
   b. 72 hours
   c. 5 days
   d. 7 days

3. Carol's decision to stay at work could cause the viruses to spread to her co-workers. Statistics tell us that colds account for _____ percent of all work absences.
   a. 10
   b. 25
   c. 30
   d. 50

4. In the United States, waves of colds tend to appear seasonally, especially in:
   a. January
   b. April
   c. September
   d. All of the above

5. Carol should know that her symptoms will last about:
   a. 2 to 4 days.
   b. 3 to 9 days.

c. 4 to 10 days.
d. 5 to 14 days.

6. Carol knows that the best treatment measures include five at-home therapies:

a. ______________________________

b. ______________________________

c. ______________________________

d. ______________________________

e. ______________________________

7. Carol calls her physician and requests an antibiotic. The physician ______________________________

____

21

Management of Patients with Chest and Lower Respiratory Tract Disorders

I. LEARNING OBJECTIVES

In addition to the learning objectives on page 422, I want my students to be able to:

1. ______________________________

2. ______________________________

3. ______________________________

II. TOP TERMS

1. Acute Respiratory Distress Syndrome
2. Air Trapping
3. Atelectasis
4. Barrel Chest
5. Bronchiectasis
6. Cor Pulmonale
7. Empyema
8. Ghon Tubercule
9. Lung Abscess
10. Pleural Effusion
11. Pneumonia
12. Pneumothorax
13. Ventilation-Perfusion Ratio

III. COLLABORATIVE LEARNING ACTIVITIES

Team Discussion Question/Seminar Topics

1. Require that students explain the pathophysiology of bacterial pneumonia from the initial inflammatory reaction to arterial hypoxemia (reference pages 426–431 and Table 21–1).
2. Ask students to describe the clinical symptoms of a hospitalized patient who is developing bacterial pneumonia (reference pages 426–434 and Table 21–1).
3. Direct students to explain the pathophysiology, clinical manifestations, diagnostic evaluation, medical management, and nursing interventions for a patient with lung cancer (reference pages 477–481).

IV. CRITICAL THINKING ACTIVITIES

In-Class Team Exercises:

Ask students to complete the following chart comparing the various types of commonly encountered pneumonias. (reference pages 426–434 and Table 21–1)

Commonly Encountered Pneumonias

Category	Bacterial Pneumonias	Responsible Organism	Incidence	Clinical Features	Treatment	Nursing Actions
Community-Acquired	Streptococcal Pneumonia					
	Haemophilus Influenza					
	Legionnaires' Disease					
	Mycoplasma Pneumonia					
Hospital-Acquired	Pseudomonas Pneumonia					

Category	Bacterial Pneumonias	Responsible Organism	Incidence	Clinical Features	Treatment	Nursing Actions
	Staphylococcal Pneumonia					
	Klevsiella Pneumonia					
Immuno-compromised	Fungal Pneumonia					
	Pneumocystitis Carinii Pneu-monia					
	Tuberculosis					

Send-Home Assignments

Tell students to read the following case study and circle the correct answers.

Case Study: Tuberculosis

Mr. Carrera, a 67-year-old retired baker and pastry chef, is admitted to the clinical area for confirmation of suspected tuberculosis. He is anorexic and fatigued and suffers with "indigestion." His temperature is slightly elevated every afternoon (reference pages 436–442).

1. Mr. Carrera's Mantoux tuberculin test yields an induration of 10 mm. This result is interpreted as indicating that:
   a. active disease is present.
   b. he has been exposed to M. tuberculosis or been vaccinated with BCG.
   c. preventive treatment should be initiated.
   d. the reaction is doubtful and should be repeated.
2. After Mr. Carrera has undergone a series of additional tests, the diagnosis is confirmed by:
   a. a chest X-ray.
   b. acid-fast bacilli in a sputum smear.
   c. a positive multiple-puncture skin test.
   d. repeated Mantoux tests that yield indurations of 10 mm or greater.
3. Mr. Carrera is started on a multiple-drug regimen. Nursing management includes observing for ototoxicity and nephrotoxicity when ___________ is used.
   a. ethambutol
   b. isoniazid
   c. rifampin
   d. streptomycin
4. Mr. Carrera needs to know that the initial intensive treatment is usually given daily for:
   a. 2 weeks.
   b. 2 to 4 weeks.
   c. 2 months.
   d. 4 to 6 months.
5. Mr. Carrera is informed that he will no longer be considered infectious when:
   a. repeat Mantoux tests are negative.
   b. serial chest X-rays show improvement.
   c. two consecutive sputum specimens are negative.
   d. all of the above parameters are met.

22

Respiratory Care Modalities

I. LEARNING OBJECTIVES

In addition to the learning objectives on page 490, I want my students to be able to:

1. ______________________________

2. ______________________________

3. ______________________________

II. TOP TERMS

1. COPD
2. Diaphragmatic Breathing
3. FiO_2
4. Hypoxemia
5. Incentive Spirometry
6. Intubation
7. IPPB
8. Lobectomy
9. Oxygen Toxicity
10. PEEP
11. Pulse Oximetry
12. SIMV
13. Tracheostomy
14. Ventilator

III. COLLABORATIVE LEARNING ACTIVITIES

Team Discussion Questions/Seminar Topics

1. Direct students to compare and contrast the purpose, use, and nursing management of intermittent positive-pressure breathing versus incentive spirometry (reference pages 494–495).
2. Ask students to explain the rationale for administering low concentrations of oxygen to patients with chronic obstructive pulmonary disease (references pages 492–494).
3. Request that students develop a patient teaching guide for a patient who needs to understand diaphragmatic breathing. Have a member of the class demonstrate the breathing technique (reference pages 498 and 515 and Plan of Nursing Care 22–1, pages 523–526).

IV. CRITICAL THINKING ACTIVITIES

In-Class Team Exercises

1. Assign the following chart comparing the various types of oxygen administration devices (reference pages 492–494 and Table 22–1).

Oxygen Administration Devices

Oxygen Device	Flow Rate	Advantages	Disadvantages	Nursing Teaching Points
Cannula				
Catheter				
Simple Mask				
Partial Rebreather Mask				
Non-Rebreather Mask				
Venturi				
Face Tent				
T-Piece Briggs				

2. Divide students into groups of six. Have one student in each group demonstrate four postural drainage positions while other team members identify the lobes being drained by each position (reference pages 496–497 and Figure 22–2).
3. Place students into four groups. Identify a team leader who will demonstrate the proper technique of percussion and vibration (reference pages 497–498 and Figure 22–3).

Send-Home Assignments

1. Assign a nursing care plan for each of the following situations, which involve managing a patient on mechanical ventilation.
   A. Richard, a 19-year-old college freshman, has been managed on a volume-controlled ventilator for several weeks after being admitted for drug overdose associated with alcohol intake. Before admission, Richard was a school athlete who was in good health and not known to use drugs or drink alcoholic beverages to extreme (reference pages 503–513).

   Nursing Diagnosis: Ineffective breathing patterns related to physiological insult to respiratory function

Goals	Nursing Actions	Rationale	Expected Outcomes

   B. Sally, a 69-year-old patient with emphysema, has been managed on a ventilator since her pneumonectomy 3 weeks ago. Sally had surgery for carcinoma of the right lung. Her emphysema was believed to be related to a history of smoking two packs of cigarettes a day for the past forty years (reference pages 503–513).

   Nursing Diagnosis: Powerlessness related to ventilator therapy dependency

Goals	Nursing Actions	Rationale	Expected Outcomes

2. Assign the following case studies. Direct students to choose one of the two options and prepare an argument to support their position. Recommend that the "Guidelines" be used in their clinical practice.

CASE STUDY: WHAT SHOULD BE THE NURSE'S ROLE IN CARING FOR PATIENTS AS LIFE-PROLONGING TREATMENTS ARE DISCONTINUED?

Situation: You have been caring for a 70-year-old man in the neurologic intensive care unit ever since his motor vehicle crash 2 weeks ago. He sustained a complete C1–C2 fracture of the neck and is a quadriplegic. Because his fracture is so high, he will be ventilator dependent for the rest of his life. From the moment he was admitted he has requested to be allowed to die. He has a living will and his wife is his durable power of attorney for health representative. He had been robust and in exceptional health, enjoying daily golf and other activities. He did not want to live the rest of his life without the ability to do the things that he enjoyed. Over the next several days he continued to request to be taken off ventilatory support so he could die. He was able to communicate via letter board and was awake, alert, and oriented. He was surrounded by his family and friends. He requested his attorneys so he could tend to his personal and financial affairs. With the loving support of his family, it was decided to remove the ventilator and medication would be given to assist him in dealing with hypoxia and anoxia. Surrounded by his family he was given sedation and the ventilator was removed.

Dilemma: Is the nurse caught in conflict between killing or letting die?

Arguments for Removing Mechanical Ventilation: The patient has an autonomous right to stop treatment. Treatment will have to be maintained for life to continue, and the patient does not desire to be maintained in this manner. The patient is competent and appears to have made a knowledge-based request.

Implications of Supporting This Position: The patient will die of his own choice to remove ventilatory support. The nurse and other health care providers are not given an opportunity to process the removal of treatments.

Arguments Against Removing Mechanical Ventilation: The patient and family made the decision to remove the ventilator quite quickly and haven't studied or considered alternatives.

Implications of Supporting this Position: The health care providers are involved in active voluntary euthanasia. Stopping treatments that sustain life is an example of how technology has induced people to make active decisions about the appropriateness of life-sustaining treatments.

Potential Compromise: Have the patient and family, along with medical and nursing staff, investigate all other possible alternatives. Maybe there is a chance that the ventilator could be removed and the patient could breathe spontaneously. Perhaps the neurologic trauma may decrease over time. Perhaps an experimental procedure could be investigated. The patient and family could be offered the opportunity for spiritual or other counseling. The family needs to be approached about care outside of the hospital. In presenting possible alternatives, the nursing staff encourages the patient and family to utilize health care services to investigate other opportunities.

Guidelines for Nursing Care:

1. Know the difference between patient assisted suicide and active or passive euthanasia.
2. Understand the institution's policies for nursing involvement in stopping treatments.
3. Know the laws of the state in which nursing is practiced.
4. Examine your own values for starting or stopping life-sustaining treatments.
5. Develop a plan of what you would do if asked to remove a ventilator and administer terminal sedation.

Bibliography

Annas, G. J. (1997). The bell tolls for a constitutional right to physician-assisted suicide. *New England Journal of Medicine 3337*(15), 1098–1103.

Battin, M. P. (1994). *The least worst death.* New York: Oxford University Press.

Emanuel, E. J. (1994). Euthanasia: Historical, ethical, and empiric perspectives. *Archives of Internal Medicine 154,* 1890–1901.

Quill, T. E. (1991). Death and dignity: A case of individualized decision making. *New England Journal of Medicine 324,* 691–694.

ETHICAL CASE STUDY: SHOULD TERMINAL PATIENTS BE SEDATED BEFORE THE VENTILATOR IS WITHDRAWN?

Patients have an ethical and legal right to refuse medical treatment, including mechanical ventilation. However, if a patient is awake and alert and extremely dependent on the ventilator, the withdrawal of the ventilator can cause extreme discomfort and distress as the patient experiences air hunger and symptoms of suffocation. Sedation effective enough to alleviate these symptoms can also virtually guarantee that the patient will not survive the ventilator's withdrawal. Should patients be sedated for comfort before ventilator withdrawal, or does such an action effectively constitute killing the patient?

Dilemma: The obligation to make the patient comfortable for a distressing procedure conflicts with the health care providers' obligation not to harm the patient (beneficence versus non-maleficence). Or, the patient's request for sedation may conflict with the obligation not to harm the patient (autonomy versus nonmaleficence).

Arguments in *Favor* of Sedation Before Terminal Ventilator Withdrawal: Health care providers have an obligation to anticipate distressing symptoms and provide medication to prevent the patient from suffering. The obligation to make the patient comfortable is more important than the provider's fear of harming the patient. It would be cruel not to sedate patients who might experience severe symptoms. Patients for whom ventilator withdrawal symptoms would be severe would probably not survive the ventilator withdrawal. The patient who dies after sedation and ventilator withdrawal dies of his or her own lung or neurological disease, not from the sedation and the ventilator withdrawal. Ventilator withdrawal allows the patient to die of the disease; sedation helps to keep the patient comfortable. Sedation and ventilator withdrawal is not the same as killing the patient.

Implications of Choosing This Position: Patients will be sedated at the time of death. Health care workers may feel guilty that they contributed to the patient's death by sedating him or her. Sedation may contribute to the patient's death or to the time of death. Patients will not experience distressing symptoms of air hunger and suffocation when their ventilators are withdrawn. Patients who might survive their ventilator withdrawal are more likely to die if given sedation.

Arguments *Against* Sedation Before Terminal Ventilator Withdrawal: Sedation before ventilator withdrawal is more like killing the patient than allowing him or her to die, because the sedation will prevent the patient from breathing electively. Health care providers should not be required to assist in what may cause a patient's death. Sedation can be given to a patient after the ventilator is withdrawn if and only if distressing withdrawal symptoms develop.

Implications of Choosing This Position: Patients may experience distressing symptoms when ventilators are withdrawn. Health care professionals may feel guilty if the patient dies after suffering through symptoms of air hunger and suffocation. Patients will be more likely to be able to talk and converse without sedation. Patients who expire without sedation after their ventilators are withdrawn are certain to have died because of their disease process and not from any sedation. Patients who survive their ventilator withdrawal are more likely to survive without sedation. Sedation given after distressing symptoms occur may be less likely to provide relief.

Potential Compromise: Provide sedation only for those patients considered likely to experience severe withdrawal symptoms. Discuss the pros and cons of sedation with the patient and family and arrive at a joint decision.

Implications of Choosing This Position: Health care professionals may still feel that the sedation caused the patient's death. The patient may decide against sedation and suffer distressing symptoms. The patient and family will know what to expect after the ventilator is withdrawn.

Guideline for the Nurse Involved in the Ventilator Withdrawal of a Terminally Ill Patient

1. Assess if the patient has made an informed choice for the ventilator withdrawal. If you believe that the patient has not made an informed consent, discuss this with the physician and supervisor and consult with the bioethics committee.
2. Assess the patient's reliance on the ventilator by reviewing the chart for the patient's disease process, course of treatment, and goals for treatment. Determine the amount of support that the patient receives from the ventilator. In your clinical judgment, is the patient likely to experience symptoms of air hunger and suffocation once the ventilator is removed?
3. If you believe the patient might suffer distressing symptoms upon removal of the ventilator, discuss the issue of sedation with the physician. Develop a plan with the physician for handling the symptoms.

4. Have the physician discuss the issue of sedation with the patient. All persons involved should agree to a plan of care. If a plan of care is not agreed upon, consult with your supervisor and consider a bioethics committee consultation.
5. If the nurse agrees to the plan of care but feels uncomfortable in giving the prescribed sedation, the nurse should inform the physician and ask the physician or another nurse to administer the sedation.

Bibliography

Devettere, R. J. (1991, Summer). Sedation Before Ventilator Withdrawal: Can It Be Justified by Double Effect and Called "Allowing a Patient to Die?" *Journal of Clinical Ethics,* 2(2): 122–125.

Basile, C. M. (1998). Advance Directives and Advocacy in End-of Life Decisions. *Nurse Practitioner,* 23(5): 44–46, 54, 57–60.

Edwards, B. S., & Ueno, W. (1991, Summer). Sedation Before Ventilator Withdrawal. *Journal of Clinical Ethics,* 2(2): 118–122.

Gordon, S. (1997). Life Support. *Medical Surgical Nursing,* 6(3): 162–165.

Truog, R. D. et al. (1991, Summer). Sedation Before Ventilator Withdrawal: Medical and Ethical Consideration. *Journal of Clinical Ethics,* 2(2): 127–129.

Twibell, R. S. (1995). Family Coping During Critical Illness. *Dimensions in Critical Care Nursing,* 17(2): 100–112.

Wilson, W. C., et al. (1992, February 19). Ordering and Administration of Sedatives and Analgesics During the Withholding and Withdrawal of Life Support from Critically Ill Patients. *Journal of the American Medical Association,* 267(7): 949–953.

INSTRUCTIONAL IMPROVEMENT TOOL FOR UNIT 5

Student feedback/evaluation indicated that I need to improve my classroom presentation by:

Adding Content

1. ______________________________

2. ______________________________

3. ______________________________

Deleting Content

1. ______________________________

2. ______________________________

3. ______________________________

Emphasizing/Deemphasizing the Following Content

1. ______________________________

2. ______________________________

3. ______________________________

Questions students asked that I need to research for the future are:

1. ______________________________

2. ______________________________

3. ______________________________

UNIT 6
CARDIOVASCULAR, CIRCULATORY, AND HEMATOLOGIC FUNCTION

23
Assessment of Cardiovascular Function

I. LEARNING OBJECTIVES

In addition to the learning objectives on page 531, I want my students to be able to:

1. ______________________________

2. ______________________________

3. ______________________________

II. TOP TERMS

1. Atrioventricular Node
2. Cheyne-Stoke Respirations
3. Crackles
4. Depolarization
5. Friction Rub
6. Gallop Sound
7. Murmurs
8. PMI
9. Sinoatrial Node
10. Wheezes

III. COLLABORATIVE LEARNING ACTIVITIES

Team Discussion Questions/Seminar Topics

1. Ask students to explain why it is important to assess the apical pulse. Identify on each other the two anatomical areas that must be palpated to accurately identify the location of the apex of the heart (reference pages 547–548 and Figure 23–8).
2. Divide students into four teams. Each team, assigned one of the four cardiac sounds (gallops, friction rub, murmurs, and clicks/snaps), is directed to compare and contrast each sound relative to timing, intensity, duration, and radiation. Students should explain what each sound means (reference pages 548–550 and Figures 23–9 and 23–10).

IV. CRITICAL THINKING ACTIVITIES

In-Class Team Exercises

Direct students to compare and contrast the characteristics of chest pain specific to pericarditis, pulmonary pain, and esophageal pain. Use pages 538–544 and Table 23–2 as a guideline.

Chest Pain Characteristics

	Pain Character, Location, Duration, and Radiation	Precipitating Events	Nursing Measures
Pericarditis			
Pain of Pulmonary Origin			
Esophageal Pain			

Send-Home Assignments

Tell students to read the following case study and circle the correct answers.

Case Study: Cardiac Assessment for Chest Pain

Mr. Anderson is a 45-year-old executive with a major oil firm. Lately he has experienced frequent episodes of chest pressure that are relieved with rest. He has requested a complete physical examination. The nurse will assist with the cardiac assessment (reference pages 538–544 and Chart 23–1 and Table 23–3).

1. The nurse takes a baseline blood pressure measurement after the patient has rested for 10 minutes in a supine position. The reading that reflects a reduced pulse pressure is:
   a. 140/90
   b. 140/100.
   c. 140/110.
   d. 140/120.
2. Five minutes after the initial blood pressure measurement was taken, the nurse assesses additional readings with the patient in a sitting and then a standing position. The reading indicative of an abnormal postural response would be:
   a. lying, 140/110; sitting, 130/100; standing, 135/106.
   b. lying, 140/110; sitting, 135/112; standing, 130/115.
   c. lying, 140/110; sitting, 130/100; standing, 120/90.
   d. lying, 140/110; sitting, 130/108; standing, 125/108.
3. The nurse returns Mr. Anderson to the supine position and measures for jugular vein distention. The finding that would initially indicate an abnormal increase in the volume of the venous system would be obvious distention of the veins with the patient at:
   a. 15 degrees.
   b. 25 degrees.
   c. 35 degrees.
   d. 45 degrees.

24

Management of Patients with Dysrhythmias and Conduction Problems

I. LEARNING OBJECTIVES

In addition to the learning objectives on page 564, I want my students to be able to:

1. ______________________________

2. ______________________________

3. ______________________________

II. TOP TERMS

1. Bigeminy
2. Cardioversion
3. Chronotropic
4. Chryoablation
5. Defibrillation
6. Dysrhythmia
7. Fibrillation
8. Pacemaker
9. Purkinje Network
10. QRS Complex
11. Refractory Period
12. Repolarization

III. COLLABORATIVE LEARNING ACTIVITIES

Team Discussion Questions/Seminar Topics

1. Ask students to explain the differences and related significance between atrial and ventricular dysrhythmias (reference pages 568–579 and Chart 24–2).
2. Direct students to distinguish between the procedure and nursing implications for cardioversion and defibrillation (reference pages 580–583).

IV. CRITICAL THINKING ACTIVITIES

In-Class Team Exercises

1. Divide students into four groups. Assign an ECG strip to each group. Ask each group to explain the dysrhythmia, expected associated symptomatology, and appropriate medical and nursing interventions (reference pages 569–579). To complete the following exercises, please refer to Figures 24–7 and 24–8 (page 571), Figure 24–10 (page 572), and Figure 24–13 (page 574).
2. For each of the following pathophysiological responses, ask students to graphically illustrate a dysrhythmia that reflects the altered cardiac functioning (reference pages 569–598 and Figures 24–9, 24–13, 24–17, and 24–19).
   A. Cardiac tissue ischemia
   B. Cardiac muscle injury
   C. Infarcted tissue

IV. CRITICAL THINKING ACTIVITIES

Send-Home Assignments

1. Ask each student to draw on a graphic sheet the depolarization-repolarization sequence that illustrates the electrical conduction system of the heart.
2. Tell students to read the following case study and fill in the blanks with the correct answers.

Case Study: Permanent Pacemaker

Mr. Woo is a 58-year-old Asian male who is scheduled for permanent pacemaker insertion as treatment for a tachydysrhythmia that doesn't respond to medication therapy. He will have an endocardial implant. Direct students to answer the following questions based upon their knowledge of pacemaker management. (reference pages 583–589).

1. Mr. Woo's pacemaker is set at 72 beats/min. His heart rate is 76. Is this expected? (Yes/No) Explain the rationale for your answer.
2. Nursing care includes incision site assessment for three complications: (a) ________________, (b) ________________, and (c) ________________.
3. The most common postoperative complication is ___________, which can be prevented by ________________________.
4. List six things about the pacemaker that must be noted on a patient's chart:
   a. ________________________________
   b. ________________________________
   c. ________________________________
   d. ________________________________
   e. ________________________________
   f. ________________________________
5. Describe nursing interventions and expected outcomes that should be used to meet the three major goals of patient care.

Goals: (a) ____

(b) ____

(c) ____

Nursing Interventions: (a) ____

(b) ____

(c) ___________________________

Expected Outcomes: (a) ___________________________

(b) ___________________________

(c) ___________________________

6. List assessment criteria that should be used to determine if expected outcomes of care are achieved.

Expected Outcomes

a. Freedom from Infection
b. Adherence to a Self-Care Program
c. Maintenance of Pacemaker Function

Assessment Criteria

1. ___________________________
2. ___________________________
3. ___________________________

25

Management of Patients with Coronary Vascular Disorders

I. LEARNING OBJECTIVES

In addition to the learning objectives on page 593, I want my students to be able to:

1. ______________________________

2. ______________________________

3. ______________________________

II. TOP TERMS

1. Afterload
2. Angina Pectoris
3. Atheroma
4. Atherosclerotic Coronary Heart Disease
5. Cardiac Output (CO = HR × SV)
6. Cardiac Tamponade
7. Coronary Artery Bypass Graft Surgery (CABG)
8. Coronary Artery Revascularization
9. Myocardial Infarction
10. Pericardial Effusion
11. Percutaneous Transluminal Coronary Angioplasty (PTCA)
12. Preload
13. Prinzmetal's Angina
14. Streptokinase
15. Transmyocardial Revascularization
16. Troponin

III. COLLABORATIVE LEARNING ACTIVITIES

Team Discussion Questions/Seminar Topics

1. Divide students into six teams. Each team should compare and contrast the etiology, clinical manifestations, diagnostic evaluation, medical management, and nursing interventions for a patient with angina pectoris and one with a myocardial infarction (reference pages 597–602 and 628–635).
2. Ask students to provide a physiologic rationale for modifying specific risk factors associated with heart disease (reference pages 594–597).

3. Choose a team to present the scientific rationale for specialized diets for individuals with heart disease. Opinions that support a controversial approach to dietary management should also be presented (reference pages 594–597).

IV. CRITICAL THINKING EXERCISES

In-Class Team Exercises:

1. Organize a discussion about the formation of atheromatous plaques in an artery, using the following terms in the discussion: atheroma, blood clots, lumen, and tunica intima (reference pages 594–595).
2. For each of the drug classifications commonly used to treat angina pectoris, have students outline specific actions, rationales, and associated nursing implications (reference pages 598–600).

Common Drugs for Angina Pectoris

	Action	**Rationale**	**Nursing Implications**
Nitrates			
Beta-Adrenergic Blockers			
Calcium Ion Antagonists			

Send-Home Assignments

Assign the following ethical case studies. Direct students to choose one of the positions and prepare an argument to support their position. Encourage discussion about the role of the nurse as outlined in the first case study. Recommend that the "Guidelines" presented in the second case study be used in the student's clinical practice.

ETHICAL CASE STUDY: WHEN IS IT APPROPRIATE TO CONSIDER WITHHOLDING OR WITHDRAWING LIFE SUPPORT?

Life support can include an intra-aortic balloon pump, ventilators, vasoactive infusions, CPR, and antibiotics. Patients receiving these treatments include acutely, chronically, and terminally ill patients. Often, when dependent on life support, a patient may be unable to make decisions about his or her own care, and the family may be in crisis. At what point is it appropriate to raise the delicate issue of withholding or withdrawing life support?

Dilemma: The patient's right to choose or refuse treatment conflicts with the obligation to do what is best for the patient (autonomy versus beneficence). Or, the patient's right to choose or refuse treatment conflicts with the obligation not to harm the patient with threatening or inappropriate questions at the wrong time (autonomy versus nonmaleficence).

Arguments That Discussions About the Limitations of Life-Supporting Treatment Should Be Held When Patients Are Admitted to the Hospital: All patients would have the opportunity to discuss the possible treatment options open to them and to express their opinions and reservations about different treatment goals and therapeutic measures. Formalized requirements to have such discussions on admission would ensure that patients' treatment preferences would be addressed and documented.

Implications of Choosing This Position: Not all patients are able to maintain a coherent and detailed discussion on admission (such as those who are confused or comatose on admission). Patients who are admitted to the hospital in relatively good health (such as for childbirth or elective surgery) may express treatment preferences that might conflict with those that they would choose if they became critically ill. Patients might experience circumstances (such as life-supporting treatment) differently than they had anticipated. Some patients who are acutely ill at admission may find a discussion about limiting life support threatening, frightening, and inappropriate.

Arguments That Discussions About the Limitations of Life-Supporting Treatment Should Be Done Only When Certain Circumstances Arise: Patients are deemed to have consented to treatment to sustain life unless certain circumstances occur that would cause either the patient or the caregivers to question if life support should be withheld or withdrawn. Some widely supported circumstances under which discussions of limiting life-supporting should occur are (1) when the patient's death is imminent; (2) When a cardiac or respiratory arrest is anticipated and the patient is either unlikely to survive resuscitation or it is likely that if he or she survives he or she will suffer a poor outcome, such as neurological impairment; (3) when life supporting treatment is not or is unlikely to achieve the treatment goals for the patient; (4) when the patient is suffering; or (5) when the patient raises questions about the appropriateness of treatment.

Implications of Choosing This Position: The timing of discussions is crucial; use of the above criteria may result in delay of discussion until the patient has deteriorated too far and is no longer able to express preferences about treatment. Patients may suffer greatly before discussions about withholding or withdrawing life support treatment are initiated.

Potential Compromise: Maintain open lines of communication with all patients about their treatment goals and preferences before hospital admission and throughout the hospital stay. Each conversation with the patient about treatment goals and preferences should be documented.

Implications of Choosing This Option: All patients will have the opportunity to discuss their treatment preferences under varied and changing circumstances. Discussions can be timed to occur at appropriate times for the patient. Staff work requirements will be increased when patients require numerous detailed discussions.

Guidelines for the Nurse in Discussion About the Withholding or Withdrawing of Life Support:

1. Familiarize yourself with all aspects of the patient's case. Review the chart for the patient's history, reason for admission, course of treatment, treatment goals, documentation of previous discussions about limiting treatment, and the existence of any advance directives.
2. Be present for all discussions between the patient and the physician.
3. Act as a patient advocate during discussions about treatment choices. Encourage the patient to speak up and ask questions or state desires about treatment. Document all conversations about treatment preferences.
4. Facilitate a patient care conference if necessary to enhance communication and resolve a disagreement about withholding and withdrawing life support.

5. If a patient care conference fails to produce an agreement about a plan of care, inform your supervisor and consult with the bioethics committee.
6. Use your nursing judgment about the patient's condition to plan the urgency and timing of the above interventions.

Bibliography

Abrams, F. R. (1987, May). Withholding Treatment When Death Is Not Imminent. *Geriatrics,* 42(5): 77–84.

Iwersen, E. (1988, May). Life at What Cost? *American Journal of Nursing,* 88(5): 639.

Meisel, A. (1991, August). Legal Myths About Terminating Life Support. *Archives of Internal Medicine,* 151: 1497–1502.

Ruark, J. E., & Raffin, T. A. (1988, January 7). Initiating and Withdrawing Life Support: Principles and Practice in Adult Medicine. *New England Journal of Medicine,* 318(1): 25–30.

Tomlinson, T., & Brody, H. (1988, January 7). Ethics and Communication in Do-Not-Resuscitate Orders. *New England Journal of Medicine,* 318(1): 43–46.

Zugar, A. (1989, December 1). High Hopes. *Journal of the American Medical Association,* 262(21): 2988.

ETHICAL CASE STUDY: WHAT DOES DNR MEAN?

At the time of its inception in the early 1960s, CPR was intended only for patients with unexpected cardiac arrest who stood a good chance for recovery. Thirty years later, all patients admitted to a hospital are deemed to have consented to full resuscitation measures unless a Do Not Resuscitate (DNR) order has been written for the patient. DNR orders are most often written for critically ill or terminally ill patients. Does the DNR order therefore refer only to actions concerning cardiac or respiratory arrest, or does a DNR order imply that a nonaggressive care plan has been instituted for a patient? Patients, physicians, and nurses may have different ideas about what DNR means, ranging from "do not start CPR" to "keep the patient comfortable" to "do not notify MD of abnormal laboratory results" to "do not admit to the ICU."

Dilemma: The patient and various practitioners have different ideas about what the DNR order means and what is best for the patient.

Arguments That a DNR Order is the *Same Thing* as a Nonaggressive Care Plan: DNR orders are often written for critically ill and terminally ill patients. If such patients would not survive a cardiac or respiratory arrest or would not want resuscitation measures performed, then they probably would not want other invasive, aggressive treatment as well (such as vasopressors or an intra-aortic balloon pump). Keeping someone comfortable does not include invasive, aggressive measures.

Implications of Choosing This Position: There will be confusion among caregivers as to what interventions are and are not required. For example, is dopamine prescribed for the purpose of promoting renal perfusion considered to be aggressive therapy? Patients might not receive interventions that might benefit them if these are considered aggressive. Physicians might avoid writing DNR orders for fear that appropriate interventions would not be initiated for their patients and that nurses would not notify them of acute changes in their patients' conditions.

Arguments That a DNR Order is *Not* the Same Thing as a Nonaggressive Care Plan: A DNR order does not address any other situations other than a cardiac or respiratory arrest. To imply that it does creates confusion. DNR patients can appropriately receive high-tech life supportive measures and aggressive treatment for symptomatic control (such as a ventilator for shortness of breath) or to treat the underlying disease (chemotherapy to treat a tumor). The aggressiveness or nonaggressiveness of the pain of care can be addressed outside of the DNR order. DNR orders are appropriate for different patients for different reasons. Not all DNR patients are alike.

Implications of Choosing This Position: There is less confusion about treatment that is covered and not covered by the order. Some patients may be treated more aggressively than they may desire.

Potential Compromise: Decisions about DNR status should also include decisions about how to handle other acute patient changes, for example: "DNR—for shortness of breath page MD stat" or, "DNR—notify MD for systolic blood pressure less than 100," or "DNR—keep patient comfortable, use morphine as prescribed."

Implications of Choosing This Position: There will be less confusion about what is required for patient care. The discussion and decisions required for a simple DNR order will be more complicated and time consuming. Physicians may avoid writing DNR orders if too many other decisions are required at the same time.

Guidelines for the Nurse Caring for a Patient Whose Status Is DNR:

1. Verify DNR status by checking the chart for the original order.
2. Review the chart for the patient's history, reason for admission, course of treatment, current care plan, and treatment goals. Distinguish DNR order from care plan and treatment goals of the patient. Assure yourself that the DNR order is in accordance with the patient's wishes and the patient's condition.
3. If, in your nursing judgment, you anticipate a deterioration in the patient's condition, notify the physician and discuss the plan of care for the patient, including specifics as to what patient conditions (e.g., changes in lab values or vital signs) the physician does and does not want to act upon. Document this information in the nurses' notes and on the physician order sheet. Communicate this information accurately at the change of shift.
4. Assure the patient and the physician that you will provide the patient with expert and vigilant nursing care.
5. In the absence of a well-documented plan to the contrary, inform the physcian of all acute changes in the patient's condition just as you would for any other patient.
6. As death approaches for a patient with a nonaggressive care plan, use nursing interventions to promote patient comfort. Consult with the physician as appropriate for medical interventions that may help to provide comfort. Provide emotional support for the patient and the family. Allow the family liberal visiting privileges. Provide for privacy as possible. Consider chaplaincy support as appropriate.

Bibliography

Council on Ethical and Judicial Affairs, American Medical Association. (1991, April 10). Guidelines for the Appropriate Use of DNR Orders. *Journal of the American Medical Association,* 265(.14): 1868–1875.

Edwards, B. S. (1990, September). Does the DNR Patient Belong in the ICU? *Crit Care Nurs Clin North Am,* 2(3): 473–480.

The Hastings Center. (1989). *Guidelines of the Termination of Life-Sustaining Treatment and the Care of the Dying* (pp. 48–52). Briarcliff Manor, NY: Author.

Lipton, H. L. (1986, September). Do-Not-Resuscitate Decisions in a Community Hospital: Incidence, Implications and Outcomes. *Journal of the American Medical Association,* 256(9): 1164–1169.

Martin, D. A., & Redland, A. R. (1988, March). Legal and Ethical Issues in Resuscitation and Withholding of Treatment. *Crit Care Nurse Quarterly,* 10(4): 1–8.

Nolan, K. (1987, October/November). In Death's Shadow: The Meanings of Withholding Resuscitation. *Hastings Center Report,* 17(5): 9–14.

Sulmasy, D. P., et al. (1992, February). The Quality of Mercy: Caring for Patients with Do-Not-Resuscitate Orders. *Journal of the American Medical Association,* 267(5): 682–686.

Youngner, S. J. (1987, February). Do Not Resuscitate Orders: No Longer a Secret But Still a Problem. *Hastings Center Report,* 17(1): 2433.

26

Management of Patients with Structural, Infectious, or Inflammatory Cardiac Disorders

I. LEARNING OBJECTIVES

In addition to the learning objectives on page 637, I want my students to be able to:

1. ______________________________

2. ______________________________

3. ______________________________

II. TOP TERMS

1. Aortic Stenosis
2. Cardiomyopathy
3. Chordoplasty
4. Commissurotomy
5. Endocarditis
6. Mitral Valve Prolapse
7. Myocarditis
8. Pericarditis
9. Valvuloplasty
10. Vegetations

III. COLLABORATIVE LEARNING ACTIVITIES

Team Discussion Question/Seminar Topics

1. Divide students into two groups and tell them to compare and contrast infective endocarditis to rheumatic endocarditis relative to pathophysiology, clinical manifestations, nursing and medical management, and prevention (reference pages 650–652).
2. Place students in separate groups and have them discuss the nursing care activities for patients with congestive, hypertrophic and restrictive cardiomyopathies (reference pages 645–648).

IV. CRITICAL THINKING ACTIVITIES

In-Class Team Exercises

1. Direct students to complete the following chart comparing the valvular disorders of the heart for the mitral and aortic valves (reference pages 638–645 and Figure 26–3).

	Pathophysiology	Clinical Manifestations	Management	Nursing Interventions
Mitral Valve				
Prolapse				
Stenosis				
Regurgitation				
Aortic Valve				
Stenosis				
Regurgitation				

2. Distribute Figure 26–3 to the class. Ask students to examine the picture of the heart and to describe the procedure commonly used in mitral and aortic valve stenosis. Students should also describe implications for postoperative nursing care activities (reference pages 641–645).

Send-Home Assignments

1. Tell students to draft a nursing care plan for preoperative and postoperative nursing interventions for a patient undergoing valvuloplasty (reference pages 641–645).
2. Tell students to read the following care study and fill in the blanks or circle the correct answers.

Case Study: Acute Pericarditis

Mrs. Russell is a 46-year-old Caucasian who developed symptoms of acute pericarditis secondary to a viral infection. Diagnosis was based on the characteristic sign of a friction rub and pain over the pericardium (reference pages 653–655).

1. Based on your knowledge of pericardial pain, you suggest the following body position to relieve the pain symptoms.
   a. Flat in bed with feet slightly higher than the head.
   b. Fowler's.
   c. Right side-lying.
   d. Semi-Fowler's.

2. Based on assessment data, choose the major nursing diagnosis: ___________
3. Initial nursing intervention includes maintenance of bed rest until the following symptom(s) disappear:
   a. fever
   b. friction rub
   c. pain
   d. all of the above
4. Identify three drug classifications that are commonly prescribed for management/treatment:
   a. ______________________________
   b. ______________________________
   c. ______________________________
5. Draw the chest wall and name the anatomical landmarks used to auscultate for a pericardial friction rub.
6. List the two major expected patient outcomes for nursing management of a patient with pericarditis.
   a. ______________________________
   b. ______________________________

27

Management of Patients with Complications from Heart Disease

I. LEARNING OBJECTIVES

In addition to the learning objectives on page 656, I want my students to be able to:

1. ______________________________

2. ______________________________

3. ______________________________

II. TOP TERMS

1. Afterload
2. ACE Inhibitors
3. Cardiogenic Shock
4. Congestive Heart Failure
5. Dyspnea on Exertion (DOE)
6. Preload
7. Pulmonary Artery Capillary Pressure
8. Pulmonary Edema
9. Pulsus Paradoxus
10. Stroke Volume

III. COLLABORATIVE LEARNING ACTIVITIES

Team Discussion Questions/Seminar Topics

1. Divide students into four groups. Each group should compare and contrast the benefits and risks of a medical management approach used to treat pulmonary edema (reference pages 657–662).
2. Organize a discussion about the priorities of nursing interventions used to manage pulmonary edema. Rationales for each intervention should be provided (reference page 662)

IV. CRITICAL THINKING ACTIVITIES

In-Class Team Exercises

Tell students to read the following case study and circle the correct answers.

Case Study: Pulmonary Edema

Mr. Wolman is to be discharged from the hospital to home. He is 79 years old, lives with his wife, and has just recovered from mild pulmonary edema secondary to congestive heart failure (reference pages 657–662).

1. The most common cause of pulmonary edema is: ________________________

2. You know that the sequence of pathophysiological events is triggered by:
   a. elevated left ventricular end-diastolic pressure.
   b. elevated pulmonary venous pressure.
   c. increased hydrostatic pressure.
   d. impaired lymphatic drainage.

3. The nurse advises Mr. Wolman to rest frequently at home. Her advice is based on the knowledge that rest:
   a. decreases blood pressure.
   b. increases the heart reserve.
   c. reduces the work of the heart.
   d. does all of the above.

4. The nurse reminds Mr. Wolman to sleep with two pillows to elevate his head about 10 inches. This position is recommended because:
   a. preload can be increased, thus enhancing cardiac output.
   b. pulmonary congestion can be reduced.
   c. venous return to the lungs can be improved, thus reducing peripheral edema.
   d. all of the above can help relieve his symptoms.

5. Mr. Wolman takes 0.25 mg of digoxin once a day. The nurse should tell him about signs of digitalis toxicity, which include:
   a. anorexia.
   b. bradycardia and tachycardia.
   c. nausea and vomiting.
   d. all of the above.

6. Mr. Wolman also takes Lasix (40 mg) twice a day. He is aware of signs related to hypokalemia and supplements his diet with foods high in potassium, such as:
   a. bananas.
   b. raisins.
   c. orange juice.
   d. all of the above.

Send-Home Assignments

Assign the following chart. Students should compare commonly used diuretics for pulmonary edema. At least 10 of the 18 found in Table 27–2 and reference pages 658–663, should be used.

Diuretics for Pulmonary Edema

Diuretic	Classification	Purpose	Normal Dosage	Significant Nursing Assessments

28

Assessment and Management of Patients with Vascular Disorders and Problems of Peripheral Circulation

I. LEARNING OBJECTIVES

In addition to the learning objectives on pages 679, I want my students to be able to:

1. ________________________________

2. ________________________________

3. ________________________________

II. TOP TERMS

1. Ankle-Arm Index
2. Bruit
3. Buerger's Disease
4. Doppler Ultrasonography
5. Hemodynamic Resistance
6. Intermittent Claudication
7. Ischemia
8. Lymphedema
9. Magnetic Resonance Angiography
10. Rest Pain
11. Thrombophlebitis
12. Varicose Veins

III. COLLABORATIVE LEARNING ACTIVITIES

Team Discussion Questions/Seminar Topics

1. Divide the class into two groups and ask students to compare and contrast the differences in alterations in blood flow in veins, arteries, and lymph vessels (reference pages 680–681).
2. Ask groups of students to present opposing theories of the pathogenesis of atherosclerosis. Ask each group to defend its theory with scientific facts (reference pages 688–690).

IV. CRITICAL THINKING ACTIVITIES

In-Class Team Exercises

1. Direct students to draw a capillary and label the arterial and venous ends. The microcirculation between the blood and the interstitial fluid depends on the equilibrium between the hydrostatic and oncotic forces of the blood and the interstitium. Tell students to depict the direction of fluid movement and explain the fluid dynamics, using symbols instead of the exact pressures in millimeters of mercury. A supplementary physiology textbook will be needed as a reference if the students wish to label their drawing with exact pressures (reference pages 680–683).
2. Assign a team of students to demonstrate Buerger-Allen exercises and defend their action with scientific rationales (reference pages 693–695 and Figure 28–9).
3. Divide the students into teams. Have them examine Figure 28–18 and explain the pathophysiology, clinical manifestations, and nursing implications for management of varicose veins (reference pages 712–715).

Send-Home Assignments

Tell students to read the following case study and circle the correct answers.

Case Study: Thrombophlebitis

Hazel seeks medical attention for left calf pain and tenderness, which seems to be relieved with rest. Hazel is 38 years old and recently delievered her seventh child (reference pages 705–709).

1. Hazel's medical diagnosis is superficial thrombophlebitis. The nurse knows that Hazel's thrombus development could be associated with the antecedent factors of:
   a. altered blood coagulation.
   b. blood stasis.
   c. vessel wall injury.
   d. all of the above
2. Clinical manifestations specific for deep venous thrombosis that are associated with Hazel's diagnosis include all of the following *except:*
   a. a positive Homan's sign.
   b. local tenderness and induration.
   c. redness and warmth.
   d. swelling and pain in the involved area.
3. Hazel is hospitalized and heparin is started by intermittent infusion. Her daily dose is calculated by measuring the:
   a. circulation time
   b. partial thromboplastin time.
   c. prothrombin time.
   d. thrombin clotting time.
4. While monitoring Hazel's response to heparinization, the nurse recalls that anticoagulant therapy cannot:
   a. delay the clotting time of the blood.
   b. dissolve a thrombus that has already formed.
   c. forestall the extension of a thrombus once it has formed.
   d. prevent the formation of a thrombus.
5. Nursing measures for heparin administration include making sure that the antagonist to heparin is available, which is:
   a. phytonadione solution or tablets.
   b. pilocarpine nitrate.
   c. promethazine hydrochloride.
   d. protamine sulfate.

29

Assessment and Management of Patients with Hypertension

I. LEARNING OBJECTIVES

In addition to the learning objectives on page 716, I want my students to be able to:

1. ______________________________

2. ______________________________

3. ______________________________

II. TOP TERMS

1. Dyslipidemia
2. Hypertensive Emergency
3. Hypertensive Urgency
4. Monotherapy
5. Nephropathy
6. Primary Hypertension
7. Rebound Hypertension
8. Secondary Hypertension

III. COLLABORATIVE LEARNING ACTIVITIES

Team Discussion Questions/Seminar Topics

1. Divide students into two groups. Assign each group one of two conditions responsible for hypertension, either increased cardiac output or increased peripheral resistance. Use Figure 29–1 and reference pages 717–720 as a guide.
2. Assign students to research one of the five hypotheses supporting the causality of hypertension. Ask students to explain the pathophysiology of the identified hypothesis (reference pages 717–719).

IV. CRITICAL THINKING ACTIVITIES

Send-Home Assignments

Have students complete the following chart. For each category listed on the left, ask students to list the recommended systolic and diastolic blood pressure readings.

Blood Pressure Classifications

Category	Systolic	Diastolic
Optimal		
Normal		
High-Normal		
Hypertension		
Stage 1		
Stage 2		
Stage 3		

Reference pages 717–718, Table 29–1.

30

Assessment and Management of Patients with Hematologic Disorders

I. LEARNING OBJECTIVES

In addition to the learning objectives on page 728, I want my students to be able to:

1. ______________________________

2. ______________________________

3. ______________________________

II. TOP TERMS

1. Agranulocytosis
2. Anemias
3. Erythropoiesis
4. Hematopoietic
5. Hodgkin's Disease
6. Idiopathic
7. Phagocytosis
8. Polycythemia
9. Sickle Cell Crisis
10. Thrombocytopenia

III. COLLABORATIVE LEARNING ACTIVIES

Team Discussion Questions/Seminar Topics

1. Direct students to compare and contrast the etiology, diagnostic evaluation, clinical manifestations, medical management, and nursing care for patients with Hodgkin's disease and leukemia (reference pages 755–764).
2. Ask a student to present the disease process of sickle cell anemia. Have another student bring the latest information from an Internet search and discuss findings (reference pages 746–751).

IV. CRITICAL THINKING ACTIVITIES

In-Class Team Exercises

1. Ask students to explain the purpose and procedure involved in a bone marrow biopsy. Have each student identify the sites on a partner and describe any preprocedure instructions that should be given (reference pages 736–738).
2. Direct students to form four work groups. Ask each group to complete the following chart comparing the various types of anemia as to etiology, diagnostic evaluation, clinical manifestations, and medical and nursing management (reference pages 738–745).

Types of Anemia

Type of Anemia	Etiology	Diagnostic Evaluation	Clinical Manifestations	Medical Treatments	Nursing Care
Aplastic Anemia					
Anemias in Renal Disease					
Anemias in Chronic Diseases					
Iron-Deficiency Anemias					
Megaloblastic Anemias					
Sickle Cell Anemia					

Send-Home Assignments

Tell students to read the following case study and fill in the blanks or circle the correct answers.

Case Study: Leukemia

John is a 51-year-old accountant recently diagnosed with acute myelogenous leukemia (reference pages 755–758).

1. Acute myelogenous leukemia affects the: ______________________________
2. A bone marrow specimen is diagnostic if it shows an excess of: ______________
3. A characteristic symptom that results from insufficient red blood cell production is:
   a. bleeding tendencies.
   b. fatigue
   c. susceptibility to infection.
   d. all of the above.

4. Survival rates for those who receive treatment average:
   a. 6 months.
   b. 1 year.
   c. 2 years.
   d. 5 years.
5. The major form of therapy that frequently results in remission is:
   a. bone marrow transplantation.
   b. chemotherapy.
   c. radiation.
   d. surgical intervention.

INSTRUCTIONAL IMPROVEMENT TOOL FOR UNIT 6

Student feedback/evaluation indicated that I need to improve my classroom presentation by:

Adding Content

1. ______________________________

____

2. ______________________________

____

3. ______________________________

____

Deleting Content

1. ______________________________

____

2. ______________________________

____

3. ______________________________

____

Emphasizing/Deemphasizing the Following Content

1. ______________________________

____

2. ______________________________

____

3. ______________________________

____

Questions students asked that I need to research for the future are:

1. ______________________________

____

2. ______________________________

____

3. ______________________________

____

UNIT 7
DIGESTIVE AND GASTROINTESTINAL FUNCTION

31

Assessment of Digestive and Gastrointestinal Function

I. LEARNING OBJECTIVES

In addition to the learning objectives on page 791, I want my students to be able to:

1. ______________________________

2. ______________________________

3. ______________________________

II. TOP TERMS

1. Ampulla of Vater
2. Chyme
3. Endoscopy
4. Fiberoscopy
5. Gastric Analysis
6. Hematemesis
7. Intrinsic Factor
8. Manometry
9. Peristalsis
10. Sigmoidoscopy

III. COLLABORATIVE LEARNING ACTIVITIES

Team Discussion Questions/Seminar Topics

1. Have students describe the purpose, patient preparation, and procedure for radiographic diagnostic tests on the upper and lower gastrointestinal tract (reference pages 798–804).
2. Ask students to divide into three teams and have each team present the similarities and differences between ultrasonography, computed tomography, and magnetic resonance imaging as they pertain to the examination of the digestive system (reference pages 803–805).

IV. CRITICAL THINKING ACTIVITES

In-Class Team Exercises

1. Divide the students into three teams and have them work with Figure 31–2. Have Team A draw the innervation of the sympathetic and parasympathetic parts of the autonomic system. Have Team B draw the blood supply, paying particular attention to the superior and inferior mesenteric arteries. Team C should describe the passage of food through the colon, listing the types of colonic activity and secretions that help propel residual waste products to the rectum (reference pages 792–796).

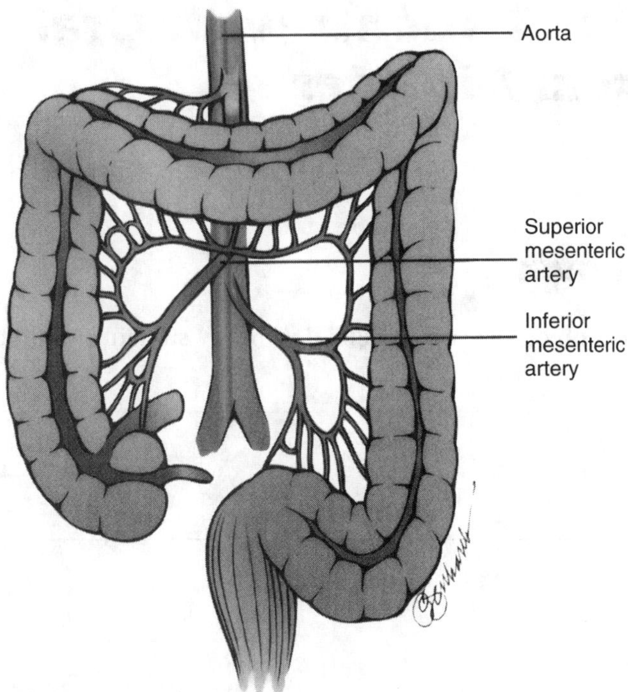

Figure 31–2. Anatomy and blood supply of the large intestine.

32

Management of Patients with Oral and Esophageal Disorders

I. LEARNING OBJECTIVES

In addition to the learning objectives on page 807, I want my students to be able to:

1. ______________________________

2. ______________________________

3. ______________________________

II. TOP TERMS

1. Achalasia
2. Diverticulum
3. Dysphasia
4. Hypoglossal
5. Odynophagia
6. Parotitis
7. Pyrosis
8. Sialolithiasis
9. Stomatitis
10. Xerostomia

III. COLLABORATIVE LEARNING ACTIVITIES

Team Discussion Questions/Seminar Topics

1. Assign students the topic, "Abnormalities of the Salivary Glands." Have students compare and contrast the differences and nursing interventions for parotitis, sialadenitis, sialothiasis, and neoplasms of the parotid (references pages 812–813).

IV. CRITICAL THINKING ACTIVITIES

In-Class Exercises

1. Dawn is a 23-year-old who has just been examined in the physician's office and diagnosed with herpes simplex on the upper lip. She was given a prescription for Acyclovir. The doctor asks you, the nurse, to

give her any health teaching information she may need before she leaves. To develop your plan, choose the information heading you believe is significant and then outline a teaching guide. Write a rationale for each action (reference pages 808–810).

Associated Data:

- Dawn has a heavy blood flow during her menstrual cycle.
- Dawn plans to work as a lifeguard at the shore beginning next month.
- She eats out frequently, especially in Mexican and Italian restaurants.
- She will be living with three roommates in a small summer cottage.
- She has limited income and is just recovering from infectious mononucleosis.

2. Compare and contrast the symptomatology of a dentoalveolar and periapical abscess. Have students develop a preventive teaching plan for young adults who use a health clinic located on a university campus. Suggest that one or more students illustrate the differences on posters that can be placed on bulletin boards near the health center (reference pages 810–811).

Send-Home Assignments

Read the following case study. Fill in the blanks or circle the correct answers.

Case Study: Cancer of the Mouth

Edith, a 64-year-old mother of two, has been a chain smoker for twenty years. During the past month she noticed a dryness in her mouth and a roughened area that is irritating. She mentioned her symptoms to her dentist, who referred her to a medical internist (reference pages 813–817).

1. Based on the patient's health history, the nurse suspects oral cancer. Describe what the nurse would expect the lesion to look like.

____

2. During the health history the nurse noted that Edith did not mention a late-occurring symptom of mouth cancer, which is:
   a. drainage.
   b. fever.
   c. odor.
   d. pain.
3. On physical examination Edith evidenced changes associated with cancer of the mouth, such as:
   a. a sore, roughened area that has not healed in 3 weeks.
   b. minor swelling in an area adjacent to the lesion.
   c. numbness in the affected area of the mouth.
   d. all of the above.
4. To confirm a diagnosis of carcinoma of the mouth, a physician would order:
   a. a biopsy.
   b. a staining procedure.
   c. exfoliative cytology.
   d. roentgenography.
5. List three therapies that are considered effective for treatment:

____

____

____

6. Edith chose to have the lesion surgically removed. A priority postoperative nursing measure is to:
   a. keep the incisional area as dry as possible.
   b. keep the mouth clean.
   c. maintain an airway.
   d. reduce the number of transient bacteria.

7. Follow-up care for Edith is based on the knowledge that:
   a. chemotherapy is a necessary part of postoperative management and should be continued for 2 to 3 years.
   b. prophylactic radiotherapy is routinely scheduled.
   c. surgical intervention in the early stages of cancer is always curative.
   d. 90% of recurrences will appear within the first 18 months.

33

Gastrointestinal Intubation and Special Nutritional Modalities

I. LEARNING OBJECTIVES

In addition to the learning objectives on page 833, I want my students to be able to:

1. ______________________________

2. ______________________________

3. ______________________________

II. TOP TERMS

1. Bolus
2. Cyclic Feeding
3. Dumping Syndrome
4. Gastrostomy
5. Hyperalimentation
6. Negative Nitrogen Balance
7. Osmosis
8. PEG Catheter
9. Total Nutrient Admixture
10. Total Parenteral Nutrition

III. COLLABORATIVE LEARNING ACTIVITIES

Team Discussion Questions/Seminar Topics

1. Have students outline and discuss the specific method for determining nasogastric tube placement. Discuss the research findings of Metheny et al. (1994 & 1998) regarding accurate assessment of tube placement (reference pages 834–840).
2. Discuss why the dumping syndrome occurs and what nursing measures can be used to prevent its occurrence (reference pages 841–843 and Table 33–3).
3. Design a nursing care plan for a patient with a gastrostomy tube. Based on the six nursing diagnoses listed on page 847, have six groups of students each design one component of the plan of care. Challenge the students to cluster related data to support their plan (reference pages 845–849).

IV. CRITICAL THINKING EXERCISES

In-Class Team Exercises

1. Bring several nasogastric and/or nasoenteric tubes to class. Based on the purposes of intubation (decompression, diagnosis, medication administration/feeding, treatment for obstruction or bleeding, or specimen collection) have students determine specific nursing interventions for teaching patients about insertion and management (reference pages 834–840).
2. Ask students to develop a patient teaching guide for a patient for home administration of an enteral feeding. Allow students to choose the patient profile (age, socioeconomic status, financial status) they want to use (reference pages 847–849).
3. Have a group of students draw a PEG catheter on sheet paper or the blackboard. Ask members of the group to explain the scientific rationale for tube placement and the use of various parts/components; e.g., the external cross-bar (reference pages 845–849 and Figures 33–6 & 33–7).

Send-Home Assignments

1. Read the following case study. Circle the correct answers.

Case Study: Total Parenteral Nutrition

Penny is 30 years old and single. She is 5 feet 7 inches tall, weighs 150 pounds, and is receiving total parenteral nutrition solution at the rate of 3 liters per day. Her postoperative condition warrants receiving nutrients by the intravenous route (reference pages 849–855 and Table 33–5).

1. The nurse knows that to spare body protein, Penny's daily calorie intake must be:
   a. about 500 calories per day.
   b. approximately 1500 calories per day.
   c. around 800 calories per day.
   d. equal to 1000 calories per day.
2. The nurse estimates Penny's caloric intake for each 1000 ml of total parenteral nutrition to yield a glucose concentration of:
   a. 500 calories.
   b. 800 calories.
   c. 1000 calories.
   d. 1500 calories.
3. Penny's parenteral nutrition infusion rate is 120 ml/hr. Her rate has slowed because of positional body changes. To compensate, the nurse could safely increase Penny's rate for 8 hours to:
   a. 100 ml/hr.
   b. 125 ml/hr.
   c. 138 ml/hr.
   d. 146 ml/hr.
4. The nurse should observe Penny for signs of rapid fluid intake, which may include:
   a. chills.
   b. fever.
   c. nausea.
   d. all of the above.
5. The nurse weighs Penny daily. After 7 days, Penny's weight gain is abnormal at:
   a. 3.5 pounds.
   b. 5 pounds.
   c. 7 pounds.
   d. 12 pounds.

2. Assign the following case study. Direct students to choose one of the two options and prepare an argument to support their position. Recommend that the "Guidelines" be used in their clinical practice.

ETHICAL QUESTION: IS IT PERMISSIBLE TO WITHHOLD OR WITHDRAW NUTRITION AND HYDRATION FROM PATIENTS WHO CANNOT EAT OR DRINK?

Discussion: It is generally agreed that patients (or their designated decision makers) can refuse life-saving treatment. Nutrition and hydration, however, are perceived as food and drink because they can be provided often by low-tech means and because withdrawing or withholding them can result in the patient becoming dehydrated or even literally starving to death. Thus, some have argued that nutrition and hydration should always be provided to every patient, regardless of the patient's preferences or the patient's condition.

Dilemma: The patient's desire to have nutrition or hydration withdrawn or withheld conflicts with others' reluctance not to harm the patient by withdrawing the food and water needed for survival (autonomy verses nonmaleficence).

Arguments AGAINST the Withholding and Withdrawing of Nutrition and Hydration: Nutrition and hydration—however administered—are symbolic of food and drink and, like nursing care, should be provided for every patient. Nutrition and hydration are relatively easy to provide with low-tech means. The withholding or withdrawing of nutrition and hydration is more like killing the patient than allowing the patient to die of his or her own disease, b e when nutrition and hydration are withdrawn, the patient will definitely die of starvation and dehydration, not of the underlying disease.

Implications of Choosing This Position: Chronically and terminally ill patients live longer in perhaps a debilitated state. Health care costs will rise due to the long-term care of these patients. Debilitated patients being maintained on nutrition and hydration may be seen as a factor in the high cost of health care. Restraints may be needed to maintain feeding in some patients. The provision of nutrition and hydration has side effects that may prove distressing to the patient (such as diarrhea or infection). The provision of nutrition and hydration becomes a special category of life support. Criteria that do not apply to the consideration of the withdrawal of other forms of life support are applied to defend the continuous use of nutrition and hydration; for example, the certainty of death that forbids the withholding of nutrition and hydration is not a factor that forbids the withdrawal of a mechanical ventilator.

Arguments in FAVOR of Withholding and Withdrawing Nutrition and Hydration: Nutrition and hydration are analogous to other life supportive means such as ventilators and should be treated as such; that is, be withheld or withdrawn when the burdens of the treatment outweigh the benefits. It is cruel to restrain patients in order to feed them forcibly. Withholding or withdrawing nutrition and hydration is not like killing the patient, because a patient's inability to sit up and eat results from the underlying disease (such as confusion or vomiting) in terminally ill patients; therefore, withdrawal of that treatment should remain an option. Debilitated patients can live for twenty years or more on artificial nutrition, which is very expensive care. Symptoms of dehydration and malnutrition after the withdrawal or withholding of nutrition and hydration can be managed through good nursing care (for example, good mouth care).

Implications of Choosing This Position: Patients may be more comfortable without artificial tubes and intravenous lines. Patients will retain their ability to choose their treatment as with other forms of life support. Patients with a low quality of life may be seen as expendable. Patients may experience symptoms of dehydration and malnutrition after nutrition and hydration are withdrawn. Money will be saved by not maintaining debilitated patients on artificial nutrition.

Guidelines for the Nurse Caring for a Patient for Whom Withholding or Withdrawal of Nutrition and Hydration Is Being Considered:

1. Assess the patient for alertness, symptoms of pain and suffering, fluid balance, nutritional state, respirator status, and gastrointestinal status. Check the most recent laboratory values. Consult with a dietician and pharmacist, as appropriate.
2. Review the patient's chart and note the reason for admission; history; course of treatment; goals of treatment; advance directives, if any; family situation; DNR order, if any; and reasons why withholding or withdrawal of nutrition and hydration is being considered.
3. Discuss the matter with the patient's physician. Be present at discussion between the patient and the physician as patient advocate.
4. Consider a patient care conference if needed to facilitate communication among those involved in the patient's care and to facilitate an agreement on a plan of care.
5. If a patient care conference does not produce an agreement about the plan of care for the patient, notify your supervisor and consult with the bioethics committee.
6. If nutrition and hydration are to be withheld or withdrawn,
   a. provide emotional support for the patient and family.
   b. provide nursing interventions for comfort.
   c. ensure that a DNR order is in place.
   d. reassess effectiveness of this plan of care and discuss with the physician and patient.
   e. decide if you are uncomfortable with this arrangement, notify your supervisor and find another RN to provide care for the patient.
7. If nutrition and hydration are to be initiated or continued,
   a. provide emotional support for the patient and family.
   b. provide nursing interventions for comfort.
   c. pay attention to fluid balance, nutrition, GI status.
   d. initiate discharge planning, if appropriate.
   e. reassess effectiveness of this plan of care and discuss with the physician and patient.

Bibliography

American Nurses' Association. (1998). *Guidelines on Withdrawing or Withholding Food and Fluid. Ethics in Nursing: Position Statements and Guidelines.* Kansas City, MO: American Nurses' Association, pp. 2–5.

Barnie, D. C. (1990, Spring). Percutaneous Endoscopic Gastrostomy Tubes: The Nurse's Role in a Moral, Ethical, and Legal Dilemma. *Society of Gastroenterology Nurses and Associates,* 250–254.

Bowers, S. (1999). Nutrition Support for Malnourished, Acutely Ill Adults. *MedSurg Nursing,* 8(3), 145–166.

Clevenger, F. W., & Rodriguez, D. J. (1995). Decision-Making for Enteral Feeding Administration: The Why Behind Where and How. *Nutrition in Clinical Practice,* 10(3), 104–113.

Kane, F. (1985, December). Keeping Elizabeth Bouvia Alive for the Public Good. *Hastings Center Report,* 15(6), 5–8.

Lynn, J. & Childress, J. F. (1983, October). Must Patients Always Be Given Food and Water? *Hastings Center Report,* 13(5), 17–21.

McCormick, R. A. (1989, Winter/Spring). The Cruzan Decision. *Midwest Medical Ethics,* 6–9.

Meilaender, G. (1989, Winter/Spring). The Cruzan Decision: A Moral Commentary. *Midwest Medical Ethics,* 6–9.

Meilaender, G. (1984, December). On Removing Food and Water: Against the Stream. *Hastings Center Report,* 14(6), 11–13.

Schmitz, P. & O'Brien, M. (1986). Observations on Nutrition and Hydration in Dying Cancer Patients. In *By No Extraordinary Means: The Choice to Forgo Life-Sustaining Food and Water.* Lynn, J. (ed). Bloomington: Indiana University Press.

34

Management of Patients with Gastric and Duodenal Disorders

I. LEARNING OBJECTIVES

In addition to learning objectives on page 857, I want my students to be able to:

1. ____________________

2. ____________________

3. ____________________

II. TOP TERMS

1. Achlorhydria
2. Antrectomy
3. *H. pylori*
4. Melena
5. Morbid Obesity
6. Peptic Ulcer
7. Pyloric Obstruction
8. Pyrosis
9. Vagotomy
10. Zollinger-Ellison Syndrome

III. COLLABORATIVE LEARNING ACTIVITIES

Team Discussion Questions/Seminar Topics

1. Compare and contrast the differences between acute and chronic gastritis according to incidence, pathophysiology, clinical manifestations, and treatment modalities (reference pages 858–860).

IV. CRITICAL THINKING EXERCISES

1. Discuss the etiology, symptomatology, diagnostic evaluation, medical management and nursing care for patients with Zollinger-Ellison Syndrome (reference pages 860–864).

In-Class Team Exercise

1. Complete the following chart by listing the major action and nursing considerations for drugs used in peptic ulcer disease (reference pages 862–864 and Table 34–2).

Drug Classification	Action	Nursing Considerations
Magnesium-Based Antacids		
Cimetidine		
Ranitidine		
Famotidine		
Sucralfate		
Misoprostal		
Omeprazole		

Send-Home Assignments

Complete the following chart by listing the description and comments for each gastric operation for peptic ulcers (reference pages 864–865 and Table 34–3).

Operation	Description	Comments
Vagotomy		
Truncal vagotomy		
Selective vagotomy		
Pyloroplasty		
Billroth I		
Billroth II		

35

Management of Patients with Intestinal and Rectal Disorders

I. LEARNING OBJECTIVES

In addition to the learning objectives on page 875, I want my students to be able to:

1. ______________________________

2. ______________________________

3. ______________________________

II. TOP TERMS

1. Borborymus
2. Crohn's Disease
3. Colonoscopy
4. Diverticulitis
5. Effluent
6. Evisceration
7. Fissure
8. Ileostomy
9. Irritable Bowel Syndrome
10. McBurney's Point
11. Megacolon
12. Peritonitis
13. Polyp
14. Regional Enteritis
15. Tenesmus
16. Valsalva Maneuver

III. COLLABORATIVE LEARNING ACTIVITIES

Team Discussion Questions/Seminar Topics

1. Discuss the physiological processes associated with the act of defecation, including the myoelectric activity (reference pages 876–877).
2. Explain the physiologic processes involved in the Valsalva Maneuver (reference page 877).
3. Locate McBurney's point on a classmate and explain the concept of "rebound tenderness" as it relates to appendicitis (reference pages 881–883 and Figure 35–2).

IV. CRITICAL THINKING ACTIVITIES

In-Class Team Exercise

Match the physical complication listed in Column II with its associated medical condition listed in Column I. An answer may be used more than once (reference pages 876–879.)

Column I	Column II
1. _______ constipation	a. megacolon
2. _______ appendicitis	b. perforation
3. _______ peritonitis	c. evisceration
4. _______ diverticulitis	d. intestinal obstruction
5. _______ abdominal hernia	
6. _______ colostomies	

Send-Home Assignments

Complete the following chart for each of the six classifications of laxatives (reference pages 876–880, Table 35–1).

Classification	Prototype	Action	Potential Side Effects	Patient Education
Bulk-Forming				
Saline Agent				
Lubricant				
Stimulant				
Fecal Softener				
Osmotic Agent				

INSTRUCTIONAL IMPROVEMENT TOOL FOR UNIT 7

Student feedback/evaluation indicated that I need to improve my classroom presentation by:

Adding Content

1. ______________________________

2. ______________________________

3. ______________________________

Deleting Content

1. ______________________________

2. ______________________________

3. ______________________________

Emphasizing/Deemphasizing the Following Content

1. ______________________________

2. ______________________________

3. ______________________________

Questions students asked that I need to research for the future are:

1. ______________________________

2. ______________________________

3. ______________________________

UNIT 8
METABOLIC AND ENDOCRINE FUNCTION

36

Assessment and Management of Patients with Hepatic and Biliary Disorders

I. LEARNING OBJECTIVES

In addition to the learning objectives on page 919, I want my students to be able to:

1. ______________________________

2. ______________________________

3. ______________________________

II. TOP TERMS

1. Ascites
2. Asterixis
3. Canaliculi
4. Cholecystectomy
5. Encephalopathy
6. Fetor Hepaticas
7. Gluconeogenesis
8. Glycogen
9. Hepatocytes
10. Kupffer Cells
11. Lithotripsy
12. Portacaval Anastomosis
13. Spider Telangiectasis
14. Urobilinogen

III. COLLABORATIVE LEARNING ACTIVITIES

Team Discussion Questions/Seminar Topics

1. Select a group of students to present the pathophysiologic processes that result in the body retaining increased amounts of ammonia, which leads to hepatic coma (reference pages 936–938).
2. Assign several students to explain the process of extracorporeal shock-wave lithotripsy, including a patient teaching plan for pretreatment preparation (reference page 966).
3. Encourage a discussion of the factors that put individuals at risk for Hepatitis B and suggest that a team of students present a list of preventive measures (reference pages 942–944).

IV. CRITICAL THINKING EXERCISES

In-Class Team Exercises

1. List in numerical order the sequence of events leading from portal hypertension to varicoid vessel formation and bleeding esophageal varices (reference pages 946–954 and Figures 36–8, 36–9, & 36–11)
   a. Development of venous collaterals
   b. Varices rupture causing hemorrhage
   c. Formation of abnormal varicoid vessels
   d. Vessels begin bleeding
   e. Obstruction to the flow of portal venous blood
   f. Portal hypertension and increased portal venous inflow
   g. Development of pressure gradient

   (1) _____
   (2) _____
   (3) _____
   (4) _____
   (5) _____
   (6) _____
   (7) _____

2. Next to each of the abnormal liver function studies (normal values found on textbook pages 923–925), list a possible rationale for each reading and any associated clinical manifestations (reference page 969 and Table 36–1).

Abnormal Study	Rationale	Clinical Manifestations
Total serum bilirubin of 1.8 mg/dl		
Alkaline phosphatase of 6.5 ul/dl (Bodansky method)		
Blood ammonia level of 100 mg/dl		
Total serum protein of 5.5 gm/dl		
Serum glutamic-oxaloacetic transaminase (SGOT) of 60 units		
Serum glutamic-pyruvic transaminase (SGPT) of 60 units		

Send-Home Assignments

1. Complete the following chart comparing five types of Hepatitis (A–E), including implications for patient education (references pages 939–945, Table 36–3, and Chart 36–1).

	Hepatitis A	Hepatitis B	Hepatitis C	Hepatitis D	Hepatitis E
Etiololgy					
Transmission					
Incubation					
Immunity					
Patient Teaching Guidelines					

2. Compare and contrast the following three types of jaundice with respect to etiology, pathophysiology, and clinical manifestations (reference pages 924–934).

Jaundice	Etiology	Pathophysiology	Clinical Manifestations
Hemolytic			
Hepatocellular			
Obstructive			

3. Assign the following case study. Direct students to choose one of the two options and prepare an argument to support their position. Recommend that the "Guidelines" be used in their clinical practice.

ETHICAL QUESTION: SHOULD PATIENTS WITH LIVER DISEASE RESULTING FROM LIFE-STYLE CHOICES RECEIVE A LIVER TRANSPLANT?

Situation: Mr. J., a 43-year-old known alcoholic, has cirrhosis of the liver. He was admitted to the hospital with liver failure, probably because he continues to drink large quantities of alcohol. To survive, he needs a new liver. He has repeatedly vowed that he will no longer drink alcohol.

Dilemma: Conflict between autonomy of the patient (request a scarce resource) and justice (fair and equal access for anyone)

Arguments for Approving Transplantation: The patient has a right to the liver because he has a great need. He also has said that he would take care of the new liver and refrain from lifestyle activities that would harm it.

Implications for Approving Transplantation: The liver will be transplanted into someone who has not made socially acceptable use of the naturally received organ. There is no guarantee that Mr. J. will care for the transplant although this may motivate him to change his lifestyle. Giving the organ to this patient may delay meeting the needs of others who also require a liver to sustain their lives.

Arguments Against Approving Transplantation: Persons who actively choose to damage an organ should not expect society to reward this behavior.

Implications of Not Approving Transplantation: Patients with liver damage not resulting from lifestyle activities (e.g. accidents or exposures to chemical or genetic causes) might not receive this scarce resource.

Potential Compromise: Talk to the patient about potential lifestyle change and provide referrals and other support to reinforce his decisions. Give a time limit for the wait for the liver transplant. By choosing this course of action, the nurse can actively help the patient make choices that will maintain the liver and change his lifestyle.

Guidelines for Nursing Care:

1. Discuss what the organ transplant criteria are in your institution and/or state.
2. Determine the difference between a legitimate request for a scarce resource and an illegitimate request.
3. Identify the kind of help available to assist this patient in making a reasonable decision.

Bibliography

Johnson, C. D., & Hathaway, D. K. (1996). The Lived Experience of End-Stage Liver Failure and Liver Transplantation. *Journal of Transplantation Coordination,* 6(3), 130–133.

Lieber, C. S. (1995). Medical Disorder of Alcoholism. *New England Journal of Medicine,* 333(16), 1058–1060.

O'Connell, D. A. (1991, February). Ethical Implications of Organ Transplantation. *Critical Care Nurse Quarterly,* 13(4), 1–7.

Olbrish, M. E., & Levenson, J. L. (1989, May 26). Liver Transplantation for Alcoholic Cirrhosis. *Journal of the American Medical Association,* 261(20), 2958.

Omery, A., & Caswell, D. (1988, November 4). A Nursing Perspective of the Ethical Issues Surrounding Liver Transplantation. *Heart and Lung,* 260(17), 2542–2544.

Rosen, H. R., Shackleton, C. R., & Martin, P. (1996). Indications for and Timing of Liver Transplantation. *Medical Clinics North America,* 80(5), 1069–1093.

Sheets, L. (1989, December). Liver Transplantation. *Nursing Clinics of North America,* 24(4), 881–889.

Sherlock, S. (1995). Alcoholic Liver Disease. *Lancet,* 345(8944), 227–231.

Starlz, T. E. et al. (1988, November). Orthotopic Liver Transplantation for Alcoholic Cirrhosis. *Journal of the American Medical Association,* 17(6), 626–681.

37

Assessment and Management of Patients with Diabetes Mellitus

I. LEARNING OBJECTIVES

In addition to the learning objectives on page 973, I want my students to be able to:

1. ____

2. ____

3. ____

II. TOP TERMS

1. DCCT
2. Gestational Diabetes
3. Glycemia Index
4. Hypoglycemia
5. Ketoacidosis
6. Ketonuria
7. Kussmaul Respirations
8. Lipodystrophy
9. Lipohypertrophy
10. Paresthesia
11. Polyuria
12. Retinopathy
13. SMGB
14. Somogyi Effect
15. Vitrectomy

III. COLLABORATIVE LEARNING ACTIVITIES

Team Discussion Questions/Seminar Topics

1. Present an outline of the epidemiology of both types of diabetes mellitus, the third leading cause of death in the United States (reference pages 974–976).
2. Explain why exercise is not recommended for patients with diabetes whose blood glucose level is over 250 mg/dl (14 ml/L) and who have ketonuria (reference pages 984–985).

3. Describe the clinical picture of someone with hyperosmolar, nonketotoxic syndrome (HNKS) (reference pages 1007–1008).
4. Draft an outline of the current treatment protocol for diabetic retinopathy (reference pages 1011–1014).

IV. CRITICAL THINKING ACTIVITIES

In-Class Team Exercises

1. Assign a group of students to develop a patient teaching guide for a 50-year-old woman to self-administer insulin subcutaneously. Tell students to develop a teaching plan that will meet the following goals and actions (reference pages 987–992 and 998–1002, Chart 37–3, and Figure 37–3).
   a. Withdrawal of 20 units of NPH insulin from a vial
   b. Preparation of the skin
   c. Insertion of the needle, aspiration, and injection
   d. Rotation of sites
   e. Care of the equipment
2. Develop preoperative and postoperative nursing management checklists for a diabetic patient who is to undergo surgery. These would supplement the routine checklists used in clinical settings. For each area to be assessed, cite the rationale for assessment and list the expected physiological alteration (reference pages 1018–1021).

Preoperative Nursing Management

Area	Rationale	Expected Physiological Alteration

Postoperative Nursing Management

Area	Rationale	Expected Physiological Alteration

Send-Home Assignments

1. Compare and contrast the most common types of diabetes according to etiology, pathophysiology, and clinical manifestations (reference pages 974–979 and Table 37–1).

Type	Etiology	Pathophysiology	Clinical Manifestations
Type 1: Insulin-dependent diabetes mellitus			
Type 2: Non-insulin-dependent diabetes mellitus			

2. Construct a nursing care plan for a 30-year-old person with diabetes who has been insulin dependent for 16 years and needs 27 units of lente insulin daily. She is moderately active, is restricted to a 2000-calorie American Diabetic Association diet, and smokes one pack of cigarettes per day. She lives at home with her husband and two children. She is beginning to show signs of retinopathy (reference pages 987–993 and Tables 37–3, 37–4, and 37–5).

   Nursing Diagnoses: ____________________

   Goals: ____________________

Nursing Interventions	Rationale	Expected Outcomes
Type 1: Insulin-dependent diabetes mellitus		

3. Paula, a 36-year-old woman with diabetes, is using an insulin pump system (continuous subcutaneous insulin infusion). She works at home in her husband's dental office and is the mother of 8-year-old twin girls (reference pages 991–993 and Figures 37–4 and 37–5).

   a. Compare the advantages and disadvantages of an insulin pump system.

   Advantages: ____________________

   Disadvantages: ____________________

   b. Develop a teaching plan for Paula to teach her how to use an insulin pump. Use the following format:

   Specific Teaching Points: ____________________

   Rationale: ____________________

38

Assessment and Management of Patients with Endocrine Disorders

I. LEARNING OBJECTIVE

In addition to the learning objectives on page 1026, I want my students to be able to:

1. ____________________

2. ____________________

3. ____________________

II. TOP TERMS

1. Calcitonin
2. Chvostek's Sign
3. Cretinism
4. Cushing's Syndrome
5. Diabetes Insipidus
6. Euthyroid
7. Exophthalmos
8. Goiter
9. Grave's Disease
10. Oxytocin
11. Secretin
12. Thyroid Storm
13. Trousseau's Sign
14. Zollinger-Ellison Tumor

III. COLLABORATIVE LEARNING ACTIVITIES

Team Discussion Questions/Seminar Topics

1. Explain the differences in structure and function of the endocrine and exocrine glands (reference pages 1028–1031 and Table 38–1).
2. Support the following statement with a rational explanation. "The pituitary gland is the master gland of the endocrine system" (reference pages 1031–1032).
3. Explain why there is an increased incidence of angina pectoris or myocardial infarction as a response to therapy for myxedema (reference pages 1038–1040).

IV. CRITICAL THINKING ACTIVITIES

In-Class Team Exercises

1. Compare and contrast the etiology, clinical manifestations, medical management, and nursing interventions for diabetes insipidus and diabetes mellitus (reference pages 1033–1034 and Chapter 37).

	Etiology	Clinical Manifestations	Medical Management	Nursing Interventions
Diabetes Insipidus				
Diabetes Mellitus				

2. Outline the concept of the negative feedback mechanism for hypothalmic-pituitary interactions as illustrated in Figure 38–4 (reference pages 1034–1036).

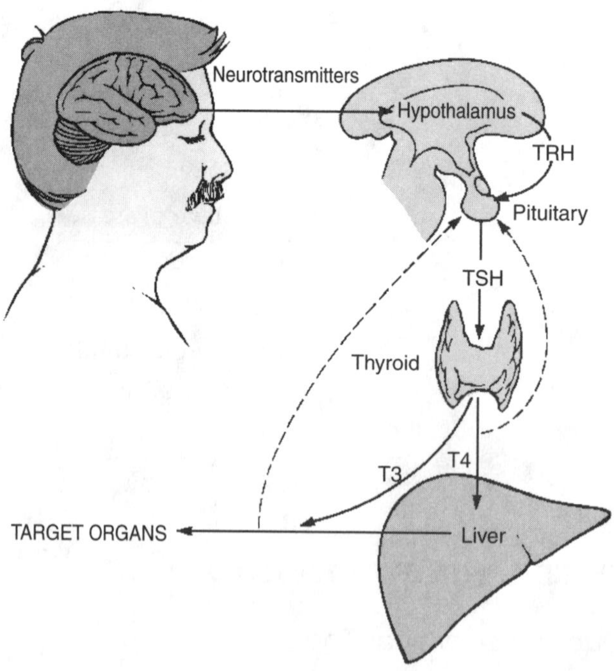

Figure 38–4. The hypothalmic-pituitary-thyroid axis.

Send-Home Assignments

Read the following case study. Fill in the blanks or circle the correct answers.

Case Study: Hyperparathyroidism

Emily is a 65-year-old who has been complaining of continued emotional irritability. Her family described her as always "on edge" and neurotic. After several months of exacerbated symptoms, Emily underwent a complete physical examination and was diagnosed with hyperparathyroidism (reference pages 1052–1054).

1. Emily's clinical symptoms are all related to an increase in serum:
   a. calcium.
   b. magnesium.
   c. potassium.
   d. sodium.

2. As a nurse, you know that the normal levels of the mineral identified above are:
   a. 8.8 to 10 mg/dl.
   b. 1.3 to 2.1 mEq/L.
   c. 3.5 to 5 mEq/L.
   d. 135 to 148 mmol/L.

3. Describe eight symptoms usually seen when hyperparathyroidism involves several body systems:
   a. ______________________________
   b. ______________________________
   c. ______________________________
   d. ______________________________
   e. ______________________________
   f. ______________________________
   g. ______________________________
   h. ______________________________

4. Name one of the most important organ complications of hyperparathyroidism: ______________________

5. A musculoskeletal symptom(s) found with hyperparathyroidism is:
   a. deformities due to demineralization.
   b. pain on weight-bearing.
   c. pathologic fractures due to osteoclast growth.
   d. all of the above.

6. The recommended treatment for primary hyperparathyroidism is:
   a. pharmacotherapy until the elevated serum levels return to normal.
   b. surgical removal of the abnormal parathyroid tissue.
   c. adrenalectomy.
   d. all of the above treatments.

7. Acute hypercalcemic crises can occur in hyperparathyroidism. The treatment would involve immediate:
   a. administration of diuretic agents to promote renal excretion of calcium.
   b. phosphate therapy to correct hypophosphatemia.
   c. dehydration with large volumes of intravenous fluids.
   d. management with all of the above modalities.

INSTRUCTIONAL IMPROVEMENT TOOL FOR UNIT 8

Student feedback/evaluation indicated that I need to improve my classroom presentation by:

Adding Content

1. ____________________

____

2. ____________________

____

3. ____________________

____

Deleting Content

1. ____________________

____

2. ____________________

____

3. ____________________

____

Emphasizing/Deemphasizing the Following Content

1. ____________________

____

2. ____________________

____

3. ____________________

____

Questions students asked that I need to research for the future are:

1. ____________________

____

2. ____________________

____

3. ____________________

UNIT 9

URINARY AND RENAL FUNCTION

39

Assessment of Urinary and Renal Function

I. LEARNING OBJECTIVES

In addition to the learning objectives on page 1083, I want my students to be able to:

1. ______________________________

2. ______________________________

3. ______________________________

II. TOP TERMS

1. ADH
2. Azotemia
3. Creatinine
4. Enuresis
5. Nephron
6. Nocturia
7. Oliguria
8. Osmolality
9. Urea
10. Uremia

III. COLLABORATIVE LEARNING ACTIVITIES

Team Discussion Questions/Seminar Topics

1. Compare and contrast the purpose and patient preparation needed for those undergoing an ultrasound, a KUB x-ray, and an MRI for kidney function assessment (reference pages 1094–1096).
2. Outline the nursing actions needed to prepare a patient for a cystoscopic examination (reference page 1096).

IV. CRITICAL THINKING ACTIVITIES

In-Class Team Exercises

For each term that describes a voiding problem, list a potential cause and associated nursing assessment activities (reference pages 1090–1092 and Tables 39–1 and 39–2).

Voiding Concern	Potential Cause	Nursing Assessment
Dysuria		
Nocturia		
Hesitancy		
Stress Incontinence		
Proteinuria		
Polyuria		

Send-Home Assignments

Develop a nursing care plan for a patient who is scheduled for a renal biopsy. Include post-biopsy nursing management guidelines (reference pages 1096–1097).

40

Management of Patients with Urinary and Renal Dysfunction

I. LEARNING OBJECTIVES

In addition to the learning objectives on page 1101, I want my students to be able to:

1. ______________________________

2. ______________________________

3. ______________________________

II. TOP TERMS

1. Arteriovenous Graft
2. CAPD
3. CAVH
4. CCPD
5. Dialysis
6. Dialysate
7. Diffusion
8. Fistula
9. Hemodialysis
10. Hemofiltration
11. Osmosis
12. Peritoneal Dialysis
13. Residual Urine
14. Shunt
15. Stress Incontinence
16. Trocar
17. Ureteral Stent
18. Urge Incontinence

III. COLLABORATIVE LEARNING ACTIVITIES

Team Discussion Questions/Seminar Topics

1. Discuss the rationale behind a liberal fluid intake with catheterization as a nursing measure for treatment of neurogenic bladder (reference pages 1107–1110).
2. Describe the procedure and patient preparation needed for a patient with suprapubic bladder drainage (reference pages 1111–1112).

IV. CRITICAL THINKING ACTIVITIES

In-Class Team Exercises

1. Describe 10 out of 18 ways nurses can prevent and control infection in catheterized patients (reference pages 1108–1110).
2. For each of the four causes of urinary incontinence, outline management interventions and nursing care activities (reference pages 1104–1107 and Chart 40–1).

Type of Urinary Incontinence	Medical Management Strategies	Nursing Interventions
Stress Incontinence		
Urge Incontinence		
Overflow Incontinence		
Reflux Incontinence		

Send-Home Assignments

1. Examine Figure 40–4. Describe the process of dialysis as illustrated in the figure, making sure to mention the principles underlying the process. Develop a nursing care plan that addresses patient teaching guidelines for management of a patient on long-term hemodialysis (reference pages 1112–1118).

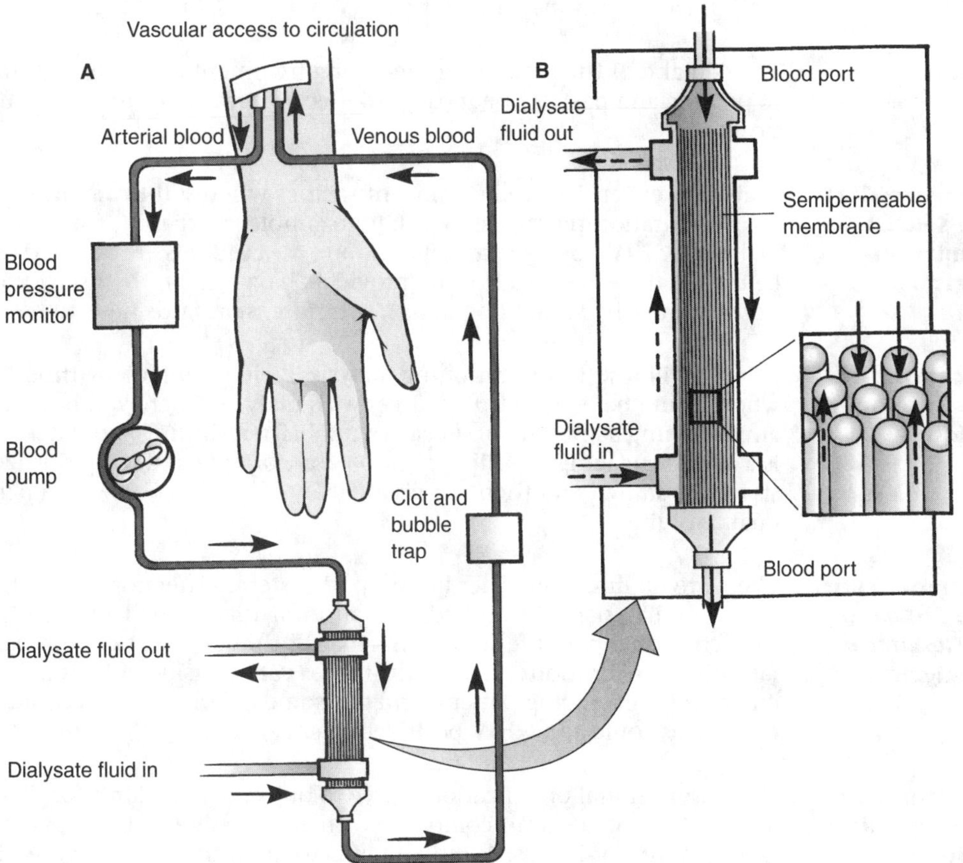

Figure 40–4

2. Assign the following case study. Direct students to choose one of the two options and prepare an argument to support their position.

ETHICAL QUESTION: SHOULD THERE BE LIMITS ON THE USE OF DIALYSIS?

Discussion: Hemodialysis is an expensive but life-saving procedure that is currently being used for more than 100,000 Americans. For some, hemodialysis allows them to live near-normal lives despite the kidney failure that would otherwise kill them. Other patients have a less optimistic outlook. Some patients with multiple system organ failure are given hemodialysis that serves to merely prolong their dying process. Since dialysis is an expensive procedure in an age when costs are being scrutinized carefully, it is reasonable to ask if dialysis should be rationed. Some ways in which dialysis can be rationed are by age, HIV status, quality of life, or ability to pay.

Dilemma: The demand of the patient for life-saving treatment conflicts with the public's need to provide and pay for the most cost-effective treatment for all (autonomy verses justice).

Arguments That There SHOULD Be Limits on Dialysis: Dialysis is expensive, and significant savings will result from rationing it. A fair means for rationing can be found; for example, no dialysis for people over 80, no dialysis for HIV positive patients. As long as standards are adhered to, everyone will be treated the same. Health care providers have shown themselves to be prone to rationing unfairly (see Bibliography); therefore, standards need to be imposed.

Implications of Choosing This Position: Savings will result from rationing dialysis. Patients will die without dialysis, some of whom could have lived fruitful lives with dialysis. There will be a public outcry over any rationing standard and negative publicity regarding those denied dialysis. There is a risk of engaging the slippery slope, for example, reducing the age at which dialysis can be started and then not giving dialysis to someone with a perceived poor quality of life.

Arguments That There SHOULD NOT Be Limits on Dialysis: There are no limits on other life-support systems. Therefore, why should there be limits for dialysis? All standards for rationing dialysis will eventually deteriorate into subjective quality of life standards—that is, the standards cannot be made fair or stay fair. Patient conditions and circumstances vary considerably; it is difficult to use one criterion for excluding patients (that is, some elderly patients could benefit from dialysis, as could some HIV positive patients).

Implications of Choosing This Position: Have professional organizations agree to objective standards for dialysis, such as an age limit, or an age limit combined with an assessment of the patient's overall degree of health or illness. Avoid attempts to quantify quality of life, though considerations of the patient's compliance with treatment may be appropriate. Government organizations should earmark monetary savings for another program such as prenatal care.

Implications of Choosing This Position: Professionally developed standards may be adhered to more successfully than governmental standards. The problems with rationing—deaths, public outcry—are still involved, as are problems with maintaining standards.

Bibliography

Forni, L. G., & Hilton, P. J. (1997). Continuous Hemofiltration in the Treatment of Acute Renal Failure. *New England Journal of Medicine,* 336(18), 1303–1309.

Gilman, C. M. (1997). Continuous Venovenous Hemofiltration: A Cost Effective Therapy for the Pediatric Patient. *American Nephrology Nurses Association Journal,* 24(3), 337–341.

Henderson, L. W. (1996). Dialysis in the 21st Century. *American Journal of Kidney Disease,* 28(6), 951–957.

National Institutes of Health. (1995, November 1–3). *Morbidity and Mortality of Dialysis*. NIH Consensus Statement, 1–33.

Scott, J. (1992, January). Ethical Issues: A Washington Perspective. *Nursing Management,* 23(1), 52–56.

Stark, J. (1997). Dialysis Choices: Turning the Tide in Acute Renal Failure. *Nursing,* 27(2), 41–46.

41

Management of Patients with Urinary and Renal Disorders

I. LEARNING OBJECTIVES

In addition to the learning objectives on page 1135, I want my students to be able to:

1. ______________________________

2. ______________________________

3. ______________________________

II. TOP TERMS

1. Bacteria
2. Cystitis
3. End-Stage Renal Disease
4. Extracorporeal Shock Wave Lithotripsy
5. Glomerulonephritis
6. Interstitial Cystitis
7. Nephrectomy
8. Nephrosclerosis
9. Pyelonephritis
10. Ureterostomy
11. Urethrovesical Reflex
12. UTI

III. COLLABORATIVE LEARNING ACTIVITIES

Team Discussion Questions/Seminar Topics

1. Draft an outline of a teaching guide to help a patient decrease the incidence of recurring urinary tract infections (reference pages 1136–1141).
2. Compare and contrast the differences between chronic and acute glomerulonephritis relative to etiology, clinical manifestations, diagnostic evaluation, medical management, and nursing interventions (reference pages 1142–1145).

IV. CRITICAL THINKING ACTIVITIES

In-Class Team Exercises

Consider a patient who has been diagnosed with renal stones. The physician has prescribed extracorporeal shock wave lithotripsy. Use the following three nursing diagnoses and develop a nursing care plan for a 46-year-old oil company executive who needs treatment away from home (reference pages 1162–1167 and Figure 41–7).

Nursing Diagnoses: (1) Pain related to inflammation, obstruction, and abrasion of the urinary tract.

(2) Knowledge deficit regarding prevention of recurrence of renal stones.

(3) Risks for loneliness related to separation from family.

Potential Complications: Infection and sepsis; obstruction of the urinary tract by a stone or edema with subsequent acute renal failure.

Send-Home Assignments

Examine Figure 41–9(A) and complete the following case study. Circle the correct answers (reference pages 1172–1181).

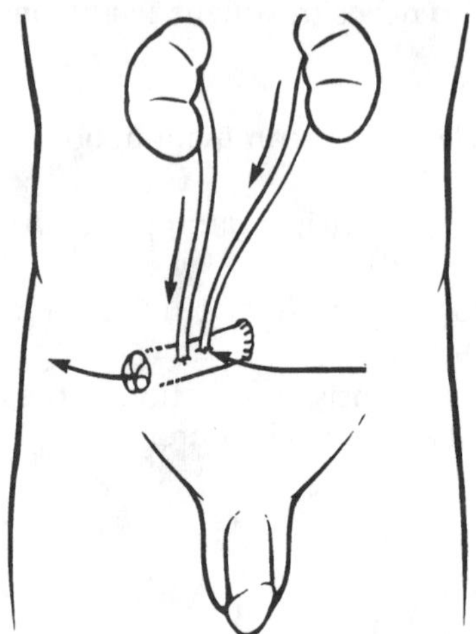

Figure 41–9(A) Ileal conduit ureters transplanted to section of ileum and brought out opening in abdominal wall.

Read the following case study. Circle the correct answers.

Case Study: Ileal Conduit

Gregory, a 69-year-old widower, has just undergone an ileal conduit. He came back to the clinical area 24 hours postoperatively.

1. In preparation for postoperative management, the nurse understands that an ideal conduit involves:
   a. bringing a detached ureter through the abdominal wall and through a skin opening.
   b. inserting a catheter into the renal pelvis through an incision into the flank.
   c. introducing the ureter into the sigmoid, thus allowing urine to flow through the colon and into the abdomen.
   d. transplanting the ureters to an isolated section of the terminal ileum and bringing one end to the abdominal wall.
2. After initial postoperative assessment, the nurse should do all of the following except:
   a. check the skin around the stoma for encrustation with dermatitis.
   b. encourage a soft, high-fiber diet for the first 3 postoperative days.
   c. inspect the stoma for bleeding.
   d. measure hourly urinary outputs.
3. The nurse frequently assesses the stomal mucosa for peristomal dermatitis, which can be avoided by maintaining a urine pH:
   a. below 6.5.
   b. around 7.0.
   c. between 7.0 and 7.5.
   d. above 8.0.
4. The nurse needs to teach Gregory to empty the ostomy appliance:
   a. before sleep so that urine does not flow backward into the abdomen.
   b. every 2 hours in an effort to control odor by frequently draining the system.
   c. twice a day, to minimize infection by decreasing the frequency of opening the valve.
   d. when it is about half full, to prevent separation of the unit from the stoma because of the increased weight caused by the urine.

5. The ostomy appliance needs to be changed every 5 to 7 days. Gregory needs to know that he should:
   a. bend over and empty the conduit before the skin is washed and dried.
   b. pat the skin dry so that the appliance will adhere.
   c. center the appliance over the stoma and apply gentle pressure to remove air bubbles and creases.
   d. do all of the above.

INSTRUCTIONAL IMPROVEMENT TOOL FOR UNIT 9

Student feedback/evaluation indicated that I need to improve my classroom presentation by:

Adding Content

1. ______________________________

2. ______________________________

3. ______________________________

Deleting Content

1. ______________________________

2. ______________________________

3. ______________________________

Emphasizing/Deemphasizing the Following Content

1. ______________________________

2. ______________________________

3. ______________________________

Questions students asked that I need to research for the future are:

1. ______________________________

2. ______________________________

3. ______________________________

UNIT **10**
REPRODUCTIVE FUNCTION

42

Assessment and Management: Problems Related to Female Physiologic Processes

I. LEARNING OBJECTIVES

In addition to the learning objectives on page 1191, I want my students to be able to:

1. ______________________________

2. ______________________________

3. ______________________________

II. TOP TERMS

1. Bartholin's Gland
2. Chadwick's Sign
3. Chandelier's Sign
4. Cystocele
5. Douches
6. Dysmenorrhea
7. Dyspareunia
8. Endometrium
9. Introitus
10. Laparoscopy
11. Luteal Phase
12. Menopause
13. Menstruation
14. Ovulation

III. COLLABORATIVE LEARNING ACTIVITIES

Team Discussion Questions/Seminar Topics

1. Compare and contrast the signs and symptoms of primary and secondary dysmenorrhea. Offer several suggestions for management of symptoms (reference pages 1209–1210).
2. Compare and contrast two sterilization methods, vasectomy and laparoscopic bilateral tubal occlusion. Outline ethical issues that might be discussed by patients prior to making these decisions. What is the scope of the nurse's role in advising (reference pages 1210–1211 and Chapter 45)?

IV. CRITICAL THINKING EXERCISES

In-Class Team Exercises

Mark 28 days on a linear graph. List five phases of endometrial changes (menstrual, follicular, ovulation, luteal, and premenstrual) over the approximate number of days. For each cycle, distinguish between the expected changes in the ovary and the endometrium, and the secretion levels of estrogen, FSH, and LH (reference pages 1194–1195, Table 42–1 and Figure 42–3).

Phase ____

Days ____

Changes ____

Send-Home Assignments

1. Keep a personal three-month menstrual cycle diary (or give the diary to someone to complete) using the form below. When the data is complete, examine the data to determine if there is any repetitive pattern. If so, then develop a teaching guide with recommendations for managing the symptoms relative to diet and exercise (reference pages 1194–1196, 1205).

Diagnostic Diary A: Evaluation of PMS Symptoms

NAME: ______________________

YEAR: ______________________

Grading of Symptoms:
0-No Symptoms ***1-Mild Symptoms*** ***2-Moderate Symptoms*** ***3-Severe Symptoms (i.e., Disabling)***

DAY OF CYCLE	1	2	3	4	5	6	7	8	9	10	11	12	13	14	15	16	17	18	19	20	21	22	23	24	25	26	27	28	29	30	31
DATE																															
MENSES																															

PSYCHOLOGICAL SYMPTOMS

Depression																															
Anxiety																															
Irritability																															
Lethargy																															
Insomnia																															
Forgetfulness																															
Confusion																															

PHYSICAL SYMPTOMS

Swelling																															
Breast tenderness																															
Abdominal bloating																															
Palpitations																															
Weight gain																															
Constipation																															
Headache																															
Rhinitis																															

PAIN SYMPTOMS (Usually NOT associated with PMS)

Menstrual cramps																															
Painful intercourse																															
Pelvic pain																															
Backache																															

Morning weight (lb)																															

Diagnostic diary for evaluation of PMS symptoms. (Chihal, H. J. *Premenstrual Syndrome: A Clinic Manual,* 2nd ed. Dallas: Essential Medical Information Systems, 1990, pp. 80–81.)

2. Assign the following case studies. Direct students to choose one of the two options and prepare an argument to support their position. Recommend that the "Guidelines" be used in their clinical practice.

ETHICAL QUESTION: SHOULD ABORTION BE LEGAL?

Discussion: At conception, a genetically unique human blueprint is formed. Allowing for the 25% of all pregnancies that will end in miscarriage, 75% of all fertilized eggs will, if allowed to grow, result in the birth of a human baby. Should the mother have the right to medical services that would allow her to terminate her pregnancy? The debate over whether the fetus is a human being and whether women should have a legal right to choose an abortion has raged for over thirty years and has dominated American laws, politics, and headlines. The debate has become so personal and fractious that it has become difficult for opposite sides to have a civilized discussion about the issue. Often the two sides cannot agree on the terminology to use in the debate. In a good ethical debate, the terminology should be neutral and the pros and cons of each position should be examined.

Dilemma: The freedom of a competent adult woman to choose whether to undergo an abortion conflicts with the life, growth, and development of the genetically unique human within her. The debate could be described as the mother's versus the baby's interest, or autonomy versus beneficence. The debate could also be characterized as the baby's interests in life conflicting with what is just and right for women in general, or autonomy versus justice. A third way of describing the debate is the mother's right versus the baby's right, or autonomy versus autonomy. Different factions characterize the debate in different ways.

Arguments FOR Abortion Being Legal: Women would be treated as less-than-competent adult citizens if they did not have the right to choose to terminate their pregnancy. The desire to terminate a pregnancy for some women is so strong that these women will resort to illegal abortions if legal abortions are not available. Thus, making abortions illegal will result in the death of women from illegal, unsterile, and unsafe abortions. The moral position of the fetus should not be held as highly as that of the mother—the fetus is not yet human because it is not yet fully developed and cannot survive outside the mother's womb, and the mother is a competent adult. Society does not provide support for pregnant women and women with children; therefore, it is a great financial burden on women to be forced to go through with a pregnancy. A woman should not be forced to carry an unwanted or deformed fetus to term.

Implications of Choosing This Position: Legal abortion services make it possible for abortion to be performed for morally disreputable reasons such as sex selection or birth control. Acceptance of legal abortions may contribute to the view that some life is expendable. There will be fewer children available for adoption. Abortions would be relatively safe, clean, and sterile. A few women would die from abortions despite legal services. The availability of abortion services might encourage some women to abort who might otherwise have carried their babies to term.

Argument AGAINST Legalized Abortion: The fetus is alive and is therefore a human life that should be respected and protected. Neither women nor men should have the right to terminate human life for reasons of convenience, sex selection, or birth control. Handicapped children are human beings and deserve to live. The unavailability of abortions will encourage women to carry their babies to term.

Implications of Choosing This Position: The numbers of abortions will be reduced. The numbers of births of normal and abnormal children will increase. There will be more children available for adoption. There will be more unwanted children. There will be an increased financial burden on women with children. Some women will resort to illegal and unsafe abortions, and some women will die from their use of these services. A black market in abortion services may arise. Women with financial resources, but not poor women, may be able to gain access to safe but illegal abortions.

Potential Compromise: Restricted abortions. Restrict abortion access to women in their first trimester only, for example.

Implications of Choosing This Position: This position does not satisfy the opinions of either side: Fetuses will still die, and some women would be denied access to safe and legal abortions. It would satisfy some requirements of each side, though, by maintaining safe, legal abortion services and reducing the number of abortions.

Guidelines for the Nurse Caring for a Woman Undergoing an Elective Abortion:

1. If you have a moral objection to abortions, you should notify your supervisor and find another nurse to care for the patient.
2. Satisfy yourself that the patient has given informed consent for the abortion and that the abortion coincides with the policies and procedures of your institution and the laws of your state. If not, notify the physician and your supervisor.
3. Provide emotional support for the patient. Avoid judgmental or political comments and trite comments or platitudes.

Bibliography

Bryan, S. (1997). One Day You're Pregnant and One Day You're Not: Pregnancy Interruption for Fetal Abnormalities. *Journal of Obstetric, Gynecologic, and Neonatal Nursing,* 26(5), 559–566.

Davis, S. E. (1989, November-December). Pro-Choice: A New Militancy. *Hastings Center Report,* 19(6): 32–33.

Glendon, M. A. (1989, July-August). A World Without Roe: How Different Would It Be? *Hastings Center Report,* 19(4): 30–37.

Kaufman, F. (1990, May-June). The Fetus's Mother. *Hastings Center Report,* 20(3): 3–4.

Kennedy, B. J. (1988, August). I'm Sorry, Baby. *American Journal of Nursing,* 88(8): 1067–1069.

Mahowald, M. E. Is There Life After Roe v. Wade? (1989, July-August). *Hastings Center Report,* 19(4): 22–29.

Nathanson, B. (1989, November-December). Operation Rescue: Terrorism or Legitimate Civil Rights Protest? *Hastings Center Report,* 19(6): 28–32.

Thomasma, D. C. (1990). *Human Life in the Balance.* Louisville, KY: Westminister/John Know Press.

ETHICAL QUESTION: SHOULD UNIMPLANTED EMBRYOS BE DISCARDED?

Discussion: Hyperstimulation of the ovaries normally precedes in-vitro fertilization (IVF) in order to obtain an optimum number of eggs. These eggs are then mixed with sperm to produce fertilized eggs for implantation into the infertile female. However, in order to avoid a multiple pregnancy, only a certain number of embryos are implanted at any one time; the rest are frozen. If the implanted embryos grow and result in a successful pregnancy, the remaining embryos may never be used by the woman. What should be done with the remaining embryos? Should they remain frozen forever? Be discarded? Be donated to another infertile couple? Be used for research? What is the status of those embryos?

Dilemma: The obligation to respect and preserve human life conflicts with the mother's right to control her family size and the destiny of her genetic material (beneficence versus autonomy).

Arguments in FAVOR of Discarding Unused Embryos: The embryos are not human life, just potential human life. There is only a very small likelihood that the embryo, even if implanted, would result in a live birth. The parents should have the right to decide about their own family size and the fate of their own genetic material.

Implications of Choosing This Position: If discarding embryos were not an option, all embryos would have to be implanted in the mother, which would put her at risk of a multiple pregnancy, which may be risky for her and for the babies. Or, if discarding embryos were not an option, unimplanted embryos would either have to be frozen forever, donated to another couple, or used for experimentation—options that may not be palatable to the parents. Embryos will be seen as expendable.

Arguments AGAINST Discarding Embryos: Embryos are equivalent to human life and should be treated as such. Embryos should be respected and protected, not discarded when their existence is of no use. When parents commit to an IVF treatment, they commit to caring for all the human life that may result. Unimplanted embryos should be kept frozen or donated to another couple.

Implications of Choosing This Position: Parents using IVF treatments would be committing potentially to a large family, when that may not be what they want at all. The problem of what to do with unused embryos still exists. A perpetually frozen existence does not seem to be a better option than discarding the embryos. Many parents may not want to donate their genetic embryos to another couple. Embryos left in limbo have resulted in custody or other legal battles.

Guidelines for the Nurse Caring for a Couple Considering IVF:

1. Assess the couple's knowledge level about IVF and initiate teaching about the procedure and its implications.
2. Encourage the physician and the couple to plan ahead for what to do with unused embryos and document this in the chart.

Bibliography

Annas, G. J. (1984, October). Redefining Parenthood and Protecting Embryos: Why We Need New Laws. *Hastings Center Report,* 14(5), 50–52.

Borum, M., et al. (1998). Women's Health Issues. *Medical Clinics of North America,* 82(2), 189–401.

The Ethics Committee of the American Fertility Society. (1990, June). Ethical Considerations of the New Reproductive Technologies: The Moral and Legal Status of the Preembryo. *Fertility and Sterility,* Special Supplement, 53(6), 34S–36S.

Grobstein, C. (1982, June). The Moral Uses of "Spare" Embryos. *Hastings Center Report,* 12(3), 5–6.

McCormick, R. A. (1991, March). Who or What Is the Pre-Embryo? *Kennedy Institute of Ethics Journal,* 1(l), 1–15.

McCormick, R. A. (1991, December). The Pre-Embryo as Potential: A Reply to John A. Robertson. *Kennedy Institute of Ethics Journal,* 1(4), 303–305.

Ozar, D. T. (1975, August). The Case Against Thawing Unused Frozen Embryos. *Hastings Center Report,* 5(4), 7–12.

Robertson, J. A. (1989, November-December). Resolving Disputes Over Frozen Embryos. *Hastings Center Report,* 19(6), 7–12.

Robertson, J. A. (1991, December). What We May Do with Pre-Embryos: A Response to Richard A. McCormick. *Kennedy Institute of Ethics Journal,* 1(4), 293–302.

43

Management of Women with Reproductive Disorders

I. LEARNING OBJECTIVES

In addition to the learning objectives on page 1225, I want my students to be able to:

1. ______________________________

2. ______________________________

3. ______________________________

II. TOP TERMS

1. Bartholin's Cyst
2. Candidiasis
3. Cystocele
4. Doderlein's Bacillus
5. Dysplasia
6. Endometriosis
7. Fibroid
8. Genital Herpes
9. Hysterectomy
10. Kegel Exercises
11. LEEP
12. Oophorectomy
13. PID
14. Rectocele
15. Toxic Shock Syndrome
16. Vaginitis
17. Vulvectomy
18. Vulvovaginal Infection

III. COLLABORATIVE LEARNING ACTIVITIES

Team Discussion Questions/Seminar Topics

1. Explain why stress increases a woman's chance of having a vaginal infection (reference pages 1226–1228).
2. Describe at least six risk factors for vulvovaginal infections and list two preventive measures for each factor (reference pages 1226–1228).
3. Compare and contrast the etiology and clinical manifestations of a cystocele versus a rectocele (reference pages 1237–1238).

4. Explain what Kegel exercises are and why they are important (reference page 1238).
5. Describe the risk factors associated with cancer of the uterus (reference pages 1247–1248).

IV. CRITICAL THINKING ACTIVITIES

In-Class Team Exercises

Read the following case studies. Fill in the blanks or circle the correct answers.

Case Study: Pelvic Inflammatory Disease (PID)

Donna is a 26-year-old graduate student who has been sexually active with multiple partners for five years. Last year she experienced several incidences of cervicitis. She now believes she has PID (reference pages 1234–1235 and Figure 43–1).

1. Based on your knowledge of PID, you know that the inflammatory condition of the pelvic cavity may involve the following five areas:

a. ______________________ d. ______________________
b. ______________________ e. ______________________
c. ______________________

2. Choose six words to describe the characteristics of the infection.

a. ______________________ d. ______________________
b. ______________________ e. ______________________
c. ______________________

3. The infection is caused by a:
   a. bacteria.
   b. fungus.
   c. parasite.
   d. virus.

4. Name the two most common causative organisms for PID.

a. ______________________ b. ______________________

5. List four disorders that can result from the PID infection.

a. ______________________ b. ______________________
c. ______________________ d. ______________________

6. Name three localized symptoms of PID and six generalized symptoms.

Localized:

a. ______________________ c. ______________________
b. ______________________

Generalized:

a. ______________________ d. ______________________
b. ______________________ e. ______________________
c. ______________________ f. ______________________

7. Develop a nursing teaching plan for Donna that addresses specific points for avoiding and controlling the illness as well as identifying and managing complications.

Case Study: Herpes Genitalis

Paige, a 37-year-old mother of one, has just been recently diagnosed with herpes genitalis (reference pages 1230–1231).

1. Herpes genitalis, a sexually transmitted disease, causes blisters on the:
   a. cervix.
   b. external genitalia.
   c. vagina.
   d. all areas described above.

2. The initial painful infection lasts ______________________________ week(s).
   a. one
   b. two
   c. four
   d. six

3. Choose the herpes virus that is accountable for the majority of genital and perineal lesions.
   a. Epstein-Barr
   b. cytomegalovirus
   c. herpes simplex Type 2
   d. varicella zoster

4. In order to acquire the infection, one must have close human contact by one of five ways. List the five possible ways:

   a. ______________ b. ______________ c. ______________

   d. ______________ e. ______________

5. The virus is killed by ______________________________.

6. The antiviral agent that can alter the course of the infection is: ______________________________.

7. List the nursing diagnoses for Paige.

   a. ______________________________

   b. ______________________________

   c. ______________________________

44

Assessment and Management of Patients with Breast Disorders

I. LEARNING OBJECTIVES

In addition to the learning objective on page 1259, I want my students to be able to:

1. ______________________________

2. ______________________________

3. ______________________________

II. TOP TERMS

1. Benign Proliferative Breast Disease
2. BRCA-1
3. BRCA-2
4. BSE
5. Fibroadenoma
6. Fibrocystic Breast Disease
7. Galactography
8. Gynecomastia
9. Lumpectomy
10. Mammoplasty
11. Mastralgia
12. Paget's Disease

III. COLLABORATIVE LEARNING ACTIVITIES

Team Discussion Questions/Seminar Topics

1. Explain the significance of the orange-peel appearance (peau d'orange) of breast tissue, which is a sign of advanced breast cancer (reference pages 1261–1263).
2. Discuss the advantage of ultrasound in conjunction with mammography as a way to diagnose breast cancer (reference pages 1264–1266).

IV. COLLABORATIVE LEARNING ACTIVITIES

In-Class Team Exercises

1. Divide the students into several teams. Have each team distinguish between the four stages of breast cancer using the TNM system. Then illustrate an example of each on a drawing of a breast (reference pages 1272–1275, Figure 44–4, and Tables 44–2 and 44–3).
2. Complete the following chart for specific chemotherapeutic drugs and hormonal therapy for breast cancer (reference pages 1277–1279 and Table 44–6).

Drug Agent	Therapeutic Goal	Side Effects	Interventions
Chemotherapy Adriamycin			
Cytoxan			
Methotrexate 5-FU Taxol			
Hormonal Therapy DES			
Tamoxin Halotestin Prednisone Nolvadex			
Megace Cytradren Arimedex			

Send-Home Assignments

Collect the following information about risk factors for breast cancer by interviewing ten women, completing the following chart for each woman. Use weighted factors. If risk factor is absent, put a "0" in the box. Summarize the results of your data and try to determine an individual's risk for developing breast cancer. Document any similarities among the women (reference pages 1270–1272).

Weight Factors	Individual Risk Factors	1	2	3	4	5	6	7	8	9	10
2	Personal history										
4	Genetic history										
1	Early menarche										
2	Child > 30										
2	Menopause > 50										
2	History of breast disease										
2	Obesity										
1	Oral contraceptives										
1	Hormone therapy										
1	Daily alcohol										
2	Radiation exposure										
	TOTAL SCORES:										

45

Assessment and Management: Problems Related to Male Reproductive Processes

I. LEARNING OBJECTIVES

In addition to the learning objectives on page 1297, I want my students to be able to:

1. ______________________________

2. ______________________________

3. ______________________________

II. TOP TERMS

1. Benign Prostatic Hyperplasia (BPH)
2. Cowper's Gland
3. Cryosurgery
4. Epididymitis
5. Hydrocele
6. Impotence
7. Orchiectomy
8. Prostate Gland
9. Prostate-Specific Antigen
10. Prostatodynmia
11. Spermatozoa
12. Testicular Cancer

III. COLLABORATIVE LEARNING ACTIVITIES

Team Discussion Questions/Seminar Topics

1. Explain and support with a scientific rationale, the medical management and patient education guidelines for a patient with acute bacterial prostatitis (reference pages 1304–1306).
2. Explain how and why DES is used for the treatment of prostatectomy (reference page 1308).

IV. CRITICAL THINKING ACTIVITIES

In-Class Team Exercises

Complete the following chart for the surgical approaches for prostatectomy (reference pages 1313–1315 and Table 45–3).

Surgical Approach	Rationale for Choice	Purpose	Preoperative Teaching Issues	Postoperative Education
Transurethral resection (TUR or TURP)				
Suprapubic approach				
Perineal approach				
Retropubic approach				
Transurethral incision (TUIP)				

Send-Home Assignments

Read the following case study. Fill in the blanks or circle the correct answers.

Case Study: The Patient Undergoing Prostatectomy

Tom is a 65-year-old college administrator who is scheduled for a prostatectomy (reference pages 1308–1313, Table 45–3, and Figure 45–3).

1. Preoperatively, two objectives to determine readiness for surgery are:

   a. ______________________________

   b. ______________________________

2. Prostatectomy must be performed *before:*

   ____

3. Choose the most commonly performed surgical procedure that is carried out through endoscopy:
   a. Perineal approach
   b. Retropubic approach
   c. Suprapubic approach
   d. Transurethral approach

4. List two possible postoperative complications of the TUR approach.

   a. ______________________________

   b. ______________________________

5. List four general postoperative complications of a prostatectomy.

   a. ______________________________

   b. ______________________________

   c. ______________________________

   d. ______________________________

6. Explain why impotence may result from a prostatectomy.

   ____

7. Choose three possible preoperative nursing diagnoses:

   a. ______________________________

   b. ______________________________

   c. ______________________________

8. Identify two nursing activities to help relieve postoperative bladder spasms:

   a. ______________________________

   b. ______________________________

9. Explain why the patient is advised not to sit for prolonged periods of time immediately after surgery.

   ____

   ____

10. Describe how you would teach a patient to do perineal exercises.

    ____

    ____

INSTRUCTIONAL IMPROVEMENT TOOL FOR UNIT 10

Student feedback/evaluation indicated that I need to improve my classroom presentation by:

Adding Content

1. ______________________________

2. ______________________________

3. ______________________________

Deleting Content

1. ______________________________

2. ______________________________

3. ______________________________

Emphasizing/Deemphasizing the Following Content

1. ______________________________

2. ______________________________

3. ______________________________

Questions students asked that I need to research for the future are:

1. ______________________________

2. ______________________________

3. ______________________________

UNIT 11
IMMUNOLOGIC FUNCTION

46

Assessment of Immune Function

I. LEARNING OBJECTIVES

In addition to the learning objectives on page 1329, I want my students to be able to:

1. ______________________________

2. ______________________________

3. ______________________________

II. TOP TERMS

1. Agglutination
2. B-Cells
3. Complement
4. Cytokines
5. Interferons
6. Lymphokines
7. Opsonization
8. Phagocytosis
9. Suppressor T-Cells
10. T-Lymphokines

III. COLLABORATIVE LEARNING ACTIVITIES

Team Discussion Questions/ Seminar Topics

1. Explain how pathologic changes occur for three disorders of the immune system: disorders related to autoimmunity, disorders related to hypersensitivity, and disorders related to gammopathies (reference page 1330, Table 46–1).
2. Design a poster for school children that explains the differences between natural and acquired immunity (reference pages 1331–1333).
3. Explain how a humoral response to an invading organism results in the production of T-lymphocytes (reference pages 1333–1335, Chart 46–1, and Figure 46–4).

IV. CREATIVE THINKING ACTIVITIES

In-Class Team Exercises

Consider each of the three variables that significantly influence the body's immunologic response. For each variable explain why it impacts on the immune system. From each rationale, develop a patient teaching guideline to help individuals minimize the impact of the variable on their body (references pages 1338–1339).

Factor Affecting Immune Response	Rationale	Prevention Guidelines
Age		
Infection		
Nutrition		

Send-Home Assignments

Complete the following chart indicating how specific medications cause immunosuppression. For each effect, suggest a patient teaching guideline to help the individual cope with or offset the negative impact of the medication (reference pages 1339–1340 and Table 46–4).

Drug Classification	Effect on Immune System	Patient Teaching Guidelines
Antibiotics (in large doses)		
Antithyroid drugs		
Nonsteroidal anti-inflammatory drugs (in large doses)		
Adrenal corticosteroids		
Antineoplastic agents (cytotoxic agents)		
Antimetabolites		

47

Management of Patients with Immunodeficiency

I. LEARNING OBJECTIVES

In addition to the learning objectives on page 1342, I want my students to be able to:

1. ______________________________

2. ______________________________

3. ______________________________

II. TOP TERMS

1. Ataxia
2. Ataxia-Telangiectasis
3. B-Lymphocytes
4. Candidiasis
5. Gamma Globulin
6. Hypogammaglobinemia
7. Job's Syndrome
8. Nezelof's Syndrome
9. Phagocytic Cells
10. T-Lymphocytes

III. COLLABORATIVE LEARNING ACTIVITIES

Team Discussion Questions/Seminar Topics

1. Compare the nursing and medical management of patients with primary immunodeficiencies to those with secondary immunodeficiencies (reference pages 1343–1347 and Table 47–1).
2. Draft a nursing care plan for a patient receiving intravenous gamma globulin at home (reference pages 1347–1348).
3. Choose nursing diagnoses and related nursing interventions for a patient with CVID (reference pages 1343–1345).

IV. CRITICAL THINKING ACTIVITIES

In-Class Team Exercises

Read each analogy. Fill in the space provided with the best response. Explain the correlation (reference pages 1343–1346 and Table 47–1).

1. Job's syndrome : phagocytic dysfunction :: Bruton's disease : __________.
2. Colony-stimulating factor : HIE syndrome :: IV gamma globulin : _________.
3. CVID : bacterial infections :: Ataxia-telangiectasia : __________________.
4. Angioneurotic edema : frequent episodes of edema :: paroxysmal nocturnal hemoglobinuria : ______________.

Send-Home Assignments

For each primary immunodeficiency disorder, identify its associated immune component, major symptoms, recommended treatments, and related patient teaching guidelines (reference pages 1343–1347 and Table 47–1).

Immuno-deficiency Disorder	Immune Component	Major Symptoms	Recommended Treatments	Related Patient Teaching Guidelines
	Phagocytic cells B-lymphocytes T-lymphocytes B & T lymphocytes Complement system			

ETHICAL QUESTION: SHOULD ALL PATIENTS BE SCREENED FOR HIV UPON HOSPITAL ADMISSION?

Discussion: The human immunodeficiency virus (HIV) causes AIDS, a still incurable and ultimately fatal disease. Many HIV-positive people are unaware that they carry the virus; this can allow the virus to spread. The virus is spread through blood and body fluids contact, contact that puts health care workers at risk for infection. A policy that would screen all patients for HIV would serve to reduce the spread of the disease and protect the health care workers who care for patients. Would this infringe on the liberty and privacy of patients?

Dilemma: The patient's right to privacy conflicts with health care workers' rights to protection from HIV infection (autonomy versus integrity of the professions). The patient's right to privacy conflicts with society's need to contain the deadly virus and stem a deadly epidemic (autonomy versus justice).

Arguments in FAVOR of Screening All Patients for HIV: Patients would be informed of their HIV status and, if HIV positive, could seek early treatment for AIDS. The spread of HIV and AIDS could be curbed if patients knew they were positive, knew the importance of changing their high-risk behavior, and notified those whom they may have exposed to HIV. Testing of all hospital patients for HIV would give definitive data on how many patients are HIV positive. Society's need to control the AIDS epidemic is more important than an individual's privacy. Health care workers would know which patients were HIV positive and would take special measures to protect themselves from infection from those patients.

Implications of Choosing This Position: There would be a very high cost for HIV testing for a very low return in numbers of HIV-positive patients. The information that a patient is HIV positive can be devastating to that patient's life, job, housing, and health insurance. Patients who thought that they might be HIV positive might avoid necessary health care if they knew they would be tested for HIV. Health care providers may be careless in using precautions against infection with patients testing HIV negative, even though they would still be at risk for hepatitis infection and the patient may have had a falsely negative test.

Arguments AGAINST Screening All Hospital Patients for HIV: A patient's privacy is more important than attempts to stem the spread of AIDS. The high cost of testing is not justified given the relatively low rate of HIV infection. The lack of testing might encourage HIV-positive patients to seek needed medical treatment. Universal precautions should serve to protect health care workers from many known and unknown infectious diseases.

Implications of Choosing This Position: An opportunity to gather scientific data about the size of the epidemic and to control the spread of the virus would be lost. Health care providers may feel threatened by possible HIV infection from their patients. Patients who are unknowingly HIV positive and remain untested will not learn that information and will not know to seek early treatment of AIDS.

Potential Compromise: Seek informed consent of HIV testing for all patients whose history indicates a risk of possible exposure to the virus. Health care providers should use universal precautions in caring for all patients.

Implications of Choosing This Position: Individual rights are respected, but patients are approached for testing who might otherwise not have been approached. Testing would be haphazard. Some health care workers will only use precautions for those whom they guess to be HIV positive.

Guidelines for the Nurse Caring for an HIV Positive Patient:

1. Practice universal precautions as you would for any patient. Avoid labeling the patient in an obvious way (such as by labeling the chart "AIDS patient," using more isolation material than is required for the patient, or using ominous warning signs outside the patient's room) so that the lay public and other hospital employees who should not have access to patient information could guess that the patient is HIV positive.
2. Help the patient and professionals distinguish between the HIV virus and the disease of AIDS.
3. Maintain confidentiality of the patient's HIV status.
4. Assess your patient's knowledge level of HIV and AIDS. Initiate teaching plan.

Bibliography

Agency for Health Care Policy and Research (AHCPR). (1994, January). *Guidelines: Evaluation and Management of Early HIV Infection.* Clinical Practice Guideline, AHCPR Publication No. 94–0572. Rockville, MD: Agency for Health Care Policy and Research, Public Health Service, U.S. Department of Health and Human Services.

American Nurses' Association Committee on Ethics. (1988). *Statements Regarding Risk versus Responsibility in Providing Nursing Care. Ethics in Nursing: Position Statements and Guidelines.* Kansas City, MO: American Nurses' Association, pp. 6–7.

Bayer, R. et al. (1986, October 6). HIV Antibody Screening: An Ethical Framework for Evaluating Proposed Programs. *Journal of the American Medical Association,* 256 (13), 1768–1774.

Freedman, B. (1988, April–May). Health Professions, Codes and the Right to Refuse to Treat HIV-Infectious Patients. *Hastings Center Report,* Special Supplement, 18(2), 20–25.

Fox, D. M. (1986, December). From TB to AIDS: Value Conflicts in Reporting Disease. *Hasting Center Report,* Special Supplement, 16(6), 2–10.

Meritt, D. J. (1986, December). The Constitutional Balance Between Health and Liberty. *Hastings Center Report,* Special Supplement, 16(6), 2–10.

Pressures Grow for AIDS Testing; Court Backs Patients' Rights. (1991, June). *Journal of Nursing,* 91(6): 96, 102.

48

Management of Patients with HIV Infection and AIDS

I. LEARNING OBJECTIVES

In addition to the learning objectives on page 1349, I want my students to be able to:

1. ______________________________

2. ______________________________

3. ______________________________

II. TOP TERMS

1. Alpha Interferon
2. Cytomegalovirus
3. Helper T-Lymphocyte
4. Human Immunodeficiency Virus
5. Human Papilloma Virus
6. Karposi's Sarcoma
7. p24 Antigen
8. Pneumocystis Carinii Pneumonia
9. Retrovir
10. Retrovirus
11. T4 Cells
12. Wasting Syndrome

III. COLLABORATIVE LEARNING ACTIVITIES

Team Discussion Questions/Seminar Topics

1. Explain how a permanent infection with HIV is established through altered RNA and DNA (reference pages 1350–1351).
2. Discuss specific nursing interventions for specific side effects of the antiretroviral agents: nucleoside reverse transcriptase inhibitors (NRTIs) (i.e., Retrovir, Videx); non-nucleoside reverse transcriptase inhibitors (NNRTIs) (i.e., Rescriptor, Viramuni); and protease inhibitors (i.e., Norvir, Crixivan) (reference pages 1361–1363 and Table 48–3).
3. Discuss and give specific examples of how health care providers can maintain "Universal Blood and Body Fluids Precautions" to prevent HIV transmission (reference pages 1352–1354 and Guidelines 48–1).

IV. COLLABORATIVE LEARNING ACTIVITIES

In-Class Team Exercises

Complete the following chart comparing various laboratory tests with findings related to the diagnosis and tracking of HIV (reference pages 1357–1360 and Table 48–2)

HIV Antibody Test	Findings Related to HIV Infection
1. HIV Antibody Tests ELISA IFA RIPA Western blot	
2. HIV Tracking PCR PMBC Quantitative plasma culture Quantitative Cell Culture B_2 Microglobulin P_{24} Antigen Branch DNA (bDNA) Nucleic acid sequence-based amplification (NASBA)	
3. Immune Status %CD_4 + Cells CD_4 : CDs ratio CD_4 cell function tests Immunoglobulin tests Skin Test-Sensitivity Reaction WBC Count	

Send-Home Assignments

Draft a nursing care plan for a 24-year-old single male who has just been diagnosed with AIDS after being admitted to an acute care facility with pneumocystis carinii pneumonia. The patient is a recent college graduate, employed full time, and engaged to be married in six months. He currently lives at home with his parents and two sisters (reference pages 1363–1376 and Plan of Nursing Care 48-I). Use the following format.

Nursing Diagnoses	Nursing Interventions	Rationale	Expected Outcome

49

Assessment and Management of Patients with Allergic Disorders

I. LEARNING OBJECTIVES

In addition to the following objectives on page 1382, I want my students to be able to:

1. ______________________________

2. ______________________________

3. ______________________________

II. TOP TERMS

1. Agglutination
2. Allergens
3. Anaphylaxis Reaction
4. Angioedema
5. Antibodies
6. Antigens
7. B-Lymphocytes
8. Epinephrine
9. Histamine
10. Immunoglobulins
11. Lymphokinines
12. Mast Cells
13. Prostaglandins
14. Rhinitis
15. Serotonin
16. T-Lymphocytes
17. Urticaria
18. Wheal

III. COLLABORATIVE LEARNING ACTIVITIES:

Team Discussion Questions/Seminar Topics

1. Compare the role of B-cells and T-cells in response to an allergic reaction (reference page 1383).
2. Distinguish between the function of primary and secondary chemical mediators in response to the function of antigens (reference pages 1384–1385).
3. Describe the physiological response that occurs with an anaphylactic reaction (reference pages 1385–1387 and Figure 49–2).

IV. CRITICAL THINKING ACTIVITIES

In-Class Team Exercises

Compare and contrast the etiology, diagnosis, clinical manifestations, medical management, and nursing teaching points for the four types of contact dermatitis (reference pages 1398–1400 and Table 49–4).

Type of Contact Dermatitis	Etiology	Diagnosis	Clinical Manifestations	Medical Management	Nursing Teaching Points
Allergic Irritant Phototoxic Photoallergic					

Send-Home Assignments

Conduct an allergy assessment on ten friends or relatives using the Allergy Assessment Form below (reference pages 1388–1389). After obtaining the data, summarize the results to see if there are any patterns of sensitivity reactions based on seasons, physical agents, habits, geographic area, or home location. Also correlate medication use with management.

Allergy Assessment Form

Name______________ Age:_________ Sex:_________ Date:________

I. Chief complaint: ____________

II. Present illness: _____________

IV. Collateral allergic symptoms: _______________

Eyes: Pruritus ________ Burning ______ Lacrimation ________
Swelling _________ Injection _________ Discharge _______

Ears: Pruritus _________ Fullness _____ Popping ________
Frequent infections _________

Nose: Sneezing ________ Rhinorrhea _______ Obstruction _____
Pruritus ______ Mouth-breathing _______ Purulent discharge______

Throat: Soreness ______ Postnasal discharge________
Palatal pruritus _________ Mucus in the morning _____________

Chest: Cough _________ Pain ____________ Wheezing _________
Sputum __________ Dyspnea ____________
Color _____________ Rest____________
Amount ____________ Exertion __________

Skin: Dermatitis ______ Eczema ___________ Urticaria_________

IV. Family Allergies: ____________

V. Previous allergic treatment or testing: ________

Prior skin testing: ____________

Medications:

Antihistamines Improved ______ Unimproved ______

Bronchodilator Improved ______ Unimproved ______

Nose drops Improved ______ Unimproved ______

Hyposensitization Improved ______ Unimproved ______

Duration ____________

Antigens ____________

Reactions ___________

Antibiotics Improved ______ Unimproved ______

Corticosteroids Improved ______ Unimproved ______

VI. Physical agents and habits: ____________________

Tobacco for ________ years	Alcohol ________	Air Conditioning ________
Cigarettes ________ packs/day	Heat ________	Muggy weather ________
Cigars ________ per day	Cold ________	Weather changes ________
Pipes ________ per day	Perfumes ________	Chemicals ________
Never smoked ________	Paints ________	Hair spray ________
Bothered by smoke ________	Insecticides ________	Newspapers ________
Cosmetics ________		

VII. When symptoms occur: ____________________

Time and circumstances of first episode: ____________________

Prior health: ____________________

Course of illness over decades: progressing ________ regressing ________

Time of year: ____________________ Exact dates: ________

Perennial: ________

Seasonal: ________

Seasonally exacerbated: ________

Monthly variations (menses, occupation): ____________________

Time of week (weekends vs. weekdays): ____________________

Time of day or night: ____________________

After insect stings: ____________________

VIII. Where symptoms occur: ____________________

Living where at onset: ____________________

Effect of vacation or major geographic change: ____________________

Symptoms better indoors or outdoors: ____________________

Effect of school or work: ____________________

Effect of staying elsewhere nearby: ____________________

Effect of hospitalization: ____________________

Effect of specific environments: ____________________

Do symptoms occur around: ____________________

old leaves ________ hay ________ lakeside ________ barns ________

summer homes ________ damp basement ________ dry attic ________

lawnmowing ________ animals ________ other ________

Do symptoms occur after eating:

cheese ________ mushrooms ________ beer ________ melons ________

bananas ________ fish ________ nuts ________ citrus fruits ________

Home: city ________ rural ________

house ________ age ________

apartment ________ basement ________ damp ________ dry ________

heating system ________

pets (how long) ________ dog ________ cat ________ other ________

Bedroom:	Type	Age	**Living room:**	Type	Age
Pillow	____	____	Rug	____	____
Mattress	____	____	Matting	____	____
Blankets	____	____	Furniture	____	____
Quilts	____	____			
Furniture	____	____			

Anywhere in home symptoms are worse? ________

IX. What does patient think makes symptoms worse? ____________________

X. Under what circumstances is patient free of symptoms? ____________________

XI. Summary and additional comments: ____________________

50

Assessment and Management of Patients with Rheumatic Disorders

I. LEARNING OBJECTIVES

In addition to the learning objectives on page 1405, I want my students to be able to:

1. ______________________________

2. ______________________________

3. ______________________________

II. TOP TERMS

1. Arthrography
2. Cytokines
3. Diarthrodial
4. Exacerbation
5. Fibromyalgia
6. Hemarthrosis
7. Leukotriene
8. Osteopenia
9. Osteophytes
10. Pannus
11. Remission
12. Scleroderma
13. Synovial
14. Tophi

III. COLLABORATIVE LEARNING ACTIVITIES

Team Discussion Questions/Seminar Topics

1. Compare and contrast the etiology, clinical manifestations, and medical management for the three types of lupus erythematosus (reference pages 1424–1426).
2. Describe several common undesirable side effects of corticosteroid therapy and list a nursing intervention for each side effect (reference pages 1413–1414 and Table 50–3).

IV. COLLABORATIVE LEARNING ACTIVITIES

In-Class Team Exercises

Identify the six major goals and strategies for treating a rheumatic disease. For each strategy, identify at least two management interventions (reference pages 1412–1419, Table 50–2, and Plan of Nursing Care 50–1).

Major Goal	**Management Interventions**
1. __________	a. __________
	b. __________
2. __________	a. __________
	b. __________
3. __________	a. __________
	b. __________
4. __________	a. __________
	b. __________
5. __________	a. __________
	b. __________
6. __________	a. __________
	b. __________

Send-Home Assignment

For each of the medication classifications for rheumatic diseases listed, identify two possible drugs in Column I, then list the drugs' action in Column II and the relevant nursing considerations in Column III (reference pages 1412–1414 and Table 50–3).

Medications Used in Rheumatic Diseases

Medications	Drug Actions	Nursing Considerations
Salicylates		
Nonsteroidal anti-inflammatory drugs (NSAIDs)		
Disease-modifying anti-rheumatic drugs (DMARDs)		
Gold-containing compounds		
Immunosuppressives		
Corticosteroids		

INSTRUCTIONAL IMPROVEMENT TOOL FOR UNIT 11

Student feedback/evaluation indicated that I need to improve my classroom presentation by:

Adding Content

1. ______________________________

2. ______________________________

3. ______________________________

Deleting Content

1. ______________________________

2. ______________________________

3. ______________________________

Emphasizing/Deemphasizing the Following Content

1. ______________________________

2. ______________________________

3. ______________________________

Questions students asked that I need to research for the future are:

1. ______________________________

2. ______________________________

3. ______________________________

UNIT 12
INTEGUMENTARY FUNCTION

51

Assessment of Integumentary Function

I. LEARNING OBJECTIVES

In addition to the learning objectives on page 1437, I want my students to be able to:

1. ______________________________

2. ______________________________

3. ______________________________

II. TOP TERMS

1. Alopecia
2. Cutaneous
3. Erythema
4. Insensible Perspiration
5. Keratin
6. Melanin
7. Petechiae
8. Pruritus
9. Sebaceous Glands
10. Telangiectasis
11. Turgor

III. COLLABORATIVE LEARNING ACTIVITIES

Team Discussion Question/Seminar Topics

1. Compare and contrast the functions of the three layers of skin: epidermis, dermis, and the subcutaneous tissues (reference pages 1441–1442).
2. Distinguish between primary and secondary skin lesions and give three examples of each. For each, describe the lesion's characteristics that aid in diagnosis (reference pages 1441–1448 and Chart 51-2).
3. Describe the six common examples of nail disorders. Examine some of your classmates' nails and determine if you can find other examples not listed in Figure 51-6 (reference pages 1445–1450 and Figure 51-6).

IV. CRITICAL THINKING ACTIVITIES

In-Class Team Exercises

Separate students into several teams. Have each team conduct a patient history on one member who has or "pretends" to have a skin disorder. Have each team record its findings and come to a diagnosis. Then each team needs to share its clusters of data and ask other teams to identify the skin disorder. Use the "Patient History Assessment: Skin Disorders" below for the outline of interview/assessment questions (reference pages 1443–1449).

Assessment
Patient History: Skin Disorders

Patient history relevant to skin disorders may be obtained by asking the following questions:

- When did you first notice this skin problem (also investigate duration and intensity)?
- Has it occurred previously?
- Are there any other symptoms?
- What site was first affected?
- What did the rash or lesion look like when it first appeared?
- Where and how fast did it spread?
- Do you have any itching, burning, tingling, or crawling sensations?
- Is there any loss of sensation?
- Is the problem worse at a particular time or season?
- How do you think it started?
- Do you have a history of hay fever, asthma, hives, eczema, or allergies?
- Who in your family have skin problems or rashes?
- Did the eruptions appear after certain foods were eaten? Which foods?
- When the problem occurred, had you recently had alcohol?
- What relation do you think there may be between a specific event and the outbreak of the rash or lesion?
- What medications are you taking?
- What topical medication (ointment, cream, salve) have you put on the lesion (include over-the-counter medications)?
- What skin products or cosmetics do you use?
- What is your occupation?
- What in your immediate environment (plants, animals, chemicals, infections) might be precipitating this problem? Is there anything new or are there any changes in the environment?
- Does anything touching your skin cause a rash?
- Is there anything else you wish to talk about in regard to this problem?
- How has this affected you (or your life)?

Send-Home Assignments

Match the description of specific lesions listed in Column II with their associated type listed in Column I (reference pages 1444–1448 and Chart 51–2).

Part I

Column I	Column II
___ 1. bulla	a. a covering formed from serum, blood, or pus drying on the skin
___ 2. crusts	b. a large vesicle or blister greater than 1 cm in diameter
___ 3. macule	c. a nonelevated discoloration of the skin
___ 4. nodule	d. a raised solid lesion larger than 1 cm in diameter
___ 5. wheal	e. a transient elevation of the skin caused by edema of the dermis and capillary dilatation

Part II

___ 6. papule	a. a lesion that contains pus, i.e., acne
___ 7. plaque	b. a small elevation of the skin that is filled with clear fluid
___ 8. pustule	c. a solid elevated lesion on the skin that is greater than 1 cm in diameter
___ 9. scales	d. a solid elevated palpable lesion that is less than 1 cm in diameter
___ 10. vesicle	e. heaped-up horny layers of dead epidermis

52

Management of Patients with Dermatologic Problems

I. LEARNING OBJECTIVES

In addition to the learning objectives on page 1452, I want my students to be able to:

1. ______________________________

2. ______________________________

3. ______________________________

II. TOP TERMS

1. Alopecia
2. Argon Laser
3. Carbuncle
4. Comedones
5. Dermabrasion
6. Dermatitis
7. Furuncle
8. Keloids
9. Keratoses
10. Lichenification
11. Melanoma
12. Pyodermas
13. Seborrhea
14. Tinea

III. COLLABORATIVE LEARNING ACTIVITIES

Team Discussion Questions/Seminar Topics

1. Discuss the etiology, increased incidence, manifestations, and treatment for the herpes zoster virus especially for those who are immunocompromised (reference page 1469).
2. Compare and contrast the etiology, clinical manifestations, diagnostic evaluation, and medical management of basal cell and squamous cell carcinoma (reference pages 1486–1488).
3. Compare and contrast the advantages of three types of laser therapy for cutaneous lesions: argon laser, carbon dioxide laser, and pulse-dye laser (reference pages 1498–1499).

IV. CRITICAL THINKING ACTIVITIES

In-Class Team Exercise

1. Design a poster outlining patient education needs for those with bacterial infections of the skin (reference pages 1467–1469).
2. Complete the following chart comparing the five types of tinea infections (reference pages 1470–1472 and Table 52–6).

Tinea Infection	Location	Clinical Manifestations	Medical Treatment	Patient Care Education
Tinea capitis Tinea corporis Tinea cruris Tinea pedis Tinea unguium				

Send-Home Assignments

Read the following case study. Fill in the blanks or circle the correct answers.

Case Study: Acne Vulgaris

Brian is a 15-year-old who has been experiencing facial eruptions of acne for about a year. The numerous lesions are inflamed and present on the face and neck. He has tried many over-the-counter medications and nothing seems to help. His father had a history of severe acne when he was a teenager (reference pages 1465–1467 and Table 52–5).

1. Based on your knowledge of acne vulgaris, you know that the skin disorder is characterized by five types of lesions:

   (a) ____________, (b)____________, (c)____________,

   (d) ____________, (e) ____________.

2. The etiology of acne stems from:
   a. genetic factors.
   b. hormonal factors.
   c. bacterial factors.
   d. an interplay of all of the above.
3. Acne, most prevalent at puberty, is the direct result of oversecretion of the ________ glands.
   a. exocrine
   b. lacrimal
   c. sebaceous
   d. mucous
4. Explain the rationale for using benzoyl peroxide:

   ____

5. Explain the rationale for using synthetic vitamin A compounds (retinoids)

   ____

6. Choose a common antibiotic that is frequently prescribed for treatment of acne:
   a. terbutaline
   b. tamoxifen
   c. tetracycline
   d. terfenadine

7. Choose the common oral retinoid that is used for acne:
   a. Accutane
   b. Acne-Aid
   c. Actinex
   d. Adalat
8. Based on assessment data, identify two collaborative problems:

   (a) ____________________ and (b) ______________

53

Management of Patients with Burn Injury

I. LEARNING OBJECTIVES

In addition to the learning objectives on page 1501, I want my students to be able to:

1. ______________________________

2. ______________________________

3. ______________________________

II. TOP TERMS

1. Biobane
2. Colloids
3. Compartment Syndrome
4. Cultured Epidermal Autografts
5. Debridement
6. Escharotomy
7. Heterograft
8. Integra
9. Ischemia
10. Keloid
11. Paralytic Ileus
12. Total Body Surface Area

III. COLLABORATIVE LEARNING ACTIVITIES

Team Discussion Questions/Seminar Topics

1. Compare and contrast the three types of wound debridement: natural, mechanical, and surgical (reference pages 1517–1520).
2. Explain exactly why carbon monoxide inhalation injuries are so fatal (reference pages 1506–1507).
3. Compare and contrast the three measures for estimating the extent of body surface injury: Rule of Nines, the Lund & Browder method, and the Palm method (reference pages 1503–1504 and Figure 53–2).

IV. CRITICAL THINKING EXERCISES

In-Class Team Exercises

Complete the following chart comparing the characteristics of the three classifications of burns according to the depth of the injury (reference pages 1503–1506 and Table 53–1).

Send-Home Assignments

Burn Classification	Layer of Skin Involved	Possible Cause	Clinical Manifestations	Treatment
Superficial Partial-Thickness (First-Degree)				
Deep Partial-Thickness (Second-Degree)				
Full-Thickness (Third Degree)				

Generating Solutions: Clinical Problem Solving

Develop a nursing care plan for each of the following two situations. Use the following format.

Nursing Diagnosis: ______________________________

Goals	Nursing Actions	Rationale	Expected Outcomes

1. Claire is 27 years old and owns an arts and crafts store. During a recent demonstration of candle making, a container of hot liquid wax (230°F) spilled over her left forearm and hand. One of her students drove her to a nearby clinic. By the time Claire arrived at the clinic, some of the wax had hardened and was falling off her arm, removing skin as it fell. She was in intense pain.

2. David, a 35-year-old single executive, was asleep when a fire began in his living room. A neighbor saw the flames and called the fire company. By the time David was rescued, he was semiconscious and had suffered smoke inhalation. He was treated by emergency technicians and transported to an emergency center.

ETHICAL QUESTION: WHAT IS ETHICAL CARE FOR PATIENTS WHO REFUSE TREATMENT?

Situation: A 32-year-old professional man is severely burned over 80% of his body in a motor vehicle crash. He is single with no dependents. He does not have a living will but states that he does not want to be treated any longer for his burns and wishes to die. He has undergone extensive therapy involving tubbing and debridement procedures for the last 2 weeks. He asks that the treatments stop because he can no longer tolerate the pain and he sees no future quality of life. His mother insists that treatment continue because it is God's will.

Dilemma: Conflict between the autonomous desires of this competent man and the wishes of his mother.

Arguments for Stopping Treatments: This man can make his own decisions and is willing to accept their consequences. He has stated that quality of life is more important to him than "being alive." The role of the health care professionals is to help the individual with life decisions (if they do not conflict with good medical care or the core values of the provider).

Implications of Stopping Treatments: If treatments stop, the man will, most likely, develop a severe infection and septicemia with increasing pain. This will result in stopping or withholding antibiotics and giving increasing amounts of narcotics. Just stopping the treatments for the burns is not the end in and of itself, but causes a whole trajectory of treatment options. Choosing this position might further increase the dissent between the man and his mother.

Arguments Against Stopping Treatment: The man cannot project what his quality of life will be after the pain resulting from tubbing and debridement subsides and the burns heal. He has an autonomous right to stop treatment but the question remains unanswered as to whether he has given the treatments an adequate trial.

Implications of Not Stopping Treatment: The patient might die when he may potentially be spared to enjoy a productive life. His autonomy may be compromised by disregarding his wishes. The relationship between his mother and him may be negatively impacted.

Potential Compromise: The nursing staff may help intervene with this patient by providing support group intervention. The patient can meet with other patients who fared well after burn therapy and the patient could be encouraged to participate in directing his own care (he can help schedule the treatments). This will give him some control of his environment. To prevent needless suffering, adequate pain medication is an absolute requirement during this painful therapy. If the patient still refuses to accept treatments then the staff needs to communicate with the patient that he is requesting assisted suicide and both staff and patient need to decide if this option is available. In pursuing these options, the care of the patient continues. The goals of treatment continue. With additional time, the patient and his mother may come to resolve their differences.

Guidelines for Nursing Care:

1. Review and understand the criteria for determining competence. Competence means that the person is able to perform a task. The definition is not global. For example the patient may be able to make decisions regarding his or her health care but not be able to drive a car. Some critieria include the following:
   a. The patient needs to know all the relevant facts.
   b. The patient needs to be able to make decisions based on the facts.
   c. The patient needs to understand the consequences that will flow from the decisions.

The concept of competence and capacity to understand go hand-in-hand with obtaining informed consent. In the case of the burn patient, pain may be so intense that the patient does not have the capacity to entertain future possibilities. The role of the nurse is to help control the pain adequately so that the patient is alert, yet pain free. To this end the nurse needs to understand the physiology of burns and the pharmacodynamics of pain management.

2. Know the institutional environment and support systems available to assist the patient in making an informed decision about his future care.
3. Use problem-solving skills and use the ethical decision-making model to determine if the patient has examined all alternatives before accepting the first decision he makes regarding his care.

Bibliography

Arnold, D. G., & Menzel, P. T. (1998). When comes 'The end of the day'? A comment on the dialogue between Dax Cowart and Robert Burt. *Hastings Center Report 28*(1), 25–27.

Cowart, D., & Burt, R. (1998). Confronting death: Who chooses, Who controls? A dialogue between Dax Cowart and Robert Burt. *Hastings Center Report 28*(1), 14–24.

INSTRUCTIONAL IMPROVEMENT TOOL FOR UNIT 12

Student feedback/evaluation indicated that I need to improve my classroom presentation by:

Adding Content

1. ______________________________

____

2. ______________________________

____

3. ______________________________

____

Deleting Content

1. ______________________________

____

2. ______________________________

____

3. ______________________________

____

Emphasizing/Deemphasizing the Following Content

1. ______________________________

____

2. ______________________________

____

3. ______________________________

____

Questions students asked that I need to research for the future are:

1. ______________________________

____

2. ______________________________

____

3. ______________________________

____

UNIT 13
SENSORINEURAL FUNCTION

54

Assessment and Management of Patients with Eye and Vision Disorders

I. LEARNING OBJECTIVES

In addition to the learning objectives on page 1539, I want my students to be able to:

1. ______________________________

2. ______________________________

3. ______________________________

II. TOP TERMS

1. Astigmatism
2. Blepharitis
3. Cataract
4. Chemosis
5. Diplopia
6. Exophthalmus
7. Glaucoma
8. Hordeolum
9. Keratitis
10. Myopia
11. Nystagmus
12. Papilledema
13. Photophobia
14. Ptosis
15. Refraction
16. Tonometry

III. COLLABORATIVE LEARNING ACTIVITIES

Team Discussion Questions/Seminar Topics

1. Compare and contrast the structure and function of the external structures of the eye (reference pages 1540–1543 and Figures 54–1 to 54–4).
2. Explain the difference between functional and visual impairment (reference pages 1546–1548 and Table 54–1).
3. Explain the five stages of deterioration for glaucoma (reference pages 1549–1552).
4. Compare and contrast the assessment, clinical manifestations, medical management and nursing interventions for retinal disorders (reference pages 1559–1561).

IV. CRITICAL THINKING ACTIVITIES

In-Class Team Exercises

1. Have a student bring the Snellen chart into class. Assign students to work in groups and assess each other's visual acuity. Record the acuity readings (i.e., 20/20) on the following chart along with each student's age and any other related conditions (corrective lens use, chronic illnesses, medications). Determine if there is a mean (average) acuity score for the class, per age group, etc. (reference pages 1543–1544).

Student	Acuity Reading	Corrective Lens	Illness	Medications
1.				
2.				
3.				
4.				
5.				
6.				
7.				
8.				
9.				
10.				
11.				
12.				
13.				
14.				
15.				
16.				
17.				
18.				
19.				
20.				

Send-Home Assignments

Read the following case study. Fill in the blanks or circle the correct answers.

Case Study: Cataract Surgery

Marcella is a 75-year-old single woman who has had progressive diminished vision and increased difficulty with night driving. Her physician suspects that Marcella has a cataract. He does a complete eye examination and history (reference pages 1554–1557, Figure 54–9, and Table 54–5).

1. As part of an oral history, the physician tries to determine if Marcella has any of the common factors that contribute to cataract development such as (a)____________, (b) ________, (c) _________, and (d)______________.
2. Marcella, during her history, told the physician that she was experiencing the three common symptoms found with cataracts: (a)_______, (b) ___________, and (c)_____________.
3. On ophthalmic examination, the physician noted the major objective finding seen with cataracts:

   ____
4. When assessing the need for surgery, the physician determined that Marcella's best corrected vision was worse than the minimal standard of:
   a. 20/15.
   b. 20/25.
   c. 20/35.
   d. 20/50.
5. The physician decided to perform ________________, the most preferred technique for cataract surgery.
6. The physician advised Marcella that there is a 25% chance that she may experience the common complication of:
   a. glaucoma.
   b. uveitis.
   c. secondary membranes.
   d. choroidal detachment.
7. Postoperatively, Marcella knows that she will need to wear an eye shield at night for about:
   a. 3 evenings.
   b. one week
   c. two weeks
   d. one month

55

Assessment and Management of Patients with Hearing and Balance Disorders

I. LEARNING OBJECTIVES

In addition to the learning objectives on page 1578, I want my students to be able to:

1. ______________________________

2. ______________________________

3. ______________________________

II. TOP TERMS

1. Acute Otitis Media
2. Cerumen
3. Cholesteatoma
4. Cochlea
5. Eustachian Tube
6. Labyrinth
7. Meniere's Disease
8. Organ of Corti
9. Otalgia
10. Otolaryngologist
11. Ototoxicity
12. Presbycusis
13. Proprioceptive System
14. Temporomandibular
15. Tinnitus
16. Tympanic Membrane
17. Vertigo

III. COLLABORATIVE LEARNING ACTIVITIES

Send-Home Assignments

1. Compare and contrast how each of the following symptoms reflects problems of the external, middle and inner ear: vertigo, tinnitus, pain, hearing loss, and discharge (reference pages 1587–1591 and 1594–1595).
2. Compare and contrast the various types of hearing aids relative to advantages, disadvantages, and range of hearing loss (reference pages 1600–1602 and Table 55–3).

IV. CRITICAL THINKING ACTIVITIES

Discussion Questions/Seminar Topics

Read the phrase that defines/explains the scrambled word. Unscramble the word (reference pages 1579–1582 and Chart 55-I)

1. AHOCELC ____________________

   A major organ of hearing

2. LIUSRRC ____________________

   Aids in collecting sound waves and passing them onto the auditory canal

3. EUECRMN ____________________

   Another name for ear wax

4. SELMUAL ____________________

   An auditory ossicle also known as the "hammer"

5. SCIUN ____________________

   The middle ossicle, also known as the anvil

6. HHIEGT ____________________

   The cranial nerve known as the cochleovestibular nerve

7. HNRBLAYIT ____________________

   Another word for the vestibular system

8. CNPYTMAI ____________________

   This membrane vibrates and transmits sound

Send-Home Assignments

Develop a nursing care plan for Julia, who is 67 years old, lives alone, and has just been diagnosed as having Labyrinthitis. She will be medically managed for her symptoms. Use the following format for development of your care plan (reference page 1596).

Nursing Diagnosis: ____________________________

Goals	Nursing Actions	Rationale	Expected Outcomes

INSTRUCTIONAL IMPROVEMENT TOOL FOR UNIT 13

Student feedback/evaluation indicated that I need to improve my classroom presentation by:

Adding Content

1. ______________________________

____

2. ______________________________

____

3. ______________________________

____

Deleting Content

1. ______________________________

____

2. ______________________________

____

3. ______________________________

____

Emphasizing/Deemphasizing the Following Content

1. ______________________________

____

2. ______________________________

____

3. ______________________________

____

Questions students asked that I need to research for the future are:

1. ______________________________

____

2. ______________________________

____

3. ______________________________

____

UNIT **14**
NEUROLOGIC FUNCTION

56
Assessment of Neurologic Function

I. LEARNING OBJECTIVES

In addition to the learning objectives on page 1607, I want my students to be able to:

1. ______________________________

2. ______________________________

3. ______________________________

II. TOPIC TERMS

1. Aphasia
2. Ataxia
3. Babinski Reflex
4. Decerebrate Posturing
5. Decorticate Posturing
6. Dyskinesias
7. Extrapyramidal System
8. Meninges
9. Paraplegia
10. Ptosis

III. COLLABORATIVE LEARNING ACTIVITIES

Team Discussion Questions/Seminar Topics

1. Explain the concept of the "blood-brain barrier" and what it means relative to pharmacotherapy (reference page 1613).
2. Explain the purpose, process, and interpretation of negative and positive Babinski responses (reference pages 1623–1625).
3. Distinguish between positron emission and single photon emission tomography (reference page 1627).
4. Explain the rationale, procedure, and nursing implications for lumbar puncture examination (reference pages 1630–1632).

IV. CRITICAL THINKING ACTIVITIES

In-Class Team Exercises

Cranial Nerve Examination

Assign students to groups of four. Each student in every group should have an opportunity to conduct a cranial nerve examination on another student. For each of the following 12 nerves, have a student document the process and the result of the clinical examination. Allot some time at the end of class for the group to share results, being sensitive to any abnormalities that might embarrass a student (reference pages 1614–1615, Table 56–2, and Figure 56–9).

Cranial Nerve	Clinical Exam Process	Results and Interpretation
1. Olfactory		
2. Optic		
3. Oculomotor		
4. Trachlear		
5. Trigeminal		
6. Abducens		
7. Facial		
8. Vestibulo-cochlear		
9. Glossopharyngeal		
10. Vagus		
11. Spinal Accessory		
12. Hypoglossal		

Send-Home Assignments

Neurologic Examination

Using the following outline, complete a neurologic examination on a relative or friend. Compare your results against the expected normal results in the textbook (reference pages 1621–1625).

Neurologic Examinations	Nursing Assessment	Results	Clinical Interpretation
1. Cerebral Function Mental status Intellectual function Thought content Emotional status Perception Motor ability Language ability Glascow Coma Scale			
2. Cranial Nerves (use form on previous pages)			
3. Motor System Muscle strength Motor power Balance & coordination The Rombergh test			
4. Reflexes Biceps Triceps Brachioradials Patellar Ankle Clonus Abdominal Babinski			
5. Sensory System Tactile sensations Pain & temperature Vibration & proprioception Position Taste & smell Tactile & visual			
6. Nursing Assessment			
7. Results			
8. Clinical Interpretation			

57

Management of Patients with Neurologic Dysfunction

I. LEARNING OBJECTIVES

In addition to the learning objectives on page 1633, I want my students to be able to:

1. ______________________________

2. ______________________________

3. ______________________________

II. TOP TERMS

1. Aphasia
2. Brain Death
3. Coma
4. Craniotomy
5. Decerebration
6. Decortication
7. Paraphasia
8. Unconscious

III. COLLABORATIVE LEARNING ACTIVITIES

Team Discussion Questions/Seminar Topics

1. Distinguish between the clinical manifestations of stupor and coma, citing the rationale for the differences in each (reference pages 1644–1646).
2. Divide the students into subgroups of four. Have each group create a different profile of an aphasic patient. Then have groups trade profiles. After a traded profile is received, each group is to draft several specific "how-to's" regarding communication with that aphasic patient (reference pages 1652–1660 and Chart 57–4).
3. Compare the purpose and clinical nursing management for a cordotomy and a rhizotomy (reference pages 1670–1672).

IV. COLLABORATIVE LEARNING ACTIVITIES

In-Class Team Exercises

Complete the following chart by documenting specific nursing interventions for a patient with increased ICP (reference pages 1634–1644, Figures 57–1, 57–3, & 57–4, and Table 57–1).

Factor Contributing to ICP	Medical Intervention	Rationale	Nursing Intervention	Patient Education

Send-Home Assignments

1. Develop a nursing care plan for Mr. Douval, a 61-year-old who suffered right-side paralysis from a stroke about one week ago. He lives with his wife and has a strong family support system (reference pages 1650–1660 and Figure 57–9).

   Nursing Diagnosis: ____________________________

Goals	Nursing Actions	Rationale	Expected Outcomes

2. Construct a list of preoperative nursing interventions and postoperative nursing interventions (with supporting rationales) for a 57-year-old lawyer who is to undergo intracranial surgery for a brain tumor. He lives in a center city townhouse with his wife, who is also a lawyer (reference pages 1661–1667 and Table 57–6).

Nursing Interventions	Rationale	Preoperative Care	Postoperative Care

3. Assign the following case study. Direct students to choose one of the two options and prepare an argument to support their position. Recommend that the "Guidelines" be used in their clinical practice.

ETHICAL QUESTION: SHOULD PATIENTS IN A PERSISTENT VEGETATIVE STATE BE USED AS ORGAN DONORS?

Discussion: The need for donated organs for transplantation has long outstripped the supply of organs from brain-dead donors. Many more patients fulfull the criteria for persistent vegetative state (PVS) than the criteria for brain death, and the recovery from a PVS is thought to be less than 1%. Many people equate the loss of higher brain functions (thought and perception) with the loss of what is essential to being human. Can the definition of death be changed to include the PVS and then free up the families of those patients to donate their organs?

Dilemma: Obligation to do what is best for the patient conflicts with the needs of the population as a whole (beneficence versus justice).

Arguments in FAVOR of Using PVS Patients as Organ Donors: The loss of higher brain function is equivalent to the loss of the human being; therefore, the PVS patient should be classified as "dead" just as brain-dead patients are classified as "dead." PVS is relatively easy to diagnose and distinguish from other conditions; therefore, only PVS patients will be considered as organ donors. The recovery from a PVS is thought to be less than 1%. The needs of many sick people for organs justify changing the current definition of death. It is very costly to maintain PVS patients on artificial nutrition in nursing homes; using PVS patients as organ donors would decrease that number, save money, and provide a source for organs for those in urgent need of them.

Implications of Choosing This Position: More organs would become available for transplant, which would help many patients on the waiting list for organs, patients who could recover from their disease with the organ transplants and contribute to society. The change in the concept of death from whole brain death to PVS would cause confusion as to what constitutes death. For example, if a spontaneously breathing, eyes-open moving patient is considered dead, why not an elderly nursing home patient with advanced Alzheimer's disease? This movement from the intended change in practice to the unanticipated, unintended result is called, in ethical terms, the *slippery slope effect.*

Arguments AGAINST Using PVS Patients as Organ Donors: The small chance of recovery from a PVS is enough to exclude the PVS patient from the category of the dead (the chance of recovery from properly diagnosed brain death is zero) The diagnosis of PVS is not as precise as that of brain death. Not everyone agrees that the loss of higher brain function is equivalent to the loss of the human being. PVS patients are people, too. PVS patients should be treated as ends and not as means to an end. The definition of death should remain restricted and tight to avoid initiating the slippery slope effect. This position is consistent with current U.S. law.

Implications of Choosing This Position: Organs for transplant will remain scarce. The concept of death will not change. Many people who consider PVS patients dead will consider it a waste of organs to either maintain PVS patients on tube feedings or to allow them to die without using their organs.

Guidelines for the Nurse Caring for a PVS Patient:

1. Review the chart for the patient's history, reason for admission, cause of PVS state, length of PVS state, current treatment, and treatment goals. See if any advance directives from the patient are included. Compare the current treatment with that specified in the advance directive.
2. Provide emotional support for the family. Consider psychiatric nurse, social work, and chaplaincy consultations for them as appropriate.
3. Discuss the plan of care with the patient's physician. If the current treatment differs from that specified in the advance directive, explore the reason for this with the physician and consult the bioethics committee if necessary.
4. Does the patient have a DNR order? If not, why not? Has this issue been explored with the family? Have they refused a DNR order? Why? Plan a patient care conference if needed to facilitate an agreement about a plan of care for the patient among the physician, family, and nursing staff.
5. If the family wants to donate the patient's organs, explain the difference between brain death and PVS. Explain that current U.S. law forbids the donation of PVS patient organs. Refer them to the physician or the local organ transplant organization if more information is desired.

Bibliography

Armstrong, P. W., & Colen, B. D. (1988, February–March). In Quinlan to Jobes: The Courts and the PVS Patient. *Hastings Center Report,* 18(1), 37–40.

Brody, B. A. (1988, February–March). Ethical Questions Raised by the Persistent Vegetative Patient. *Hastings Center Report,* 18(1), 33–37.

Chabalewski, F., and Norris, M. K. G. (1994, June). The Gift of Life: Talking to Families About Organ and Tissue Donation. *American Journal of Nursing,* 94(6), 28–33.

Cranford, R. E. (1988, February–March). The Persistent Vegetative State: The Medical Reality (Getting the Facts Straight). *Hastings Center Report,* 18(1), 27–32.

Lawrence, M. (1995). The Unconscious Experience. *American Journal of Critical Care,* 4(3), 227–232.

Ozuna, J. (1996). Persistent Vegetative State: Important Considerations for the Neuroscience Nurse. *Journal of Neuroscience Nursing,* 28(3), 199–203.

Schneiderman, L. J. (1990, May–June). Exile and PVS. *Hastings Center Report,* 20(3), 5.

Steinbock, B. (1989, July–August). Recovery from Persistent Vegetative State?: The Case of Connie Coons. *Hastings Center Report,* 19(4) 14–15.

Veatch, R. M. (1993, July–August). The Impending Collapse of the Whole-Brain Definition of Death. *Hastings Center Report,* 23(4), 18–24.

Wikler, D. (1988, February–March). Not Dead, Not Dying? Ethical Categories and Persistent Vegetative State. *Hastings Center Report,* 18(1), 41–47.

Wilke, J. C., & Andrusko, D. (1988, October–November). Pensonhood Redux. *Hastings Center Report,* 18(5), 30–33.

58

Management of Patients with Neurologic Trauma

I. LEARNING OBJECTIVES

In addition to the learning objectives on page 1674, I want my students to be able to:

1. ______________________________

2. ______________________________

3. ______________________________

II. TOP TERMS

1. Autonomic Dysreflexia
2. Concussion
3. Contusion
4. Diffuse Axonal Injury
5. Epidural Hematoma
6. Halo Vest
7. Intracerebral Hemorrhage
8. Postconcussion Syndrome
9. Spinal Cord Injury
10. Subluxation

III. COLLABORATIVE LEARNING ACTIVITIES

Team Discussion Questions/Seminar Topics

1. Compare and contrast the presenting symptoms and treatment for two types of brain injury, a concussion, and a contusion (reference pages 1676–1677).
2. Describe the cause, pathophysiology, medical management, and nursing interventions for a patient with a subdural hematoma (reference pages 1677–1679).
3. With another classmate, demonstrate how a spinal cord injury patient should be immobilized at the scene of an accident (reference pages 1687–1689).

IV. CRITICAL THINKING ACTIVITIES

In-Class Team Exercises

For each of the following spinal cord injuries, describe the area of cord damage in the brain, the resulting cord syndrome characteristics, and implications for immediate nursing intervention (reference pages 1687–1689 and Charts 58–4 and 58–5).

Spinal Cord Injury Syndrome	Area of Damage	Cord Syndrome Characteristics	Nursing Interventions
Central Cord			
Anterior Cord			
Brown-Séquard Syndrome			
Quadriplegia			
Paraplegia			

Send-Home Assignments

Develop an assessment guide for Edward, a 24-year-old who was admitted unconscious to the emergency department with a head injury sustained in a vehicular accident. Share your guide with your classmates for their comments. After developing your assessment guide for Edward, construct a nursing care plan that will emphasize the following areas: fluid and electrolyte replacement, nutritional management, restlessness, potential complications, and family education. Edward is the adopted son of a couple who are now both retired from schoolteaching. Use the format below and share it with your instructor for comment (reference pages 1679–1686 and Tables 58–1 and 58–2).

Nursing Diagnosis: ______________________________

Goals	Nursing Actions	Rationale	Expected Outcomes

1. Assign the following case study. Direct students to choose one of the two options and prepare an argument to support their position. Recommend that the "Guidelines" be used in their clinical practice.

ETHICAL QUESTION: WHAT ARE THE DIFFERENCES, IF ANY, IN OBLIGATIONS TOWARD PATIENTS IN A PERSISTENT VEGETATIVE STATE (PVS) AND PATIENTS IN A COMA?

Situation: The family of a 55-year-old woman with the diagnosis persistent vegetative state (PVS) wants to withdraw tube feedings and let the patient die. The nursing student on the unit states that the patient is not brain dead because the patient moves her eyes toward the assistant and has periods of sleep and awakening. The student has come to you as the charge nurse. She says that if the family's request to remove the feeding tube is honored, the family will be guilty of murder.

Dilemma: Conflict between the nursing student and the understanding of the obligations to the patient and the family.

Arguments for Withdrawing Nutrition and Hydration: The patient is not aware and never will recover from PVS. This is a permanent state resulting from loss of cognition and cerebral function. The brainstem is still intact and the patient only appears to arouse. The patient is not in a coma—a potentially recoverable condition. The patient can no longer function and the wishes of the family to remove the nutrition and hydration can be followed.

Implications of Withdrawing Nutrition and Hydration: The patient will die over time from dehydration. This type of death may be unpleasant if the patient is aware. This patient is not aware, but still many persons have strong cultural and religious taboos against "starving" anyone.

Arguments Against Withdrawing Nutrition and Hydration: The family might not be aware of the consequences of their request. The family needs support and guidance in making a decision.

Implications of Not Withdrawing Nutrition and Hydration: All the nursing staff should be educated on the differences between PVS and coma and what the legal decisions have been regarding obligations of care to persons in these states. If the nursing student is strongly opposed on religious grounds to stopping treatments, then perhaps he or she should receive counseling and the clinical assignment changed.

Potential Compromise: In another option, perhaps the patient could be moved, if not already in such an institution, to a long-term care facility for the PVS-type patient. Then the question of tube feedings would not be as much an issue. Patients in a PVS can be maintained for many years. The family may need financial guidance and assistance in caring for this patient.

It is unclear without further data if the family needs financial and psychological support. Having a family member in such a condition can be emotionally devastating. The institution in which the patient is housed may need to discharge the patient to an institution where the costs are not as high. If the family members have been so informed, they may think their only option is to remove the feeding tube.

Guidelines for Nursing Care:

1. Recognize the differences between patients in PVS and those in a coma.
2. Know the potential differences in outcome between the two neurologic conditions.
3. Make sure that all the nursing staff and family understand the differences between PVS and coma.
4. Assist the family in social planning by asking if talking with someone from social services or the business office will be helpful.
5. Appreciate your own values and desires with regard to stopping nutrition and hydration.

6. Know the laws of your state with regard to living wills, patient self-determination acts, and discontinuing treatment.
7. Know the policies of your institution with regard to discontinuing nutrition and hydration.
8. Read up on the US Supreme Court decision on Cruzan vs Director, Missouri Department of Health. (There is a wealth of literature on the Cruzan case as well as volumes on discontinuing treatments. See Cruzan vs Director, Missouri Department of Health and the resultant US Supreme Court decision, 110 S. Ct 2841-2890.)

Bibliography

Beauchamp, T. L., & Childress, J. F. (1994). *Principles of biomedical ethics* (4th ed.). New York: Oxford University Press.

Cantor, N. L. (1993). *Advance directives and the pursuit of death with dignity*. Bloomington, IN: Indiana University Press.

Cranford, R. E. (1988). The persistent vegetative state: The medical reality (getting the facts straight). *Hastings Center Report 18 (February-March).*

King, P. (1991). The authority of families to make medical decisions for incompetent patients after the Cruzan decision. *Law, Medicine, and Health Care 19,* 76–79.

59

Management of Patients with Neurologic Disorders

I. LEARNING OBJECTIVES

In addition to the learning objectives on page 1700, I want my students to be able to:

1. ______________________________

2. ______________________________

3. ______________________________

II. TOP TERMS

1. Akathisia
2. Amyotrophic Lateral Sclerosis (ALS)
3. Angioma
4. Ataxia
5. Bradykinesia
6. Brain Abscess
7. Chorea
8. Epilepsy
9. Glioma
10. Guillian-Barré
11. Intracranial Aneurysm
12. Meningitis
13. Migraine
14. Myasthenia Gravis
15. Myelin
16. Parkinson's Disease
17. Trigeminal Neuralgia

III. COLLABORATIVE LEARNING ACTIVITIES

Team Discussion Questions/Seminar Topics

1. Compare and contrast the different medications and treatment modalities for the various types of migraine headaches (reference pages 1702–1704).
2. Describe the etiology, pathophysiology, medical management, and nursing intervention for a patient with myasthenia gravis (reference pages 1733–1737).

3. Divide the class into two groups and ask them to compare the clinical manifestations and nursing management for patients with multiple sclerosis and those with Parkinson's disease (reference pages 1718–1730).

4. Ask students to describe emergency measures for a patient who experiences a seizure in the following environments: a hospital, a shopping mall, and a soccer field (reference pages 1738–1740).

IV. CRITICAL THINKING ACTIVITIES

Send-Home Assignments

1. For each of the following common brain tumor sites listed below, have students name as many types of tumors as possible. One example is given (reference pages 1705–1707 and Figure 59–1).

Brain Tumor Site	**Common Tumors**
Brain Stem	1. Astrocytoma 2. Glioblastoma Multiforme
Pituitary Area	1. ____________ 2. ____________ 3. ____________
Optic Chiasm	1. ____________
Corpus Callosum	1. ____________ 2. ____________ 3. ____________
Lateral Ventricle	1. ____________ 2. ____________
Cerebrum	1. ____________ 2. ____________ 3. ____________ 4. ____________
Pineal Area	1. ____________ 2. ____________
Cerebellum	1. ____________ 2. ____________ 3. ____________ 4. ____________
Fourth Ventricle	1. ____________
Third Ventricle	1. ____________

2. Develop an assessment guide for Sadie, a 19-year-old freshman nursing student at a New York university, who has just been diagnosed with bacterial meningitis. She is hospitalized and her family lives in California. Be sure to include the community perspective (reference pages 1711–1714).

Nursing Diagnosis: ____________________

Goals	Nursing Interventions	Rationale	Expected Outcomes

INSTRUCTIONAL IMPROVEMENT TOOL FOR UNIT 14

Student feedback/evaluation indicated that I need to improve my classroom presentation by:

Adding Content

1. ______________________________

2. ______________________________

3. ______________________________

Deleting Content

1. ______________________________

2. ______________________________

3. ______________________________

Emphasizing/Deemphasizing the Following Content

1. ______________________________

2. ______________________________

3. ______________________________

Questions students asked that I need to research for the future are:

1. ______________________________

2. ______________________________

3. ______________________________

60

Assessment of Musculoskeletal Function

I. LEARNING OBJECTIVES

In addition to the learning objectives on page 1763, I want my students to be able to:

1. ______________________________

2. ______________________________

3. ______________________________

II. TOP TERMS

1. Atrophy
2. Crepitus
3. Diaphysis
4. Effusion
5. Hypertrophy
6. Isometric
7. Isotonic
8. Ligaments
9. Osteoporosis
10. Periosteum
11. Sarcomere
12. Tendons
13. Tonus

III. COLLABORATIVE LEARNING ACTIVITIES

Team Discussion Questions/Seminar Topics

1. Explain the interaction between the five factors that help regulate bone formation and bone resorption: stress, vitamin D, parathyroid hormone, calcitonin, and circulation (reference pages 1764–1766).
2. Describe how blood cells are produced in the bone marrow (reference pages 1764–1766).
3. Describe some expected musculoskeletal changes that occur with aging (reference pages 1769–1771).

IV. CRITICAL THINKING ACTIVITIES

In-Class Team Exercises

Match the function of the specific bone tissue listed in Column II with its associated type of bone listed in Column I (reference pages 1764–1768).

Column I	Column II
1. Bone marrow	a. Bone formation occurs by the secretion of bone matrix.
2. Osteon	b. This membrane covers the marrow cavity of long bones.
3. Osteoclasts	c. This tissue produces red and white blood cells.
4. Endosteum	d. This membrane covers the bone.
5. Osteoblasts	e. The microscopic functioning unit of mature bone.
6. Periosteum	f. These cells help bone reabsorption and remodeling.

Send-Home Assignments

1. Complete a physical examination of the musculoskeletal system on three individuals that you know: a child under 14 years of age, an adult, and an elderly person over 70 years of age. Document differences in muscle strength, appearance, use, range of motion, and any abnormalities/deformities. Compare and contrast differences among age groups (reference pages 1771–1774).
2. For each of the five peripheral nerves listed below, document a nursing assessment test for sensation and movement. Perform each test on a family member and document findings (reference page 1774).

Nerve	Sensation	Movement
Peroneal		
Tibial		
Radial		
Ulnar		
Median		

61

Musculoskeletal Care Modalities

I. LEARNING OBJECTIVES

In addition to the learning objectives on page 1778, I want my students to be able to:

1. ____________________

2. ____________________

3. ____________________

II. TOP TERMS

1. Arthroplasty
2. Buck's Traction
3. Compartment Syndrome
4. Countertraction
5. Fasciotomy
6. Homan's Sign
7. Internal Fixation
8. Meniscectomy
9. Open Reduction
10. Orthoses
11. Spica Cast
12. Volkmann's Constructure

III. COLLABORATIVE LEARNING ACTIVITIES

Team Discussion Questions/Seminar Topics

1. Explain, demonstrate, and give the scientific rationale for the process used for turning a patient in a hip spica cast (reference pages 1780–1781).
2. Compare and contrast the nursing interventions for a patient in skin and skeletal traction (reference pages 1787–1790).
3. Explain, demonstrate, and give the scientific rationale for quadriceps and gluteal-setting exercises (reference page 1790).

IV. CRITICAL THINKING ACTIVITIES

In-Class Team Exercises

Complete the following chart for each of the following common types of cylindrical casts. (reference pages 1779–1781).

Cast Type	Area Covered	Pressure Point	Nursing Assessments	Patient Education
Short arm cast				
Long leg cast				
Walking cast				
Body cast				
Shoulder spica				
Hip spica cast				

1. Assign the following case study. Direct students to choose one of the two options and prepare an argument to support their position. Recommend that the "Guidelines" be used in their clinical practice.

Send-Home Assignments

Case Study in Professional Competency

A 35-year-old female patient is admitted to an orthopedic unit where you work as a staff RN. The patient is admitted from the recovery room after a reduction of a fibula fracture secondary to a motor vehicle crash. The patient has a cast from her thigh to her toes. The patient progresses normally on the day of the surgery, but on her first postoperative day she begins to complain of pain in her casted heel. You note that there is no drainage from the cast and that her toes have good circulation and neurological status. You provide her with the pain medication ordered for her, but this is not adequate to cover her pain. On her second postoperative day, after consultation with the physician, he discontinues the patient's oral pain medications and prescribes a patient-controlled analgesia pump for better pain management. By the third postoperative day, the patient is at the upper limit of the pain medication through the PCA pump and still complaining of severe pain in the heel. On that day, you notice a change in her condition. Her temperature has spiked to 101˚F, there is a small amount of drainage at the heel area of her cast, and her toes on the casted foot are edematous and cool.

You page the physician and report your observations. The physician becomes angry and refuses to come to the unit to examine the patient's foot. He accuses you of not knowing how to take care of orthopedic patients and then states that the only reason that the patient has pain is because she has an addictive personality and is addicted to the pain medication. As evidence he cites the fact, which is true, that the patient's blood alcohol level in the emergency room on admission was 0.12%. Before the physician hangs up on you he tells you that he does not want to hear anything more about this patient's ankle pain.

Discussion: This is not, strictly speaking, an ethical dilemma. The nursing obligation to protect the patient is clear, and there is no countering ethical obligation to protect the physician. But the pressure on the nurse not to follow through on her observations about her patient is quite real. The nurse may indeed be placing herself in an angry, confrontational battle with the physician, which could lead to some difficult working relationships in the future. Nevertheless, the nurse is ethically obligated to intervene in this situation to protect the patient. Indeed, if she does not pursue this matter, she may find herself guilty of neglect and malpractice.

Dilemma: The obligation to protect the patient is impeded by political and social pressure not to pursue the issue.

Option 1: Confront the patient with your evidence, denounce the physician as incompetent, and urge the patient to another physician.

Rationale: The patient has a right to know that she is receiving unsafe medical care.

Implications of Choosing This Option: The nurse may find herself at cross purposes with nursing administration, as the action is undoubtedly not consistent with any hospital policy. If wrong about the physician, you will have destroyed the physician–patient relationship, poorly represented the nurses on your unit, and you may find yourself sued for slander. The second physician may agree with the first physician. The patient's primary physician will be angry and you may find yourself sued for slander.

Option 2: Document your information clearly and do not pursue the issue further. The record will speak for itself.

Rationale: The documentation will help to make the case against the physician while you protect yourself.

Implications of Choosing This Option: The patient will not receive the medical attention she needs; she will undoubtedly need to suffer harm before the medical chart will be reviewed. The physician may blame you for not pursuing the issue further. You may be liable for malpractice.

Option 3: Reverify your information, consult with your peers and your supervisor. Explain to your supervisor why you believe the patient requires medical intervention. Go up the chain of command to obtain the medical care that the patient needs.

Rationale: This will produce medical and administrative backing for intervening in the patient's current care and will preserve professional relationships.

Implications of Choosing This Option: The patient will receive the medical attention that she needs and professional relationships will be maintained. The physician may be angry with you but administrative support will make it politically difficult for him to express it.

Guidelines for the Nurse Dealing with an Issue of Competency:

1. Reverify your information. Review the chart and note the patient's history, course of illness, documentation of the present problem, and the present plan of care. Consult with your peers, clinical specialist, and your supervisor to confirm or challenge your conclusions.
2. If your conclusions are verified, document them and attempt again to speak to the physician about your concerns. Document this conversation, including details about information given to the physician.
3. If the physician refuses to intervene in the way you think is necessary for the good of your patient, consult with your supervisor. Describe the information that supports your argument.
4. If the supervisor agrees with your conclusions, he or she should attempt to speak with the physician. If that fails to bring about the desired intervention, the supervisor can make contacts within the medical chain of command (medical director of the unit, chief of surgery, hospital administrator in charge of

medical staff, and so on), who can then contact the patient's physician and initiate the required treatment for the patient.

5. Other resources for the nurse in the situation are the risk manager and the bioethics committee.

Bibliography

American Nurses' Association. (1985). *Code for Nurses with Interpretive Statements.* Kansas City, MO: American Nurses' Association.

American Nurses' Association. (1988). *Ethics of Safeguarding Client Health and Safety, Ethics in Nursing Position Statements and Guidelines.* Kansas City, MO, American Nurses' Association.

Bandman, E. (1985). *Whistle-Blowers Take Risks to Halt Wrongdoing in Ethical Dilemmas Confronting Nurses* (pp. 18–22). Kansas City, MO: American Nurses' Association.

Colwell, C., & Morris, B. (1995). Patient-Controlled Analgesia Compared with Intramuscular Injection of Analgesics for the Mangement of Pain after an Orthopaedic Procedure. *Journal of Bone and Joint Surgery,* 77-A (5), 726–733.

Edwards, B. S. (1993, September). When the Physician Won't Give Up. *American Journal of Nursing,* 93(9), 34–37.

Novy, C., & Jagmin, M. (1997). Pain Management in the Elderly Orthopaedic Patient, *Orthopaedic Nursing,* 16(1): 51–57.

Sprague, J. (1998). Cast Syndrome. *Orthopaedic Nursing,* 17(4), 12–15.

62

Managing Patients with Musculoskeletal Disorders

I. LEARNING OBJECTIVES

In addition to the learning objectives on page 1806, I want my students to be able to:

1. ______________________________

2. ______________________________

3. ______________________________

II. TOP TERMS

1. Bunion
2. Carpal Tunnel Syndrome
3. Dowager's Hump
4. Dupuytren's Contracture
5. Epicondylitis
6. Ganglion
7. Hammer Toe
8. Intervertebral Discs
9. Kyphosis
10. Osteogenic
11. Osteoporosis
12. Pes Cavus

III. COLLABORATIVE LEARNING ACTIVITIES

Team Discussion Questions/Seminar Topics

1. Compare and contrast the clinical manifestations, medical management, and nursing interventions for osteomalacia and Paget's disease (reference pages 1820–1822).
2. Explain the pathophysiology of and latest management techniques for carpal tunnel syndrome and Dupuytren's contracture (reference pages 1811–1812).
3. Explain in detail the relationship between menopause and osteoporosis. (reference pages 1816–1819).

IV. CRITICAL THINKING ACTIVITIES

In-Class Team Exercises

1. Develop a patient teaching outline for a 36-year-old mother of six (children range in age from 1 year to 8 years) who suffers form acute low back pain. Make your instructions specific to her needs. She lives in a split-level house. The kitchen is on the middle level, the washer and dryer are on the lower level and the children's toy room is in a converted attic area. Try to emphasize modifications for standing, sitting, lying, and lifting (reference pages 1807–1811).
2. Construct a diet that would provide 1.5 to 2.0 gm of calcium daily for a 60-year-old woman who is moderately active and does not drink milk. The diet should be a weight-reducing diet, since this person is 5 feet 5 inches tall and is 12 pounds overweight (reference pages 1818–1820).

Send-Home Assignments

Review the pictures of common foot deformities found in Figure 62–6, pages 1814–1816. Complete the exercises.

1. Identify each foot ailment and list the associated clinical manifestations.
2. For each ailment, list associated nursing diagnoses.
3. From each diagnosis, draft a nursing plan of care.
4. Broadly explain the medical/surgical management for each ailment

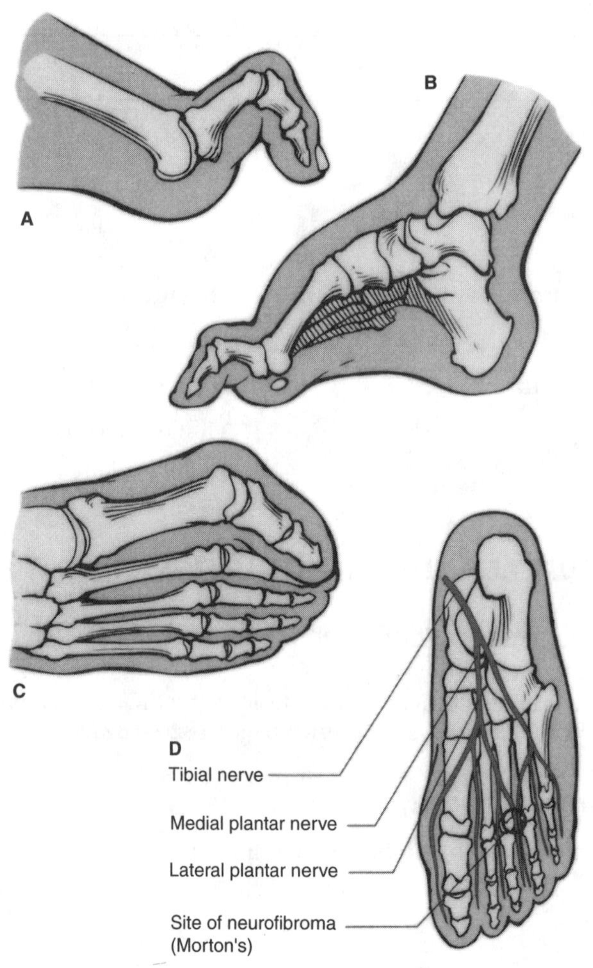

Figure 62–6 Common foot deformities.

63

Management of Patients with Musculoskeletal Trauma

I. LEARNING OBJECTIVES

In addition to the learning objectives on page 1831, I want my students to be able to:

1. ______________________________

2. ______________________________

3. ______________________________

II. TOP TERMS

1. Amputation
2. Arthroscopic
3. Dislocation
4. Ecchymosis
5. Fat Embolus
6. Hemarthrosis
7. Meniscus
8. Pseudoarthrosis
9. RICE
10. Subluxation

III. COLLABORATIVE LEARNING ACTIVITIES

Team Discussion Questions/Seminar Topics

1. Describe the concept behind the acronym RICE as it refers to the management of soft tissue injuries (reference page 1832).
2. List clinical manifestations commonly associated with fractures and identify a nursing care activity for each clinical manifestation (reference pages 1835–1837 and Chart 63–1).
3. Outline the medical management and nursing intervention for a patient with an anterior cruciate ligament injury (reference pages 1834–1835).

IV. CRITICAL THINKING ACTIVITIES

In-Class Team Exercises

1. Imagine that a classmate has experienced a fracture of the clavicle. Apply a figure 8 bandage and have one of your instructors check it for accurate placement (reference pages 1842–1843 and Figure 63–5).
2. Demonstrate for a classmate the range-of-motion exercises recommended for a patient who has sustained a clavicular fracture (reference page 1843 and Figure 63–6).

Send-Home Assignments

Complete a nursing care plan for an elderly person who has sustained a hip fracture. Divide your care plan into a preoperative section and a postoperative section. Use the format below. Share your finished paper with your instructor for comment (reference pages 1847–1850).

Nursing Diagnosis: ____________________________

Goals	Nursing Actions	Rationale	Expected Outcomes

INSTRUCTIONAL IMPROVEMENT TOOL FOR UNIT 15

Student feedback/evaluation indicated that I need to improve my classroom presentation by:

Adding Content

1. ______________________________

____

2. ______________________________

____

3. ______________________________

____

Deleting Content

1. ______________________________

____

2. ______________________________

____

3. ______________________________

____

Emphasizing/Deemphasizing the Following Content

1. ______________________________

____

2. ______________________________

____

3. ______________________________

____

Questions students asked that I need to research for the future are:

1. ______________________________

____

2. ______________________________

____

3. ______________________________

____

64

Management of Patients with Infectious Diseases

I. LEARNING OBJECTIVES

In addition to the learning objective on page 1869, I want my student to be able to:

1. ______________________________

2. ______________________________

3. ______________________________

II. TOP TERMS

1. Bacteremia
2. Chlamydia
3. Colonization
4. Emerging Infectious Diseases
5. Epidemiology
6. Gonorrhea
7. MRSA
8. Nosocomial Infections
9. OSHA
10. Portal of Entry
11. Reservoir
12. Septicemia
13. Syphilis
14. Transient Flora
15. VISA

III. COLLABORATIVE LEARNING ACTIVITIES

Team Discussion Questions/Seminar Topics

1. Discuss the purpose, location, and role of the Centers for Disease Control and Prevention (reference pages 1873–1874).
2. Explain the pathophysiology, risk factors, clinical manifestations, diagnostic findings, medical management, and nursing interventions for Legionnaires' disease (reference page 1884).
3. Design a health awareness pamphlet for Lyme's disease and post it on bulletin boards throughout your school (reference pages 1884–1885).

IV. CRITICAL THINKING ACTIVITIES

In-Class Team Exercises

Complete the following chart for each of the specific diseases or conditions (reference pages 1871–1872 and Table 64–1).

Disease or Condition	Organism	Usual Mode of Transmission	Nursing Measures for Prevention of Spread
AIDS			
Gonorrhea			
Chancroid			
Cholera			
Diarrheal disease			
Cytomegalovirus infection			
Hepatitis (bloodborne)			
Herpes simplex			
Impetigo			
Legionnaires' disease			
Hantavirus			
Meningitis			
Pneumocystis pneumonia			
Rabies			
Rubella			
Syphillis			
Tetanus			
Tuberculosis			

65

Emergency Nursing

I. LEARNING OBJECTIVES

In addition to the learning objectives on page 1900, I want my student to be able to:

1. ______________________________

2. ______________________________

3. ______________________________

II. TOP TERMS

1. Alcohol Withdrawal Delirium
2. Anaphylactic Reaction
3. Antivenin
4. Café Coronary
5. Carboxyhemoglobin
6. Endotracheal Intubation
7. Frostbite
8. Heat Stroke
9. Hypothermia
10. Near-Drowning
11. Post-Traumatic Stress Disorder (PTSD)

III. COLLABORATIVE LEARNING ACTIVITIES

Team Discussion Questions/Seminar Topics

1. Describe three symptoms that a nurse would expect to see in someone who is experiencing post-traumatic stress disorder (reference pages 1930–1931).
2. Explain what a nurse should do for both acid and corrosive poisoning, both at the scene of the accident and at the emergency room (reference pages 1919–1921).
3. List the priorities of nursing interventions with supporting rationales for the treatment of frostbite (reference pages 1914–1915).

IV. CRITICAL THINKING ACTIVITIES

In-Class Team Exercises

1. Work in teams of two. Each person needs to palpate the seven pressure points used to control hemorrhage on his or her partner (reference pages 1905–1908 and Figure 65–2).
2. For each of the drugs listed below, identify the recommended nursing interventions with supporting rationales (reference pages 1922–1925 and Table 65–1)

Drug	Nursing Interventions	Rationale
Cocaine		
Opium		
Morphine		
Seconal		
Amphetamine-type drugs		
"Ecstasy"		
Valium		

Send-Home Assignments

1. Develop a nursing care plan for a 16-year-old high school student who was brought into the emergency department by her parents. She had been raped on her way home from cheerleading practice. On admission she was withdrawn and would only talk about the situation with her mother (reference pages 1927–1929).

Nursing Diagnosis: ______________________________

Goals	Nursing Actions	Rationale	Expected Outcomes

2. Assign the following case study. Direct students to choose one of the two options and prepare an argument to support their position. Recommend that the "Guidelines" be used in their clinical practice.

ETHICAL QUESTION: SHOULD A JEHOVAH'S WITNESS PATIENT RECEIVE LIFE-SAVING BLOOD TRANSFUSIONS AGAINST HIS OR HER WISHES?

Discussion: The purpose of emergency departments is to provide life-saving treatment for patients. Jehovah's Witnesses are a sect of Christians who agree to aggressive medical treatment in case of illness or trauma, but who consistently refuse any blood or blood products because of their unique interpretation of the Bible. Should a viable and potentially salvageable Jehovah's Witness patient suffering from an acute blood loss be allowed to die because of a request based on religious beliefs if a relatively easy and accessible treatment (that is, blood transfusions) could save his or her life?)

Dilemma: The patient's right to refuse treatment conflicts with the professional obligation to help the patient (autonomy versus beneficence).

Arguments that Jehovah's Witnesses SHOULD Receive Life-Saving Transfusions Against Their Will: The professional obligation to help the patient is more important than the patient's right to refuse treatment. Religious beliefs are not as important as saving lives.

Implication of Choosing This Position: The lives of some patients who otherwise would have died without blood transfusions will be saved. Jehovah's Witnesses whose lives are saved by blood transfusions may find themselves ostracized from their church and family and may believe that they cannot go to heaven. Giving blood transfusions against the patient's will shows disrespect for minority religious beliefs. The patient may suffer side effects from the blood transfusions, including hepatitis or HIV infection. The patient may die despite the blood transfusion. The professionals who transfuse the patient over his or her objections may find themselves liable for malpractice or assault.

Arguments that Jehovah's Witnesses Should NOT Receive Blood Transfusions if They Refuse Them: The patient's right to refuse treatment is more important than the professional's desire to save the patient's life. Patients do not lose their right to make health care choices just because those choices are based on religious beliefs.

Implications of Choosing This Position: Patients will die who would have survived with blood transfusions. Professionals may feel guilty about a patient's death from lack of blood transfusions. Religious beliefs are respected. Some patients will survive despite the lack of blood transfusions.

Possible Compromise: Uphold the right of patients to refuse life-saving treatment based on religious beliefs except when minor children and pregnant women are involved, under the theory that unborn babies and children have not "chosen" the Jehovah's Witness religion. This has been the opinion of most trial courts in the United States. This exception for pregnant women, of course, raises ethical questions about the rights of pregnant women versus non-pregnant women.

GUIDELINE FOR THE NURSE CARING FOR A JEHOVAH'S WITNESS PATIENT WITH A LIFE-THREATENING NEED FOR A BLOOD TRANSFUSION:

1. Explore the issue of blood transfusion with the patient. Explain the risks and benefits of the treatment. The patient should be able to give an informed consent for blood or no blood. Document your discussion and the patient's decision clearly in the patient's chart.

2. If the patient refuses a blood transfusion, notify the physician. Encourage the physician to talk to the patient and explain again the risks and benefits of treatment with and without blood transfusions. Again, document this discussion and the patient's decision in the patient's chart.
3. Not every Jehovah's Witness will refuse blood transfusions. If the patient agrees to a blood transfusion, document this clearly in the chart and proceed with the transfusion as ordered. Keep in mind that the patient may not want to share this information with family or friends. Talk with the patient about this. You may need to curb visitors to the patient during the transfusion. Talk with the patient and physician about how to handle requests from family members about the specifics of the patient's transfusion and agree upon a plan.
4. If the patient refuses a blood transfusion, document this clearly in the patient's chart. Notify your supervisor. Consider alternative forms of treatment acceptable to the patient, for example, infusion of volume expanders or vasopressors, or both. Discuss treatment of the underlying bleeding source with the physician.
5. If the physician orders a blood transfusion despite the patient's refusal, notify your supervisor, consult with the institution's risk management office, and initiate an immediate bioethics committee consultation.

Bibliography

Dixon, J. L. & Smalley, M. G. (1981, November). Jehovah's Witnesses: The Surgical/Ethical Challenge. *Journal of the American Medical Association,* 286(21), 358–472

Jehovah's Witnesses and the Question of Blood. (1977). New York: Watchtower Bible and Tract Society of New York, Inc.

Answer Key

Based upon the individual responses to most of the exercises, specific answers are only provided for case studies, multiple-choice responses, and sample flow charts.

CHAPTER 6

Flow Chart Pathophysiologic Process:

Hypertensive Health Disease

Decreased Renal Blood Flow	=	↑ Renin ↑ Angiotensin I ↑ Angiotensin II	=	↑ Blood Pressure ↑ Aldosterone ↑ Retention of Sodium and Water	=	↑ Increased Extracellular Fluid
Increased Extracellular Fluid	=	↑ Blood flow ↑ to the Heart	=	↑ Cardiac ↑ Output	=	↑ Increased Stroke Volume
Increased Stroke Volume	=	↑ Peripheral ↑ Resistance	=	↑ Left Ventricular ↑ Emptying	=	↑ Increased Pulmonary Activity
Increased Pulmonary Activity	=	↑ Pulmonary Edema				

(pp 74–78, Figure 6–2 and Table 6–1)

CHAPTER 10

Case Study: Pressure Ulcers

1. d
2. b
3. d
4. d

(pp 135–141)

Case Study Assisted Ambulation: Crutches

1. b
2. b
3. c
4. b

(pp 132–135, Chart 10–2)

CHAPTER 13

Case Study: Postoperative Intravenous Infusion

1. a
2. a
3. d
4. d

(pp 234–242)

Three Column Matching

1. d	a. V
2. e	b. IV
3. f	c. III
4. a	d. II
5. b	e. VI
6. c	f. I

(pp 202–207)

CHAPTER 14

Flow Chart: Hypovolemic Shock

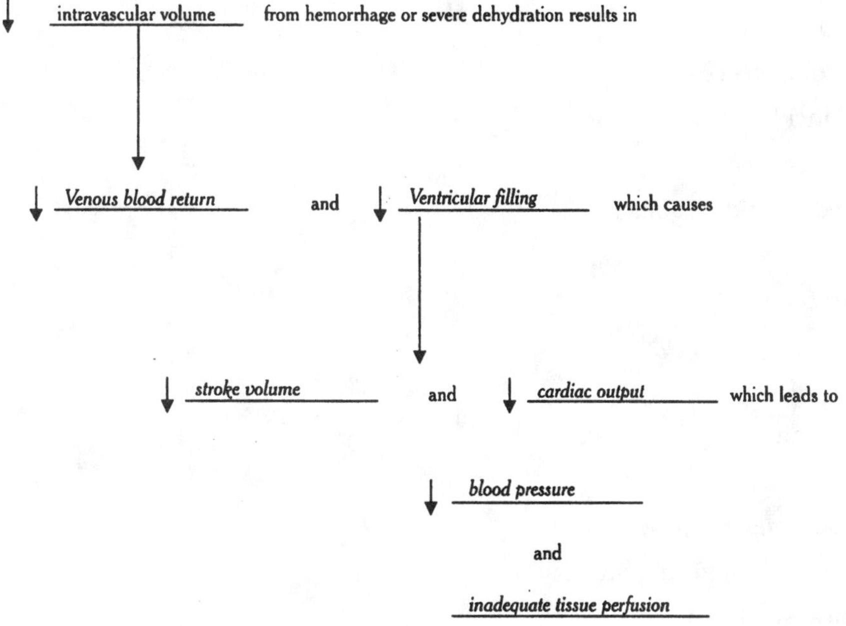

(pp 252–254 and Figure 14–3)

Case Study: Septic Shock

1. Escherichia Coli
2. 40% and 90%
3. a. urine
   b. blood
   c. sputum
   d. wound drainage
4. a. aggressive fluid replacement
   b. antibiotic pharmacotherapy
   c. crystalloids
   d. colliods
5. Cardiovasvular overload and pulmonary edema
6. 4–12 cm H_2O

(pp 257–259)

CHAPTER 15

Case Study: Cancer of the Lung

1. d
2. a. disease progression
   b. immune competence
   c. increased incidence of infection
   d. delayed tissue repair
   e. diminished functional ability
3. a. fear
   b. apprehension
   c. fatigue
   d. anger
   e. social isolation
4. c
5. a. answer questions and concerns
   b. identify resources and support persons
   c. communicate and share concerns
   d. help frame questions for the physician
6. infection
   a. Pseudomonas aeruginosa and Escherichia coli
8. b

(pp 282–290, Nursing Care Plan 15–1)

CHAPTER 17

Case Study: Spinal Anesthesia

1. d
2. d
3. d

(pp 338–342, Figure 17–2, Table 17–5)

Case Study: Malignant Hyperthermia

1. b
2. a
3. d

(pp 343–344)

CHAPTER 18

Case Study: Hypovolemic Shock

1. b
2. b
3. a
4. a
5. b

(pp 350–351, Table 18–1)

CHAPTER 20

Case Study: The Common Cold

1. a. nasal congestion
   b. sore throat
   c. sneezing
   d. cough
   e. fever
   f. chills
   g. headache
   h. muscle aches
2. a
3. d
4. d
5. d
6. a. rest
   b. adequate fluids
   c. nasal decongestants
   d. Vitamin C
   e. expectorants
7. Tells Carol that antibiotics do not affect the virus.

(pp 402–403)

CHAPTER 21

Case Study: Tuberculosis

1. b
2. b
3. d
4. b

5. c
6. c

(pp 436–442, Table 21-2, and Figure 21-4)

CHAPTER 23

Case Study: Cardiac Assessment for Chest Pain

1. d
2. c
3. d

(pp 538–544, Chart 23-1)

CHAPTER 24

Case Study: Permanent Pacemaker

1. Yes. Heart rate can vary as much as five beats above or below the preset rate.
2. a. bleeding
   b. hematoma formation
   c. infection
3. infection; maintaining a clean incision site
4. a. pacemaker model
   b. date and time of insertion
   c. stimulation threshold
   d. pacer rate
   e. incision appearance
   f. patient tolerance
5.

Goals	Nursing Activities	Expected Outcomes
a. Absence of infection	a. Sterile wound care	a. Free of infection
b. Adherance to a self-care program	b. Patient teaching	b. Adheres to a self-care program
c. Maintenance of pacemaker function	c. Patient teaching	c. Maintains pacemaker function

6. a. Normal temperature, WBC's within normal range and no evidence of redness or swelling at insertion site
   b. Understands sign and symptoms of infection and knows when to seek medical attention
   c. Assesses pulse rate at regular intervals and experiences no abrupt changes in pulse rate or rhythm

(pp 583–589)

CHAPTER 26

Case Study: Acute Pericarditis

1. a
2. Pain related to inflammation of the pericardium
3. d
4. a. Analgesics, b. Antibiotics, and c. Corticosteriods
5. Left sternal edge in the fourth intercostal space
6. a. Freedom from pain and b. Experiences absence of complications

(pp 653–655)

CHAPTER 27

Case Study: Pulmonary Edema

1. cardiac disease
2. a
3. d
4. b
5. d
6. d

(pp 657–662)

CHAPTER 28

Case Study: Thrombophlebitis

1. d
2. a
3. b
4. b
5. d

(pp 705–709)

CHAPTER 29

Schematic: Pathophysiology of Hypertension Secondary to Renal Dysfunction

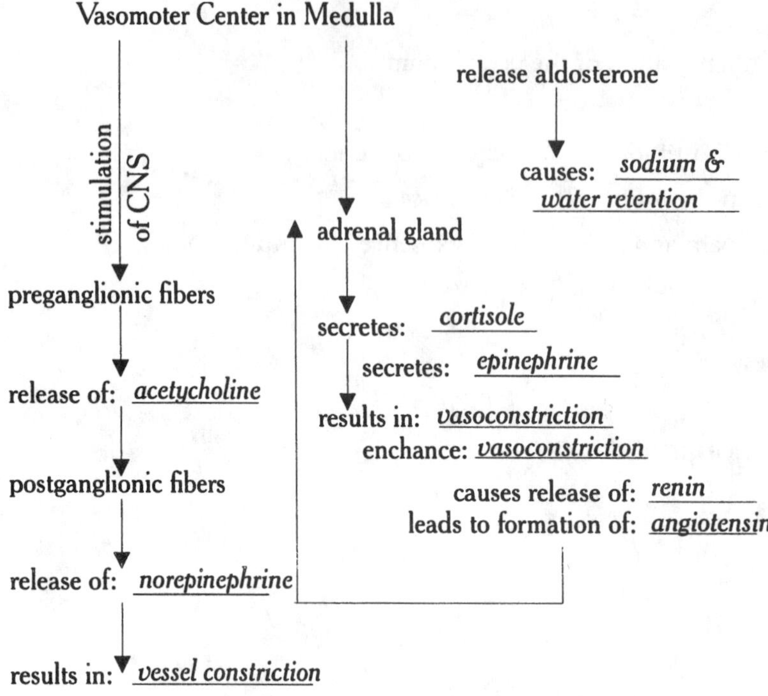

(pp 717–719)

CHAPTER 30

Case Study: Leukemia

1. hematopoietic stem cell
2. immature blast cells
3. d
4. b
5. b

(pp 755–758)

CHAPTER 32

Case Study: Cancer of the Mouth

1. The typical lesion in oral cancer is a painless, indurated (hardened) ulcer with raised edges.
2. d
3. d
4. a
5. Resectional surgery, radiation therapy and chemotherapy are considered effective.
6. c
7. d

(pp 813–817)

CHAPTER 33

Case Study: Total Parenteral Nutrition

1. b
2. c
3. c
4. d
5. d

(pp 849–855 and Table 33–5)

CHAPTER 35

Matching

1. a
2. b
3. c
4. b
5. d
6. b

(pp 876–879)

CHAPTER 36

In-Class Exercise

1. e
2. f
3. g
4. a
5. c
6. d
7. b

(pp 947–955, Figures 36–8 & 36–9)

CHAPTER 38

Case Study: Hyperparathyroidism

1. a
2. a
3. a. apathy
   b. fatigue

   c. muscular weakness
   d. nausea
   e. vomiting
   f. constipation
   g. hypertension
   h. cardiac dysrhythmias
4. kidney stones
5. d
6. b
7. c

(pp 1052–1054)

CHAPTER 41

Case Study: Illegal Conduit

1. d
2. b
3. a
4. d
5. d

(pp 1172–1181, Figure 41–9)

CHAPTER 43

Case Study: Pelvic Inflammatory Disease

1. (a) uterus, (b) fallopian tubes, (c) ovaries, (d) pelvic peritoneum, and (e) pelvic vascular system
2. (a) acute, (b) subacute, (c) recurrent, (d) chronic, (e) localized, and (f) widespread
3. a
4. Gonorrhea and Chlamydia
5. (a) ectopic pregnancy, (b) inferility, (c) recurrent pelvic pain, and (d) recurrent disease
6. Localized: (a) vaginal discharge, (b) lower abdominal pain, (c) and tenderness after menses. Generalized: (a) fever, (b) general malaise, (c) anorexia, (d) nausea, (e) headache, and (f) vomiting.
7. Use as a guide the "Home Care Teaching Checklist"

(pp 1234–1236, Figure 43–1)

Case Study: Herpes Genitalis

1. d
2. a
3. c
4. (a) mouth, (b) oropharynx, (c) mucosal surface, (d) vagina, and (e) cervix

5. drying at room temperature
6. Acyclovir
7. (a) Pain related to the presence of genital lesions, (b) risk for recurrence of infection or spread of infection, and (c) anxiety and distress related to embarrassment

(pp 1230–1231)

CHAPTER 45

Case Study: The Patient Undergoing Prostatectomy

1. Assessment of general health status and establishment of optimum renal function.
2. Acute urinary retention develops and damages the urinary tract and collecting system.
3. d
4. Stricture formation and retrograde ejaculation
5. Hemorrhage, clot formation, catheter obstruction, and sexual dysfunction
6. Damage to the pudendal nerves may cause impotence
7. Anxiety related to the inability to void, pain related to bladder distention, and knowledge deficit about factors related to the problem and the treatment protocol
8. Warm compresses to the pubis and sitz baths can help relieve spasms
9. Prolonged sitting increases intra-abdominal pressure and increases the possibility of bleeding
10. Teach the patient to tense the perineal muscles by pressing the buttocks together, holding the position for 15–20 seconds and then relaxing.

(pp 1308–1318)

CHAPTER 47

Primary Immunodeficiency Disorder

1. B-lymphocyte
2. CVID
3. Progressive neurological deterioration
4. Excess occurrences of lysis of erythrocytes

(pp 1343–1346 and Table 47–1)

CHAPTER 51

Matching

Part I	Part II
1. b	6. d
2. a	7. c
3. c	8. a
4. d	9. c
5. e	10. b

(pp 1444–1448 and Chart 51–2)

CHAPTER 52

Case Study: Acne Vulgaris

1. open comedones, closed comedones, erythematous papules, imflammatory pustules, and inflammatory cysts
2. d
3. c
4. Benzoyl Peroxide has an antibacterial effect because it suppresses Propionibacterium acnes, depresses sebum production and helps breakdown comedone plugs.
5. Vitamin A clears up the keratin plugs from the pilosebaceous ducts by speeding up cellular turnover and forcing the comedone out of the skin.
6. c
7. a
8. scarring and infection

(pp 1465–1467 and Table 52–5)

CHAPTER 54

Case Study: Cataract Surgory

1. smoking, diabetes mellius, alcohol abuse, and inadequate intake of antioxidant vitamins over time
2. painless blurring of VISION, glare and functional impairment due to loss of VISION
3. a grayish pearly haze in the pupil
4. d
5. extracapsular extraction
6. c
7. c

(pp 1554–1557, Table 54–5, and Figure 54–9)

CHAPTER 55

In-Class Exercise: Unscramble the Words

1. | C | O | C | H | L | E | A |
2. | A | U | R | I | C | L | E |
3. | C | E | R | U | M | E | N |
4. | M | A | L | L | E | U | S |
5. | I | N | C | U | S |
6. | E | I | G | H | T | H |
7. | L | A | B | Y | R | I | N | T | H |
8. | T | Y | M | P | A | N | I | C |

(pp 1579–1582 and Chart 55–1)

SECTION 2

CRITICAL THINKING EXERCISES

UNIT I BASIC CONCEPTS IN NURSING PRACTICE

CHAPTER 1 Healthcare Delivery and Nursing Practice

1. Your clinical assignment is on a medical-surgical unit in an acute care hospital. Identify a patient care issue (e.g., patient education) that could be improved. Describe the mechanism that is available within the hospital to address such quality improvement issues.
   - Discusses QA or CQI program in terms of structure
   - Identifies persons involved in the program discussed
   - For QA program: Refers to objective and measurable indicators used to monitor, evaluate, and communicate the quality and appropriateness of care delivered
   - For CQI program: Refers to analysis of problem identified, use of representatives from multiple areas of facility and their focus on identifying and streamlining all the processes involved to effect an improved outcome
2. You are caring for an elderly patient who has several chronic medical conditions and is soon to be discharged. A case manager has been assigned to this patient. How would you explain the role of the case manager to the patient and her daughter?
   - Refers to common themes of case management: responsibility and accountability
   - Describes the goals of decreased cost of care associated with decreased length of stay along with quality, appropriateness, and timeliness of services
   - Identifies the collaboration with nurses and other members of the health team who care for the patient
   - Points out the inpatient as well as outpatient aspects of management
3. You are assigned to care for a patient whose health care is covered by a managed health care plan. How have managed health care plans affected nursing care delivery in acute care hospitals and outpatient settings? How might this specific patient's care be affected?
   - Regarding effects on nursing care delivery in acute care hospitals and outpatient settings, refers to:
     - Dramatic reduction in inpatient hospital day
     - Declining revenues
     - Declining number of patients
     - More severely ill patients
     - Shorter lengths of stay
     - Continuing expansion of ambulatory care
     - Increased demand for home care and community-based services
   - Regarding effects on specific patient's care, refers to:
     - Prenegotiated payment rates
     - Mandatory precertification
     - Utilization review
     - Limited choice of provider
     - Fixed-price reimbursement

CHAPTER 2 Community-Based Nursing Practice

1. Identify several discharge planning situations in which you have been involved. Evaluate the effectiveness of the processes used to accomplish the goals. What changes could have been made that would have improved the processes and the outcomes?
   - Describes the time when discharge planning began
   - Identifies level of formality (e.g., verbal communication, completion of forms, consults)
   - Describes agencies involved in discharge planning
   - Comments on needs assessment, planning, implementation, and evaluation in terms of discharge planning
   - Refers to essential requirement for communication with and cooperation of the patient and family
2. An elderly man was referred for home care after discharge from the hospital. During the initial visit, the patient's daughter asks how often home care visits will be made and for how long. What assessment criteria will you use to develop answers to these questions? What factors affect the patient's eligibility for home care services versus ambulatory health services?
   - Assessment criteria—Refers to:
     - Current health status
     - Home environment
     - Levels of self-care abilities
     - Levels of nursing care needed
     - Prognosis
     - Patient education needs
     - Mental status
     - Level of adherence
   - Eligibility for home care services versus ambulatory health services:
     - Refers to assessment criteria (as stated above)
     - Denotes that as progress is made, use of ambulatory health services may supplant home care services

CHAPTER 3
Critical Thinking, Ethical Decision Making

1. How does the approach to critical thinking differ among nursing practice settings (i.e., acute care, ambulatory, extended care, home care, and community settings)?
   - Points out that regardless of setting, each patient is viewed as unique and dynamic
   - Notes that unique factors that the patient and nurse bring to the health care situation are considered, studied, analyzed, and interpreted
   - Refers to the interpretation of information presented, allowing the nurse to focus on the factors most relevant and significant to situation
   - Identifies the plan of action as developing from decisions about what to do and how to do it
2. You have just completed the physical assessment of your assigned patient. How would you develop the patient's nursing diagnoses? Describe the kind of resources that are available to help you identify these diagnoses.
   - Development of nursing diagnoses:
     - Refers to assessment component serving as basis for identifying nursing diagnoses
     - Describes identifying commonalities among assessment data, noting problem areas by comparing the patient's data base to normal findings
     - Identifies characteristics of the problem as well as etiology
     - Points out difference between nursing diagnosis and collaborative problems
   - Resources:
     - Refers to NANDA-Approved Nursing Diagnoses
     - Refers to specialty texts, such as L.J. Carpenito, *Nursing diagnosis: Application to clinical practice,* as well as comprehensive texts such as medical-surgical nursing textbooks
3. You have developed a plan of nursing care for your assigned patient, who is terminally ill. The next day you note a "do not resuscitate" order on the chart. Describe how you use critical thinking skills to develop the plan of care. How do you integrate your critical thinking into the nursing process? What changes might you make in your plan of care considering the DNR order? What ethical problems or dilemmas might you anticipate?
   - Reviews features of critical thinking
   - Points out that a patient with a DNR order is the same person evaluated initially
   - Identifies hospital policy regarding DNR order, noting specifically actions to be taken and those to NOT be taken
   - Ethical problems or dilemmas may relate to the patient's competence, the patient's wishes—as understood by the nurse prior to the DNR order, the appropriateness of nursing interventions used
4. A family member of your patient tells you information about the patient that the patient has not revealed. How would you determine if you should communicate this information to the patient's primary nurse?
   - Considers relationship of family member providing information in relation to the patient
   - Evaluates patient's competence to provide information
   - Considers issues of reliability and credibility of family member
   - Evaluates the pertinence of the information to the patient's care
   - Refers to the obligations of the nurse described in the *ANA Code for Nurses*

CHAPTER 4
Health Education and Promotion

1. You are developing a patient teaching plan for a patient with diabetes mellitus. Describe the strategies you would develop to promote adherence to the therapeutic regimen. Indicate the possible variables that could influence the patient's willingness or ability to follow instructions.
   - Strategies to promote adherence—refers to:
     - Stimulating patient motivation
     - Promoting choice of method for teaching
     - Establishment of mutual goals
     - Quality of patient-provider relationship
     - Usefulness of learning contracts
     - Frequent, positive reinforcement
   - Variables to be considered as influencers of patient adherence—refers to:
     - Number of chronic illnesses demonstrated
     - Age and educational level
     - Ability to adjust to change and stress
     - Financial considerations
     - Forgetfulness
     - Support systems
     - Lifetime habits
     - Visual and hearing impairments
     - Mobility limitations

2. You are assigned to teach an elderly patient about the medications that she will be taking at home. How would you assess this patient's condition and psychosocial situation to determine how best to instruct her about her medications?
   - Refers to evaluation of patient's learning readiness:
     - Culture
     - Personal values
     - Physical and emotional status
     - Past experience in learning
   - Describes importance of identifying a learning environment suited to the patient's needs:
     - Lighting
     - Temperature
     - Noise level
     - Timing
   - Describes selection of teaching techniques and methods appropriate to the individual's needs:
     - Lectures, groups, demonstrations, discussion
     - Group versus individual teaching
     - Teaching aids (books, pamphlets, pictures, films, slides, audio and video tapes, models, programmed instruction, computer-assisted learning models
     - Indicates importance of reverse demonstration, reinforcement, and follow-up sessions
3. A neighbor tells you that he has heard about a health fair that is being offered at a nearby civic center. He asks you if you think that he should attend. Describe the reasons you might give for why he should attend.
   - Opportunity to learn
   - Opportunity to ask questions
   - Likelihood of print materials that may be taken home for future reference
   - Increased awareness
   - Opportunity to develop/reinforce prudent health living strategies

CHAPTER 5
Health Assessment

1. Compare the approaches you would use in assessing a patient who is experiencing severe acute pain; is blind or hard of hearing; is mentally retarded; is from a culture with very different values from yours.
   - Severe acute pain patient: Emphasis is on essential information and focuses assessment in regard to the severe acute pain
   - Blind patient: Complete assessment requires detailed verbal description and warning and explanation prior to any contact with the patient
   - Hard of hearing patient: Privacy must be protected although volume of verbal interaction will be increased; repeat information as necessary
   - Mentally retarded patient: Gain information within the limits demonstrated by the patient's ability to understand questions and respond; use resource persons to gain additional information; inform and support patient during examination
   - Patient from different culture: Review typical beliefs of patient's culture and conduct assessment with respect and attention given to patient's differences
2. Your nutritional assessment reveals that your patient has an inadequate protein intake. How would you develop dietary instructions for the patient who is a vegetarian? For the elderly patient on a fixed income? For the patient who has an intolerance for dairy foods?
   - Vegetarian: Emphasize the protein value of legumes and nuts (eggs and dairy products may be considered for intake by some vegetarians)
   - Elderly patient on a fixed income: Refer to nutritional guide for less expensive sources of protein
   - Patient with intolerance for dairy foods: Emphasize the protein value of meat, poultry, fish, dry beans, eggs, and certain nuts
3. The findings of your physical and nutritional assessment of an 18-year-old college student suggest to you that she may have an eating disorder. How would you further assess this patient and develop a plan of management for her?
   - Assess her attitude toward food
   - Assess her self-concept, self-esteem
   - Ask her to perform a 24 hour diet recall
   - Ask her to keep a food diary
   - Seek consultation with individual experienced in treating eating disorders
   - Refer patient appropriately
4. You have received a referral for home care for a 72-year-old patient who lives in a single room on the third floor of a boarding house. He is malnourished and requires daily injections of antibiotics for treatment of osteomyelitis. What factors would you include in your initial assessment on your first home visit?
   - Current health status
   - Home environment
   - Level of self-care abilities
   - Level of nursing care needed
   - Prognosis
   - Patient education needs
   - Mental status
   - Level of adherence

UNIT 2 BIOPHYSICAL AND PSYCHOSOCIAL CONCEPTS

CHAPTER 6 Homeostasis, Stress, and Adaptation

1. Think back to a time when you had an acute illness. Describe the illness-related stressors you experienced. How did you cope with these stressors? What evidence was there that your coping ability was successful or unsuccessful?

   - Illness-related stressors
     - Physical
     - Psychological
     - Emotional
     - Social
     - Financial/economic
   - Coping mechanisms
     - Tolerance
     - Distraction
     - Avoidance
     - Use of support systems (social, spiritual)
     - Acceptance
     - Self-Talk
   - Evidence of success of coping
     - Resolution of illness
     - Increased energy
     - Improved attitude
     - Evidence of learning

2. Think back to a time when you had an injury. How was homeostasis maintained or disrupted and what compensatory mechanisms were evident?

   - Homeostasis maintained (examples)
     - Diaphoresis after elevated temperature
     - Development of scar tissue after injury
     - Laying down of callus formation at site of fracture
     - Increased reticulocyte count after blood loss
   - Compensatory mechanisms (examples)
     - Inflammatory response to invading microorganism in skin breakdown
     - Healing of tissue by first intention

3. Select a patient to whom you are assigned who has an acute illness or injury. Describe the manner in which homeostasis has been maintained or disrupted and the compensatory mechanisms that are evident. How does the patient's medical treatment support the compensatory mechanisms? How do you determine the nursing interventions that are appropriate for promoting the healing process?

   - Homeostatis maintenance and compensatory mechanisms (refer to Question 2)
   - Medical treatment that supports compensatory mechanisms (examples)
     - Intravenous hydration
     - Cooling blankets
     - Transfusions of blood components
     - Oxygen therapy
   - Nursing interventions (examples):
     - Promoting adequate dietary and fluid intake
     - Monitoring prescribed treatments
     - Providing health teaching

4. You are caring for a patient in his home. Describe how you would assess the patient's health status and lifestyle to determine health-promotion activities that should be explored with the patient and his family. How would your plans vary between a patient who is weak and debilitated versus a patient who is recuperating according to schedule; or has failing eyesight; or is alone most of the day?

   - Assessment of health status
     - How well is the patient progressing?
     - How serious are the present signs and symptoms?
     - Has the patient shown signs of progressing as expected, or does it seem that recovery will be delayed?
   - Assessment of lifestyle
     - Is patient active, sedentary, or inactive?
     - In what types of activities does the patient participate?
     - What are his resources and limitations?
     - Fundamental premise: Assess the patient to determine where he is (in terms of abilities to undertake health promotion activities) and guide patient accordingly
   - Failing eyesight: SAFETY is the most vital consideration to any health-promotion activities suggested
   - Alone most of the day: Determine resources available from family, community, church, social organizations to assist in providing health-promotion activities

CHAPTER 7 Individual and Family Considerations

1. The wife of a patient who is dying from bone cancer tells the nurse that she is prepared for the death of her partner. Her distress is based on family members who tell her that she is an

"uncaring, cold person" because she is not openly crying and expressing other outward signs of being emotionally distraught. In counseling this family member what would you say to her? How could the wife's behavior be explained to other family members?

- Points out that all people experience loss in the form of change, growth, and transition.
- Informs the individuals that people grieve in different ways, and there is no timeline for completing the grief process
- Suggests that the wife, who possibly knows her partner better than anyone else, believes that she can best support her partner by remaining strong and stoic

2. The nurse is working with a family to develop therapeutic interventions for a member who has a cocaine and alcohol addiction problem. One family member tells the nurse she will never be able to support the plan decided on by the rest of the family. How would you approach this person? What strategies would be useful for this person and for the entire family?

   - Discuss the role that family plays in the life of a patient
   - Review functions of the family
   - Promote coping skills through direct care, communication skills, and education
   - Consider health team conference for:
     - Comprehensive family assessment
     - Development of interventions tailored to hand the identified stressors specific to the family
     - Facilitating construction of social support systems

3. The nurse notices that a patient has pain and exacerbation of symptoms after the family visits. The patient tells the nurse that he is letting his family down and he feels like a failure because he can no longer provide for them in the way that he promised. During visits, his spouse and children complain to him about financial, social, and other problems. What strategies would be useful in talking to the patient? How could the nurse approach the entire family to tell them about the patient's distress and request that they change their behavior? What referrals could be helpful to this family?

   - Strategies useful in talking to patient:
     - Listen actively
     - Allow patient to describe his fears, frustration, anger, and despair
     - Discuss roles of family members, functions of family
   - Talk with family:
     - Present information in positive manner
     - Address impact of family behavior on patient's well-being
     - Discuss alternative coping mechanisms
     - Allow family to ventilate regarding fears and frustrations
   - Consider:
     - Social work consult
     - Health team conference, including family members
     - Chaplaincy referral
     - Behavioral counseling consult

CHAPTER 8 **Perspectives in Transcultural Nursing**

1. You are assigned to care for a hospitalized young adult whose cultural background is very different from yours. Describe how you would assess his cultural beliefs and practices in developing a nursing care plan. Explain why it is important to examine your own feelings about his cultural beliefs and practices.

   - General guidelines to assess culture:
     - What is the patient's country of origin? How long has he or she lived in this country?
     - What is the primary language and literacy level?
     - What is the patient's ethnic background? Does he or she identify strongly with others from the same cultural background?
     - What is the patient's religion, and how important is it to his or her daily life?
     - Does the patient participate in cultural activities such as dressing in traditional clothing and observing traditional holidays and festivals?
     - Are there any food preferences or restrictions?
     - What are the patient's communication styles? Is eye contact avoided? How much physical distance is maintained? Is the patient open and verbal about symptoms?
     - Who is the head of the family, and is he or she involved in decision making about the patient?
     - What does the patient do to maintain his or her health?
     - What does the patient think caused the current problem?
     - Has the advice of traditional healers been sought?
     - What kind of treatment does the patient think will help? What are the most important results he or she hopes to get from this treatment?
     - Are there religious rituals revealed to sickness, death, or health that the patient observes?

- Important for nurse to examine own feelings because:
  - Own cultural attitudes, values, beliefs, and practices may be source of conflict
  - Potential for effects of ethnocentrism to impact care delivery

2. An elderly patient who does not speak English is hospitalized after elective surgery. Even though he is progressing well and his discharge has been planned, his family insists on staying with him for as many hours as possible, refusing to leave when visiting hours are over. How can you help the nursing staff to explore the meaning of the family's behavior and to understand their own feelings about this behavior? Devise a strategy that you think will help resolve this situation.
   - Review culturally mediated factors affecting behavior
   - Identify sources of nursing staff conflict
   - Identify impact of family's behavior on delivery of nursing care
   - Communicate with family, respect family's beliefs, and attempt to gain family assistance in achieving balance between family's culturally based needs and goals of nursing care

3. You are preparing for a home visit to provide care for an elderly patient who is of foreign origin. The record indicates that she does not speak English and lives in a neighborhood where most of the residents are from the same ethnic background as herself. Describe how you would plan for this visit to ensure that you can communicate with the patient and family while providing the necessary nursing care. Explore other aspects of the patient's and family's background that you would want to assess before making the visit and while you are at the home.
   - Identify resource persons who may accompany the nurse on the home visit
   - Refer to general guidelines to cultural assessment (Question 1, above)

CHAPTER 9
Chronic Illness

1. A 24-year-old woman has just been diagnosed with lupus. She is very upset about the diagnosis, concerned about her potential for childbearing, and refusing to listen to teaching about illness management. How would you respond to her reaction to the diagnosis?
   - Encourage the patient to continue to communicate regarding her concerns
   - Provide factual information to refute misconceptions
   - Accept the patient's right to make her own choices
   - Make referrals as indicated

2. A 46-year-old man has developed complications from a chronic health problem that he has had but largely ignored for the past twenty years. Describe how you would determine what factors and psychological reactions to consider in developing a teaching plan to assist the patient in dealing with complications.
   - Elicit from the patient his understanding of his current health needs
   - Determine the patient's choices regarding goals for care
   - Incorporate elements of patient education to facilitate a teaching plan for the patient:
     - Motivators
     - Learning abilities (strengths and limitations)
     - Learning environment
     - Teaching techniques
     - Reinforcement
     - Rewards

3. How would the learning needs of a patient with a newly diagnosed chronic condition differ from those of a patient with a chronic condition that has been stable for many years, and from those of a patient who has experienced progressive deterioration in health status? Describe those factors that would be the focus of your assessment in these three patients to assess their needs for patient education.
   - Newly diagnosed chronic condition—focus of assessment
     - Abilities to alleviate and manage symptoms
     - Abilities to adapt to illness
     - Knowledge level re: preventing and managing crises and complications
     - Resources to support normalizing individual and family life
   - Chronic condition stable for many years—focus of assessment
     - Knowledge level re: preventing, adapting to, and managing disabilities
     - Knowledge level re: preventing and managing crises and complications
   - Progressive deterioration in health status—focus of assessment
     - Resources and support networks
     - Status re: adapting to repeated identity threats and progressive loss of function
     - Dying with dignity and comfort

4. A 55-year-old patient with continuous severe pain has been informed by his physician that he has cancer, that he is likely to survive for no longer than 6 months, and that no medical treatment is likely to increase the length of his survival. How would you address the patient's goals to maintain his quality of life and to "get his affairs in order"

in the time he has remaining? What resources would you consider in helping him to accomplish his goals?

- Identify resources and establish networks of support
- Obtain chaplaincy consult
- Obtain social work consult
- Utilize community organizations (e.g., Make Today Count)
- Prepare patient and family for effects of disease
- Instruct patient and family regarding bodily function changes with death

CHAPTER 10 Principles and Practices of Rehabilitation

1. You are caring for a patient who is recovering from a stroke. You are discussing the patient's level of functioning with the physical rehabilitation team. Describe the kinds of self-care activities that you would assess to determine the rehabilitation plan for the patient.
   - Degree of independence while eating
   - Degree of independence while dressing
   - Time taken for activities of daily living
   - Mobility, coordination, endurance
   - Amount of assistance required for ambulating
   - Joint motion and muscle strength
   - Cardiovascular status (vital signs, pulse, respiration—sitting, standing, reclining)
   - Neurological status
2. An elderly patient who has limited mobility and ambulation abilities is to be discharged to his home and cared for by his family. His family members express particular concern about how to prevent pressure ulcers. Describe the instructions you would give them. How might your strategies differ if family members converse primarily in their native tongue, which is not English?
   - Change the patient's position frequently to relieve and redistribute pressure
   - Position the patient laterally, prone, and dorsally in sequence unless not tolerated or contraindicated
   - Inspect skin at each position change and assess for temperature elevation (redness or heat; or if patient complains of discomfort, pressure on the area must be relieved)
   - Use pillows to bridge body parts and protect bony prominences
   - Use commercial heel and elbow protectors
   - Encourage patient to remain active and ambulated whenever possible
   - Use active and passive range of motion exercises
   - Monitor patient's nutritional status
   - Reduce friction and shear
   - Keep skin dry
3. You are caring for a young man who was injured in a motor vehicle crash. He is to return home to continue his rehabilitation as an outpatient. You accompany the home health nurse who is conducting an assessment of the patient's home environment in anticipation of his discharge. Compare the types of safety factors that might be considered if the patient lives in a single-story house, in a two-story house, in a two-room apartment, in a high-rise building, or on a farm.
   - Number of exits of dwelling; presence of stairs; handicapped-accessible modifications
   - Access to emergency assistance (neighbors, ambulance, hospital)

CHAPTER 11 Health Care of the Older Adult

1. Your clinical assignment is in an adult day care center. Based on your knowledge of the aging process and theories about aging, describe the strategies and goals you would devise to enhance communication with the elderly patients.
   - Assess each patient as an individual according to level of vision, hearing, cognition, and short-term memory
   - Provide diffuse, glare-free lighting
   - Minimize background noise
   - Face each patient while communicating
   - Use written forms of communication to complement, enhance, and facilitate verbal communication
2. A neighbor whose wife has recently been diagnosed with Alzheimer's disease approaches you expressing concern about his wife. He appears quite distraught and expresses anxiety about how he will be able to continue to care for her. Drawing on your knowledge about the course of this condition and the problems it presents to both the afflicted person and the caregiver, describe the guidance you would offer.
   - Support cognitive function (e.g., provide predictable environment, regular routine; limit environmental stimuli; make instructions and explanations simple; use memory aids and cues; prominently display calendars and clocks)
   - Promote physical safety (e.g., supervise smoking; lock doors; remove hazards)

- Reduce anxiety and agitation (e.g., keep environment simple, familiar, and noise free; identify and eliminate stressors)
- Improve communication (e.g., use lists and simple instructions; reduce noise and distractions)
- Promote independence in self-care activities (e.g., simplify daily activities by organizing them into short, achievable steps)
- Provide for socialization and intimacy needs (e.g., visits should be brief, nonstressful, and limit visitors to 1 or 2 at a time)
- Promote adequate nutrition (e.g., offer one dish at a time; assist with intake; keep mealtime calm)
- Promote balanced activity and rest (e.g., promote exercise and discourage long periods of daytime sleep)
- Identify family support groups, respite care, and day care resources

3. You are caring for an elderly patient in the home setting. Describe the focus of your assessment to determine if any changes need to be made in the patient's home environment and support systems to better meet his physical and psychosocial needs.
   - Safety and comfort
   - Personal space

UNIT 3 CONCEPTS AND CHALLENGES IN PATIENT MANAGEMENT

CHAPTER 12 Pain Management

1. Your patient has cancer and is nearing the end of his life. He is in severe discomfort, rating his pain as 9 on a visual analogue scale, but he is not receiving the maximum dose of opioids he could potentially receive. On discussing this with his sister, who is caring for him at home, it comes apparent that she fears he is becoming addicted. She also knows that, in her words, "He is strong enough to take it." Describe the strategies you would use to ensure that your patient receives pain relief.
   - Talk with her regarding common concerns and misconceptions regarding pain
   - Describe the pain of cancer
   - Review that the patient is terminal
   - Describe pain in terms of its physiologic basis
   - Provide the nurse's assessment of and experience with terminal cancer pain

2. Earlier in your shift, you sent Ms. Jones to surgery for an exploratory laparotomy related to abdominal pain. She returns to the unit 4 hours later with a PCA pump for postoperative pain. The postanesthesia care unit nurse reports that while the patient was in the PACU, she received unusually large doses of an opioid analgesic but was never pain-free. Now she is screaming in pain. When asked the level of her pain, she indicates that it is off the pain scale. The patient's husband is yelling at you to do something. What assessment data would you collect, and what actions would you anticipate?
   - Assessment data:
     - Blood pressure, pulse, respirations
     - Auscultation and palpation of abdomen
     - Inspection of dressing and drainage sites
   - Actions:
     - Report pain unrelieved by medication at current dosage to surgeon
     - Implement comfort measures
     - Review all medications for "break-through" pain coverage
     - Decrease environmental stimuli
     - Observe patient very closely

CHAPTER 13 Fluid and Electrolytes: Balance and Disturbances

1. Your patient is an 89-year-old man in a coma. His serum sodium level is 190 mEq/L; his serum glucose level is 100 mg/dL. What IV solution do you anticipate will be prescribed for him? Provide a rationale for its use and discuss the nursing actions relevant to its administration.
   - 5% dextrose in water is used in treatment of hypernatremia and dehydration, normal serum sodium levels range between 135 and 145 mEq/L
   - Nursing actions:
     - Monitor intake and output
     - If enteral feedings are given, sufficient water must be administered

2. A 29-year-old patient has been admitted to the emergency department with a history of laxative

abuse in an effort to lose weight. Laboratory values in the emergency department are as follows: serum sodium, 140 mEq/L; serum chloride, 90 mEq/L; serum bicarbonate, 34 mEq/L; serum potassium, 3.1 mEq/L; serum glucose, 120 mg/dL; blood urea nitrogen, 30 mg/dL; arterial blood gases: pH, 7.48: PCO2, 47; HCO3, 34. What is the acid-base disorder? What treatments and relevant nursing actions related to the underlying disorder and its treatment should the nurse anticipate?

- Metabolic alkalosis
- Nursing treatments and actions:
  - Intravenous fluid monitoring
  - Potassium administration
  - Repeat blood gas analyses and serum electrolytes
  - Counseling regarding purging disorder

3. An elderly woman has been hospitalized with gastroenteritis and dehydration. While obtaining the patient's history, you learn that she intentionally avoids drinking liquids because of her fear of incontinence. Explain the potential fluid and electrolyte disorders that could occur as a result of her failure to consume an adequate fluid intake. What approaches would you use in teaching the patient about the potential risks and about strategies to prevent them?
   - Disorder: Fluid volume deficit
   - Potential risks: Decreased mental function; decreased peripheral perfusion; acute cardiopulmonary decompensation
   - Strategies:
     - Identify interventions to deal with incontinence
     - Protective clothing or devices
     - Pace fluid intake
     - Seek evaluation by urologist to identify cause of incontinence and potential methods for treating disorder

CHAPTER 14
Shock and Multisystem Failure

1. A patient in septic shock arrives in the emergency department. How would you explain septic shock to the patient's family? How might your approach differ if the family members are distraught and crying? If they do not speak English well?
   - Explanation of septic shock
     - Role of overwhelming infection
     - Body changes that take place in reaction to the infection
   - Approach if family members are distraught and crying
     - Emphasis on fact that family member is getting treatment
     - Refrain from false reassurance
     - Respond to questions family members have
     - Refer to chaplaincy or social work for support
   - Approach if family members do not speak English well
     - Assess level of English understood
     - Use simple sentences to convey essential information
     - Seek assistance from hospital resources or family resources (e.g., church, community) for interpreter

2. You are on duty as the occupational health nurse for a large farm equipment manufacturer when an accident occurs in the plant. One worker is seriously injured and is bleeding profusely when you are notified. Describe the measures you would take at the scene to prevent or reduce the severity of shock and describe your reasons for these measures.
   - Measures to prevent/reduce severity of shock:
     - Apply pressure to hemorrhage sites (control bleeding)
     - Keep patient warm, but refrain from causing patient to diaphorese (promote tissue perfusion)
     - Apply MAST trousers, if indicated (maintain circulation to vital organs)
     - Initiate two IV lines (per protocol) and begin fluid resuscitation (provide fluid volume)
     - Initiate oxygen therapy (decrease demand on heart)

3. A patient has experienced second- and third-degree burns over 50% of his body. You know you must be alert for different types of shock that can occur during various phases of burn management. How would you assess for the various types of shock at different management stages, and how would the management of the different types of shock differ?
   - Initial stage: Hypovolemic shock as fluid shifts into damaged tissues
     - Assess: Blood pressure, pulse, respirations, urine output, lab values
   - Healing stage: Septic shock may occur if overwhelming infection takes place
     - Assess: Same signs as above. In addition, culture and sensitivity reports of any wound cultures taken

4. How would you distinguish anaphylactic shock from other forms of shock?

- Anaphylactic shock is caused by the immune system. Severe allergic reactions take place, producing overwhelming systemic vasodilation and relative hypovolemia.

CHAPTER 15
Oncology: Nursing Management in Cancer Care

1. A 45-year-old woman with a history of breast cancer developed irreversible lower extremity paralysis and urinary incontinence as a result of a spinal cord compression. She is otherwise in relatively good health and has no other areas of organ or tissue metastasis. On completion of radiation therapy, she would like to continue her job as a high school teacher. She is married and has two children ages 17 and 15 years. Identify this patient's learning needs in relation to radiation therapy, ongoing monitoring, and altered mobility. Describe the assessment, planning, and potential interventions needed to facilitate her continued roles as wife, mother, and teacher.
   - Learning needs in relation to radiation therapy:
     - Needs must be focused regarding TYPE of radiation therapy instituted
     - Effects of radiation (cell death)
     - Skin care and general health measures
   - Learning needs in relation to ongoing monitoring:
     - Spread of disease and implications
     - Continued serum testing and physical assessment by MD to track disease
   - Learning needs in relation to altered mobility:
     - Irreversible nature of paralysis and loss of bladder control
     - Methods of transfer to and from wheelchair
     - Delegation of family responsibilities to daughters
     - Support of daughters to accept altered mobility of mother
     - Support of mother to accept irreversible altered mobility
   - Assessment, planning, and potential interventions:
     - Knowledge level (provide patient education)
     - Emotional reaction—stage of loss (provide support, consider referral)
     - Resources for support (e.g., family, community)
     - Coping skills (consider referral)
     - Psychological impact (role changes—consider referral to social work, counselor, support group)
2. One of your home care patients, a 64-year-old man with end-stage metastatic lung cancer, has been experiencing uncontrolled pain for which he has been taking a nonopioid analgesic. Both the patient and his spouse have refused to consider opioid analgesics because of a fear of addiction. The patient's wife confides that using "strong drugs for pain" signals a loss of hope and a desire to die. They both fear that hospitalization will be needed if other analgesics are used. What course of action would you take? What educational needs should be addressed?
   - Establish rapport with patient and wife
   - Instruct regarding pain (physiologic basis)
   - Instruct regarding opioid necessity and indications for use
   - Counsel regarding loss and grief
   - Counsel regarding fear of dying
   - Explore receptiveness to in-home hospice and refer accordingly
3. A female patient in the clinic has been given the choice of standard treatment for a malignant brain tumor or enrollment in a clinical trial of investigational therapy. She is concerned about the potential "unknowns" of the clinical trial, but is eager to support the physician's desire to participate in research activities. How would you assist her in the decision-making process?
   - Assist patient in differentiating her needs from her desire to support MD's suggestion
   - Determine whether patient has adequate information regarding the advantages and disadvantages of each form of treatment
   - Assist patient in identifying impact of "unknowns" on her daily life
   - Determine coping skills of patient—for either method selected
   - Refer patient for identified needs (e.g., knowledge—physician; emotional support—social work, chaplaincy, psychiatry)

UNIT 4
PERIOPERATIVE CONCEPTS AND NURSING MANAGEMENT

CHAPTER 16
Preoperative Nursing Management

1. During the preoperative assessment of a patient scheduled for a major surgical procedure, the

patient's responses suggest to you that he does not understand the procedure and the effect it will have on his ability to function postoperatively. What further assessment is indicated and what actions are warranted?

- Identify preoperative medications, if any, that may have been given
- Identify central nervous system depressants that may have been given
- Speak with family members and assess their knowledge as well as their interpretation of the patient's knowledge
- Refer to informed consent form signed by patient
- Refer to progress note signed by surgeon indicating explanations provided to patient
- If patient does not understand the changes to his functioning postoperatively, the surgeon must be informed prior to surgery
- Staff nurse should report finding to immediate supervisor and seek direction and support

2. A patient with a long history of severe asthma is scheduled for major surgery. What effect would this information have on your preoperative care of this patient?
   - Any indication that a patient may have respiratory difficulty postoperatively (general anesthesia is used for most major surgeries) must be reported to physician and thoroughly assessed
   - Surgeon or anesthesiologist may require pulmonary function studies or seek consultation from pulmonologist
   - Indication for use of steroids must be considered, surgeon or anesthesiologist may seek consultation from internist
   - Patient must be instructed regarding patient's role in maintaining ventilatory function postoperatively (e.g., incentive spirometry, deep breathing)
3. Two patients are admitted to the same-day surgery unit for hip replacements. One patient is 40 years old and the other is 72 years old. How would your assessments and preoperative preparation differ for these two patients?
   - Basic assessment of each is the same
   - Focused assessment would likely occur for the aged patient in terms of medical history, prior surgeries and experience with anesthesia, daily medications, and functioning of the non-affected hip joint as well as other joints

CHAPTER 17 Intraoperative Nursing Management

1. A patient in the holding area awaiting surgery indicates that he had not received instructions not to take his usual medications (i.e., antihypertensive agent, diuretic, digoxin, potassium chloride, and insulin injection); as a result, he took them a few hours ago. What implications does this have for the patient's care and well-being while awaiting surgery, during surgery, and in the immediate postoperative period?
   - Awaiting surgery:
     - Diuretic may result in need for urination
     - Type of insulin must be assessed (if injection was REGULAR insulin, the nurse anticipates signs of hypoglycemia)
     - Measurement of blood glucose level is indicated, regardless of type of insulin injected
     - Measurement of electrolyte levels is indicated
   - During surgery:
     - Nurse must be certain that anesthesiologist is aware of medications taken since anesthesiologist will be monitoring the patient's bodily functions intraoperatively
   - Immediate postoperative period:
     - Monitor vital signs
     - Measure blood glucose level
     - Focus assessment on signs of untoward effects of medications taken
2. What are the differences in responsibility for the operating room nurse for care of patients who receive general anesthesia, conscious sedation, spinal anesthesia, and regional anesthesia?
   - Role of nurse will vary with the presence or absence of anesthesiologist
     - Anesthesiologist present: Nursing activities will be supportive to patient needs and surgeon requests
     - Anesthesiologist absent: Nursing activities will include monitoring of vital signs, pulse, respirations, respiratory status, level of sedation, level of oxygen saturation, in addition to patient needs and surgeon requests
3. While she is being assisted in transfer from the cart to the operating table, a patient indicates that she is very anxious about her surgery because of previous negative experiences. What assessment and interventions are indicated at this time?
   - Review of central nervous system depressants and anti-anxiety agents administered preoperatively
   - Review of physician progress notes regarding history

- Acceptance of patient's status
- Emotional support and reassurance
- Refrain from leaving patient alone—maintain contact

CHAPTER 18
Postoperative Nursing Management

1. Your patient has a history of esophageal cancer. After undergoing ambulatory surgery to insert a gastric feeding tube, he is to be discharged from the PACU to home. Describe a teaching plan for the patient and his family. How would you modify the plan if the patient lives alone?
   - Teaching plan should include
     - Methods to relieve pain; symptoms to report
     - Methods to ensure adequate respiration; signs and symptoms to report
     - Need for ambulation; signs and symptoms regarding DVT to report
     - Need for activity
     - Need to return to self-care to extent possible
     - Tube site care and methods to prevent infection; signs and symptoms to report
   - Patient who lives alone must be considered candidate for home visit(s) and managed accordingly
2. A patient who has undergone a lumbar fusion reports severe pain and as a result is unable to cough, deep breathe, or turn. When you check the patient's chart, you find that medication cannot be given for another hour. What assessment would you carry out at this time? How would you deal with this situation?
   - Assessment:
     - Wound site for indications of bleeding, hematoma formation
     - Vitals signs, pulse, respiration
   - Nursing actions:
     - Comfort measures
     - Spend time with patient to determine role of anxiety and fear in pain perception
     - Identify medication such as anti-inflammatory that may be given and provide some pain relief
     - SEVERE PAIN must be reported to physician
3. Your patient is a 72-year-old woman with poor nutritional status who has undergone emergency surgery. How would you modify your assessment, nursing care, and plans for home care management because of her poor nutritional status?
   - Consult with social work to determine financial constraints
   - Consult with dietician to identify patient likes, dislikes, and methods for intervening
   - Teach patient and family member of need for high-protein meals that provide sufficient fiber, calories, and vitamins
   - Suggest use of nutritional supplements, if indicated

UNIT 5
GAS EXCHANGE AND RESPIRATORY FUNCTION

CHAPTER 19
Assessment of Respiratory Function

1. After a thoracentesis for diagnostic purposes, your patient reports shortness of breath and appears anxious. Based on your knowledge of the risks associated with thoracentesis, how would you focus your assessment because of those risks?
   - Risk: Punctured lung—development of tension pneumothorax
   - Focus assessment: Listen to breath sounds; measure pulse oximetry; obtain vital signs
   - Notify physician who performed thoracentesis
   - Notify respiratory therapy for potential supplemental oxygen needs
   - Have emergency equipment available in the event of mediastinal shift due to tension pneumothorax resulting in cardiopulmonary arrest
2. Your patient is scheduled for pulmonary function tests before heart surgery. You know that a patient who understands the purposes of the tests and what to expect during the procedures will be able to cooperate more during the tests. What teaching points would you emphasize when explaining the procedure to this patient? What types of details would you include?
   - Teaching points:
     - Need for accurate measurements of volumes to guide anesthesiologist, pulmonologist
     - Patient's role in testing and ability to assist
     - Signs and symptoms to communicate to technician doing testing
   - Details:
     - Requests technician will make to obtain volumes (e.g., forced exhalation after normal exhalation)

- Need for patient to communicate any discomfort, any request for change of position, etc.

3. Based on your understanding of clinical conditions, discuss at least one condition that would affect ventilation, diffusion, and perfusion.
   - Condition within the lungs (e.g., obstructive or restrictive disease)
   - Condition outside lungs affecting lung function (e.g., pulmonary embolus, congestive heart failure)

CHAPTER 20
Management of Patients with Upper Respiratory Tract Disorders

1. You are caring for a patient who is scheduled for a complete laryngectomy for cancer of the larynx. In anticipating the altered speech that will result from this surgery, describe the information you would share with the patient about methods of communicating in the early postoperative period, as well as in the long term.
   - Methods of communicating (early postoperatively):
     - Magic slate
     - Letter board (to spell out words)
     - Hand bell or call bell
     - Picture-word-phrase board
     - Hand signals
   - Methods of communicating (long term)
     - Esophageal speech
     - Voice replacement methods
2. You are making the first home visit to a patient who has just been discharged from the hospital following a laryngectomy. What will be the focus of your initial home visit? What aspects of assessment and nursing management are key at this point of your patient's rehabilitation?
   - Focus of initial home visit
     - Tracheostomy and stoma care
     - Hygiene and safety measures
     - Continuing care needs
   - Key points
     - Airway clearance; humidification
     - Stoma and tracheostomy care
     - Protective cloth at stoma site
     - Avoiding cold air to prevent airway irritation
     - Safe technique in changing laryngectomy tube
     - Signs and symptoms of infection and response to same
     - Wearing medical identification information
     - Fluid and caloric needs
     - Mouth care
     - Alternative communication methods
     - Support groups and agency resources
     - Need for regular check-ups and reporting of any problems to MD immediately.
3. A 20-year-old college student is diagnosed with acute viral pharyngitis and possible strept throat. What assessment and treatment should the nurse anticipate? What teaching and management strategies should be discussed with the patient?
   - Comfort and treatment measures
   - Contacts/spread of disease
   - Need for taking all prescribed medication
   - Complications of strept throat
4. A 26-year-old man who has been hit in the face with a baseball comes to the urgent care center for treatment for a bleeding nose. What are the initial measures you would use to stop the bleeding? What other options are available if the bleeding does not stop within a reasonable period of time?
   - Apply direct pressure
     - Patient sits upright with head tilted forward
     - Patient is directed to pinch the soft outer portion of nose against midline septum continuously for 5 to 10 minutes
   - Upon physician's order:
     - Insertion of cotton tampon
     - Gauze packing with petrolatum or antibiotic ointment
   - Physician intervention
     - Cautery (silver nitrate or electric)
     - Surgical intervention (ligation of artery)

CHAPTER 21
Management of Patients with Chest and Lower Respiratory Tract Disorders

1. Use of an MDI has been prescribed for the first time for your patient, a 35-year-old with asthma. Describe the teaching approach you would use to ensure correct use of the MDI. How would your approach differ if the patient had a learning disability or did not speak English?
   - Refers to home teaching checklist provided in chart form in Chapter 21
   - Notes that nurse would observe patient performing metered-dose inhalation
   - Learning disability:
     - Assess need for supervision and methods to meet need
     - Use simple instructions

    - Provide reinforcement
  - Non–English-speaking patient:
    - Identify family or community support
    - Seek assistance from interpreter

2. Your patient has a diagnosis of COPD and is short of breath. Oxygen is prescribed at 2L/min. His family wants the oxygen flow increased to relieve his shortness of breath. How would you explain to the patient and family the need to keep the oxygen at the prescribed rate? What actions would you take to assist in decreasing the patient's breathlessness?
   - Family instruction:
     - Explain respiratory drive of COPD patient as different from normal person (normal drive comes from increased CO_2; COPD patient's drive comes from decreased O_2)
     - Inform family the increasing oxygen level may cause patient to QUIT breathing
   - Actions:
     - Stay with patient—employ techniques to promote relaxation
     - Decrease stimuli
     - Use medication, as indicated

3. During a home visit to a patient with advanced lung cancer, the patient says he cannot do anything except sit in a chair because of shortness of breath with any exertion. Describe the strategies you would plan with the patient to minimize his shortness of breath, improve his comfort level, and improve the quality of his life.
   - Minimize shortness of breath:
     - Keep frequently used articles close at hand
     - Ensure easy communication by patient (e.g., hand bell and telephone within easy reach)
     - Assess other indicators of ways to decrease exertion
   - Improve comfort level:
     - Positioning and support for eased respirations (e.g., high Fowler's with arms supported on over-bed or over-chair table)
     - Refrain from wearing constricting clothing
     - Maintain room temperature according to patient's need
   - Quality of life:
     - Communicate with patient to determine his or her determination of needs
     - Work with resources to meet needs
     - Provide emotional support and reassurance

4. Your patient, a 54-year-old employee at a homeless shelter, has just been diagnosed with active TB. She has been started on treatment at home, with specific instructions about her medication. She cannot take time off from work and has close contact with the adults and children in the shelter. What are the public health concerns, and what strategies will you provide to the patient and to those who live and work at the shelter?
   - Public health concerns: Prevention of spread of disease; early detection and treatment
   - Strategies should incorporate CDC recommendations provided in chart form in Chapter 21

5. You are working on a surgical unit. Your patient is a 75-year-old man who had colon surgery 2 days ago for cancer. He is drowsy and reluctant to move in bed or mobilize to the chair, and he uses his patient-controlled analgesia pump on a regular basis. The family does not want him disturbed so that he can rest. What are the potential postoperative pulmonary complications? What information would you provide to the patient and family regarding care? What interventions would you implement to prevent pulmonary complications in this patient?
   - Potential postoperative complications:
     - Atelectasis
     - Pneumonia
   - Information:
     - In order to decrease potential for pneumonia and other complications of immobility, patient must be urged to move, deep breathe, and increase independence in self-care
   - Interventions:
     - Ensure adequate hydration to liquefy secretions
     - Encourage deep breathing and change of position, at least every 2 hours
     - Use incentive spirometry to guide patient's effort to deep breathe
     - Request patient to deep breathe and cough AFTER pain medication has been used

CHAPTER 22
Respiratory Care Modalities

1. An elderly patient with COPD is receiving oxygen by nasal cannula. His family believes that the oxygen flow rate is too low and keeps insisting that it can be increased because the patient reports being short of breath. What assessments and interventions are indicated in this situation? What explanations are appropriate for the patient and family about the administration of oxygen?
   - Differentiate the normal ventilatory drive (increased CO_2) from the COPD patient's ventilatory drive (decreased O_2)

- Answer family questions and enforce potential for patient to QUIT breathing if oxygen administration level is increased

2. Your 55-year-old patient is to be sent home on mechanical ventilation in the care of his wife. Develop a checklist to use in teaching the patient and his family about care in the home. Identify resources that would be helpful to this family in providing care of the patient in the home.
   - Refers to content of Chapter 22 charts, which describe:
     - Assessment criteria for successful home ventilator care
     - Home teaching checklist for ventilator care
     - Resources (e.g., home care nurse visits, community agency support, support group support)

3. A patient is returning to the nursing unit after chest surgery with an endotracheal tube, a chest tube, and two intravenous lines in place. Identify the priorities of assessment and interventions for this patient.
   - Priorities of assessment:
     - Adequacy of respirations
     - Endotracheal tube placement
     - Need for suctioning
     - Chest tube functioning
     - Underwater seal drainage system intact
     - Attachment of suction to drainage system, if ordered
     - Notation of fluctuation and bubbling in underwater seal chamber
   - Intravenous infusions:
     - Correct fluid, flow rate
     - Site appearance (e.g., no signs of infiltration or phlebitis)

4. A patient who has had a tracheostomy tube inserted 12 hours ago becomes confused and removes the tracheostomy tube. What are the immediate actions that are indicated in this situation? What nursing assessments and nursing interventions are needed once the immediate situation has been corrected?
   - If educated to do so, place obturator (which should be taped to head of bed or wall above head of bed) into tube and attempt to reinsert tube
   - Ensure adequate ventilation
   - Notify physician/surgeon immediately
   - Prepare for potential code situation if respirations are completely obstructed
   - Once situation corrected, ensure that patient will not remove tube
   - Sitter or family member at bedside
   - Monitor vigilantly to determine changes in behavior
   - Monitor oxygen saturation (hypoxemia may be cause of agitation)
   - Seek order for restraint (e.g., chemical or physical) if other measures fail

UNIT 6
CARDIOVASCULAR, CIRCULATORY, AND HEMATOLOGIC FUNCTION

CHAPTER 23
Assessment of Cardiovascular Function

1. Your patient is an elderly woman who has just been discharged from the local hospital's cardiac telemetry unit. This is her second hospitalization within the last 6 weeks for CHF. As her home care nurse, you are in the process of identifying her home care needs. What questions will you include in this patient's health history to help you identify potential causes for her frequent hospitalizations?
   - Knowledge and understanding of diet, medication, and exercise guidelines
   - Financial constraints on dietary needs and medication requirements
   - Compliance with guidelines
   - Sources of emotional support
   - Need for attention—and how the need is met or not met
   - Patient's reaction to and feelings regarding frequent hospitalizations

2. During rounds, the physician tells your patient that she will need a stress test. She has limited range of motion of both her upper and lower extremities. Based on these findings, what type of a stress test and radionuclide imaging technique do you anticipate the physician will order? What implications will this have for patient preparation?
   - Pharmacologic stress test (using vasodilating agents or sympathetic sympathomimetic agents)
   - Myocardial perfusion imaging with Tahllium 201 is used with stress testing to assess changes

immediately after exercise (pharmacologic injection, in this instance)
- Implications for patient preparation:
  - Vasodilators may cause chest discomfort, dizziness, headache, flushing, and nausea—but the effects should not be long-lasting
  - With sympathomimetics, patient may note increased heart rate
  - Patient should inform physician conducting studies of any untoward effects experienced

3. You are called into the room of a middle-aged man who had an MI 2 days ago. He tells you that he is experiencing chest pain. Keeping in mind the common causes of chest pain, what history and physical assessment information will you elicit from this patient to determine the source of his chest pain?
   - Character, location, and radiation of chest pain
   - Similarity to or difference from that experienced 2 days prior (MI)
   - Duration of the pain
   - Precipitating events
   - Any palpitations, dizziness, shortness of breath, loss of consciousness

CHAPTER 24
Management of Patients with Dysrhythmias and Conduction Problems

1. You are working in a clinic when a patient enters complaining of dizziness and fatigue. She tells you that she has been diagnosed as having an atrial dysrhythmia. How would you focus your assessment of this patient, and what key assessment factors would you highlight in reporting to the primary care provider?
   - Focused assessment/key factors:
     - When diagnosis made
     - What medications prescribed
     - Any procedures performed (e.g., cardiac ablation)
     - Time of onset of symptoms (duration)
     - Names and amounts of medications taken on day of clinic appearance
     - Level of consciousness (mental status)
     - Precipitating events

2. You are caring for a patient who is being prepared for cardioversion. He indicates that he is very anxious about the procedure because it is the same as the "defibrillation" that his brother had when he died. In offering an explanation to the patient, how would you describe the difference in the two treatments?
   - Cardioversion is a planned procedure; defibrillation is always performed as an emergency procedure.
   - The clinical problem indicating need for cardioverson is under the control of the physician; the clinical problem indicating need for defibrillation is not under the control of the health care provider.
   - Cardioverson uses lower joules of electricity than defibrillation.

CHAPTER 25
Management of Patients with Coronary Vascular Disorders

1. You are caring for a patient who was admitted to the hospital 6 hours earlier with angina pectoris. He complains of chest pain and states that he has received no relief from three nitroglycerin tablets. How would you determine what actions to take? How would your actions differ if this is a patient in a walk-in clinic?
   - Refer to protocol—and anticipate actions, such as:
     - Morphine injection
     - Obtaining EKG
     - Obtaining serum enzymes
     - Notifying physician
   - Walk-in clinic:
     - Alert emergency medical system for transport to acute care facility (per American Heart Association Guidelines)
     - Institute measures per protocol as identified previously

2. You are caring for a patient who is scheduled to have a CABG surgery. He appears quite anxious and states that he is afraid of the pain after surgery. His wife tends to minimize the significance of his concerns about pain. How would you respond to this patient and his wife? How might your response differ if the wife shares her husband's concerns?
   - Discuss pain as a unique personal experience and educate both individuals regarding the significance of pain
   - Identify potential sources of pain (chest, leg)
   - Use teaching materials that describe the use of pain medications postsurgery
   - If wife shares concerns, indicate how she will be able to support and comfort husband postsurgery

3. You are caring for an elderly patient who underwent open-heart surgery 4 days ago and is progressing well. After ambulating in the corridor with his daughter, he returns to his room and

bumps his nose, which begins to bleed profusely. His daughter is visibly upset. Explain what your first action will be and why. If your initial actions are not successful in decreasing the bleeding, how would you proceed? How would you explain the episode to the daughter to help her understand the bleeding?

- First actions:
  - Protect patient safety—return to bed or chair
  - Have patient tilt head forward and apply pressure to the soft tissue of nose against the septum continuously for 5–10 minutes
  - Determine if patient is taking anticoagulant, if so, obtain most recent lab values regarding clotting times
- Initial actions unsuccessful:
  - Notify surgeon
  - Ensure patent intravenous access
  - Anticipate using medications to reverse effects of anticoagulant and frequent blood sampling to gauge level of anticoagulation
- Explanation to daughter:
  - Anticoagulant therapy results in even minor trauma causing profuse bleeding
  - Patient is being monitored and anticoagulation therapy can be controlled

4. The wife of a patient who is preparing for discharge after an MI approaches you and expresses concern about what to do if her husband suffers another heart attack. How might you instruct her in preparation for such an event? How would your instructions vary if the wife is in her 40s versus her late 60s, or lives in a rural community versus a suburban community?

   - Instructions for preparation:
     - Early detection (e.g., changing patterns of angina)
     - Use of nitroglycerin
     - Contacting EMS at first indications of heart attack (e.g., avoid denial)
     - Recognize that early detection and treatment provide opportunity to provide early intervention and minimize damage
   - Wife in 40s versus late 60s:
     - Wife in late 60s may have health problems and must identify stressors that may affect her health
     - Wife in late 60s should be advised to have written list of EMS number, physician number, and numbers of close family members or neighbors who could be contacted in the event wife believes husband is having another MI
   - Rural community:
     - In addition to previously stated information, have directions written out in order to provide SPECIFICs to EMS driver (county roads, state roads, etc.)—time spent with driver getting lost is costly

CHAPTER 26
Management of Patients with Structural, Infectious, or Inflammatory Cardiac Disorders

1. One of your neighbors has just had a mitral valve replacement and says he does not understand why he has been instructed to take antibiotics before undergoing any dental work. How would you explain the rationale for these instructions?

   - Dental work generally results in opening of oral tissue and exposing the blood to microorganisms contained within the mouth.
   - Because of the potential for the circulation carrying the microorganisms, the risk for infection of the valve is significant, and prophylactic treatment with antibiotics is indicated.

2. Discharge plans are being made for a middle-aged man with cardiomyopathy. His wife says she is prepared to care for him at home; she expects that he will be unable to participate extensively in his care. Based on your knowledge about developmental tasks of the middle years, how would you explain the husband's emotional and physical needs to the wife and the ways she can address these needs, as well as her own?

   - Major development tasks of middle-aged adults:
     - Reassessing life accomplishments and goals
     - Adjusting to role changes
     - Accepting physical, emotional, and social changes associated with middle age
     - Planning for retirement
     - Strengthening relationships with spouse, family, friends, companions
     - Adjusting to responsibilities of aging parents
     - Developing skills, hobbies, or activities that provide satisfaction
   - Instructions to wife:
     - Comparison of husband's response to tasks without disease; with disease
     - Impact of limitations superimposed by disease
     - Identify sources of strength and support for husband, wife
     - Identify resources from family, church, community, support groups

3. A patient recovering from heart transplantation says he feels he has "a new lease on life" and is "looking forward to a normal life." What further

information about the patient will be helpful in identifying his teaching and discharge planning needs? Another patient who has undergone the same operation seems depressed and apprehensive. How would you explain the different reactions, and how would your teaching strategies for these two patients differ?

- Methods to balance risk of rejection with risk of infection
- Diet, medication, activity guidelines
- Follow-up studies (essential)
- Clinic visits (essential to keep contact with health care providers)
- Positive response versus depressed response:
  - Assess knowledge level, coping skills, support systems
  - Assess educational level, financial resources
  - Identify changes required by transplant (e.g., employment, residence)
  - Identify lifestyle changes
  - Support as indicated
  - Seek referral of depressed patient for evaluation and treatment

4. You are caring for a patient with pericarditis. His systolic blood pressure begins to fall and heart sounds cannot be heard. Describe the actions you would take and why.
   - Fall in systolic blood pressure and diminished heart sounds indicate that the pericarditis is restricting cardiac motion and functioning.
   - Physician must be contacted immediately.
   - Nurse must prepare for code situation.
   - Nurse must ensure patient IV access.

CHAPTER 27
Management of Patients with Complications from Heart Disease

1. A patient who had a myocardial infarction 2 days ago begins to complain of shortness of breath and coughing. Describe the assessment data you would gather in preparing to report this development.
   - Intake and output for prior 24 hours
   - Weight (2 days ago, yesterday, today)
   - Breath sounds
   - Rate of breath
   - Vital signs and pulse
   - Medications
   - Current lab reports
   - History of smoking or lung disease
2. A patient is readmitted for cardiac failure for the third time in 2 months. Describe how you would assess for the factors that contribute to the patient's readmission.
   - Compliance with taking medications as prescribed
   - Compliance with dietary guidelines
   - Compliance with exercise guidelines
   - Smoking history (?restarted)
   - Stress level at home
   - Home environment (pleasant/unpleasant; live alone vs. with others; cares for self with or without help)
   - Emotional well-being (fear of dying)
   - Desire to live life without following mediation, diet, and exercise guidelines

CHAPTER 28
Assessment and Management of Patients with Vascular Disorders and Problems of Peripheral Circulation

1. You are assigned to a medical clinic where many elderly patients receive care. Two patients, both with peripheral vascular disease, are overheard comparing their symptoms and their medical management. When they realize that many of their symptoms are similar, but their medical management is distinctly different, they question you about this. What further information will be helpful in determining an accurate explanation to give to these two patients?
   - Ages
   - History of surgeries
   - Co-morbidities (e.g., diabetes mellitus, hypertension, coronary artery disease)
   - Smoking history
2. Your patient has been diagnosed with a calf vein deep vein thrombosis. The physician gives the patient two treatment options: hospitalization with intravenous heparin therapy, or home treatment with low molecular-weight heparin. How would you direct your assessment to identify the factors that might affect the patient's decision?
   - Assessment:
     - Home situation (role, support, dependents)
     - Patient ability to comply with home treatment (knowledge level, coping abilities)
     - Indicators of patient's attitude toward compliance with home treatment
     - Insurance coverage of either form of therapy
3. You are visiting a patient with a known venous ulceration of the right leg. During your home visit, she complains of right ankle swelling,

constant pain in the right fourth and fifth digits of the foot, and pain that is worse when she tries to sleep at night. Physical examination reveals cyanotic digits and no palpable dorsalis pedis pulse. There is a 3-cm shallow weeping ulcer in the medial malleolus region. Analyze these findings, indicate what you think the possible causes may be for these findings, and describe the actions you would take, and explain why.

- Comparison of typical signs and symptoms of venous ulceration versus arterial ulcerations
- No pulse, cyanosis, and pain indicate arterial insufficiency
- Nurse must report findings to attending physician and seek evaluation and treatment of arterial disorder immediately

CHAPTER 29
Assessment and Management of Patients with Hypertension

1. You are a nursing student assigned to a hypertension clinic. One of the patients is a 58-year-old telemarketer. During the physical assessment, the patient, who is 5 foot 6 inches tall and weighs 180 lb asks you why a complete physical examination is performed at every clinic visit. How would you answer this patient's question? Identify what additional data you needed to gather to support your answer.
   - Hypertension is a disease that affects all body systems and early detection of a particular problem allows early treatment and opportunity to minimize damage
   - Review patient's past history, identify problems that have been detected or indicators of need for vigilant observation
2. You are a home care nurse. One of your patients is an elderly man who lives alone and who has hypertension along with other health problems, including congestive heart failure. In one of your visits with him, you learn that he has difficulty taking his medications as directed. What questions come to mind as you consider the situation? How will you direct your assessment to identify factors contributing to this problem? Using the factors identified, develop a sample follow-up home care teaching plan for this patient.
   - Questions:
     - Explain difficulty (e.g., opening containers, remembering to take medications, difficulty swallowing, side effects)
     - Determine if patient has ideas regarding ways to resolve difficulty
     - Contact physician for possibility for changes (e.g., ability to take one long-acting vasodilator as opposed to "t.i.d" medication)
   - Plan:
     - Outlines problem areas, potential measures to resolve problems (goals), specific instructions to patient, and methods for evaluating success or need for further teaching

CHAPTER 30
Assessment of Patients with Hematologic Disorders

1. An elderly patient who is anemic says she believes that the anemia is due to her age, and she asks why she must have so many tests performed. What explanation would you give this patient about the rationale for the diagnostic tests?
   - Aging does not cause anemia; however, anemia may occur due to physiologic changes that occur with aging
   - There are several types of anemia, and tests are needed to identify which type patient demonstrates
   - Treatment varies with type of anemia
2. You are caring for a young adult patient who has had repeated hospitalizations for sickle cell crisis. What factors should be assessed to determine the patient's educational, coping, and pain management needs?
   - Education:
     - Formal education attained
     - Experience with the disease
     - Observations of family members' experiences with SCD
   - Coping:
     - Assess coping skills
     - Identify resources for support
     - Consider referral if symptoms indicate clinical depression
   - Pain management:
     - Assess pain experience
     - Assess methods for pain relief
     - Ascertain ability to obtain and take medications as prescribed
     - Instruct patient
     - Keep warm
     - Maintain adequate hydration
     - Avoid stressful situations
3. You are caring for a patient diagnosed with leukemia. The family members are very concerned about the patient's risk for infection at home. What instructions should they be given about decreasing the risks for infection?

- Refer to Chapter Chart: Home Care Teaching Checklist: The Patient at Risk for Infection
- Wash hands thoroughly
- Perform total body hygiene
- Maintain skin integrity
- Avoid fresh flowers, plants, garden work
- Avoid birdcages and litterboxes
- Avoid fresh salads and unpeeled fruits and vegetables
- Maintain high-calorie, high-protein diet and intake of 3,000 cc/day (unless fluids restricted)
- Avoid people with infections
- Avoid crowds
- Perform deep breathing exercises every 4 hours while awake
- Avoid anal intercourse
- Provide adequate lubrication with gentle vaginal manipulation in intercourse

4. You are caring for a patient who is septic and is now receiving a transfusion of 2 units of packed RBCs. The patient spikes a temperature to 38.5° Centigrade after half of the second unit has been transfused. What are the possible causes of the fever? What are the appropriate nursing interventions?

- Possible cause: Febrile, nonhemolytic reaction
  - Fever more than one degree Centrigrade elevated
  - Prior transfusion
- Actions:
  - Stop transfusion, maintaining intravenous line with normal saline at slow rate of infusion
  - Assess patient: Vital signs; respiratory status; mental status
  - Notify MD of assessment findings
  - Notify blood bank
  - Send blood container and tubing to blood bank

UNIT 7 DIGESTIVE AND GASTROINTESTINAL FUNCTION

CHAPTER 31 Assessment of Digestive and Gastrointestinal Function

1. You are caring for a patient who is to have a barium enema. The patient received a clear liquid diet and a laxative the evening before the test. On the morning of the test, she indicates that the laxative had caused her to have diarrhea during the night, and she refuses to have a cleansing enema. Based on your knowledge of intestinal physiology, how would you explain to this patient what has happened and why? Describe what the goals would be in this situation and the interventions that could be implemented to achieve them.

- The laxative may have resulted in hyperactivity of the bowel causing diarrhea
- Although patient has had diarrhea, cleansing enema is indicated to assure clear return
- Success of barium enema relies on adequate bowel preparation
- Goals/interventions:
  - Offer explanations to promote patient understanding and compliance
  - Administer enema solution only until return is clear
  - Promote patient safety (e.g., inability to retain solution; leakage of solution on floor increasing risk for fall)

2. You accompany your patient to the endoscopy suite, where he is to have a colonoscopy. You notice that emergency equipment is readily available. After the procedure is completed, the nurse who assisted with the procedure must now assist with another procedure and asks you to monitor the patient's vital signs. You agree to carry out this function because you have a thorough understanding of the complications that can occur. Describe the changes in vital signs that you might detect as an indication that complications are developing, and the reasons these changes may occur.

- Potential complications:
  - Cardiac dysrhythmias (due to medications and vagal stimulation) indicated by irregular rhythm upon auscultation of patient's apical pulse
  - Respiratory depression (due to medications used to sedate patient) indicated by decreased rate and/or depth of medications
  - Circulatory problems (due to too much or too little fluid administration) indicated by increased or decreased pulse, urine output
  - Decreased oxygen saturation (due to vasovagal reaction or medications) demonstrated through pulse oximetry

CHAPTER 32 Management of Patients with Oral and Esophageal Disorders

1. You are interviewing a patient in the medical clinic who has been treated in the clinic previously for gastroesophageal reflux. He

complains that his symptoms are worse but that he has been taking his medications as prescribed. He states that he has tried many different kinds of antacids but none of them are helping him. Describe how you would continue to assess this patient to obtain the additional information that is needed. Speculate as to the different causes that may underlie this patient's inability to obtain relief.

- Assess patient for compliance with instructions to:
  - Eat a low-fat, high-fiber diet
  - Avoid caffeine, tobacco, carbonated beverages
  - Avoid eating or drinking 2 hours before bedtime
  - Maintain normal body weight
  - Avoid tight clothes
  - Elevate head of bed on 6- to 8-inch blocks
  - Determine if physician has prescribed antacid or if antacid may be retarding absorption of medications

2. You are caring for two postoperative patients. One patient is being treated for cancer of the mouth and the other for cancer of the esophagus. How will the nutritional care of these two patients differ?

- Nutritional care may differ according to method used to provide nutrition
- Oral feedings versus enteral feedings versus gastrostomy feeding
- Both patients require adequate nutrition to meet metabolic demands of disease and treatment.
- Nutritional consultation would be indicated for both patients

CHAPTER 33
Gastrointestinal Intubation and Special Nutritional Modalities

1. You are caring for a patient with an NG feeding tube. Before administering the medications, you must confirm that the tube is placed correctly. Based on research findings, how will you check to make sure that the tube is properly placed?

- Detect souffle (sound of air going into stomach upon being injected into NG tube with syringe)
- Ask conscious, oriented patient to speak
- Withdraw gastric contents

2. A patient receiving NG tube feedings begins to have diarrhea. Explain what you think might be causing the diarrhea, describe the assessment data important in determining its possible causes, and discuss ways to control it.

- Refer to Chapter 33 Chart on complications of enteral therapy and selected nursing interventions

3. When conducting a home visit with a patient receiving nightly 10-hour parenteral nutrition feedings, you find that the patient has chills, diarrhea, and a fever of 100° Farenheit. The patient's sister states that the previous evening's feeding solution looked "funny" and that she sped up the rate of the feeding so it would finish early. Analyze this situation and determine the actions you would take, explaining the reasoning behind your decision.

- Analysis:
  - Feeding may have been contaminated
  - Sister does not understand safety features of TPN
- Actions/reasoning:
  - Contact physician to report observations, situation, and signs and symptoms of infection (e.g., MD may wish to examine patient or send patient to acute care facility for diagnostic testing, hydration, management of symptoms, prevention of further complications)
  - Assess sister's understanding of TPN administration, provide teaching regarding TPN administration, indications of problems, and actions to be taken when she believes the solution looks "funny"
  - Emphasize that TPN rate is NEVER increased without physician instruction to do so because of potential for fluid overload with cardiac complications

CHAPTER 34
Management of Patients with Gastric and Duodenal Ulcers

1. You are visiting a resident of a retirement community. She tells you that she has begun to have symptoms of a peptic ulcer just like she had many years ago and that she is treating the ulcer as she did before, with a bland diet and antacids. Based on your knowledge of current theories about peptic ulcers, how would you advise her? If she is skeptical of your explanations, how might you convince her?

- Current theory: Infection with gram-negative Helicobacter pylori; seek physician evaluation and treatment as soon as possible
- Peptic ulcers treated with antibiotics to eradicate H. pylori have a 10% recurrence rate; those not treated have a 95% recurrence rate.

2. You are caring for a patient who has had a gastrectomy to treat gastric cancer. The patient's wife says she is eager for him to return home so that she can give him all of his favorite foods and help him regain the weight he has lost. Describe the conclusions you would draw from these statements and explain how you would devise an instructional program that you believe would be helpful for this couple.

   - Conclusion: Wife does not understand disease process or prognosis
   - Instructional program features:
     - Small, frequent portions of nonirritating foods to decrease gastric irritation
     - Food supplements high in calories, vitamins A and C, and iron to enhance tissue repair
     - Monitor weight, intake, and output
     - Signs of dehydration
     - Use of antiemetics

CHAPTER 35
Management of Patients with Intestinal and Rectal Disorders

1. You are visiting a resident in an extended care facility. She complains that she has had pain throughout her abdomen for the past day. She has not had a bowel movement in 4 days, and she complains of loss of appetite. Physical examination reveals that her abdomen is distended and rigid and that bowel sounds are absent. Analyze these findings, indicate what you think possible causes may be, and explain the actions you would take and why.

   - Possible causes: Medications, rectal or anal disorder, obstruction, disease process
   - Actions:
     - Because perception of pain in the elderly patient is limited by deterioration of afferent nerve fibers, pain must be evaluated by physician
     - Contact MD for indications
     - Reassure patient that early treatment of bowel problems with conservative measures is indicated and may achieve relief of symptoms

2. During a conversation with an elderly gentleman at a community center for senior citizens, he tells you he cannot have a bowel movement without taking a laxative each day. He asks if this is acceptable, given that he also takes "blood pressure medicine, a heart pill, and aspirin" each day. Explain how you would advise this patient and give the rationale behind your advice.

   - Advise patient that taking daily laxative is not recommended since it affects absorption of his other medications and does not allow his bowel to function normally
   - Referring to Chapter Table on Preventing Constipation, teach patient methods for enhancing bowel function

3. You are caring for a patient who has been treated medically for ulcerative colitis for 5 years. The patient underwent a total colectomy and ileostomy yesterday. What are the similarities and differences between the care of this patient and that of a patient who had a colon resection and colostomy? Explain how you would meet the emotional and health education needs of the patient with an ileostomy and the patient with a colostomy.

   - Both patients are at risk for development of infection because the bowel has been entered during surgery, and must be monitored vigilantly for early signs
   - Both will require teaching regarding ostomy care
   - Patient with ileostomy cannot establish bowel habits because the contents of the ileum are fluid and are discharged continuously
   - Patient with colostomy may be able to institute bowel management program to promote control over defecation of formed stool
   - Emotional needs of both require:
     - Assessment of coping skills
     - Identification of support systems
     - Identification of resources (family, community, support group)

UNIT 8
METABOLIC AND ENDOCRINE FUNCTION

CHAPTER 36
Assessment and Management of Patients with Hepatic and Biliary Disorders

1. A 60-year-old patient is admitted to the hospital with a diagnosis of cirrhosis and impending liver failure. What diagnostic workup and treatment would you anticipate, and what are the implications for nursing care of this patient?

- Diagnostic Workup Anticipated: Refer to Chapter 36 Table: Liver Function Studies and Additional Studies
- Nursing interventions:
  - Providing rest
  - Improving nutritional status
  - Providing skin care
  - Reducing risk of injury
  - Monitoring for and managing potential complications
  - Teaching patients self-care
  - Making referrals for continuing care

2. A 78-year-old patient is scheduled for a laparoscopic cholecystectomy. What postoperative care is indicated for this patient? What factors would you consider in preparing her for discharge? How would your care differ if she lived alone?

- Postoperative care:
  - Observation of puncture sites
  - Managing postoperative pain
  - Reporting signs and symptoms of intra-abdominal complications:
  - Loss of appetite
  - Vomiting
  - Pain
  - Distention of the abdomen
  - Temperature elevation
  - Preparation for discharge
  - Instruction regarding aforementioned information
- If patient lived alone, nurse must consider and use resources to ensure that patient has assistance at home during first 24–48 hours.
  - Social work referral
  - Identification of resources and support systems (family, church, community)

3. A 20-year-old college student has ben diagnosed with hepatitis B. What teaching is warranted for this patient to prevent transmission to others and to reduce the risk of complications?

- To prevent transmission:
  - Use condom when engaging in sexual intercourse
  - Do not share razors, fingernail tools, toothbrushes, or any personal care item that may come into contact with blood or body fluids
  - Demonstrate understanding that hepatitis B is transmitted through contact with contaminated blood or body secretions
- To reduce risk of complications:
  - Adhere to guidelines regarding stress, diet, exercise, rest, and medications
  - Report any signs or symptoms of deterioration to physician

4. A 64-year-old man with a long history of alcohol abuse is admitted to the hospital with possible bleeding esophageal varices. Describe the possible treatments for this patient and the nursing implications of different treatment and strategies with liver biopsy.

- Treatment for bleeding esophageal varices:
  - Close monitoring of vital signs as well as overt signs of bleeding
  - Prepare equipment (Sengstaken-Blakemore tube, IV fluids, medications)
  - Review procedure for room-temperature saline lavage
  - Prepare patient for immediate transfer to ICU or surgery, as indicated
- Nursing implications re: liver biopsy
  - Refer to Chapter 36 Chart: Assisting with Liver Biopsy, Items 9, 10, 11

CHAPTER 37
Assessment and Management of Patients with Diabetes Mellitus

1. A diabetic diet has been prescribed for a newly diagnosed diabetic patient. Compare and contrast the modifications that would be made in the diet in the following situations: (a) The patient is a pregnant woman; (b) the patient is a devout Muslim; (c) the patient is a 55-year-old woman with osteoporosis.

- Goals of nutritional management:
  - Providing all the essential food constituents
  - Achieving and maintaining a reasonable weight
  - Meeting energy needs
  - Preventing wide daily fluctuations in blood glucose levels with blood glucose levels as close to normal as it safe and practical
  - Decreasing serum lipid levels, if elevated
- Pregnant patient:
  - Increased calorie requirements
  - Controlled weight gain
- Devout Muslim:
  - Consideration of food restrictions
  - Consideration of impact of observation of holy days and fasting requirements
- 55-year-old woman with osteoporosis:
  - Increased intake of calcium and Vitamin D
  - Exercise requirements influencing diet

2. A patient is brought to the emergency department by his coworkers because he has become drowsy and has developed slurred speech over the last hour. You learn that he has diabetes and takes insulin, but no other medical information is available. Describe how you would gather additional assessment data to help you

distinguish between hypoglycemia and hyperglycemia. Before conducting an in-depth history and physical examination, the physician administers glucose to the patient. How would you explain the rationale for administering glucose before the definitive cause of the patient's symptoms is identified?

- Perform Accu-chek or another form of blood glucose measurement
- Check patient for medic-alert tags
- Contact family to obtain history of patient's onset and management of disease
- Rationale for administration of glucose: Patients can survive with elevated glucose levels; dangerously low blood glucose may result in seizuring, brain damage, and death

3. Your patient has had diabetes for many years and has not adhered to a treatment regimen as prescribed. He states to you, "What's the use? I'm going to die from the complications of diabetes anyway." What is your response to him? What is the next step for him?

- Response: By following treatment guidelines, blood glucose levels near normal can be maintained in many patients and complications minimized (Refer to Chapter Chart: Misconceptions Related to Diabetes and its Treatment)
- Next step:
  - Counseling regarding feelings and attitudes
  - Instruction regarding the disease and prevention of complications
  - Identification of support systems
  - Identification of resources (family, church, community)

4. Your patient has diabetes and is recommended to do blood glucose monitoring. What areas of assessment are important in choosing a blood glucose monitoring system for him? Determine a plan for teaching blood glucose monitoring to him.

- Patient's cognitive abilities
- Patient's comfort with securing his own blood specimen
- Patient's visual acuity and fine motor coordination
- Patient's comfort with technology
- Patient's willingness to learn
- Cost
- Plan: Employ fundamental patient education methods integrating content referring to blood glucose monitoring
  - Indications/times prescribed
  - Safety considerations
  - Quality control methods for machine used
  - Record-keeping
  - Reports to physician

CHAPTER 38
Assessment and Management of Patients with Endocrine Disorders

1. During a home visit to a patient with recently diagnosed diabetes mellitus, you observe that the patient's grandmother is slow to respond to others, seems depressed and lethargic, and is wearing a heavy coat in the warm house. You suspect that she might have a severe hypothyroid condition. Describe how you would proceed in this situation, how you would determine what actions to take, and how you would prioritize your actions.

- Perform complete assessment providing emotional support and reassurance
- Review current medications ordered
- Determine patient compliance with therapeutic regime
- Determine date of last physician's visit and next visit
- Contact health care provider reporting observations and determining course of action

2. Your patient is beginning antithyroid mediation to control her hyperthyroidism. Her husband has been very concerned about her irritability, rapid mood swings, and weight loss. How would you explain to him the reasons for his wife's symptoms and the rationale for the medication being prescribed?

- Reasons for wife's symptoms are the disease—oversecretion of thryoid hormone and its effects
- Rationale for medication being prescribed:
  - Suppression of thyroid gland activity
  - Provision for symptomatic relief

3. Your patient has been receiving corticosteroids for treating a chronic disease. She has been admitted for an emergency hysterectomy. Based on your knowledge of the effects of the long-term use of corticosteroids, how would you focus your assessment and management strategies of this patient in the postoperative period?

- Be certain physician is aware of status; intravenous steroids may be required to prevent steroid-induced adrenal insufficiency
- Observe patient closely for signs of steroid-induced adrenal insufficiency
- Observe patient closely for signs of infection
- Refer to Chapter 38 Table: Side Effects of Corticosteroid Therapy and Implications for Practice

4. Corticosteroids have been prescribed for your patient, and it is expected that she will take them

for at least 1 month. How would you instruct her to minimize complications of corticosteroid use?

- Take medication as prescribed and at time prescribed
- Follow guidelines for tapering medication
- Be certain to have an adequate supply so she does not miss a dose
- Contact physician for untoward signs/symptoms

5. A 57-year-old patient has a history of alcoholism and cirrhosis. He is admitted to your unit with a diagnosis of acute pancreatitis. Describe nursing care for this patient and compare and contrast care with and without the additional diagnosis of pancreatitis.

- Observe closely for signs of delirium tremens
- Relieve pain and discomfort
- Improve breathing pattern
- Improve nutritional status
- Improve skin integrity
- Monitor and manage potential complications:
    - Fluid and electrolyte disturbance
    - Hemorrhage
    - Septic shock
    - Multisystem organ failure

UNIT 9
URINARY AND RENAL FUNCTION

CHAPTER 39
Assessment of Urinary and Renal Function

1. After a closed renal biopsy for diagnostic purposes, your patient reports a backache. You also notice the patient's urinal contains about 300 ml of bright red blood. Based on your knowledge of the risks associated with renal biopsy, explain how you would focus your assessment and nursing care.

- Backache and hematuria are anticipated findings post renal biopsy.
- Patient must be monitored vigilantly for the first hour after biopsy to detect early sings of abnormal bleeding
- Symptoms such as sharp flank pain, shoulder pain, dysuria, anorexia, vomiting, and the development of a dull, aching discomfort in the abdomen should be reported to the urologist immediately

2. Your patient is scheduled for a series of urodynamic tests as part of a workup for incontinence. You know that a patient who understands the purpose of the test and what to expect during the procedure will be able to cooperate more while the test is being down. Describe how you would teach this patient, and discuss the details of the explanations you would give.

- Refer to Chapter 39 Chart: Patient Education and Homecare Before and After Urodynamic Testing

CHAPTER 40
Management of Patients with Urinary and Renal Dysfunction

1. A 65-year-old woman comes to the clinic complaining that she dribbles urine whenever she coughs. She wears a pantyliner every day because she is not sure when an accident may occur. She asks if there is anything that can be done to help this problem. Discuss your response to the patient. Include what she can anticipate regarding a diagnostic workup, treatment plan, and patient education strategies.

- Refer to urodynamic testing (Chapter 39)
- Inform patient that successful management depends on type of incontinence and its causes
- Inform patient that behavioral strategies are tried first
- Program of timed or habit voiding
- Bladder retraining
- Biofeedback
- Kegel exercises
- Vaginal cone retention exercises
- Refer to Chapter 40 Chart: Patient Education and Home Care: Strategies for Managing Urinary Incontinence
- Pharmacologic therapy
- Surgical correction, if behavioral strategies and pharmacologic therapy are not successful

2. You are a staff nurse at an outpatient dialysis facility. The local nephrologist is sending a young man to the clinic today who will need dialysis in the near future. The physician has asked you to teach the patient and his wife about his dialysis options. Describe how you would develop a teaching plan to explain the different types of dialysis, their goals, and the level of involvement on the part of the patient and family. How would you modify your approach if the patient is so

distraught that he cannot seem to hear what you are saying?

- Teaching plan:
  - Compare and contrast Hemodialysis with Peritoneal Dialysis
  - Identify goal of adequate filtration of blood
  - Refer to Chapter 40 Charts: Home Care Teaching Checklist: Hemodialysis; Peritoneal Dialysis (CAPD or CCPD)
- If patient is too distraught, recognize such and limit instruction to facts/basics:
  - Arrange future time for more detailed discussion
  - Provide print media covering choices

3. A patient who is treated with hemodialysis is admitted to the hospital for an elective nephrectomy in preparation for a kidney transplantation. How would your preoperative and postoperative care be modified by the patient's renal failure and the need for dialysis? What differences in your plan of care would be appropriate if the patient is treated with CAPD?

- Nursing management:
  - Protecting vascular or peritoneal access sites
  - Taking precautions during intravenous therapy
  - Monitoring symptoms of uremia
  - Detecting cardiac and respiratory complications
  - Controlling electrolyte levels and diet
  - Managing discomfort and pain
  - Monitoring blood pressure
  - Preventing infection
  - Caring for the catheter site
  - Administering medications
  - Providing psychological support

4. You are the evening charge nurse in an extended care facility. An elderly woman is admitted from the local hospital after fracturing her hip. The staff nurse admitting the patient tells you the patient has urinary incontinence. The nurse intends to contact the physician to get an order for an indwelling catheter. What would be an appropriate response to the staff nurse? Describe the plan of care you would recommend for this patient.

- Response: Time-voiding pattern introduction as opposed to catheterization—urinary catheter is invasive and may cause infection; pain associated with the hip fracture will prohibit moving patient on and off bedpan.
- Plan of care:
  - Promote comfort
  - Provide vigilant skin care
  - Seek discontinuation of catheter as soon as patient is able to tolerate movement of the broken hip (under pain medication)
  - Establish time-voiding pattern

CHAPTER 41
Management of Patients with Urinary and Renal Disorders

1. Your patient tells you that she is very discouraged because she has had repeated episodes of UTI during the past 3 years. How would you focus your assessment to assist in uncovering factors associated with these infections? Describe the teaching program you would devise to help the patient reduce the incidence of infection.

- Evaluate patient in terms of risk factors (see Chapter 41 Chart: Risk Factors for Urinary Tract Infection)
- Provide teaching (see Chapter 41 Chart: Patient Education and Homecare: Preventing Recurrent Urinary Tract Infections)

2. You are working in the emergency department and are caring for a patient who has a severe renal colic from a kidney stone. Discuss nursing care of this patient, including pain management strategies. The patient passes the kidney stone and is going to be discharged home. Describe the teaching program you would devise to help the patient obtain the necessary follow-up treatment and prevent recurrence of any kidney stones.

- Nursing care of patient with severe renal colic from kidney stone:
  - Administer analgesics and NSAIDS as ordered
  - Provide hot baths or moist heat to flank areas
  - Allow patient to assume position of comfort
  - Assist patient to ambulate, if desired
- Teaching program: Follow-up treatment
  - Signs and symptoms of: obstruction, infection, renal hematoma, hypertension
  - Signs and symptoms of stone formation and need to report such promptly
- Teaching program: Preventing recurrence (see Chapter 41 Chart Nutrition: Dietary Recommendations for Prevention of Kidney Stones)

3. Your patient is scheduled for a cystectomy and urinary diversion. Describe how you would meet the emotional and health education needs of the patient if (a) the patient is a 32-year-old woman who has recently married; (b) the patient is a 74-year-old man with limited vision and poor hygiene habits.

- Young, recently married woman:
  - Include spouse
  - Provide factual information
  - Promote competence in caring for stoma
  - Identify support systems and resources
  - Address issues of self-esteem, altered body image
  - Explore sexuality issues
  - Refer for counseling as indicated

- Aged male:
  - Evaluate cognitive ability, visual acuity, and fine motor coordination
  - Identify support systems and resources
  - Refer for home care assistance
  - Address impact on self-esteem, altered body image
  - Explore sexuality issues
  - Refer for counseling, as indicated

4. You are caring for two patients in the same room. One is a diabetic patient in an acute intrinsic renal failure after receiving intravenous contrast dye. The other patient has ESRD from hypertension. Compare and contrast management of each patient and discuss your different priorities of care for each.

- Acute renal failure (ARF) may be reversible; ESRD is irreversible
- Interventions may prevent ARF (refer to Chapter 41 Chart: Health Promotion and Illness Prevention: Interventions to Prevent Acute Renal Failure)
- Priorities with ARF:
  - Monitoring fluid and electrolyte balance
  - Reducing metabolic rate
  - Promoting pulmonary function
  - Preventing infection
  - Providing skin care
  - Providing emotional support
- Priorities with ESRD—Identification and treatment of:
  - Electrolyte imbalances
  - Anemia
  - Bone disease
- Providing emotional support:
  - Promoting comfort
  - Providing skin care

UNIT 10 REPRODUCTIVE FUNCTION

CHAPTER 42 Assessment and Management: Problems Related to Female Physiologic Processes

1. A 35-year-old woman is having a complete physical examination for the first time since she was sexually assaulted 4 years ago. She is very apprehensive about pelvic exams. How would you approach the history and physical examination with her?

- History:
  - Establish rapport
  - Allow patient to narrate event
  - Demonstrate openness, support, and remain nonjudgmental
- Physical examination:
  - Use calm manner
  - Provide explanations and teaching
  - Instruct patient to void before examination
  - Provide for privacy

2. You are a nurse practitioner in a neighborhood health clinic. Upon performing a pelvic examination of a 15-year-old, you discover that she is pregnant. Her father, who has brought her for the examination because she has missed two menstrual periods, asks you the results of the examination. How would you respond to the patient's father if he insists that his daughter is not sexually active? How would you discuss the results of the examination with the patient?

- Balance rights of father of a minor with privacy rights of a female
- Consider potential for domestic abuse
- Consult with other nurse practitioners or physicians regarding situation
- To discuss results with fifteen year old:
  - Establish rapport
  - Promote discussion of pregnancy
  - Determine daughter's needs
  - Identify resources and support systems
  - Report finding according to agency policy and state law

3. A 47-year-old woman tells you that she believes she is perimenopausal. She has read a great deal about menopause, its effect on health, and the risks associated with hormone replacement therapy. She asks you for your advice and recommendations about measures to maintain health, including the use of hormone therapy. How would you respond to her request? How would you modify your recommendation if she had a strong family history of breast cancer?

- Review the research findings of the Postmenopausal Estrogen/Progestin Interventions (PEPI) trial as well as other studies
- Assist patient in identifying the benefits and risks of HRT (hormone replacement therapy)
- Point out that HRT is generally contraindicated in women with history of breast cancer (family history of breast cancer adds to woman's risk of the disease)
- Encourage patient to speak with her gynecologist regarding specific medical concerns

4. A 23-year-old woman has been admitted to the hospital with possible ectopic pregnancy. What emergency management strategies would you

anticipate and which nursing measures would you plan for the patient's hospital stay and long-term recovery? Include the rationale for your decisions.

- Vaginal examination, ultrasonography, colposcopy, serum analyses of beta hCG
- Potential pharmacologic interventions (Metroxate)
- Surgical management, with potential for loss of tube and ovary on affected side
- Nursing measures:
  - Relieving pain (abdominal pain is anticipated, ranging from cramping to severe continuous pain)
  - Support the grieving process (conception did occur)
  - Manage potential complications (patient is at risk for hemorrhage, infection)

5. During a checkup at the clinic where you work, a 35-year-old lesbian patient tells you that she has met a new partner and is not concerned about sexual risks of STDs because of her sexual orientation. How would you address the educational needs of this patient?

- Determine educational level and cognitive abilities
- Ascertain patient's understanding of transmission of STDs (intimate contact with persons or fomites)
- Review incubation periods for STDs (particularly HIV)
- Point out the implications of herpes genitalis outbreaks

CHAPTER 43
Management of Women with Reproductive Disorders

1. Your 24-year-old patient has received a diagnosis of genital HPV and is very upset, stating that her boyfriend lied to her when he told her that she was his first sexual partner. What approach would you take to assist her in learning about HPV and coping with her feelings related to her relationship?
   - Describe modes of transmission, incidence, and risk factors
   - An individual may be an unknowing carrier—may have no symptoms
   - Incubation period can be long
   - Condoms prevent some but not all transmission, because transmission occurs during skin-to-skin contact in areas not covered by condoms.
   - Acknowledging the emotional distress that occurs when an STD is diagnosed is often helpful to patients
   - Refer for counseling, if indicated

2. How would you explain Kegel exercises to a woman? How would your explanation differ if the woman understands little English?

   - Kegel exercises may be explained by informing the female to begin voiding and then stop the flow. Muscles used to stop the flow are the muscles that should be contracted to perform Kegel exercises.
   - For a woman who understands little English, the nurse may use pictures or may seek assistance of close family member or friend who speaks patient's language.

3. Your 54-year-old patient is scheduled for surgery to treat cervical cancer. In discussing with her the strategies to prevent postoperative complications, you realize that her husband believes they will never be able to have sexual relations again. What approach would you take in discussing this with the patient and her husband?

   - Provide fact-driven explanation of the surgery. Usually, total abdominal hysterectomy is performed to treat cervical cancer. The external genitalia and vagina are not affected.
   - Approach:
     - Establish rapport
     - Protect privacy concerns
     - Use texts and pictures to communicate type of surgery being performed and structure remaining intact
     - Encourage dialogue regarding concerns
     - Address questions nonjudgmentally and informatively
     - Refer patient and wife to physician or to counselor, as indicated

4. During a routine pelvic examination, a suspicious vulvar lesion is detected in a 70-year-old patient. What treatment options are likely, and what are the implications for the preoperative and postoperative phases of nursing care and for home care?

   - Treatment options:
     - Excision
     - Radiation
   - Preoperative care: Relieve anxiety, prepare skin for surgery
   - Postoperative care:
     - Relieve pain
     - Improve skin integrity
     - Support positive sexuality and sexual function
     - Monitor and manage potential complications (infection, hemorrhage, DVT)

CHAPTER 44
Assessment and Management of Patients with Breast Disorders

1. Your 35-year-old patient has just been diagnosed with breast cancer. Her mother, aunt, and one of her sisters have all had breast cancer. She is very worried about her own children's well-being and future. Describe the teaching program you feel is indicated for this patient and her children.
   - Refer to Chapter 44 Chart: Risk Factors for Breast Cancer
   - Encourage breast self-examination
   - Encourage annual examinations by physician and mammography
2. A 42-year-old woman reports to you that she has never had a mammogram and is afraid to have one done. How would you respond to her, and what teaching would you provide?
   - Refer to Chapter 44 Chart: Risk Factors for Breast Cancer
   - Advise her to check with her physician regarding age at which to obtain mammogram
   - Describe the procedure
   - Address questions with factual explanations
   - Provide print media and other teaching resources
   - Refer for counseling, if indicated
3. Two of your patients have undergone surgery for the treatment of breast cancer. One had a lumpectomy and axillary lymph node dissection; the other had a modified radical mastectomy. How would your nursing assessment and management of these two patients differ?
   - Assessment and management would not differ; both would require:
     - Observation during recovery from anesthesia
     - Pain relief interventions
     - Psychological support
   - Monitoring for potential complications:
     - Infection
     - Hematoma formation, seroma formation
     - Explanation of paresthesias due to nerve trauma
4. A 40-year-old woman is scheduled for a modified radical mastectomy and indicates that she is confused about the various types of breast reconstruction procedures. How would you instruct her about the differences, including the advantages and disadvantages of each and the postoperative course?
   - Refer to Chapter 44 Table: Surgical Treatment of Breast Cancer
   - Refer to Chapter 44 Chart: Contraindications to Breast Conservation Treatment
   - Refer to response to Exercise 3
5. When you ask your patient about her pattern of doing BSE, she states that she does not know how to do it. Describe the teaching approach you would use to teach her. How would your approach differ if the patient did not speak English? What modifications would you make if the patient previously had a mastectomy?
   - Provide print media describing BSE
   - Note importance of performing BSE after menses (day 5 to day 7 counting first day of menses as day 1)
   - Demonstrate BSE to patient
   - Ask for return demonstration
   - For non-English speaking individual, use films or videos in her native language; use illustrations; seek assistance of close family member; seek interpreter
   - Previous mastectomy: Emphasize need to examine both affected and unaffected sides monthly

CHAPTER 45
Assessment and Management: Problems Related to Male Reproductive Processes

1. A 49-year-old man tells you he has been informed by is physician that he has an elevated PSA level but that he does not understand its significance or what action he should take. How would you respond to his statement? What factors would you consider in formulating your response?
   - Response:
     - PSA is a substance produced and secreted by prostate tissue
     - Its elevation is an indicator of prostate tissue, but does not necessarily indicate malignancy
     - The gentleman must follow up with his physician for digital rectal examination as well as additional studies, as indicated
   - Factors to consider:
     - Educational level and cognitive ability
     - Understanding of anatomy
     - Financial implications of follow-up care
     - Emotional impact of information
2. One of your patients, a 50-year-old man with longstanding diabetes, asks you about Viagra. What information and teaching approach would you give to him about Viagra? How would your approach differ if the patient is a 32-year-old

patient with a spinal cord injury? If you patient is a 68-year-old man with coronary artery disease?

- Refer to Chapter 45 Chart: Patient Education and Homecare: Questions and Answers About Viagra

3. You are caring for two patients who have undergone prostatectomy. One has had a TUR; the other has undergone an open surgical approach to remove the prostate. How would your care differ for these two patients? How would your assessment be directed to detect possible complications?

   - Refer to Chapter 45 Chart: Comparing Surgical Approaches for Prostatectomy with Nursing Implications

UNIT 11 IMMUNOLOGIC FUNCTION

CHAPTER 46 Assessment of Immune Function

1. A 20-year-old college student who has been sexually active for 3 years asks if you think it is a good idea for her to be tested for HIV infection. How would you respond to her, and what recommendations would you give and why?

   - Response:
     - Is she in a high risk category?
     - Has she used protection?
     - Has she had multiple partners?
   - Recommendations:
     - If high risk, multiple partners, no protection—testing is indicated
     - Since the period for incubation is up to 10 years, repeat testing is indicated
     - Review strategies to reduce risk for HIV infection if sexually active

2. Your patient is a 68-year-old woman who is hospitalized with a fractured hip. Her long-standing rheumatoid arthritis has been treated with anti-inflammatory medications and corticosteroids periodically for the last 30 years. Describe the parameters you would use to assess her immune function. How would altered immune function affect your care?

   - Review Chapter 46 Chart: Assessment: Indications of Immune Dysfunction
   - Affect of altered immune function on nursing care: Strong emphasis on prevention and early detection of infection

3. A 28-year-old man is seeking treatment for his sixth episode of STD. In addition to assisting with medical management and follow-up, what other interventions would you consider for this patient?

   - Review risk factors, methods of prevention
   - Consider referral for psychiatric counseling

4. During a routine physical examination, a 23-year-old man indicates that he does not perform TSE and does not know how to do so. Develop a teaching plan to instruct him in this examination. How would you modify the plan and approach if the patient is unable to understand English? If the patient has severely impaired vision?

   - Refer to Chapter 45 Chart: Patient Education and Homecare: Testicular Self-Examination
   - For non-English speaking patient:
     - Use print media with diagrams
     - Seek assistance from close family member, spouse, or friend
     - Seek assistance of interpreter
   - For vision-impaired person:
     - Develop audiotape with instructions recited

CHAPTER 47 Management of Patients with Immunodeficiency

1. Gamma-globulin infusions have been prescribed for your patient, who has an immunodeficiency. He tells you that he is very fearful that he may contract HIV infection or AIDS from the infusion. How would you respond to these fears and concerns?

   - Gamma globulin is recovered from pooled human plasma. It is purified and processed for intravenous administration.
   - IV preparations have been shown to be safe by the FDA
   - Refer to Chapter 47 Chart: Pharmacology: Managing a Gamma-Globulin Infusion

2. During a home care visit to a patient who is immunocompromised, you note spoiled food in the kitchen, dirty dishes and countertops, an unclean bathroom, and the presence of several cats and dogs. Explain the course of action you

would take to ensure a safe environment for your patient.

- Assess family members' understanding of significance of being immunocompromised, providing correction and instruction
- Refer to Chapter 47 Chart: Home Care Teaching Checklist: Infection Prevention for the Patient with Immunodeficiency

3. Describe the teaching plan you would use to instruct a patient with an immunodeficiency disorder about prevention and management of infection. How would you modify your approach if the patient understood little English? If the patient was unable to read?

   - Refer to Chapter 47 Chart: Home Care Teaching Checklist: Infection Prevention for the Patient with Immunodeficiency
   - For patient who understood little English:
     - Use diagrams and pictures
     - Speak in simple sentences
     - Seek assistance of family member or friend who speaks English
     - Seek assistance from interpreter
     - Identify resources (family, church, community)
   - Patient unable to read:
     - Provider verbal instruction
     - Prepare audiotape of instruction

CHAPTER 48
Management of Patients with HIV Infection and AIDS

1. A patient tells you that he and his sexual partner are both HIV positive. He informs you that because they both have HIV infection already, they do not practice safe sex. How would you respond to this, and what approach would you use to educate the patient and his partner?

   - Response: potential for infection of others must be considered
   - Approach:
     - Establish rapport
     - Encourage dialogue and open communication
     - Teach both about disease transmission through contact with items soiled by body fluids (by family members, friends, service workers, etc.)
     - Refer to Chapter 48 Plan of Nursing Care: Nursing Diagnosis: Knowledge deficit related to means of preventing HIV transmission

2. You are making a home visit to a patient with HIV encephalopathy. Describe the aspects of the home environment you would assess to ensure safety and adequate care.

   - Refer to Chapter 48 Chart: Guidelines for Care of the Patient with HIV Encephalopathy

3. You are the nurse manager of a medical-surgical unit. A new graduate working on your unit accidentally sticks herself with a needle during a resuscitation effort. She tells you that she is frightened about the possible consequences of this. What actions should you take as nurse manager? What do you tell the new graduate about possible risks and consequences related to her needlestick?

   - Actions taken:
     - Listen to nurse regarding fears
     - Provide factual information as indicated regarding disease transmission
     - Offer counseling, as indicated
     - Follow agency policy regarding follow-up care and testing after needlestick
     - Provide teaching regarding use and disposal of needles
   - Potential risks include infection with bloodborne diseases as well as local cellulitis from the stick
   - Encourage new grad to always report and seek treatment for needlesticks

4. The wife of a patient hospitalized with AIDS asks you directly, "Does my husband have AIDS?" Explain how you would respond to her and why you decided on this course of action.

   - Review agency policy regarding disclosure of HIV status and act accordingly
   - Recognize that nurses are responsible for protecting patient's right to privacy by safeguarding confidential information
   - Ask wife if she has discussed issue with husband—encourage open communication

5. You are caring for a 24-year-old woman who is HIV positive. During your conversation with her, she tells you that she and her husband are considering having a child. She asks you what you think of this idea. How would you respond to her? What information would you consider in your response?

   - Response: What matters is what the patient, her husband, and her treating physician think about a potential pregnancy
   - Recent research indicates that fewer babies born to HIV mothers are demonstrating posi-

tive HIV status—primarily due to medications being taken by the mother

CHAPTER 49
Assessment and Management of Patients with Allergic Disorders

1. During a patient's hospital admission procedure, you inquire about allergies. The patient reports that he is allergic "to everything." Describe the additional information you would obtain from him and how you would document this information on the patient's medical record.
    - Refer to Chapter 49 Chart: Assessment: Allergy Assessment Form
    - Review hospital policy to identify chart and bedside locations for documenting allergies
    - Method for providing allergy information on the patient's body (e.g., wristband)
2. Your patient has had a skin test done before a diagnostic test because of the possibility that she is allergic to the contrast agent that will be used for the test. She reports pruritis, tightness in the throat and chest, and a feeling of anxiety. How would you respond to this situation? Describe the medical management you would anticipate and the nursing strategies you expect to carry out.
    - Reported signs and symptoms indicate allergic reaction and physician should be notified
    - Medical management depends on the severity of the reaction
    - Anticipate need for:
        - Oxygen
        - Patent IV site
        - Epinephrine (1:1000 dilution) for intravenous administration
        - Aminophylline
        - Corticosteroids
        - Vasopressors
        - Glucagon
        - Close observation/monitoring
3. A patient is undergoing extensive diagnostic studies to identify the allergens that are causing her allergic symptoms. What recommendations would you give to her about her home environment? How might you modify those instructions if the patient lives near an industrial area? On a farm? Has small children, each of whom has a favorite pet?
    - Refer to Chapter 49 Chart: Home Care Teaching Checklist: Allergy Management

CHAPTER 50
Assessment and Management of Patients with Rheumatic Disorders

1. You are caring for a 46-year-old woman after a second knee replacement because of RA. She depends on other family members for assistance with most activities because her hands, hips, and knees are severely affected. She tells you that she does not want to be a burden on her family any longer. Explore possible strategies you could suggest she try during her hospitalization and when she is recovering at home.
    - Refer to Chapter 50 Chart: Plan of Nursing Care: Care of the Patient with a Rheumatic Disease: Nursing Diagnosis: Impaired physical mobility related to decreased range of motion, muscle weakness, pain on movement, limited endurance, lack of or improper use of ambulatory devices
2. As a nurse in an immunology clinic, you receive a call from a young woman who has just been informed that her sister has been diagnosed with SLE. She is very concerned about her own risks and those of her children for developing this disorder. How would you respond to her concerns and fears?
    - Response:
        - SLE is a result of disturbed immune regulation that causes an exaggerated production of autoantibodies
        - SLE is brought about by some combination of genetic, hormonal, and environmental factors
3. An elderly woman is admitted for surgery to treat suspected cancer of the colon. She has a history of OA. How would you modify your care of this patient because of the OA?
    - Refer to Chapter 50 Chart: Plan of Nursing Care: Care of the Patient with a Rheumatic Disease: Nursing Diagnosis: Pain and impaired physical mobility
4. An NSAID has been prescribed for your patient because of RA. What instructions and recommendations would you give to the patient to ensure safe administration of this medication? If the patient tells you that she has a hard time remembering whether she has taken her medication, how would you modify or focus you instructions?
    - Instructions/recommendations: Refer to Chapter 50 Table: Medications Used in Rheumatic Diseases—NSAIDS: Action, Use, Indication and Nursing Considerations

- To promote recall:
  - Provide calendar
  - Provide written instructions or audiotaped instructions
  - Include family member, friend, or caregiver in teaching
- 30-year-old mother of two small children:
  - Suggest MD evaluation
  - Instruct regarding bathing, nutrition, hydration, lotions

UNIT **12**
INTEGUMENTARY FUNCTION

CHAPTER 51
Assessment of Integumentary Function

1. An elderly, debilitated patient is to be discharged home to be cared for by her daughter. You know that skin trauma and pressure ulcers can occur if proper care is not carried out. How would you instruct the daughter in preventing these skin problems, especially in someone as old as her mother?
   - Change position
   - Protect bony prominences
   - Avoid shear and friction
   - Ensure skin is kept dry
   - Ensure adequate hydration and nutrition
   - Attend to toileting needs; implement time-void schedule and bowel program
   - Seek MD attention at first sign of increased temperature of skin over bony prominences
2. An elderly patient complains of very dry, itching skin. Based on your knowledge of the skin changes that occur in the elderly, how would you proceed to instruct and guide this patient? What if the patient were a 30-year-old mother of two small children? How would you assess this situation, and what factors might you surmise could be causing the dry, itchy skin in a person of this age?
   - Instruction/guidance:
     - With aging, skin produces less lubrication
     - Apply lotions locally to increase skin moisture
     - Avoid scratching skin
     - Increase hydration
     - Decrease bathing frequency while maintaining hygiene
     - Ensure adequate nutrition
     - Use fabric softener—avoid "scratchy" clothing

CHAPTER 52
Management of Patients with Dermatologic Problems

1. A corticosteroid cream has ben prescribed for a patient at a dermatology clinic. The patient expresses relief that he now has a medicine that he can use to relieve his symptoms whenever they occur. How would you caution this patient about the use of this medication, and how would you explain the reasons for these precautions?
   - Indicate that the medication must be used as prescribed
   - Point out that topical application has systemic effects
   - Prolonged skin use of steroids can result in thinning of skin
2. You are caring for a young man who has had surgery. You notice that his face, arms, and torso are very tan. He states that he does yard work during summer breaks from school and spends time at the beach whenever he can. What type of precautions would you suggest in view of the harmful effects ultraviolet rays can have on skin?
   - Explain damage to all skin layers by ultraviolet rays
   - Describe relationship between ultraviolet ray damage and subsequent development of skin cancers
   - Indicate that damage that occurs at a young age may result in dermatological problems with aging
   - Suggest covering head with hat and using UV-blocking agents
3. A teenage patient requests a diet to control his acne. How would you explain to this patient the nutritional and dietary considerations associated with acne? What other factors might need to be assessed in counseling this patient?
   - Although food restrictions may be recommended, diet does not play a major role in therapy
   - Other factors to consider:
     - Skin hygiene
     - Family history
     - Hormonal factors
     - Bacterial factors
4. A patient in a home for senior citizens has an ill-defined red patch on her face, which she says has

been present for at least 6 months and bleeds when she washes her face. She tells you that the area is painful, and that she has been applying a hydrocortisone cream to it but it is not getting better. How would you assess this situation to determine what course of action to take? Explain your reasoning for deciding how to proceed.

- Because a red patch on the skin is characteristic of a number of disorders—and application of hydrocortisone cream has not improved the patch over time—the patient must be evaluated by a physician or dermatologist
- Report findings to health care provider and seek referral

CHAPTER 53
Management of Patients with Burn Injury

1. A 62-year-old patient is being treated for partial- and full-thickness burns over 20% of her body. She received these burns in her home 3 days ago. She is becoming confused, is refusing to eat or drink fluids, and is not cooperating with dressing changes. She is afebrile and her vital signs have not changed significantly from her baseline values. Analyze these data and explain why you think these cognitive changes have occurred. Based on your analysis, explain the assessment and management strategies you would implement at this time, and describe the patient outcomes that would indicate your interventions have been successful.
   - Cognitive changes may be due to:
     - Electrolyte imbalances
     - Hypoxemia
     - Reaction to medication
     - Assessment and management strategies must be directed to identifying cause, if possible
   - Patient outcomes indicative of successful intervention:
     - Decreased confusion
     - Ability to eat and drink
     - Cooperation with dressing changes
2. An 18-year-old has suffered severe burns of the head and neck, necessitating a tracheostomy. It is expected that the burned areas will require extensive skin grafting. Describe the physical and developmental issues you would consider important in the immediate care of this patient and explain how you would expect these issues to change during the different phases of burn care.
   - Immediate care:
     - Physical issues take priority
     - Refer to Chapter 53 Chart: Plan of Nursing Care: Care of the Patient During the Emergent/Resuscitative Phase of Burn Injury
   - Acute phase:
     - Physical and psychological developmental issues arise (identity, altered body image, self-esteem)
     - Refer to Chapter 53 Chart: Plan of Nursing Care: Care of the Patient During the Acute Phase of Burn Injury
   - Rehabilitative Phase:
     - Developmental issues both psychological (see above) and physical occur (restrictions, limitations, permanent damage, time for regeneration of tissue, spacing of plastic surgeries)
3. Your patient is expected to be discharged from the hospital after 1 month of treatment for severe burns of the legs. What instructions and recommendations would you give to the patient and family to ensure that his recovery will continue? If this patient lived alone, how would you modify your teaching and discharge planning?
   - Refer to Chapter 53 Chart: Home Care Teaching Checklist: The Patient with a Burn Injury
   - If patient lived alone, refer for home visit and evaluation of home situation. Identify resources and support systems (personal and community) available.

UNIT 13
SENSORINEURAL FUNCTION

CHAPTER 54
Assessment and Management of Patients with Eye and Vision Disorders

1. During a follow-up telephone call with a nurse after cataract surgery, the patient reports that his eye that was operated on is red and painful and that he cannot see clearly. He states that acetaminophen does not relieve the pain, particularly in the last 12 hours, that the redness has increased over the last 24 hours, and that is vision is hazy and blurred compared with the morning after surgery. What are the implications of these signs and symptoms? What nursing actions are appropriate?

- Refer to Chapter 54 Chart: Potential Complications of Cataract Surgery (Early postoperative complications)
- If the nurse is employed by the opthalmologist, he or she must report the observations immediately
- If the nurse is employed by an institution, such as a hospital or clinic where cataract surgeries are performed, the nurse instructs the patient to contact the opthalmologist immediately

2. A patient who has sustained an eyelid laceration is seen by the emergency department staff and found to have decreased peripheral vision and IOPs of 34 and 38 mm Hg. The ophthalomologist informs the patient of the significance of these findings and arranges for follow-up with a glaucoma specialist. The patient informs the nurse he has been on glaucoma medication for 3 years but stopped taking it 5 months ago because he could not afford the medication. He does not see the need to go to a specialist for follow-up. What nursing actions are appropriate?
   - Social work referral to determine sources of financial support available for the patient
   - Patient education focusing on the complications that will occur when glaucoma is not treated

CHAPTER 55
Assessment and Management of Patients with Hearing and Balance Disorders

1. An elderly patient in an extended care facility appears withdrawn and distrustful of others. She does not participate in conversations with other residents. You suspect that she has a hearing loss. Describe the strategies you would use to assess this patient's hearing. What intervention strategies would you implement if your assessment confirms that the woman has a hearing loss? If your assessment indicates that she does NOT have a hearing loss?
   - Assessment strategies:
     - Otoscopic inspection
     - Whisper test
     - Watch tick test
   - Hearing loss:
     - Seek physician consult for evaluation and treatment
   - No hearing loss:
     - Complete physical assessment
     - Review of prescribed medications (considerations: overdosage, interactions)
     - Seek physician consult for evaluation and treatment

2. An antiemetric and a tranquilizer have been prescribed for a patient with Meniere's disease. You realize that safety precautions are indicated. Devise a teaching plan for this patient and explain the reasons behind each part of the plan.
   - Refer to Chapter 55 Chart: Plan of Nursing Care: Care of the Patient with Vertigo
   - Implement patient education principles regarding motivation, readiness, learning environment, and teaching techniques
   - Point out focus on promoting independence in daily living

3. The daughter of an elderly patient complains that her father refuses to use his hearing aid. How would you focus your assessment to gather other pertinent information in determining a plan of action? Describe the patient outcomes you anticipate your interventions will achieve.
   - Refer to Chapter 55 Chart: Hearing Aid Problems
   - Implement strategies to resolve identified problems
   - Provide patient education for father and daughter regarding hearing aid problems and how to resolve them using patient education principles

UNIT 14
NEUROLOGIC FUNCTION

CHAPTER 56
Assessment of Neurologic Function

1. Your patient is scheduled to have a lumbar puncture (spinal tap), and says she is afraid that she may end up paralyzed as a result of the procedure. Based on your knowledge of the anatomy and physiology of the CNS, how would you structure your explanation to reassure the patient and dispel her fears?
   - Establish rapport
   - Assess patient's education level and cognitive ability, tailoring instruction accordingly
   - Provide instruction, referring to textbook pictures, if possible to point out the spinal cord and the fluid surrounding the cord
   - Explain to the patient that the needle is advanced very slowly, and the physician observes the needle for outflow of spinal fluid with each adjustment; therefore, the needle is advanced no further than the fluid space

- Further, the needle is inserted between the third, fourth, or fifth lumbar vertebra—and the spinal cord divides into a sheath of nerves at the first lumbar vertebrae
- Paralysis would occur if the spinal cord were damaged by the needle—emphasizing why patient positioning and cooperation are essential to the examination
- Refer to Chapter 56 Chart: Guidelines for Assisting with a Lumbar Puncture

2. Your patient is to have MRI. How would you explain the test to the patient and the precautions that are needed before the procedure? How would you adjust your approach if the patient has difficulty understanding English? If the patient is elderly and has severe skeletal deformities?

- Explanation and precautions:
  - MRI uses a magnetic field to obtain images of different areas of the body
  - All metal objects and credit cards must be removed before patient enters room where MRI is to be performed
  - Patient must be assessed for any INTERNAL metal objects (e.g., aneurysm clips, orthopedic hardware, pacemakers, artificial heart valves, intrauterine devices) because internal medial objects may be dislodged, could malfunction, or may heat up as they absorb energy
  - Scanning process is painless—but patient hears loud thumping of the magnetic coils as the magnetic field is being pulsed
- Patient who has difficulty understanding English:
  - Use pictures, diagrams
  - Use simple sentences
  - Seek assistance from family member, friend, or interpreter
  - Identify community resources that may be of assistance
- Patient with skeletal deformities:
  - Patient lies on a platform during the procedure and may require preprocedure medication to allay anxiety
  - May require medication during procedure to be able to tolerate pain associated with lying on the platform
  - May require supervised recovery from medications given postprocedure

CHAPTER 57
Management of Patients with Neurologic Dysfunction

1. Your patient had symptoms of an ischemic stroke approximately 2 hours ago and is undergoing a confirmatory CT scan in 30 minutes. You know t-PA must be administered within 3 hours of the symptoms. What actions would you take? What is your rationale for these actions?

- Actions:
  - Review MD notes or confirm with MD that patient is a candidate for t-PA since multiple criteria must be met (not just time limitation)
  - Determine from MD who will administer t-PA, confirm MD's interpretation of time constraints, and seek his or her counsel regarding facilitation of the procedure
  - Refer to hospital policy and procedure regarding administration of t-PA

2. After undergoing cranial surgery, your patient has had elevated ICP for 15 minutes. Mannitol, an osmotic diuretic, was administered, but the ICP remains unchanged. The patient is receiving sedation and pain medication. Describe some other interventions that may be initiated.

- Refer to Chapter 57 Chart: Increased ICP and Interventions

3. Your patient is admitted with hemorrhagic stroke and exhibits homonymous hemianopsia. How would you explain this phenomenon to the patient and family? Describe ways that the patient and family may work together to compensate for this problem.

- Homonymous heminopsia (loss of half of the visual field) may be temporary or permanent
- The affected side of vision corresponds to the paralyzed side of the body
- Refer to Chapter 57 Chart: Neurologic Deficits of Stroke: Manifestations and Nursing Implications—Visual Field Defects

4. A 50-year-old patient is scheduled for several diagnostic tests (MRI, evoked potentials, and lumbar puncture) to determine the cause of a recent onset of sensory and motor symptoms. After the tests, he is expected to go home. He tells you that he lives alone in a small apartment; he knows none of his neighbors. What teaching would be indicated for him? What resources may be needed to enable him to go home as scheduled?

- Teaching (both verbal and written):
  - Postlumbar puncture: Potential for development of headache (managed by bed rest, analgesics, and hydration)
  - Complications (temporary voiding problems, slight elevation of temperature, backache or spasms, and stiffness of the neck)
  - Signs and symptoms to report
- Resources:
  - Home care nurse
  - Family or friend to make frequent contact post procedure (hours to days)
  - Community (e.g., church, social organizations)

CHAPTER 58
Management of Patients with Neurologic Trauma

1. A patient has been brought to the emergency department after a fall on his head at work. He says he was knocked out for about 10 minutes but now seems alert and oriented. What type of injury has he most likely sustained? What discharge instructions are warranted for this patient's family? How would you modify your discharge instructions if the patient lives alone?
   - Most likely injury: concussion
   - Discharge instructions: Return to ED or notify MD or clinic if patient demonstrates:
     - Difficulty in awakening
     - Difficulty in speaking
     - Confusion
     - Severe headache
     - Vomiting
     - Weakness on one side of body
   - If patient lives alone:
     - Contact family member or friend to stay with patient overnight
     - If no other individual is available, speak with MD and seek social work consult to hospitalize patient overnight for observation
     - Refer to Chapter 58 Chart: Home Care Teaching Checklist: The Patient with a Head Injury
2. A patient with a T4 SCI has just returned to the nursing unit from physical therapy. He reports a severe, pounding headache and nausea. His blood pressure is very elevated and his pulse is slow. What are the possible causes of these signs and symptoms? What immediate actions should you take? What medical treatments can you anticipate? What teaching is warranted, and why?
   - Patient is exhibiting signs of autonomic hyperreflexia, an acute emergency that occurs as a result of exaggerated autonomic responses to stimuli that are innocuous in normal people
   - Actions/anticipated medical treatments:
     - Place patient in sitting position
     - Perform rapid assessment to identify and alleviate cause
     - Empty bladder via urinary catheter; assure patency if catheter is in place
     - Examine rectum for fecal mass; if so, insert topical anesthetic prior to attempting to remove
     - Examine skin for areas of pressure, irritation, or breakage
     - Observe environmental stimuli that may be affecting patient (draft of cold air, object on the skin)
     - If hypertension is not relieved, anticipate administration of Apresoline
     - Label patient's medical record regarding risk for autonomic hyperreflexia
   - Teaching regarding autonomic hyperreflexia :
     - Is provided to every patient with SCI above T6
     - Emergency nature of problem is emphasized
     - Preventive and management strategies must be understood by patient and family
     - Written as well as verbal instruction should be given

CHAPTER 59
Management of Patients with Neurologic Disorders

1. Your patient has been informed that she has MS. She is distraught and believes that MS is the same as ALS, which caused rapid deterioration and death in a family friend. How would you explain the differences between MS and ALS to her, and how would you devise a program to help her adjust to the diagnosis? Describe the patient behaviors that would indicate a successful outcome.
   - Differences:
     - MS is chronic degenerative neurologic disorder affecting myelin sheath covering brain and spinal cord; ALS is disease of lower motor neuron death
     - MS is a disease that can be controlled and remains stable in many patients; ALS is a disease that cannot be controlled
   - Program: Refer to Chapter 59 Chart: Home Care Teaching Checklist: The Patient with Multiple Sclerosis
   - Patient behaviors demonstrating successful outcome:
     - Adapts to impaired mobility and spasticity
     - Avoids injury
     - Attains or maintains improved bladder and bowel control
     - Participates in strategies to improve speech
     - Compensates for cognitive dysfunction
     - Demonstrates improved coping strategies
     - Adapts to changes in sexual function
2. A patient who is experiencing frequent migraine headaches is being treated at a local clinic. She does not understand the relationship between her headaches and the recommended dietary restrictions. How would you explain this relationship and the reasons for the dietary restrictions? What assessment parameters would you expect were explored to determine other factors that would precipitate her headaches?

- Refer to Chapter 59 Chart: Home Care Teaching Checklist: The Patient with Migraine Headaches

3. While you are in the grocery store, another shopper experiences a grand mal seizure. How would you respond to this event, and why would you take these actions? If the shopper had a 3-year-old with her, how might you address this additional consideration?

- Response: Protect patient from injury (remove articles in the area of the seizure) and contact EMS (Refer to Chapter 59 Chart: Guidelines for Care of the Patient Having a Seizure)
- While seizure may be self-limiting, status epilepticus can result in death.
- Oxygen therapy, intravenous access, and transport to emergency room should be available to the patient
- 3-year-old child:
  - Console and reassure child
  - Stay with child until official authorities take custody of the child

4. You have a patient with epilepsy who develops status epilepticus. Based on your knowledge of this disorder, describe the medical management you would anticipate to control the seizures and the nursing measures that are indicated. Identify the patient outcomes that would indicate that the goals have been achieved.

- Medical management anticipated:
  - Airway maintenance (potential ET tube insertion)
  - Oxygenation
  - Establishment of intravenous line
  - Intravenous Valium, Ativan, Cerebrex
  - Continuing monitoring of vital signs and neurologic signs
  - Blood studies to determine serum levels of medications
- Nursing measures:
  - Side-lying position
  - Ongoing assessment
  - Suction equipment available
  - Maintenance of IV line (may become dislodged during seizuring)
  - Refer to Chapter 59 Chart: Guidelines for the Care of a Patient Having a Seizure
- Patient outcomes:
  - Patient demonstrates adequate respiratory function (oxygen saturations)
  - Seizure activity subsides
  - Patient recovers from seizure activity

5. A patient assigned to your care has been admitted to the hospital for control of myasthenic crisis. Describe the differences between myasthenic crisis and cholinergic crisis. Explain how your nursing actions would differ for myasthenic and cholinergic crisis and what the underlying rationale would be for these interventions.

- Differences:
  - Myasthenic crisis is the sudden onset of muscular weakness in patients with MG and usually the result of undermedication or no cholinergic medication at all
  - Cholinergic crisis occurs in the patient with MG when that patient is overmedicated with cholinergic or anticholinesterase agents
  - Symptoms of either crisis require medical intervention
  - Intravenous edrophonium is used to differentiate the type of crisis
- Nursing interventions:
  - Providing adequate ventilatory assistance in the management of myasthenic crisis
  - Follow MD evaluation of patient response to edrophonium closely
- Anticipate:
  - ABGs and serum electrolyte evaluations
  - Daily weight and intake and output
  - NG tube feedings if patient is unable to swallow
  - AVOID sedatives and tranquilizers

UNIT 15 MUSCULOSKELETAL FUNCTION

CHAPTER 60 Assessment of Musculoskeletal Function

1. A young man who has a cast applied to his fractured arm expresses concern that he will lose muscle strength because he cannot exercise his arm. How would you respond to him and address his concern? If the patient were an elderly woman who had broken her arm in a fall and now was fearful of falling again, how would your approach differ in addressing this patient's concerns?

- Response to young man: While disuse does result in atrophy, isometric exercises can be performed while cast is in place to decrease the effects of immobility
- Elderly patient response: Isometric exercises must be cleared with physician because they are contraindicated in patients with hyperten-

sion, a disease often affecting the elderly. In addition:
- Fear of falling in the elderly demonstrates recognition of a daily threat
- Patient should be taught safety precautions, such as:
  - Rise from sitting or reclining positions slowly
  - Wear nonslip footwear
  - Allow sufficient time for toileting needs
  - Have vision checked, at least annually
  - Seek assistance with ambulation
  - Use handrails
  - If gait becomes unstable, seek physician evaluation and referral for physical therapy instruction and assistive devices

3. The son of an elderly patient asks why his mother is "so much shorter than she used to be." How would you explain this phenomenon to him? How might you incorporate preventive measures related to his mother's musculoskeletal condition into a teaching session?
   - Explanation: Loss of height with aging is due to:
     - Osteoporosis
     - Kyphosis
     - Thinned intervertebral discs
     - Flexion of the knees and hips
   - Instruct son regarding his mother's need for:
     - Adequate diet
     - Adequate intake of calcium
     - Exercise
     - Follow-up care with physician (regarding hormone replacement therapy)
4. After arthroscopy, a patient complains that the dressing on his knee is too tight. He begins to loosen it. How would you react to his actions and why? If the patient had removed the dressing during the night without being detected and you discovered the fact early the next morning, how would the patient's situation have changed, and how would you respond to this different set of circumstances?
   - Nurse observes patient removing dressing:
     - Reinstruct patient that the dressing is a compression dressing used to control swelling postarthroscopy
     - Advise patient that nurse will monitor neurovascular status to prevent complications from compression
     - Inform patient that analgesics are available for discomfort
   - Patient unwraps dressing—undetected by nurse until early next morning:
     - Perform complete assessment—with particular observation of compromised neurovascular status due to swelling
     - Inform surgeon, provide report of status, and seek direction regarding reapplication of compression dressing

CHAPTER 61
Musculoskeletal Care Modalities

1. You are caring for two patients in the same room. One patient has had a knee replacement. The other patient has had a hip replacement. Both patients are experiencing pain. How would you compare and contrast pain management strategies for each patient? How would you describe the differences in general care related to their respective mobility limitations?
   - Pain management strategies:
     - Multiple approaches are used and will vary according to patient's age, procedure, and surgeon (PCA; intermittent IV, IM, and oral analgesics)
     - While the leg may be elevated and ice may be applied to control the pain of the patient with TKA (total knee arthroplasty), the same strategies are not used with the patient with THA (total hip arthroplasty)
   - General care:
     - Patient with TKA has restriction of affected leg only
     - Patient with THA must be instructed and observed closely to prevent hip dislocation (sitting, bending, any adduction of affected hip joint)
2. A patient who was in a motor vehicle crash has a cast on his leg. He complains that the cast feels tight and that the pain medication is not relieving his pain. What do you think is happening? What actions would you take and why?
   - Primary concern: Compartment syndrome
   - Nursing should report increasing and uncontrollable pain to the orthopedic surgeon for evaluation
   - Neurovascular status must be assessed very frequently
3. A patient who has had internal fixation of the hip complains about her elastic stockings and requests that they be removed. How would you respond to this request, and how would you explain the purpose of the stockings? The patient does not understand English and keeps trying to remove the stockings. Describe two different strategies you could follow in this circumstance and the pros and cons of each intervention.
   - Elastic stockings (anti-embolic stockings):
     - Stockings should be removed daily for inspection of skin and hygiene with reapplication
     - Purpose: To promote venous return and prevent stagnation of blood in leg veins (predisposing to thrombus formation)
   - Non-English-speaking patient:
     - Seek assistance from family member or close friend

- Request assistance from interpreter
- Strategy: Inform physician of patient's behavior and seek order to remove stocking
  - Physician may not grant order
  - Patient may develop DVT and pulmonary embolus
- Strategy: Use analgesic or sedative medication
  - Medication, in this instance, would be used as chemical restraint and may have legal implications for nurse
  - Complications resulting from sedation (inadequate respiration, immobility) may occur

4. You are caring for two patients in the same room. One patient has skeletal traction applied to his leg, and the other has skin (Buck's) traction. The patients ask you why their traction setups are different. How would you explain the differences to them? Describe the different priorities of care for each of these patients.

- Different types of fractures and their treatment require different types of traction
- Skeletal traction is applied directly to the bone
- Skin traction is used to control muscle spasm and to immobilize an area prior to surgery
- Different priorities:
  - Patient with skeletal traction will have pin insertion sites that require inspection and daily care—they may be source of infection
  - Patient with skin traction may develop skin breakdown

5. You are making a home visit to a patient who had experienced an open fracture of the lower leg. The fracture is being managed with an external fixator. What would you include in your assessment of the fixator and the pin sites? During your assessment, the patient states that the pin in the foot is tender, and it is loose on examination.

- Refer to Chapter 61 Chart: Home Care Teaching Checklist: The Patient with an External Fixator
- Tenderness in the foot may indicate development of infection, nerve pressure, or neurovascular compromise and should be reported to the physician.
- Any change in the appliance must be reported to the physician for evaluation

CHAPTER 62
Management of Patients with Musculoskeletal Disorders

1. A classmate who has a small child states that she has been having low back pain for several months. She asks for your advice. Describe how you would assess this situation, indicate the questions you would ask, and explain the kind of information you are seeking and why. How would your thinking redirect your assessment if the woman is (a) overweight, (b) jogs regularly, and (c) is expecting another child?

- Ask classmate to:
  - Describe discomfort (location, severity, duration, characteristics, radiation, associated weakness in the legs)
  - Describe how pain occurred (e.g., with specific action)
  - Describe how she has dealt with pain
  - Describe how back pain has affected lifestyle
- Refer to Chapter 62 Chart: Health Promotion and Illness: The Patient with Low Back Pain
- Refer to Chapter 62 Chart: Patient Education and Homecare: Activities to Promote a Healthy Back

2. You volunteer to help with a health fair in your community. You are asked to participate in the booth that will offer information about osteoporosis. How would your advice differ when you are talking to (a) teenagers, (b) older adults, and (c) elderly people? Explain the reasons for your modifications.

- Refer to Chapter 62 Chart: Home Care Teaching Checklist: Osteoporosis

3. You are visiting with a patient in an extended care facility. The patient's daughter states that her mother has osteoarthritis and her aunt has osteoporosis. She asks if these conditions are the same because her mother and aunt got them late in life and both are debilitated. What explanations do you feel would be helpful to her? How would the care of people with these two disorders differ? How would the care be similar?

- Differences:
  - Osteoarthritis is a degenerative disease believed to be related to wear and tear on joints over time
  - Osteoporosis is a disorder to decrease in total bone mass and change in bone structure
  - Care would differ in terms of pain management (osteoarthritis is associated with joint pain and aching; osteoporosis is not associated with pain); diet (intake of calcium and vitamin D may delay effects of osteoporosis; diet is not known to directly affect osteoarthritis); exercise (exercise is indicated for treatment of osteoporosis; exercise may cause extreme pain in osteoarthritis)
- Care would be similar in terms of:
  - Potentially altered mobility
  - Safety considerations

CHAPTER 63 Management of Patients with Musculoskeletal Trauma

1. A classmate tells you that she is going to start jogging and that her goal is to run in a marathon in several months. Describe the kind of advice you would give her and explain your rationale for making these suggestions.
   - Sports-related injuries (contusions, strains, and sprains) can be prevented by:
     - Using proper equipment (e.g., running shoes)
     - Effectively training and conditioning the body
     - Using a warm-up routine followed by slow, gradual stretching (stretch is held for 10 to 20 seconds before relaxing and repeating the stretch
     - After exercise, cool-down should take place wherein activity changes and decreased stress takes place gradually (e.g., if running or jogging, continue to walk, slowly decreasing pace)
2. A middle-aged patient who has been hospitalized for 3 days with a fractured pelvis is making plans for discharge. His wife approaches you and expresses concern that he has become very irritable and that he "just doesn't seem to be himself." Analyze this information and speculate as to the possible causes for this behavior. Describe the additional kinds of information you would seek in a further assessment of the situation. What findings would confirm you initial speculation? What findings would lead to a different conclusion.
   - Nurse's suspicion: Fat embolism syndrome
   - Assessment should include:
     - Vital signs, temperature, pulse, respirations
     - Pulse oximetry
     - Mental status examination
     - Auscultation of breath sounds
     - Inspection for pallor and petechiae
     - Suspicion should be reported to physician
   - Nurse anticipates:
     - Arterial blood gas evaluation
     - Establishing patent IV site
     - Respiratory support with oxygen in high concentration
     - Vasoactive medications
     - Accurate intake and output monitoring
     - Medication to treat pain and anxiety
   - Suspicion confirmed by:
     - Hypoxia, tachypnea, tachycardia, ABG value of PO_2 below 60 mm Hg with an early respiratory alkalosis
   - Suspicion disconfirmed by:
     - Not finding previously described signs and symptoms
3. You witness a person falling on a patch of ice and you offer assistance. She does not seem to be seriously injured, but she complains that her left elbow is sore and her left hand feels weak. She indicates that she thinks she can drive herself home and will then decide if she needs to seek medical attention. What conclusions would you draw from the complaints she described. Based on that conclusion, how would you advise her and why?
   - Complaints described indicates that at a minimum, she has soft tissue injury, and she may have a fracture
   - Weakness in hand suggests nerve trauma may have occurred
   - Advise her to visit ED or clinic since early treatment can prevent permanent damage
4. You are visiting an elderly gentleman who is in an extended care facility recovering from a below-the-knee amputation. He expresses satisfaction that he has progressed to the point that he has the stamina to sit in his wheelchair from breakfast time until after dinner. How would you advise him to modify his daily routine and why? Describe the plan of care you would devise for him and the outcomes you hope to have him achieve through this plan.
   - While the patient's desire to be active is to be commended, the nurse must caution the patient about the complications from sitting in one position for so many hours as well as the sitting position resulting in flexion of the knee joint.
   - The leg must be straightened and elevated periodically to promote venous return and prevent breakdown of the incision line.
   - Plan:
     - Up in chair for two hours, maximum
     - Supine or dorsal recumbent position for 45 minutes to one hour
     - Flexion and extension exercise of knee joint
   - Outcomes:
     - No pressure sores
     - No breakdown of incision line
     - Ability to flex and extend knee joint

UNIT 16 OTHER ACUTE PROBLEMS

CHAPTER 64 Management of Patients with Infectious Diseases

1. A nurse who is returning to nursing after 10 years is being oriented to your nursing unit. She is assigned to take care of a patient with AIDS. She questions why the patient is not isolated. What conclusions might you draw from the comment? To ensure appropriate care for this patient, how would you explain to the nurse the best way to approach AIDS patients when giving care?
   - Conclusion:
     - Orienting nurse does not understand the disease, particularly modes of transmission
     - Orienting nurse requires teaching regarding the disease as well as CDC and hospital guidelines regarding universal precautions
   - Explanation:
     - Virus is very weak, cannot survive for long outside the body, and is transmitted through body fluids and secretions
     - Universal precautions (reviewed in detail) provide protection in working with the AIDS patients
     - Approach to AIDS patient should be nonjudgmental, courteous, and attentive
2. You are supervising a patient care technician who is changing the bed of a postoperative patient. There is fresh blood on the patient's sheet from a venipuncture that was performed. The technician is not wearing gloves as she disposes of the linen. How would you evaluate the situation, and what action would you take? Explain the rationale for your decision.
   - Evaluation: The technician has not been instructed about communicable disease transmission, has forgotten concepts and techniques of reducing risk of contracting communicable diseases in the hospital setting, or knows of the potential risks and complications and has chosen not to wear gloves while changing soiled linen.
   - Action:
     - Inquire as to technician's understanding of direct skin contact with fresh blood (to establish basis for additional interventions)
     - Provide teaching as indicated
     - Provide reinforcement of instruction as indicated
     - Review hospital policy and procedure
     - Send tech to health center for evaluation of potential exposure risks and necessary precautions or potential prophylaxis
3. An elderly patient with cardiac disease questions you about why her physician suggested that she received an influenza vaccination. She states the she received the vaccination years ago and then got the flu from the vaccine. How would you respond to her and explain the situation? Describe the line of reasoning you would follow to convince her to get the vaccine. If she rejects your explanation, examine the different courses of action you could take and the pros and cons of each strategy.
   - Response/Explanation:
     - Establish rapport
     - Offer facts to substantiate benefits of vaccine: Vaccine does not cause flu — probably, exposure had taken place prior to vaccination; vaccine prevents flu in the majority of individuals; if a vaccinated patient becomes infected with the flu, the vaccine will decrease the severity of the illness; vaccination results in preventing pneumonia and hospitalization in the elderly patient who becomes infected 50%–70% of the time and is 80% effective in preventing death
     - Because of her cardiac disease, patient is at increased risk of cardiac complications from the flu
   - Different courses of action:
     - Accept patient's refusal of vaccine: Pro—recognizes patient's right to refuse illness; con—patient may not survive influenza infection:
     - Report patient's resistance to MD: Pro—MD may be able to convince patient; con—MD may inform nurse to TELL patient she is GOING to take the vaccine (ethical dilemma)

CHAPTER 65 Emergency Nursing

1. A young man arrives at the ED by ambulance after a car crash. He is immobilized on a backboard with a cervical collar. An oxygen mask is in place. You note shallow, slow respirations and no movement of the left chest wall. His scalp is bleeding, and his left leg is angulated. How would you prioritize the patient's needs? Generate an assessment strategy and describe the patient's treatment needs.

- Priority:
  - Chest Xray to determine potential rib fractures, collapsed left lung, and pneumothorax
  - Since respiratory functioning is not satisfactory, assuring adequate ventilation is priority
  - Cause for deficient function must be established and remedied
  - Scalp wound can be covered with pressure dressing and leg can be immobilized pending patient stabilization

2. A homeless man comes to the ED for treatment of frostbite of his feet. He insists that his feet be placed in a pan of hot water. Describe how you would respond and the explanation you would give to this patient. How would you proceed with managing this patient? Describe the discharge planning issues to be addressed for a homeless person.

   - Response: Hot water would cause tissue damage; passive rewarming with the use of warm blankets is indicated
   - Nurse must use therapeutic communications techniques to assess patient's understanding of and experience with frostbite
   - Nurse must assess educational level and cognitive abilities and provide instruction accordingly
   - Discharge planning:
     - Make social work referral to determine community resources that may provide support to homeless persons
     - Provide written instruction as well as verbal instruction regarding treatment and follow-up care

3. A young woman with a toddler in her arms waits her turn in line at the triage desk of the ED. The child is crying and rubbing her eyes and face. You overhear the mother telling another patient that the child has had an allergic reaction to her first soft-cooked egg, which the child smeared on her face. Analyze this information and explain the conclusion you would draw and why. Then describe the action you would take and the rationale for your decision.

   - Conclusion: Child is not manifesting symptoms of allergic reaction (Refer to Chapter 65 Chart: Assessment Signs and Symptoms of Anaphylaxis)
   - Although eggs are recognized as potentially allergenic to many people, the child reportedly did not ingest the eggs—she smeared them on her face
   - Child may be crying because she rubbed egg into her eyes as well
   - Actions:
     - Calm child and mother
     - Cleanse face and rinse eyes with water
     - Ask mother to describe, with detail, events that had transpired
     - Monitor child for untoward signs/symptoms

4. An elderly patient is brought to the ED by her son. She is complaining of pain in her hip, and the son says that she tripped over a child's toy and fell. Upon initial assessment you notice that the patient has many bruises on her body in varying stages of resolution. What conclusions might you draw from these findings and how might you proceed to evaluate the situation to determine your course of action?

   - Conclusions:
     - None at this time—insufficient information
     - Suspicion for elder abuse
     - Obtain additional information from son and from patient separately
     - Medications being taken (specifically, anticoagulants, antiplatelet medications, NSAIDs, salicylates)
     - Nature of fall (when, where, what kind of toy, circumstances leading to toy being in patient's path, etc.)
     - Medical history
     - Perform complete physical assessment
     - Discuss findings with nurse practitioner or MD
     - Review institutional policy and procedure regarding reporting of suspected elder abuse

SECTION 3

TESTBANK

UNIT 1
BASIC CONCEPTS IN NURSING PRACTICE

CHAPTER 1
Health Care Delivery and Nursing Practice

1. A nurse is caring for a homeless client at a shelter. According to Maslow's hierarchy of needs, before the client can achieve his safety needs, he must first meet his need for
   A. affection.
   B. self-esteem.
   *C. food.
   D. belonging.

   Rationale: Before a client can address his need for safety and shelter, physiologic needs must be met first. These needs include food and water.

   Reference: p. 4

   Descriptors:
   1. 01 2. 01 3. Application
   4. IV–3 5. Nursing Process 6. Moderate

2. A primary goal of health care providers today is to
   *A. promote positive behaviors in clients.
   B. reduce the number of adolescent pregnancies.
   C. provide chronic illness care to the elderly.
   D. decrease acuity of hospitalized clients.

   Rationale: Wellness has been defined as being the equivalent of health. With this in mind, a primary goal of health care providers today is to promote wellness, or positive behaviors in clients.

   Reference: p. 5

   Descriptors:
   1. 01 2. 01 3. Application
   4. IV–3 5. Nursing Process 6. Moderate

3. The population in the United States is changing, and these changes will affect health care in the future. Health care providers of the future will be influenced by
   A. increasing numbers of newborns and toddlers.
   B. migration of middle-income families to the cities.
   C. increasing numbers of middle-aged men in the population.
   *D. increasing numbers of senior citizens who require health care.

   Rationale: The birth rate is declining while the life span is increasing. There will be an increased number of senior citizens who require health care, and this may influence costs.

   Reference: p. 5

   Descriptors:
   1. 01 2. 02 3. Comprehension
   4. IV–1 5. Nursing Process 6. Easy

4. Population demographics have an effect on health care and health care providers. One of the fastest growing segments of the population are individuals over the age of
   *A. 85 years.
   B. 50 years.
   C. 20 years.
   D. 10 years.

   Rationale: Those individuals over 85 years constitute one of the fastest-growing segments of the population. Women are expected to outnumber men.

   Reference: p. 6

   Descriptors:
   1. 01 2. 02 3. Knowledge
   4. II–1 5. Nursing Process 6. Moderate

5. Changing illness patterns will affect health care of the present and the future. The illnesses that have been increasing in the population in the United States include
   A. accidental injuries.
   *B. chronic conditions.
   C. childhood infectious diseases.
   D. mental deterioration.

   Rationale: Almost 50% of the population has one or more chronic conditions. Health care will be focused on providing care to older individuals with these chronic illnesses, e.g., arthritis.

   Reference: p. 6

   Descriptors:
   1. 01 2. 02 3. Application
   4. IV–3 5. Nursing Process 6. Moderate

6. Because of concerns over spiraling health care costs, the federal government altered the Medicare program to pay providers based on
   A. length of hospital stays.
   B. acuity of the client's condition.
   C. need for technology to provide care.
   *D. diagnostic related groups.

   Rationale: Spiraling health care costs and wide variations in charges among providers led the federal government to alter Medicare payments based on diagnostic related groups and the prospective payment system.

   Reference: pp. 6–7

   Descriptors:
   1. 01 2. 02 3. Knowledge
   4. IV–1 5. Nursing Process 6. Moderate

7. Unlike Quality Assurance programs that focus on individual incidents, Continuous Quality Improvement programs focus on
   A. decreasing length of hospital stays.
   *B. the processes used to provide care.
   C. alternative medical therapies.
   D. providing minimal expectations for care.

Rationale: Quality Assurance programs, which were developed by JCAHO, focused on individual incidents or errors and minimal expectations. Continuous Quality Improvement Programs focus on the processes used to provide care with the aim of improving quality by improving the processes.

Reference: p. 7

Descriptors:
1. 01 2. 01 3. Comprehension
4. IV–1 5. Nursing Process 6. Difficult

8. One common feature of managed health care includes
   A. designated copayments by the client.
   *B. prenegotiated payment rates.
   C. use of physician assistants.
   D. wide variety of health care providers.

Rationale: Common features of managed care include prenegotiated payment rates, mandatory precertification, limited choice of provider, and fixed price reimbursement.

Reference: p. 8

Descriptors:
1. 01 2. 0-3 3. Comprehension
4. IV–1 5. Nursing Process 6. Moderate

9. Managed care has resulted in
   A. increased length of treatment.
   B. increased resources.
   *C. more severely ill clients.
   D. less competition among providers.

Rationale: Managed care has resulted in more severely ill clients, shorter hospital stays, increased home care, and more competition among providers.

Reference: p. 9

Descriptors:
1. 01 2. 03 3. Knowledge
4. IV–1 5. Nursing Process 6. Moderate

10. A nurse is employed by a hospital focusing on managing a client caseload with fractured hip and total hip replacements. This nurse serves as a
   *A. case manager.
   B. client advocate.
   C. nursing supervisor.
   D. team leader.

Rationale: Case managers focus on managing a caseload of clients with certain diagnoses. They collaborate care with other nurses and promote coordination for home care following hospitalization.

Reference: p. 9

Descriptors:
1. 01 2. 03 3. Application
4. IV–1 5. Nursing Process 6. Moderate

11. A nurse researcher is conducting a study about the effects of noise on client pain levels while hospitalized. The primary purpose of nursing research is to
   A. involve clients in their care while hospitalized.
   *B. contribute to the scientific base of nursing practice.
   C. draw conclusions about the quality of client care.
   D. explain ongoing medical studies to clients.

Rationale: Nursing research may be conducted by direct care providers or nurse researchers. The primary purpose of nursing research is to contribute to the scientific base of nursing and improve nursing practice based on evidence.

Reference: p. 11

Descriptors:
1. 01 2. 04 3. Application
4. I–1 5. Nursing Process 6. Difficult

12. A nurse is employed in an acute care setting and provides care to the client during the client's entire hospital stay and has 24-hour accountability for the client's care. The nurse is functioning as a
   A. team leader.
   B. nursing supervisor.
   C. critical path manager.
   *D. primary nurse.

Rationale: Primary nursing pertains to individualized care provided by the same nurse during the entire hospital stay. The nurse has 24-hour accountability for the client's care. Most institutions view this as too costly and have moved to case management.

Reference: p. 12

Descriptors:
1. 01 2. 05 3. Application
4. IV–1 5. Nursing Process 6. Moderate

13. The practice setting for nursing that is becoming the largest area is
   A. intensive care nursing.
   B. emergency room nursing.
   C. pediatric nursing.
   *D. home health nursing.

Rationale: As a result of decreased hospital stays and more critically ill clients being released to home, home health care is becoming one of the largest practice areas for nursing.

Reference: p. 12

Descriptors:
1. 01 2. 06 3. Application
4. I–1 5. Nursing Process 6. Moderate

14. A nurse who provides primary health care to specific clients, collaborates with other health professionals, and has prescriptive authority is termed a
   A. nurse generalist.
   B. clinical nurse specialist.
   C. independent practice nurse.
   *D. nurse practitioner.

Rationale: Nurse practitioners are prepared as generalists, usually for a specific population, and provide primary health care. Many states allow prescriptive authority. Clinical nurse specialists practice within a circumscribed area of care, e.g., cardiac, and most practice in acute care (secondary) settings.

Reference: p. 13

Descriptors:
1. 01 2. 06 3. Application
4. I–1 5. Nursing Process 6. Moderate

15. A nurse is employed in an acute care setting within a decentralized structure and the nurse and the physician jointly make clinical decisions. The nurse is functioning in a
*A. collaborative practice model.
B. coopertive agreement model.
C. team model.
D. traditional model.

Rationale: The nurse–physician collaborative practice model requires the nurse and the physician to function collaboratively in making clinical decisions.

Reference: p. 13

Descriptors:
1. 02 2. 06 3. Application
4. I–1 5. Nursing Process 6. Moderate

CHAPTER 2
Community-Based Nursing Practice

1. More medical surgical nurses are needed in community-based settings, primarily due to
A. decreased employment opportunities in acute care settings.
*B. decreased length of hospital stays for most clients.
C. increased need for primary health care services.
D. proliferation of nursing-based centers in most communities.

Rationale: There is a greater need for skilled medical surgical nurses in community-based settings because of the decreased length of hospital stays for most clients. Intravenous therapies, ventilators, and alternate feeding devices are now common in home care.

Reference: p. 16

Descriptors:
1. 02 2. 01 3. Application
4. I–1 5. Nursing Process 6. Moderate

2. A nurse has instructed a group of high school seniors on the topic of healthy lifestyles. This type of preventive care is termed
*A. primary prevention.
B. secondary prevention.
C. tertiary prevention.
D. complementary prevention.

Rationale: Primary prevention centers on health promotion and protection from health problems and would include health teaching related to healthy lifestyles.

Reference: p. 16

Descriptors:
1. 02 2. 01 3. Application
4. IV–3 5. Nursing Process 6. Moderate

3. Home care nursing services are used most frequently by
A. families with chronically ill children.
B. newly delivered first-time mothers.
C. clients with private insurance.
*D. elderly clients on Medicare.

Rationale: The elderly who are receiving Medicare funding are the most frequent users of home care services.

Reference: p. 17

Descriptors:
1. 02 2. 01 3. Application
4. I–1 5. Nursing Process 6. Easy

4. A nurse is planning a home visit to a postoperative client who needs a dressing change and wound assessment. When the nurse provides care in the home,
A. the nurse retains full decision-making authority.
B. cleanliness standards similar to the hospital must be maintained.
*C. the client maintains control over his or her care.
D. supplies are similar to what is used in the hospital.

Rationale: In a home care setting, the client maintains control over his or her care. This can cause conflict for the nurse. Improvisation may be necessary as supplies may not be similar to that of the acute care setting and cleanliness may not be the same.

Reference: p. 17

Descriptors:
1. 02 2. 02 3. Analysis
4. I–1 5. Nursing Process 6. Moderate

5. An adult client has just been admitted from the emergency room following an automobile accident. Discharge planning for this client should begin
A. on the day before anticipated discharge.

B. when the client and family are ready to discuss discharge plans.
*C. soon after the client is admitted to the hospital.
D. several hours before the actual discharge of the client.

Rationale: Discharge planning should begin soon after the client's admission to the agency. Waiting until the day before or the day of discharge may not allow enough time to coordinate the various services that may be needed once the client is discharged.

Reference: p. 18

Descriptors:
1. 02 2. 03 3. Application
4. IV–3 5. Nursing Process 6. Moderate

6. A nurse is preparing to discharge a well-functioning postoperative client following cardiac surgery, and a home health nurse will be making visits to the client. It is the nurse's responsibility to
A. ask the physician for an order for appropriate community resources.
B. ask the social worker to contact the client and family once the client is home.
*C. provide the client and family with information related to community resources.
D. contact the cardiac rehabilitation support group for the client and family.

Rationale: During initial and subsequent visits to the client at home, the home health nurse should provide the client and family with information about other available community resources to meet their needs. The nurse may make the initial contact if the client or family is unable to do so.

Reference: p. 18

Descriptors:
1. 02 2. 04 3. Application
4. IV–4 5. Nursing Process 6. Moderate

7. A nurse is preparing to make a home visit to a client following a total right hip replacement. Before initiating a home visit to the client, the nurse should
A. notify the client and family of the supplies that are needed.
B. tell the client which date the nurse will be making the visit.
C. schedule the visit when the family can be present.
*D. be familiar with the agency policies related to the nurse's role.

Rationale: Becoming familiar with the agency's policies is an essential step before initiating a home visit to a client. The nurse should know the agency's policies and state laws for unusual situations, such as finding the client dead in the home or unsafe living conditions.

Reference: p. 18

Descriptors:
1. 02 2. 05 3. Application
4. I–1 5. Nursing Process 6. Moderate

8. The home health nurse has received a referral from a social worker for a client who needs a home visit. After reviewing the referral form, the first step before making the home visit is to
A. validate Medicare payment.
B. contact the referral agency.
*C. call the client to obtain permission.
D. locate the general area where the client lives.

Rationale: After receiving a referral, the first step is to call the client and obtain permission to make the visit. Then the nurse should schedule the visit and verify the address.

Reference: p. 18

Descriptors:
1. 02 2. 05 3. Application
4. I–1 5. Nursing Process 6. Moderate

9. A nurse is preparing to make a home visit for the first time to a postoperative client. Personal safety precautions that the nurse should take when providing home care to a client include
A. parking the car well away from the client's home.
B. carrying a personal weapon or Mace for self-defense.
C. entering the client's home if the door is ajar.
*D. letting the agency know the daily schedule and phone numbers of the clients.

Rationale: Nurses are not expected to put their own safety at risk when making home visits. The nurse should park the car close to the home and lock it, let the agency know the daily schedule and phone numbers of the clients, and never enter a home uninvited. The nurse should schedule visits only in the daytime and leave the area if it is not safe.

Reference: p. 19

Descriptors:
1. 02 2. 06 3. Application
4. IV–3 5. Nursing Process 6. Moderate

10. Documentation is important for reimbursement of home health care visits. During the initial visit, the nurse should plan to document
A. whether Medicare will pay for the services.
*B. expected client outcomes and actions for attaining the outcomes.
C. possible health hazards in the client's home.
D. the family's ability to provide skilled nursing care.

Rationale: Documentation should include medical diagnosis and specific detailed information about the functional limitations, expected client outcomes and actions for attaining the outcomes, and nursing diagnoses and interventions.

Reference: p. 19

Descriptors:
1. 02 2. 05 3. Analysis
4. I–1 5. Nursing Process 6. Moderate

11. A nurse is caring for a homebound client following abdominal surgery and who continues to receive stomach feedings. When the nurse considers the need for future home visits, the nurse should consider which of the following factors? The client's
A. significant others.
*B. current health status.
C. costs of the visits.
D. relationship with the physician.

Rationale: Factors to consider when the nurse evaluates the need for subsequent visits include the client's current health status, home environment, level of self-care, level of nursing care needed, prognosis, and mental status.

Reference: p. 19

Descriptors:
1. 02 2. 05 3. Analysis
4. IV–3 5. Nursing Process 6. Moderate

12. A nurse who has achieved advanced education in primary care for a gerontologic population and who is employed in an ambulatory care clinic is functioning in the role of a
*A. nurse practitioner.
B. case manager.
C. clinical nurse specialist.
D. clinic supervisor.

Rationale: Nurse practitioners, educated in primary care, often practice in ambulatory care centers with a focus on gerontology, pediatrics, family or adult health, or women's health.

Reference: p. 20

Descriptors:
1. 02 2. 07 3. Application
4. IV–3 5. Nursing Process 6. Moderate

13. A nurse working in a local industry setting is often responsible for
A. vision screening examinations.
B. nutrition counseling of the cafeteria staff.
C. making referrals to home health agencies.
*D. conducting health education programs for the industry staff.

Rationale: Occupational health nurses may provide direct care to clients who are ill, conduct health education programs for the industry staff, or set up health programs. The nurse must also be familiar with OSHA regulations and other legislation.

Reference: p. 20

Descriptors:
1. 02 2. 07 3. Application
4. IV–3 5. Nursing Process 6. Moderate

14. A nurse is working as an elementary school nurse for a local community. One of the leading health problems for school-age children that the nurse must treat is/are
A. mental stressors.
B. fatigue-related symptoms.
C. obesity.
*D. injuries.

Rationale: Leading health problems of school-age children include injuries, infections, malnutrition, dental disease, and cancer.

Reference: p. 20

Descriptors:
1. 02 2. 07 3. Application
4. IV–4 5. Nursing Process 6. Moderate

15. A nurse is working as a volunteer in a homeless shelter along with several other health professionals. One of the major problems in providing health care to homeless clients is that
*A. they seek health care late in the course of the illness.
B. they are afraid of authority figures and do not seek care.
C. alcohol and drug abuse problems interfere with health-seeking behaviors.
D. many refuse to visit homeless shelters because there is a chance of infection.

Rationale: Because of many obstacles to the health care system, homeless clients seek health care late in the course of the illness and deteriorate more quickly than other clients. Much of this is due to their homeless environment.

Reference: pp. 20–21

Descriptors:
1. 02 2. 08 3. Application
4. I–1 5. Nursing Process 6. Moderate

CHAPTER 3
Critical Thinking, Ethical Decision Making, and the Nursing Process

1. Critical thinking includes the examination of one's own thought processes while thinking, which is termed
A. analysis.
B. independent thought.
C. judgment making.
*D. metacognition.

Rationale: The examination of one's own reasoning or thought processes while thinking is termed metacognition and is a process that helps to strengthen and refine thinking skills.

Reference: p. 23

Descriptors:
1. 03 2. 01 3. Comprehension
4. I–1 5. Nursing Process 6. Moderate

2. One of the characteristics of a nurse who is a critical thinker is that the nurse is
A. egocentric.
*B. fair.
C. ethnocentric.
D. mentally stimulated.

Rationale: Some characteristics of critical thinkers include having a sense of fairness and integrity, the courage to question personal ethics, and the perseverance to strive continuously to minimize the effects of egocentricity, ethnocentricity, and other biases on the decision-making process.

Reference: p. 23

Descriptors:
1. 03 2. 02 3. Comprehension
4. I–1 5. Nursing Process 6. Moderate

3. Ethics can best be defined as
A. informal personal values.
B. social good.
C. doing right or wrong.
*D. study of moral beliefs.

Rationale: Ethics is the formal, systematic study of moral beliefs, while morality is adherence to informal personal values.

Reference: p. 24

Descriptors:
1. 03 2. 03 3. Knowledge
4. I–1 5. Nursing Process 6. Moderate

4. A nurse is working in the emergency room following a tornado disaster that caused a tremendous amount of damage and injury to the population. Using the utilitarian ethical theory, the nurse should attempt to
A. care for only the clients that are likely to need surgery.
B. perform nursing procedures that are morally neutral.
*C. provide the greatest good for the greatest number of individuals.
D. use higher-level moral principles if there is a conflict.

Rationale: The utilitarian ethical theory asserts that the nurse should provide the greatest good for the greatest number. The deontological approach argues that moral standards exist independently of the ends or consequences.

Reference: p. 24

Descriptors:
1. 03 2. 03 3. Application
4. I–1 5. Nursing Process 6. Moderate

5. A nurse has witnessed a client's signature on a consent form for surgery. When the nurse questions whether the client has signed a truly informed consent form, the nurse is practicing
*A. metaethics.
B. applied ethics.
C. medical ethics.
D. deontological ethics.

Rationale: When a question arises as to whether the client has been truly informed about a consent for surgery, the nurse is practicing metaethics or understanding the concepts used in ethics.

Reference: p. 25

Descriptors:
1. 03 2. 03 3. Application
4. IV–3 5. Nursing Process 6. Moderate

6. The ethical term *nonmaleficence* involves the nurse's duty to
A. do only good acts.
B. keep facts confidential.
C. treat all clients alike.
*D. do no harm to the client.

Rationale: The duty not to inflict as well as prevent and remove harm is termed *nonmaleficence. Beneficence* is the duty to do good.

Reference: p. 25

Descriptors:
1. 03 2. 03 3. Application
4. I–1 5. Nursing Process 6. Moderate

7. An example of paternalism in a health care situation exists when the physician
A. allows the client to complete advance directives.
B. maintains the client on fluid therapy even though the client is comatose.
*C. decides what is best for the client rather than providing the client with options.
D. allows the client to decide whether he wants resuscitation if necessary.

Rationale: Paternalism is the intentional limitation of another's autonomy. Paternalism exists when the physician decides what is best for the client rather than providing the client with options.

Reference: p. 25

Descriptors:
1. 03 2. 03 3. Application
4. I–1 5. Nursing Process 6. Moderate

8. When the nurse practices fidelity, there is a commitment to
A. do only good and promote kindness.
*B. keep all promises made.
C. tell the truth at all times.
D. respect the client's autonomy.

Rationale: Fidelity requires the nurse to keep promises made and to be faithful to one's commitments.

Reference: p. 25

Descriptors:
1. 03 2. 04 3. Application
4. I–1 5. Nursing Process 6. Moderate

9. The ethical principle where the nurse has the obligation to tell the truth to a client and not to lie or deceive is termed
A. fidelity.
B. nonmaleficence.
C. beneficence.
*D. veracity.

Rationale: The obligation to tell the truth and not lie or deceive others is termed veracity.

Reference: p. 25

Descriptors:
1. 03 2. 04 3. Application
4. I–1 5. Nursing Process 6. Moderate

10. One frequently encountered ethical dilemma with confused, elderly clients in long-term care settings is the
A. determination of mental competency.
*B. use of restraints to prevent falls.
C. use of pain medication.
D. client's right to privacy.

Rationale: Because there are safety risks involved when not using restraints on elderly confused clients, this is a common ethical problem in long-term care settings, as well as other health care settings. Restraints limit the individual's autonomy.

Reference: p. 26

Descriptors:
1. 03 2. 04 3. Application
4. I –2 5. Nursing Process 6. Difficult

11. A terminally ill client has identified another individual to make decisions on her behalf. When a decision about the client's care arises, the nurse should consult the client's records for the
*A. power of attorney.
B. living will.
C. benefactor of the client.
D. doctor of record.

Rationale: A power of attorney is said to be in effect when a client has identified another individual to make decisions on her behalf.

Reference: p. 28

Descriptors:
1. 03 2. 05 3. Application
4. I–1 5. Nursing Process 6. Easy

12. A client is admitted to the hospital and provides the nurse with a copy of her living will for the client's records. One of the drawbacks of a living will is that the
A. state may not believe the client was competent.
B. physician may disagree with the client's desires for treatment.
*C. client may nullify the living will during the illness.
D. power of attorney may change while the client is hospitalized.

Rationale: Since living wills are often written when the person is in good health, it is not unusual for the client to nullify the living will during illness.

Reference: p. 28

Descriptors:
1. 03 2. 05 3. Application
4. I–1 5. Nursing Process 6. Moderate

13. Nursing ethics is concerned with
A. metaethics.
B. general ethics.
*C. applied ethics.
D. medical ethics.

Rationale: Nursing ethics may be considered a distinct form of applied ethics because it addresses many moral situations that are specific to the nursing profession.

Reference: p. 25

Descriptors:
1. 03 2. 04 3. Application
4. I–1 5. Nursing Process 6. Moderate

14. Which of the following best describes the diagnosis phase of the nursing process?
A. A decision is made that prioritizes the clients problems.
B. Data is collected continuously to determine if the problem can be resolved.
*C. Client's nursing problems are defined through analysis of client data.
D. Nurse–physician collaboration is used to formulate a diagnostic label for the client.

Rationale: In the diagnostic phase of the nursing process, the client's nursing problems are defined through analysis of client data. Implementation of care is based on the client's nursing diagnoses.

Reference: pp. 28–29

Descriptors:
1. 03 2. 06 3. Application
4. I–1 5. Nursing Process 6. Moderate

15. When the nurse administers an injectable pain medication to a client who is suffering from post-operative pain at the incision site, the phase of the nursing process accomplished by the nurse is the
A. assessment phase.
B. analysis phase.
*C. implementation phase.
D. evaluation phase.

Rationale: Carrying out a plan of care through nursing interventions is the implementation phase.

Reference: p. 29

Descriptors:
1. 03 2. 06 3. Application
4. IV–1 5. Nursing Process 6. Moderate

16. One hour after the administration of aspirin to a client with a fever, the nurse determines that the medication has been effective and documents this in the client's record. This phase of the nursing process is termed
A. analysis.
*B. evaluation.
C. assessment.
D. diagnosis.

Rationale: Determination of the client's responses to nursing interventions and the extent to which outcomes have been achieved is termed the evaluation phase of the nursing process.

Reference: p. 29

Descriptors:
1. 03 2. 06 3. Application
4. I–1 5. Nursing Process 6. Moderate

17. An important difference between nursing diagnoses and collaborative problems is that nursing diagnoses
*A. can be managed by independent nursing actions.
B. require input from the entire health team.
C. are treated with physician-prescribed orders.
D. require goals and outcomes to be identified.

Rationale: An important difference between nursing diagnoses and collaborative problems is that nursing diagnoses are actual or potential problems that can be managed by independent nursing actions. Collaborative problems involve physician-prescribed orders.

Reference: p. 29

Descriptors:
1. 03 2. 06 3. Application
4. IV–1 5. Nursing Process 6. Difficult

18. After the health history and health assessment data are completed, the information should be documented in the client's permanent record. Besides planning and continuity of care, the client's record
A. contains the nursing care plan.
B. identifies the religious contact person for the client.
*C. serves as a legal record for the health care agency.
D. can be taken with the client when he leaves the agency.

Rationale: Besides planning and continuity of care, the client's record serves as the business and legal record for the health care agency and for the professional staff responsible for the client's care.

Reference: p. 30

Descriptors:
1. 03 2. 06 3. Application
4. I–1 5. Nursing Process 6. Moderate

19. When the nurse chooses a nursing diagnosis for a particular client, the nurse must first
A. collaborate with the client's physician.
B. collect data from the client's family.
C. review the client's past medical history.
*D. identify the commonalities among the assessment data collected.

Rationale: When choosing the nursing diagnosis for a particular client, the nurse must first identify the commonalities among the assessment data collected. These common features lead to the categorization of the data that reveal the existence of a problem.

Reference: p. 31

Descriptors:
1. 03 2. 06 3. Application
4. I–1 5. Nursing Process 6. Difficult

20. During an initial assessment interview, a good method for getting the client to talk is for the nurse to use open-ended questions. An example of an open-ended question that the nurse can use to begin the interview is
*A. "How have you been doing since your last hospitalization?"
B. "What time do you usually have breakfast?"
C. "Have you been having trouble sleeping at night?"
D. "Do you have any drug or food allergies?"

Rationale: An open-ended question allows the client to verbalize and encourages the client to continue. The open-ended question "How have you been doing since your last hospitalization?" allows the client to verbalize and continue the discussion.

Reference: p. 31

Descriptors:
1. 03 2. 06 3. Application
4. IV–1 5. Nursing Process 6. Moderate

21. A 75-year-old client is admitted to the hospital following a fall that resulted in a fractured tibia. The client has rheumatoid arthritis and is scheduled for surgery. An appropriate nursing diagnosis for the client is
A. Stiffness and pain related to rheumatoid arthritis and impending surgery.
B. Fractured tibia related to fall and rheumatoid arthritis stiffness.
C. Surgical repair of fractured tibia related to a fall.
*D. Impaired physical mobility related to pain and stiffness with joint movement.

Rationale: Nursing diagnoses are not medical diagnoses or treatments. The appropriate nursing diagnosis for this client is impaired physical mobility related to pain and stiffness with joint movement.

Reference: p. 33

Descriptors:
1. 03 2. 07 3. Analysis
4. IV–1 5. Nursing Process 6. Moderate

22. During the planning phase of the nursing process, the nurse should
    *A. establish priorities in collaboration with the client and family.
    B. analyze the physical assessment data and document these in the client's record.
    C. perform a physical assessment of the client and record deviations.
    D. collaborate with the physician to determine nursing diagnoses.

Rationale: Assigning priorities to the nursing diagnoses and collaborative problems is carried out in the planning phase of the nursing process. This is a joint effort between the nurse and the client and family.

Reference: p. 34

Descriptors:
1. 03 2. 07 3. Application
4. IV–1 5. Nursing Process 6. Difficult

23. A nurse is caring for a diabetic client with a nursing diagnosis of knowledge deficit related to the client's prescribed diet. An immediate goal for the client is that the client will
    A. adhere to a prescribed diabetic diet and exercise routine throughout the stay.
    B. plan meals and exercise for two weeks based on diabetic exchange list.
    C. refrain from eating high carbohydrate foods for a period of two weeks.
    *D. demonstrate oral intake and tolerance of 1500 calorie diabetic diet spaced in three meals and one snack.

Rationale: Immediate goals are those that can be reached in a short period of time. An appropriate immediate goal for this client is that the client will demonstrate oral intake and tolerance of 1500 calorie diabetic diet spaced in three meals and one snack.

Reference: p. 34

Descriptors:
1. 03 2. 07 3. Application
4. IV–3 5. Nursing Process 6. Difficult

24. A nurse is performing an independent nursing intervention when the nurse
    *A. provides a back rub to a restless client to help her sleep.
    B. irrigates a wound with hydrogen peroxide.
    C. administers pain medication to a postoperative client.
    D. withholds food and fluid after midnight for a client scheduled for surgery in the morning.

Rationale: Irrigating a wound, administering pain medication, and withholding food and fluid after midnight are interdependent nursing actions and require a physician's order. An independent nursing action occurs when the nurse provides a back rub to a restless client to help her sleep.

Reference: p. 36

Descriptors:
1. 03 2. 07 3. Application
4. I–1 5. Nursing Process 6. Difficult

25. During the evaluation phase of the nursing process, the nurse should
    *A. document whether the client's pain medication was effective.
    B. record the observations made during the client's dressing change.
    C. provide the client with a pamphlet on a diabetic diet.
    D. Teach the client about turning, coughing, and deep breathing after surgery.

Rationale: During the evaluation phase of the nursing process, the nurse determines the client's response to nursing interventions. An example of this is when the nurse documents whether the client's pain medication was effective.

Reference: p. 36

Descriptors:
1. 03 2. 07 3. Application
4. IV–1 5. Nursing Process 6. Easy

CHAPTER 4
Health Education and Promotion

1. Nurses play an important role in providing health education to clients. The population that is most in need of health education today is
    A. newly delivered first-time mothers.
    B. student athletes.
    *C. clients with chronic illnesses.
    D. clients who will undergo surgery.

Rationale: People with chronic illnesses are among those most in need of health education today. As the elderly population grows, the number of people with such illnesses will also increase.

Reference: p. 41

Descriptors:
1. 04 2. 01 3. Application
4. I–1 5. Teaching/Learning 6. Moderate

2. One variable that appears to influence the degree of adherence to a prescribed therapeutic regimen is
    *A. gender.
    B. motivation.
    C. wellness state.
    D. competency of the nurse.

Rationale: Variables that appear to influence the degree of adherence to a prescribed terapeutic regimen include gender, race, education, illness, complexity of the regimen, intelligence, attitudes toward health professionals, and religious and cultural practices.

Reference: p. 42

Descriptors:
1. 04 2. 02 3. Application
4. I–1 5. Teaching/Learning 6. Moderate

3. Nonadherence to a therapeutic regimen is a significant problem for elderly people. One of the common reasons for the nonadherence of the elderly is
 A. lack of time.
 B. religious practices.
 C. childlike beliefs.
 *D. inadequate financial resources.

Rationale: Some of the common reasons for the nonadherence of the elderly include increased sensitivity to medications, lack of support systems, inadequate financial resources, visual and hearing impairments, and mobility limitations.

Reference: p. 42

Descriptors:
1. 04 2. 03 3. Application
4. I–1 5. Teaching/Learning 6. Difficult

4. A nurse is preparing to teach a client how to ambulate using crutches. One of the major variables that influences a client's readiness to learn is
 A. age.
 B. gender.
 C. medications.
 *D. culture.

Rationale: One of the major variables that influences a client's readiness to learn is the client's culture, because it affects how a person learns and what information gets learned. Other variables include illness states, values, emotional readiness, and physical readiness.

Reference: p. 42

Descriptors:
1. 04 2. 04 3. Application
4. I–1 5. Teaching/Learning 6. Difficult

5. A nurse is preparing to teach a 65-year-old client how to change his ostomy bag. One of the best methods to teach the client this skill is by
 *A. demonstration.
 B. lecture.
 C. discussion.
 D. group teaching.

Rationale: Demonstration and practice are essential ingredients of a teaching program, especially when skills are to be learned.

Reference: p. 43

Descriptors:
1. 04 2. 05 3. Application
4. IV–4 5. Teaching/Learning 6. Easy

6. When the nurse plans to teach a 75-year-old client about her diabetic diet, the nurse can enhance the client's ability to learn by
 A. using high-pitched speech.
 B. excluding family members from the session.
 C. using color-coded materials.
 *D. making the information relevant.

Rationale: Studies have shown that older adults can learn and remember if the information is paced appropriately, relevant, and followed by appropriate feedback.

Reference: p. 44

Descriptors:
1. 04 2. 05 3. Application
4. IV–1 5. Teaching/Learning 6. Moderate

7. Assessment in the teaching/learning process is similar to a nursing process assessment when the nurse
 A. assigns priorities to the diagnoses.
 B. specifies the expected outcomes.
 *C. analyzes the data collected.
 D. documents the goals.

Rationale: Assessment in the teaching/learning process is directed toward the systematic collection of data about the person's learning needs. It is similar to a nursing process assessment when the nurse organizes and analyzes the data collected.

Reference: p. 44

Descriptors:
1. 04 2. 06 3. Application
4. IV–1 5. Teaching/Learning 6. Difficult

8. Teaching is an integral intervention implied by all nursing diagnoses. For which of the following nursing diagnoses is education a primary nursing intervention?
 A. Risk for impaired mobility related to arthritis.
 B. Stress incontinence related to surgical repair of bladder.
 C. Altered health maintenance related to financial restraints.
 *D. Risk for ineffective management of therapeutic regimen.

Rationale: For some nursing diagnoses, education is a primary nursing intervention. These diagnoses include: risk for ineffective management of therapeutic regimen, risk for impaired home management, health seeking behaviors, and decisional conflict.

Reference: p. 44–48

Descriptors:
1. 04 2. 06 3. Application
4. IV–1 5. Teaching/Learning 6. Difficult

9. The nurse concludes the planning component of the teaching/learning process when the nurse
 *A. formulates the teaching plan.

B. documents the client's readiness to learn.
C. establishes priorities for health education.
D. specifies long-term goals for the client.

Rationale: The entire planning phase of the teaching/learning process concludes when the nurse formulates the teaching plan. This teaching plan should be communicated to all members of the nursing team.

Reference: pp. 44–45

Descriptors:
1. 04 2. 06 3. Application
4. IV–1 5. Teaching/Learning 6. Difficult

10. A nurse has taught a diabetic client how to administer his daily insulin. The nurse should evaluate the teaching learning process by
A. determining the client's motivation to learn.
*B. deciding if the learning outcomes have been achieved.
C. allowing the client to practice the skills learned.
D. documenting the teaching session in the client's record.

Rationale: Evaluation of the teaching/learning process determines how effectively the person has responded to the teaching strategies and to what extent the goals or outcomes have been achieved.

Reference: p. 45

Descriptors:
1. 04 2. 06 3. Application
4. IV–2 5. Teaching/Learning 6. Difficult

11. Which of the following is an example of a health-promotion teaching project?
A. Demonstrating an injection technique to a diabetic client.
B. Explaining the side effects of a medication to an adult client.
*C. Discussing the importance of exercise to a group of fourth-grade students.
D. Instructing a middle-aged client about a low salt diet to control hypertension.

Rationale: Health promotion encourages people to live a healthy lifestyle and to achieve a high level of wellness. Discussing the importance of exercise to a group of fourth-grade students is the best example of a health-promotion teaching project.

Reference: p. 46

Descriptors:
1. 04 2. 08 3. Application
4. IV–3 5. Teaching/Learning 6. Difficult

12. A nurse is using the health belief model to assess a client. Using this model, the nurse should begin to understand what
A. resources the client needs to improve his lifestyle.
B. motivates the client to learn new behaviors.
C. effects the health delivery system has on the client's health patterns.
*D. made some healthy people choose actions to prevent illness.

Rationale: The health belief model was devised to foster understanding of what made some healthy people choose actions to prevent illness while others refuse to engage in these protective recommendations.

Reference: p. 47

Descriptors:
1. 04 2. 09 3. Application
4. IV–1 5. Teaching/Learning 6. Difficult

13. The nurse is caring for a hospitalized client on the second postoperative day. The nurse should explain to the client that the single most significant factor in determining health and longevity is
*A. good nutrition.
B. exercising daily.
C. use of herbal medicines.
D. health risk screenings.

Rationale: It has been suggested that the single most significant factor in determining health and longevity is good nutrition. A balanced diet that uses few artificial ingredients and is low in fat, caffeine, and sodium constitutes a healthy diet.

Reference: p. 47

Descriptors:
1. 04 2. 10 3. Application
4. IV–3 5. Teaching/Learning 6. Moderate

14. A nurse is caring for a client when the client tells the nurse that she has been undergoing a great deal of stress from her job in recent weeks. The nurse should explain to the client that excessive stress levels can lead to
A. osteoporosis.
*B. infectious diseases.
C. weight gain.
D. mental deterioration.

Rationale: Excessive stress levels have been associated with infectious diseases because of a decreased immune response, traumatic injuries, such as automobile accidents, and some chronic illnesses.

Reference: p. 47

Descriptors:
1. 04 2. 10 3. Application
4. IV–3 5. Teaching/Learning 6. Moderate

15. A nurse is planning a health-promotion presentation for a group of senior students at a local high school. Which of the following should be included in the teaching plan?
A. Need for vision screenings annually.
B. Exercise physiology.
C. Coping with asthma.
*D. Reducing risky sexual behaviors.

Rationale: Adolescence is a time for experimentation and risk taking. The negative results of practices such as smoking, risky sexual behaviors, and alcohol and drug abuse are appropriate topics for adolescents.

Reference: p. 48

Descriptors:
1. 04 2. 11 3. Application
4. IV–3 5. Teaching/Learning 6. Moderate

16. Nurses play a vital role in health promotion because of their
   A. need for self-actualization.
   *B. expertise in health and health care.
   C. desire to help others.
   D. ability to provide illness care.

Rationale: Nurses, by virtue of their expertise in health and health care and their long-established credibility with consumers, play a vital role in health promotion.

Reference: p. 49

Descriptors:
1. 04 2. 12 3. Comprehension
4. IV–3 5. Teaching/Learning 6. Easy

CHAPTER 5
Health Assessment

1. A nurse admits a disoriented client to an acute care facility. The nurse interviews the client's wife about the client's past medical history. In this situation, the client's wife is acting as the
   A. substitute.
   B. matriarch.
   C. power of attorney.
   *D. informant.

Rationale: The informant, or the person providing the information, may not always be the client, as in the case of a disoriented or unconscious client.

Reference: p. 52

Descriptors:
1. 05 2. 01 3. Comprehension
4. I–1 5. Nursing Process 6. Easy

2. The nurse is interviewing a newly admitted client. The client's medical history and nursing assessments form the foundation for the client's
   A. medical diagnosis.
   B. teaching plans.
   *C. health history.
   D. kardex.

Rationale: The format of the health history has traditionally been a combination of the medical history and the nursing assessments, although other frameworks are also available.

Reference: p. 54

Descriptors:
1. 05 2. 01 3. Comprehension
4. V–1 5. Nursing Process 6. Moderate

3. A nurse is preparing to conduct a health history interview on a newly admitted adolescent client. Before beginning, the nurse should explain to the client
   *A. how the information will be used.
   B. who specifically will have access to the client's records.
   C. where the health record will be maintained.
   D. what treatments the client will undergo.

Rationale: Before beginning a health history and interview, the nurse should explain to the client what the examination is, how the information will be obtained, and how it will be used. The client's records should always be maintained in a safe place.

Reference: p. 53

Descriptors:
1. 05 2. 02 3. Comprehension
4. V–1 5. Caring 6. Moderate

4. A nurse has conducted a physical examination of an adult client diagnosed with a probable tumor. When the nurse documents the client's skin as appearing jaundiced, the nurse has used the skill of
   A. palpation.
   B. percussion.
   *C. inspection.
   D. auscultation.

Rationale: Documentation of the client's skin as appearing jaundiced involves the nurse's using the skill of inspection.

Reference: p. 58

Descriptors:
1. 05 2. 04 3. Comprehension
4. IV–1 5. Nursing Process 6. Easy

5. While interviewing a newly admitted adult client, the nurse observes that the client prefers to sit upright because "lying flat makes me short of breath." The nurse suspects that the client is experiencing symptoms of
   *A. cardiac disease.
   B. stress-related reactions.
   C. peritonitis.
   D. cancer.

Rationale: Clients who have breathing difficulties (dyspnea) secondary to cardiac disease may prefer to sit upright and may report feeling short of breath lying flat for even a short time.

Reference: p. 58

Descriptors:
1. 05 2. 04 3. Analysis
4. V–1 5. Nursing Process 6. Difficult

6. A nurse is conducting a health history interview with a 65-year-old male. The nurse observes that

the client prefers to sit upright with his arms forward and laterally onto the edge of the bed. The nurse suspects that the client is experiencing symptoms of

A. chronic rheumatoid arthritis.
B. abdominal distention.
C. meningeal irritation.
*D. emphysema.

Rationale: When the nurse observes that the client prefers to sit upright with his arms forward and laterally (tripod position) onto the edge of the bed, The nurse should suspect that the client is experiencing symptoms of emphysema. This position places accessory respiratory muscles at an optimal mechanical advantage.

Reference: p. 58

Descriptors:

1. 05	2. 04	3. Analysis
4. IV–3	5. Nursing Process	6. Moderate

7. While interviewing a newly admitted client, the nurse observes that the client speaks in a very hoarse voice. The nurse suspects that the client is experiencing symptoms of

*A. damage to the recurrent laryngeal nerve.
B. multiple sclerosis.
C. cerebral vascular accident.
D. brain tumor.

Rationale: Damage to the recurrent laryngeal nerve will result in the client's speech being very hoarse. Halting, slurred, or interrupted speech may be indicative of CNS disorders.

Reference: p. 58

Descriptors:

1. 05	2. 04	3. Analysis
4. IV–1	5. Nursing Process	6. Difficult

8. When the nurse assesses a newly admitted client's lymph nodes, the nurse should use the technique of

A. inspection.
B. auscultation.
*C. palpation.
D. percussion.

Rationale: The nurse should use the technique of palpation to assess the lymph nodes of a client.

Reference: p. 59

Descriptors:

1. 05	2. 04	3. Application
4. V–1	5. Nursing Process	6. Easy

9. When the nurse prepares to examine a client's abdomen, auscultation is performed before palpation in order to

A. obtain a more thorough history.
*B. avoid altering bowel sounds.
C. prevent excessive blood flow to the area.
D. hear thrills more clearly.

Rationale: Auscultation of the client's abdomen is performed before palpation and percussion in order to avoid altering bowel sounds.

Reference: p. 59

Descriptors:

1. 05	2. 04	3. Application
4. V–1	5. Nursing Process	6. Difficult

10. A nurse is planning to percuss the lungs of a newly admitted adult client diagnosed with emphysema. The nurse should be able to detect the client's

A. tympanny.
B. dull sounds.
C. flat sounds.
*D. hyperresonance.

Rationale: The nurse should be able to detect the client's hyperresonance, which is audible when one percusses over inflated lung tissue. Dull sounds are associated with liver palpation and flat sounds with percussion of the thigh.

Reference: p. 59

Descriptors:

1. 05	2. 04	3. Application
4. V–1	5. Nursing Process	6. Difficult

11. In order to assess whether an adult client has a diastolic heart murmur, the nurse should use the

*A. bell of the stethoscope.
B. fingers to palpate the heart area.
C. eyes to inspect the client's color.
D. diaphragm of the stethoscope.

Rationale: In order to assess whether an adult client has a diastolic heart murmur, the nurse should use the bell of the stethoscope, since this is a very low-frequency sound. The diaphragm of the stethoscope is used to assess high-frequency sounds.

Reference: p. 59

Descriptors:

1. 05	2. 04	3. Application
4. I–1	5. Nursing Process	6. Moderate

12. A nurse is assessing the anthropometric measurements of an adult male client who has a medium frame and is 5 feet 6 inches tall. The client's ideal body weight is

A. 132 pounds.
*B. 142 pounds.
C. 158 pounds.
D. 168 pounds.

Rationale: An adult male with a medium frame should weigh 142 pounds. Allow 106 pounds for each 5 feet of height and add 6 pounds for each additional inch.

Reference: p. 60

Descriptors:

1. 05	2. 06	3. Application
4. IV–3	5. Nursing Process	6. Moderate

13. A 67-year-old female client tells the nurse that she has lost 2 inches of height over the last several years. The nurse suspects that the client may be experiencing symptoms of
    A. premature aging.
    B. rheumatoid arthritis.
    C. leukemia.
    *D. osteoporosis.

    Rationale: Osteoporosis should be suspected in a postmenopausal female when there is a loss of height of 2 to 3 inches.

    Reference: p. 61

    Descriptors:
    1. 05 2. 06 3. Analysis
    4. IV–3 5. Nursing Process 6. Moderate

14. A nurse has admitted a malnourished elderly client to the acute care facility after a fractured hip. The nurse anticipates that this client's assessment will reveal
    A. a body mass index greater than 27.
    *B. decreased serum albumin and transferrin levels.
    C. elevation of lymphocytes.
    D. increased antibody synthesis.

    Rationale: Decreased serum albumin and transferrin levels are associated with severe malnutrition and protein deficits. Body mass index would be less than 24, and lymphocytes and antibody synthesis would be decreased.

    Reference: pp. 62–63

    Descriptors:
    1. 05 2. 06 3. Analysis
    4. V–1 5. Nursing Process 6. Difficult

15. A nurse has admitted a 78-year-old male who appears malnourished. The nurse should explain to the client and his family that nutritional problems in older adults often occur or are precipitated by such illnesses as
    A. hip fractures.
    *B. pneumonia.
    C. peritonitis.
    D. biliary tumors.

    Rationale: Nutritional problems in older adults often occur or are precipitated by such illnesses as pneumonia or urinary tract infections. Medications and financial constraints can also affect the nutritional patterns of the older adult.

    Reference: p. 65

    Descriptors:
    1. 05 2. 07 3. Application
    4. IV–3 5. Nursing Process 6. Difficult

UNIT 2 BIOPHYSICAL AND PSYCHOSOCIAL CONCEPTS IN NURSING PRACTICE

CHAPTER 6 Homeostasis, Stress, and Adaptation

1. Dubos (1965) believed that two complementary concepts were necessary for balance in human beings. These concepts included homeostasis and
    A. regulation.
    B. reaction.
    C. exchanges.
    *D. adaptation.

    Rationale: Dubos (1965) believed that two complementary concepts, homeostasis and adaptation, were necessary for balance in human beings. Adaptive processes resulted in structural or functional changes over time.

    Reference: p. 72

    Descriptors:
    1. 06 2. 01 3. Comprehension
    4. III–1 5. Nursing Process 6. Moderate

2. For human beings, the type of stressor that has been shown to have the greatest health impact is the
    A. chronic, enduring stressor.
    B. major life event.
    C. stressor sequence.
    *D. day-to-day hassle.

    Rationale: Daily hassles, which are less dramatic, but cause frustration and irritation, have been shown to have a greater health impact because of their cumulative effect over time.

    Reference: p. 73

    Descriptors:
    1. 06 2. 02 3. Comprehension
    4. III–1 5. Nursing Process 6. Moderate

3. A primary source of stress for clients who are hospitalized in a surgical intensive care unit includes
    *A. immobilization.
    B. fear of pain.
    C. spiritual distress.
    D. lack of family support.

    Rationale: Sources of stress for clients who are hospitalized in a surgical intensive care unit include immobilization, isolation, orientation, and sensory deprivation, according to a study by Ballard (1981).

Reference: p. 74

Descriptors:
1. 06 2. 03 3. Application
4. III–1 5. Nursing Process 6. Difficult

4. Psychological stress is defined as a
   A. generalized state of anxiety involving psychoneuroendocrine activity.
   B. constant ongoing process that occurs along a continuum.
   *C. state produced by a situation that a person perceives as threatening.
   D. change that evokes an adaptive response.

Rationale: After the recognition of a stressor, the individual will consciously or unconsciously react to manage the situation. Psychological stress is defined as a state produced by a situation that a person perceives as threatening or challenging.

Reference: p. 74

Descriptors:
1. 06 2. 03 3. Comprehension
4. III–1 5. Nursing Process 6. Moderate

5. According to Lazarus, secondary appraisal occurs when the individual
   *A. evaluates what might and can be done.
   B. changes his or her mind about the stressor based on new information.
   C. identifies the stressor as causing harm to the individual.
   D. decides that the stressor may result in gain.

Rationale: Secondary appraisal is an evaluation of what might and can be done. This includes assigning blame and thinking about whether one can do something about the situation. Primary appraisal occurs when an individual views the stressor as causing harm or resulting in a gain.

Reference: p. 74

Descriptors:
1. 06 2. 03 3. Comprehension
4. III–3 5. Nursing Process 6. Difficult

6. In human beings, the physiologic response to a stressor is best defined as a/an
   A. way for the person to view the stressor.
   *B. adaptive mechanism to maintain the homeostatic balance.
   C. long-term reaction to physiologic changes.
   D. short-acting response that is resolved.

Rationale: The physiologic response to a stressor can occur whether the stressor is psychological or physiological and is a protective and adaptive mechanism to maintain the homeostatic balance of the body.

Reference: p. 74

Descriptors:
1. 06 2. 03 3. Comprehension
4. III–3 5. Nursing Process 6. Easy

7. In the sympathetic-adrenal-medullary response to stress, the sympathetic nervous system stimulates the adrenal gland to release
   A. corticotropin-releasing factor.
   B. ACTH.
   C. glucocorticoids.
   *D. epinephrine.

Rationale: In the sympathetic-adrenal-medullary response to stress, the sympathetic nervous system stimulates the adrenal gland to release epinephrine and norepinephrine. Corticotropin-releasing factor, ACTH, and glucocorticoids are released in the hypothalamic-pituitary response to stress.

Reference: p. 75

Descriptors:
1. 06 2. 04 3. Comprehension
4. III–3 5. Nursing Process 6. Difficult

8. In the hypothalamic-pituitary response to a stressor, the hypothalamus secretes
   A. ADH.
   *B. corticotropin-releasing factor.
   C. growth hormones.
   D. endorphins.

Rationale: In the hypothalamic-pituitary response to a stressor, the hypothalamus secretes corticotropin-releasing factor, which stimulates the anterior pituitary to produce ACTH.

Reference: p. 76

Descriptors:
1. 06 2. 04 3. Comprehension
4. III–1 5. Nursing Process 6. Moderate

9. In human beings, the immune system can become depressed when the body secretes high levels of
   *A. glucocorticoids.
   B. endorphins.
   C. ACTH.
   D. cortisol.

Rationale: The immune system can become depressed when the body secretes high levels of glucocorticoids, resulting in a reduction in the inflammatory response to injury or infection.

Reference: p. 77

Descriptors:
1. 06 2. 04 3. Comprehension
4. III–1 5. Nursing Process 6. Moderate

10. In Selye's General Adaptation Syndrome, the second stage of the stress response is termed the
   A. alarm stage.
   B. noxious stage.
   *C. resistance stage.
   D. exhaustion stage.

Rationale: In Han Selye's General Adaptation Syndrome, the second stage of the stress response is termed the resistance stage, where adaptation to the noxious stressor occurs.

Reference: p. 75

Descriptors:
1. 06 2. 05 3. Comprehension
4. III–1 5. Nursing Process 6. Difficult

11. An adult client visits the clinic for a routine examination. The client tells the nurse that "his wife has just filed for a divorce." In planning care for the client, the nurse should include interventions designed to
 A. prevent the stress response.
 B. distract the client from the source of stress.
 *C. assist the client to cope with the situation.
 D. ignore the daily stressors and focus on the divorce.

Rationale: For this client, the nurse should include interventions designed to assist the client to cope with the situation and appraise the situation adequately.

Reference: p. 77

Descriptors:
1. 06 2. 12 3. Application
4. III–2 5. Nursing Process 6. Moderate

12. Negative feedback mechanisms throughout the body monitor the internal environment and restore homeostasis when conditions shift out of normal range. One example of a function regulated through such compensatory mechanisms includes
 *A. blood pressure.
 B. pupillary reaction.
 C. melanin in skin.
 D. hearing.

Rationale: Examples of functions regulated through such compensatory mechanisms is blood pressure, acid-base balance, blood glucose levels, and fluid and electrolyte balances.

Reference: p. 79

Descriptors:
1. 06 2. 06 3. Comprehension
4. III–1 5. Nursing Process 6. Moderate

13. The large muscles in the legs of an avid jogger are an example of
 A. atrophy.
 B. hyperplasia.
 C. metaplasia.
 *D. hypertrophy.

Rationale: Compensatory hypertrophy is the result of an enlarged muscle mass and commonly occurs in skeletal and cardiac muscle that experiences a prolonged workload.

Reference: p. 79

Descriptors:
1. 06 2. 07 3. Comprehension
4. III–1 5. Nursing Process 6. Easy

14. A client visits the clinic and the nurse observes that the client has an enlarged thyroid. An enlarged thyroid when there is a deficit of thyroid hormone is an example of
 A. hypertrophy.
 *B. hyperplasia.
 C. metaplasia.
 D. dysplasia.

Rationale: Hyperplasia is an increase in the number of new cells in an organ or tissue. An enlarged thyroid when there is a deficit of thyroid hormone is an example of hyperplasia.

Reference: p. 79

Descriptors:
1. 06 2. 07 3. Application
4. III–1 5. Nursing Process 6. Moderate

15. The most common cause of cellular injury is
 *A. hypoxia.
 B. genetic defects.
 C. malnutrition.
 D. psychogenic factors.

Rationale: The most common causes of cellular injury include hypoxia, chemical injury, and infections. These injuries may arise from the external or internal environment.

Reference: p. 80

Descriptors:
1. 06 2. 08 3. Knowledge
4. III–1 5. Nursing Process 6. Moderate

16. The most common cause of hypoxia in the human body is a
 A. ventilation/perfusion or respiratory problem.
 B. deficiency in the cellular enzyme system.
 *C. decrease in blood supply to the area.
 D. deficiency in the immune response.

Rationale: The usual cause of hypoxia, or inadequate cellular oxygenation is ischemia or a decrease in the blood supply to the area.

Reference: p. 81

Descriptors:
1. 06 2. 08 3. Comprehension
4. III–1 5. Nursing Process 6. Moderate

17. An adult client is seen in the emergency room and is diagnosed with hyperthermia. The nurse anticipates that the client will exhibit
 A. clot formations.
 B. sluggish blood flow.
 *C. an increased heart rate.
 D. a subnormal glucose level.

Reference: p. 81

Rationale: Clients diagnosed with hyperthermia, or high fever, have an increase in their metabolism and thus an increased heart rate. Clot formations, sluggish blood flow, and a subnormal glucose level are not symptoms associated with hyperthermia.

Descriptors:
1. 06 2. 08 3. Comprehension
4. III–1 5. Nursing Process 6. Moderate

18. Down syndrome, sickle cell disease, and hemophilia are considered to be what type of disorder?
A. Immune.
B. Infectious.
*C. Genetic.
D. Psychogenic.

Rationale: Genetic disorders include Down syndrome, sickle cell disease, hemophilia, and cystic fibrosis.

Reference: p. 82

Descriptors:
1. 06 2. 08 3. Comprehension
4. III–1 5. Nursing Process 6. Moderate

19. A client has just been stung by a bee and visits the emergency care center. One of the five cardinal signs of an inflammatory response is
A. pallor.
B. perspiration.
C. numbness.
*D. swelling.

Rationale: The five cardinal signs of inflammation include redness, swelling, heat, pain, and loss of function.

Reference: p. 82

Descriptors:
1. 06 2. 09 3. Comprehension
4. IV–4 5. Nursing Process 6. Moderate

20. Cells such as epithelial cells of the skin that have the ability to regenerate are termed
*A. labile.
B. permanent.
C. neurological.
D. stable.

Rationale: The ability of cells to regenerate depends on whether they are labile, permanent, or stable. Labile cells, such as epithelial cells, multiply constantly.

Reference: p. 83

Descriptors:
1. 06 2. 10 3. Comprehension
4. IV–4 5. Nursing Process 6. Moderate

21. A nurse is conducting a health risk appraisal for a group of middle-aged adults. After assessment of the clients' responses, the nurse recognizes that the single most important factor for determining health status is the client's
*A. social class.
B. occupation.
C. age.
D. weight.

Rationale: The single most important factor for determining health status is the client's social class, and within a social class the research suggests that the major factor influencing health is the level of education.

Reference: p. 84

Descriptors:
1. 06 2. 13 3. Comprehension
4. IV–4 5. Nursing Process 6. Moderate

22. A nurse is using Benson's Relaxation Response to assist a client to reduce her stress levels. The nurse should instruct the client to
A. tense and relax each major muscle group.
B. focus mentally on a pleasant scene.
*C. combine meditation with relaxation.
D. include music therapy in her daily routine.

Rationale: Benson's Relaxation Response combines meditation with relaxation. Along with a repeated word or phrase, a passive attitude is essential.

Reference: p. 85

Descriptors:
1. 06 2. 14 3. Comprehension
4. IV–4 5. Nursing Process 6. Moderate

23. An elderly client who is grieving over the loss of her husband visits the clinic for a routine examination. The nurse encourages the client to join a support group because social networks can reduce stress by providing the individual with
A. improved immune responses.
*B. a positive social identity.
C. extra coping outlets.
D. someone with whom to share meals.

Rationale: Social networks can reduce stress by providing the individual with a positive social identity, emotional support, material aid, information, and new social contacts.

Reference: p. 86

Descriptors:
1. 06 2. 15 3. Comprehension
4. III–2 5. Nursing Process 6. Moderate

CHAPTER 7
Individual and Family Considerations Related to Illness

1. One of the reasons that clients seek care from a holistic health care practitioner is the
A. lack of access to traditional therapies.

*B. feeling of depersonalization from traditional medicine.
C. greater access to health information.
D. emotional state of the client.

Rationale: Some of the reasons that clients seek care from a holistic health care practitioner include the feeling of depersonalization and depolarization from traditional medicine and a lack of focus on the individual client.

Reference: p. 90

Descriptors:
1. 07 2. 01 3. Comprehension
4. I–1 5. Nursing Process 6. Moderate

2. A nurse is caring for a postoperative client following cardiac surgery. The nurse should explain to the client that an individual's coping ability is strongly influenced by the client's
A. immune system.
B. ability to respond to stressors.
C. hormonal levels.
*D. genetic factors.

Rationale: An individual's coping ability is strongly influenced by genetic and biologic factors, physical and emotional growth and development, learning, and family and childhood experiences.

Reference: p. 90

Descriptors:
1. 07 2. 02 3. Application
4. III–1 5. Nursing Process 6. Moderate

3. One of the primary variables that influences a client's ability to cope and is associated with mental disorders is
*A. severe anxiety.
B. family adjustment.
C. financial resources.
D. nutritional impairments.

Rationale: Variables that influence a client's ability to cope and are associated with mental disorder include severe anxiety, severe depression, ineffective coping strategies, helplessness, and extreme negative thoughts.

Reference: p. 92

Descriptors:
1. 07 2. 03 3. Application
4. III–1 5. Nursing Process 6. Moderate

4. According to Wright and Leahy, one of the first functions of a family is to
A. assist the members towards self-actualization.
*B. make decisions about resources.
C. socialize the members to society.
D. provide family support to the members.

Rationale: Wright and Leahy (1994) have identified five family functions. The first function I management or making decisions about resources. The other functions include boundary setting, communication, education and support, and socialization.

Reference: p. 92

Descriptors:
1. 07 2. 06 3. Comprehension
4. III–1 5. Nursing Process 6. Moderate

5. A nurse is caring for a client who has just been diagnosed with cancer of the colon. After hearing this news, the nurse anticipates that the client will most likely initially experience
A. depression.
B. confusion.
C. frustration.
*D. anxiety.

Rationale: Following unwelcome news about a diagnostic test, most clients will initially experience anxiety, which may be manifested in various ways.

Reference: p. 93

Descriptors:
1. 07 2. 04 3. Application
4. III–1 5. Nursing Process 6. Moderate

6. A nurse is caring for a client who has been diagnosed with posttraumatic stress disorder. The nurse anticipates that this client will manifest this disorder by
*A. excessive vigilance.
B. numbness.
C. decreased urinary epinephrine levels.
D. decreased body metabolism.

Rationale: Clients with posttraumatic stress syndrome have difficulty sleeping, an exaggerated startle response, excessive vigilance, increased urinary epinephrine levels, and increased body metabolism.

Reference: p. 94

Descriptors:
1. 07 2. 04 3. Application
4. III–1 5. Nursing Process 6. Moderate

7. A client visits the clinic and tells the nurse that "he has been extremely depressed lately." The nurse should instruct the client that clinical depression differs from everyday sadness by severity and
A. feelings of loss.
B. loss of self control.
*C. duration of the sadness.
D. difficulty sleeping.

Rationale: Clinical depression differs from everyday sadness by severity and duration of the sadness, which is usually for a least a two-week period or longer.

Reference: p. 94

Descriptors:
1. 07 2. 04 3. Application
4. III–1 5. Nursing Process 6. Moderate

8. A nurse is caring for a female client who is codependent on her alcoholic husband. The nurse plans care for the client based on the client's
 A. desire to end her relationship.
 *B. need to control others.
 C. sense of isolation.
 D. desire to be in a social group.

Rationale: Codependents struggle with a need to be needed, the urge to control others, and a willingness to remain involved and suffer with a person who has a drug problem.

Reference: p. 96

Descriptors:
1. 07 2. 07 3. Application
4. III–1 5. Nursing Process 6. Difficult

9. A nurse is caring for a terminally ill client who says to the nurse "I've been praying to God for a few more months to live." The nurse assesses this client to be in the stage of grief termed
 A. denial.
 B. anger.
 C. depression.
 *D. bargaining.

Rationale: The client's prayers to God for a few more months to live reflect the bagaining stage of grief.

Reference p. 98

Descriptors:
1. 07 2. 05 3. Analysis
4. III–1 5. Nursing Process 6. Moderate

10. A nurse is caring for a 26-year-old male who has been admitted with multiple injuries following an automobile accident. The developmental task that will have an impact on how this client copes with his illness and hospitalization is
 *A. developing a career.
 B. establishing financial security.
 C. reviewing life's accomplishments.
 D. launching children.

Rationale: Developmental stages and tasks of young adulthood that can have an impact on how this client copes with his illness and hospitalization include establishing independence, establishing a lifestyle, developing a career and intimate relationships, and marrying and starting a family.

Reference: p. 92

Descriptors:
1. 07 2. 08 3. Application
4. II–1 5. Nursing Process 6. Moderate

11. When a nurse enters an adult client's hospital room, the nurse observes that the client is praying with a minister. The nurse is aware that the foundation of spirituality is
 A. acceptance.
 B. love.
 *C. faith.
 D. charity.

Rationale: The foundation of spirituality is faith, or a belief in something the person cannot see. Illness and loss can result in a loss of faith.

Reference: p. 99

Descriptors:
1. 07 2. 09 3. Comprehension
4. III–1 5. Nursing Process 6. Moderate

12. A nurse is caring for a family in which the husband has sustained multiple injuries and will face months of rehabilitation. The nurse can assist this family to cope with this crisis by focusing on the family's
 *A. communication skills.
 B. support strategies.
 C. financial resources.
 D. physical needs.

Rationale: Communication skills and spirituality have been found to be the most useful traits that enhance coping of family members (Burr et al., 1994). Other strengths include cognitive abilities, use of community resources, relationship capabilities, and individual strengths.

Reference: p. 99

Descriptors:
1. 07 2. 10 3. Comprehension
4. III–1 5. Nursing Process 6. Moderate

13. A nurse is caring for a client who is severely anxious following the news that she must have surgery on her back. The nurse should
 A. discuss his or her own experiences with surgery.
 B. tell the client to calm herself down.
 *C. listen actively and focus on the client's personal feelings.
 D. tell the client that the surgeon is very skilled.

Rationale: When caring for a client who is severely anxious, the nurse should listen actively and focus on the client's personal feelings. Other interventions include positive remarks, appropriate use of touch, and use of coping strategies.

Reference: p. 94

Descriptors:
1. 07 2. 10 3. Application
4. III–1 5. Nursing Process 6. Moderate

CHAPTER 8
Perspectives in Transcultural Nursing

1. The major purpose of culturally competent nursing care is to enable the nurse to
 A. be cognizant of his or her own cultural beliefs.
 *B. provide care in a culturally sensitive manner.

C. change his or her own beliefs to meet the client's needs.
D. refrain from making judgments when the client's beliefs are wrong.

Rationale: Culturally competent care is defined as providing effective care in cross-cultural situations. The major purpose of culturally competent nursing care is to enable the nurse to provide care in a culturally sensitive manner.

Reference: p. 103

Descriptors:
1. 08 2. 01 3. Comprehension
4. I–1 5. Cultural Awareness 6. Moderate

2. The nursing theorist that has developed a theory of comprehensive research-based theory called Culture Care Diversity is
A. Sister Callista Roy.
B. Betty Newman.
C. Margaret Mead.
*D. Madeleine Leininger.

Rationale: Leininger's theory of Culture Care Diversity includes providing culturally congruent care through culture care accomodation and culture care restructuring.

Reference: p. 103

Descriptors:
1. 08 2. 01 3. Comprehension
4. I–1 5. Cultural Awareness 6. Moderate

3. A nurse is interviewing a newly admitted client who speaks only limited English. The nurse should
A. greet the client by his first name.
B. refrain from using family members as interpreters.
*C. repeat and summarize frequently.
D. ask the client about his discomforts.

Rationale: The nurse should greet the client by using his last name and repeat and summarize frequently. Family members can interpret for the client.

Reference: p. 105

Descriptors:
1. 08 2. 04 3. Application
4. I–1 5. Cultural Awareness 6. Moderate

4. When the nurse stands very close to a hospitalized client to perform a nursing procedure, the nurse should be aware that some culturally diverse clients may find this threatening. Which cultural group would find the nurse's closeness threatening?
A. Latin American.
B. Mexican American.
C. Iranian.
*D. Canadian.

Rationale: Research reveals that clients from the United States, Great Britain, and Canada require the most personal space between themselves and others.

Reference: p. 105

Descriptors:
1. 08 2. 02 3. Application
4. I–1 5. Cultural Awareness 6. Moderate

5. When the nurse is caring for an Asian American, the nurse should be more cautious when touching the client's
A. chest.
B. legs.
C. hands.
*D. head.

Rationale: For many Asian Americans, it is impolite to touch the client's head because the spirit is believed to reside in the head.

Reference: p. 105

Descriptors:
1. 08 2. 04 3. Application
4. I–1 5. Cultural Awareness 6. Difficult

6. When planning the nutritional needs of a client who is a Mormon, the nurse should be aware that certain food and drinks are prohibited, including
A. milk.
B. pork.
*C. coffee.
D. shellfish.

Rationale: Mormons are typically prohibited from drinking caffeinated drinks such as coffee and colas. In addition alcohol and tobacco use is also prohibited. Jews abstain from pork, while Seventh Day Adventists abstain from pork and shellfish.

Reference: p. 106

Descriptors:
1. 08 2. 04 3. Application
4. I–1 5. Cultural Awareness 6. Moderate

7. A nurse is caring for a client from Jamaica who tells the nurse that his family practices voodoo. The nurse determines that this client's world view is termed
*A. magico-religious.
B. hot/cold.
C. yin/yang.
D. holistic.

Rationale: Individuals who believe in the magico-religious world view believe that there are magical causes of illness, such as voodoo or witchcraft.

Reference: p. 107

Descriptors:
1. 08 2. 01 3. Analysis
4. I–1 5. Cultural Awareness 6. Moderate

8. A nurse is caring for a Native American client who has a world view that human life is only one aspect of nature. The nurse assesses that this client has a world view that is considered

A. biomedical.
B. scientific.
C. magico-religious.
*D. naturalistic.

Rationale: In a naturalistic or holistic world view, human life is only one aspect of nature. The forces of nature must be kept in natural balance or harmony.

Reference: p. 106

Descriptors:
1. 08 2. 02 3. Application
4. I–1 5. Cultural Awareness 6. Moderate

9. A nurse is caring for an Asian American client who believes in the naturalistic world view of yin and yang. The nurse is aware that yin energy represents
*A. darkness.
B. warmth.
C. positive feelings.
D. maleness.

Rationale: Yin energy represents female and negative forces, such as emptiness, darkness, and cold. Cold foods are eaten when there is a "hot" illness, such as a fever.

Reference: p. 106

Descriptors:
1. 08 2. 03 3. Analysis
4. I–1 5. Cultural Awareness 6. Moderate

10. A nurse is caring for a client who has recently immigrated to the United States from Albania. Which of the following would be appropriate to include when assessing the client's culture? The client's
A. age.
B. marital status.
*C. religious practices.
D. support systems.

Rationale: Assessment of a client's culture should include the client's country of origin, language, food preferences or restrictions, health maintenance practices, and religious preferences and practices.

Reference: p. 107

Descriptors:
1. 08 2. 02 3. Application
4. I–1 5. Cultural Awareness 6. Moderate

CHAPTER 9
Chronic Illness

1. Chronic illness is best defined as a
*A. health problem that requires long-term management.
B. curable illness that has a slow onset.
C. congenital defect that is present at birth.
D. medical or psychological condition resulting from a traumatic injury.

Rationale: Chronic conditions are best defined as medical conditions or health problems with associated symptoms or disabilities that require long-term (3 months or longer) management. Congenital defects at birth are an example of a chronic condition.

Reference: p. 111

Descriptors:
1. 09 2. 01 3. Comprehension
4. I–1 5. Self-Care 6. Easy

2. In developing countries, chronic conditions have become the major cause of health related problems due to
A. comprehensive prenatal care available at community health clinics.
B. slow treatment of acute conditions such as myocardial infarction.
*C. a decrease in mortality rates from infectious diseases.
D. increasing automobile accidents due to population increases.

Rationale: In developing countries, chronic conditions have become the major cause of health-related problems due to a decrease in mortality rates from infectious diseases, longer life spans, improved screening and diagnostic procedures, and prompt and aggressive management of acute conditions such as myocardial infarction.

Reference: p. 113

Descriptors:
1. 09 2. 02 3. Comprehension
4. IV–3 5. Self-Care 6. Moderate

3. When planning care for a client who has been diagnosed with chronic rhematoid arthritis, the nurse should
A. focus on the medical problems of the disability.
B. rely on health care members to provide care in the home.
*C. recognize that the socioeconomic status of the client may impact treatments.
D. explain to the client that chronic illness follows a distinct, slow pattern.

Rationale: The implications of a chronic illness have an impact on the client in that the socioeconomic status may impact treatments, family members may experience role changes, managing chronic illness involves more than just the medical problems, and individuals and their families must assume major responsibility for day-to-day management of the disease.

Reference: p. 113

Descriptors:
1. 09 2. 03 3. Application
4. IV–3 5. Self-Care 6. Moderate

4. A nurse is caring for an elderly female diagnosed with diabetes mellitus. The client has not been adhering to her prescribed diet. The nurse's response to the client's behavior should be guided by an understanding that the
   A. client must follow the prescribed diet in order to continue receiving medical care.
   B. client's family has a responsibility to monitor the client's dietary practices.
   C. client may be noncompliant in order to get attention from the health care system.
   *D. client has the right to make her own decisions regarding health care.

Rationale: Although it may be difficult for nurses and other health care providers to stand by while clients make unwise decisions about their health, they must accept the fact that the client has the right to make his or her own choices and decisions about lifestyle and health care.

Reference: p. 114

Descriptors:

1. 09	2. 03	3. Application
4. IV–3	5. Self-Care	6. Moderate

5. A nurse is caring for a client who was diagnosed with sickle cell disease three years ago. The client has been hospitalized with extreme joint pain and immobility. The nurse would assess this phase of the client's chronic condition to be
   *A. acute.
   B. trajectory.
   C. unstable.
   D. comeback.

Rationale: During the acute phase, there is a sudden onset of severe or unrelieved symptoms, which is what this client is experiencing.

Reference: p. 114

Descriptors:

1. 09	2. 04	3. Analysis
4. IV–3	5. Self-Care	6. Difficult

6. An adult client is undergoing diagnostic testing to determine if he has osteoarthritis. The nurse determines that the phase of chronic illness that this client is in is the
   A. acute.
   B. crisis.
   *C. trajectory.
   D. stable.

Rationale: The trajectory phase is characterized by the onset of symptoms and is the phase in which diagnostic tests are performed.

Reference: p. 114

Descriptors:

1. 09	2. 04	3. Analysis
4. IV–3	5. Self-Care	6. Moderate

7. A nurse is caring for a client who has been diagnosed with multiple sclerosis. The nurse establishes a nursing diagnosis of Fatigue related to symptoms of multiple sclerosis. The nurse should then
   A. identify the trajectory phase of the chronic condition.
   B. implement nursing interventions to improve the client's fatigue.
   *C. validate the nursing diagnosis with the client.
   D. identify barriers that will affect implementation of the care plan.

Rationale: Once the nurse has formulated the nursing diagnosis based on the assessment data collected, the nurse should validate and prioritize the diagnosis with the client.

Reference: p. 115

Descriptors:

1. 09	2. 05	3. Application
4. I–1	5. Self-Care	6. Moderate

8. A nurse is caring for a client diagnosed with rheumatoid arthritis. Once the client has been located within the trajectory and nursing diagnoses have been established, the nurse should next
   *A. establish the goals of care with the client.
   B. establish a plan for meeting the client's goals.
   C. discuss methods for the client to accomplish self-care activities.
   D. identify barriers to attainment of goals established.

Rationale: Once the client has been located within the trajectory and nursing diagnoses have been established, the nurse should next establish the goals of care with the client.

Reference: p. 115

Descriptors:

1. 09	2. 05	3. Application
4. I–1	5. Self-Care	6. Moderate

9. A nurse is caring for a client following a myocardial infarction. It is important for the nurse and client to identify barriers to goal attainment of the client's goals because these factors
   A. will predict how likely the client will be able to follow the plan of care.
   B. can be used by the nurse to determine how long it will take to achieve the goals.
   *C. can influence the nurse's suggestions to develop strategies to improve self-care.
   D. help to determine what phase of the chronic illness the client is experiencing.

Rationale: It is important for the nurse and client to identify barriers to goal attainment of the client's goals because these factors can influence the nurse's suggestions to develop strategies to improve self-care and enhance goal achievement.

Reference: p. 116

Descriptors:

1. 09	2. 05	3. Application
4. IV–3	5. Self-Care	6. Difficult

10. A nurse is making the third home visit to a client following a total hip replacement due to arthritis. In evaluating the effectiveness of the nursing interventions, the nurse should keep in mind that for clients with a chronic illness, effectiveness is oftendetermined by
    A. the relief of the client's symptoms.
    B. how quickly the client is discharged from home care.
    C. the need to redefine the client's goals.
    *D. the amount of progress made toward a change in behaviors.

Rationale: For clients with a chronic illness, effectiveness is often determined by the amount of progress made toward a change in behaviors. If no progress is made, there may be a need to redefine the goals.

Reference: p. 116

Descriptors:
1. 09 2. 05 3. Application
4. IV–3 5. Self-Care 6. Moderate

11. An adult client who was diagnosed with chronic obstructive pulmonary disease three years ago visits the clinic for a routine examination. Although the client has managed his condition at home for three years, the nurse should
    A. recognize that the client is very knowledgeable about his condition.
    B. motivate the client by discussing what happens with poor management.
    *C. reassess the client's learning needs as these may change over time.
    *D. determine if the client understands what this condition involves.

Rationale: Because of changes in the client's learning needs over time and personal life changes, the nurse should reassess the client's learning needs. The nurse should not assume that a client who has had an illness for a number of years has all of the knowledge needed to manage the illness.

Reference: p. 117

Descriptors:
1. 09 2. 05 3. Application
4. IV–3 5. Self-Care 6. Moderate

CHAPTER 10
Principles and Practices of Rehabilitation

1. A nurse is caring for a client following an automobile accident that resulted in numerous injuries. The nurse should explain to the client that one of the goals of rehabilitation is to
    A. maintain the client's former lifestyle.
    B. identify the client's strengths and weaknesses.
    C. minimize the client's disabilities.
    *D. restore the client to independence.

Rationale: The goal of rehabilitation includes restoring the client to independence or to the pre-illness or pre-injury level of functioning in as short a period of time as possible. If this is not possible, the aims of rehabilitation are maximal independence and quality of life acceptable to the client.

Reference: p. 119

Descriptors:
1. 10 2. 01 3. Comprehension
4. IV–3 5. Self-Care 6. Moderate

2. Principles of rehabilitation apply to clients
    *A. during the initial contact with the health care delivery system.
    B. with diagnoses that are not terminal.
    C. with major physical defects such as paralysis.
    D. who are younger than 70 years of age.

Rationale: The principles of rehabilitation apply to clients during the initial contact with the health care delivery system because every major illness or injury has a threat of disability.

Reference: p. 119

Descriptors:
1. 10 2. 01 3. Application
4. I–1 5. Self-Care 6. Moderate

3. A client is undergoing rehabilitation following a total right hip replacement. The key member of the rehabilitation team is the
    A. case manager.
    B. nurse.
    C. physical therapist.
    *D. client.

Rationale: The client is the key member of the rehabilitation team because the client is the one who determines the final outcome of the process.

Reference: p. 120

Descriptors:
1. 10 2. 02 3. Application
4. IV–3 5. Self-Care 6. Moderate

4. A nurse is caring for a client during rehabilitation following an automobile accident. When the nurse coordinates the client's total rehabilitative plan of care, the nurse is functioning as a
    A. team leader.
    B. caregiver.
    *C. case manager.
    D. client advocate.

Rationale: When the nurse coordinates the client's total rehabilitative plan of care, the nurse is functioning as a case manager. The nurse must coordinate services provided by all of the team members.

Reference: p. 120

Descriptors:
1. 10 2. 02 3. Comprehension
4. I–1 5. Nursing Process 6. Easy

5. An adult client has just been diagnosed with paralysis due to an automobile accident that injured the spinal cord. The nurse can anticipate that emotionally, the client will
   A. go through all stages of grief before adaptation takes place.
   B. progress sequentially through the grief process.
   C. need to be "cheered up" at times.
   *D. respond to grief in an individualistic manner.

Rationale: Not all clients experience all stages of grief. Grief over lost function is a normal response and clients handle their grief in an individualistic manner. The nurse should not blithely encourage the client to "cheer up," but should actively listen to the client's emotional statements.

Reference: p. 120

Descriptors:
1. 10 2. 03 3. Comprehension
4. IV–3 5. Self-Care 6. Moderate

6. A nurse is caring for a client with a self-care deficit of ADLs. The nurse plans to record the client's daily performance of these activities in order to
   *A. motivate the client to continue to improve.
   B. determine if self-care devices are needed.
   C. identify whether a support group is needed.
   D. suggest better ways of achieving the goals.

Rationale: Recording the client's performance provides data for evaluating the progress and may be used as a source of motivation and morale building.

Reference: p. 122

Descriptors:
1. 10 2. 05 3. Application
4. I–1 5. Self-Care 6. Moderate

7. A nurse is assessing a client with limited mobility following a stroke. In order to assess the client for contractures, the nurse should assess the client's
   A. coordination.
   B. muscle tone.
   C. muscle strength.
   *D. range of motion.

Rationale: Each joint of the body has a normal range of motion. To assess a client for contractures, the nurse should assess whether the client can complete the full range of motion activities.

Reference: p. 123

Descriptors:
1. 10 2. 04 3. Application
4. I–1 5. Nursing Process 6. Moderate

8. A client is hospitalized following a stroke that has impaired the client's mobility. To prevent outward rotation of the client's hip when the client is in the supine position, the nurse should
   A. place a bed cradle over the client.
   B. align the head with the spine and support it with a pillow.
   C. support the back with a small pillow.
   *D. place trochanter rolls under the greater trochanter.

Rationale: A trochanter roll extending from the crest of the ilium to the midthigh prevents outward rotation of the client's hip.

Reference: pp. 124–125

Descriptors:
1. 10 2. 04 3. Application
4. IV–3 5. Nursing Process 6. Moderate

9. While assisting a client with limited mobility to perform range of motion exercises, the nurse plans to assess the client's abduction of his arm, which is the client's ability to
   *A. move the limb away from the midline of the body.
   B. bend the joint so that the angle of the joint diminishes.
   C. turn the limb towards the center of the body.
   D. rotate the forearm so that the palm of the hand is down.

Rationale: Abduction is movement away from the midline of the body. Flexion is the bending of the joint. Pronation is rotation of the forearm. Adduction is moving the limb toward the midline of the body.

Reference: p. 126

Descriptors:
1. 10 2. 04 3. Analysis
4. IV–3 5. Nursing Process 6. Moderate

10. A nurse is caring for a client who has limited mobility following paralysis from a stroke. To prepare the client for ambulation, the nurse should instruct the client in strengthening his
   A. biceps muscles.
   B. shoulder extensor muscles.
   C. wrist muscles.
   *D. quadriceps muscles.

Rationale: Prior to ambulation, the quadriceps and gluteal muscles should be strengthened through exercises that are repeated hourly.

Descriptors:
1. 10 2. 06 3. Application
4. IV–3 5. Self-Care 6. Moderate

Reference: pp. 131–132

11. A nurse is preparing to assist an adult client to stand following abdominal surgery. The nurse should
   A. place his or her arms and hands under the client's shoulders.

*B. firmly grasp the client's rib cage with the hands.
C. position the client's feet at right angles.
D. instruct the client to push off the bed with her wrists.

Rationale: To assist an adult client to stand following abdominal surgery, the nurse should instruct the client to push into the bed with the elbows, then position the client's feet so that they will be well grounded. Then the nurse should firmly grasp the client's rib cage with the hands. Finally, the nurse should rock the client forward to a standing position.

Reference: p. 132

Descriptors:
1. 10 2. 06 3. Application
4. I–2 5. Nursing Process 6. Moderate

12. A nurse is planning to instruct an adult client in crutch walking. The nurse should plan to instruct the client to
A. wear soft shoes such as slippers to avoid injuries.
B. keep using the crutches even when fatigued to strengthen the muscles.
*C. support his weight on the hand pieces of the crutches.
D. support his weight on the axillae of each arm.

Rationale: When instructing the client how to use crutches for the first time, the client should be wearing sturdy, well-fitting shoes. The nurse should then plan to instruct the client to support his weight on the hand pieces of the crutches to prevent injury to the brachial plexus nerves. The client should rest when fatigue occurs.

Reference: p. 133

Descriptors:
1. 10 2. 06 3. Application
4. IV–3 5. Self-Care 6. Moderate

13. A client is being assessed for the need of an orthosis. The nurse should explain to the client that an orthosis is
A. an adapted eating utensil.
B. a grab bar.
C. elastic stockings.
*D. a neck brace.

Rationale: Orthoses include braces, splints, collars, or corsets and are used to provide support or correct deformities.

Reference: p. 135

Descriptors:
1. 10 2. 06 3. Application
4. IV–3 5. Self-Care 6. Moderate

14. A nurse has just admitted an elderly client following a fractured tibia. The client appears malnourished. To assess the client for protein deficiency, the nurse should assess which of the following laboratory findings?
*A. Serum albumin.
B. White blood cells.
C. Hematocrit.
D. Liver enzymes.

Rationale: Serum albumin is a sensitive indicator of protein deficiency. Albumin levels of less than 3 g/mL are indicative of hypoalbuminemia.

Reference: p. 136

Descriptors:
1. 10 2. 07 3. Application
4. IV–3 5. Nursing Process 6. Moderate

15. A nurse is planning to assess an immobilized client for impaired skin integrity due to shear and friction. The nurse should plan to assess the client's
*A. sacrum.
B. elbows.
C. toes.
D. neck.

Rationale: The sacrum and the heels are the most susceptible areas for skin breakdown due to shear and friction.

Reference: p. 136

Descriptors:
1. 10 2. 07 3. Application
4. IV–3 5. Nursing Process 6. Moderate

16. A nurse assesses a client's heels for skin breakdown and notes that both heels have a blister with slight necrosis. The nurse should document the presence of a pressure ulcer in stage
A. I.
*B. II.
C. III.
D. IV.

Rationale: When both heels have a blister or a break in the skin with slight necrosis, the nurse should document the presence of a pressure ulcer in stage II. Stage III extends into the subcutaneous tissue, while Stage IV extends into the muscle or bone.

Reference: p. 137

Descriptors:
1. 10 2. 07 3. Application
4. IV–3 5. Nursing Process 6. Difficult

17. To prevent a pressure ulcer from forming on a client hospitalized with limited mobility and a draining wound, the nurse should
A. offer the client foods that are high in vitamin D.
B. use baby powder on the client's skin.
C. use alcohol wipes to keep the skin dry.
*D. apply a bland lotion to skin after thorough drying.

Rationale: Drying agents and powders should be avoided. A bland lotion can be applied to the skin or petroleum jelly may be used. The client should be encouraged to eat foods high in protein, carbohydrates, and vitamins A, B, and C.

Reference: p. 140

Descriptors:
1. 10 2. 07 3. Application
4. IV–3 5. Nursing Process 6. Moderate

18. A nurse is caring for a paralyzed client who has been diagnosed with reflex incontinence. The nurse should explain to the client that reflex incontinence is the term used when the client
   A. has a strong perceived need to void.
   B. has weakened perineal musles that allow leakage of urine.
   C. has a psychological impairment and cannot control excreta.
   *D. has no sensory awareness of the need to void.

Rationale: Reflex incontinence is associated with a spinal cord lesion that interrupts cerebral control, resulting in no sensory awareness of the need to void. Total incontinence occurs in clients with a psychological impairment when they cannot control excreta.

Reference: p. 141

Descriptors:
1. 10 2. 08 3. Application
4. I–1 5. Nursing Process 6. Moderate

19. An elderly female client visits the clinic because she has been experiencing stress incontinence. The nurse should instruct the client to
   A. keep a record of voiding "accidents" for one week.
   B. sterile intermittant catherization.
   *C. perform Kegel exercises 4 to 6 times per day.
   D. attempt suprapubic tapping to stimulae the void reflex.

Rationale: For cognitively intact women who experience stress incontinence, the nurse should instruct the client to perform Kegel exercises 4 to 6 times per day to strengthen the pubococcygeus muscle. A record can be kept for 48 hours to determine patterns.

Reference: p. 142

Descriptors:
1. 10 2. 08 3. Application
4. IV–3 5. Nursing Process 6. Difficult

20. A nurse is working as a volunteer with a group of severely disabled individuals. The nurse should explain to the group that there is a growing trend for severely disabled individuals toward
   A. extended rehabilitation care.
   *B. independent living alone or in groups.
   C. long-term nursing home care.
   D. state institutions that provide care for life.

Rationale: There is a growing trend toward independent living for severely disabled clients, either alone or in groups. The goal is integration into the community.

Reference: p. 146

Descriptors:
1. 10 2. 09 3. Application
4. IV–3 5. Nursing Process 6. Moderate

CHAPTER 11
Health Care of the Older Adult

1. By the year 2030, the U.S. Census Bureau predicts that the number of people over the age of 65 years will outnumber people who are
   *A. 18 years of age.
   B. 30 years of age.
   C. 40 years of age.
   D. 50 years of age.

Rationale: The older segment of the population is growing faster than the rest of the population. The U.S. Census Bureau predicts that the number of people over the age of 65 years will outnumber people who are 18 years of age and that people will live to be "very old."

Reference: p. 148

Descriptors:
1. 11 2. 02 3. Comprehension
4. I–1 5. Caring 6. Moderate

2. For the elderly population, hospitalizations have increased in recent years, particularly for clients experiencing
   A. gallstones.
   B. cancer.
   *C. cardiovascular disease.
   D. renal disease.

Rationale: An increase in utilization of hospital services by the elderly population has been observed, particularly for clients experiencing end stage cardiovascular disease, musculoskeletal disease, frailty, and nosocomial events.

Reference: p. 149

Descriptors:
1. 11 2. 02 3. Comprehension
4. I–1 5. Caring 6. Moderate

3. A nurse is assessing an 80-year-old client who tells the nurse that he continues to enjoy golf and hiking and maintaining an active lifestyle. The nurse determines that this client is exhibiting a theory of aging termed
   A. ego integrity.
   B. self actualization.
   *C. activity.
   D. continuity.

Rationale: The client is exhibiting the activity theory proposed by Havighurst (1972), which proposes that life satisfaction in normal aging involves maintaining the active lifestyle of middle age.

Reference: p. 150

Descriptors:

1. 11	2. 01	3. Analysis
4. I–1	5. Caring	6. Moderate

4. The leading cause of death for clients over the age of 65 years is
   *A. cardiovascular disease.
   B. chronic obstructive pulmonary disease.
   C. malignant neoplasms.
   D. Alzheimer's disease.

Rationale: As of 1995, the leading cause of death for clients over the age of 65 years continues to be cardiovascular disease. Malignant neoplasms are the second leading cause.

Reference: p. 150

Descriptors:

1. 11	2. 02	3. Comprehension
4. IV–3	5. Caring	6. Moderate

5. The nurse visits a 90-year-old client in her home. The client has been diagnosed with benign senescent forgetfulness. The nurse determines that the client will exhibit memory loss that is
   A. stored.
   *B. short-term.
   C. long-term.
   D. frequent.

Rationale: Benign senescent forgetfulness is the term used when an elderly client has short-term and recent memory loss. The nurse can aid the client through the use of mnemonics or link new information with familiar information.

Reference: p. 151

Descriptors:

1. 11	2. 03	3. Analysis
4. I–1	5. Nursing Process	6. Difficult

6. A nurse is planning to teach an 80-year-old client about his dressing change. The client has exhibited short-term memory loss. The nurse should plan to
   A. set long-term goals with the client.
   B. provide bright glaring lighting in the room.
   C. keep visual cues to a minimum.
   *D. keep teaching periods short.

Rationale: To assist the elderly client with short-term memory loss, the nurse should keep teaching periods short, provide glare-free lighting, link new information with familiar information, use visual and auditory cues, and set short-term goals with the client.

Reference: p. 151

Descriptors:

1. 11	2. 03	3. Application
4. IV–3	5. Self-Care	6. Moderate

7. A 65-year-old client has been diagnosed with essential hypertension. The nurse should explain to the client that this means that the
   *A. diastolic pressure is greater than or equal to 90 mm Hg.
   B. systolic pressure is greater than 140 mm Hg.
   C. hypertension can be attributed to an underlying cause.
   D. hypertension is transient and will decrease over time.

Rationale: Essential hypertension is the diagnosis given when the diastolic pressure is greater than or equal to 90 mm Hg regardless of the systolic pressure. Secondary hypertension can be attributed to an underlying cause, and isolated systolic hypertension is said to be present when the systolic pressure is greater than 140 mm Hg.

Reference: p. 151

Descriptors:

1. 11	2. 03	3. Application
4. I–1	5. Nursing Process	6. Moderate

8. A 75-year-old client is hospitalized following a fractured tibia. The client has very dry skin. The nurse should instruct the client to
   A. bathe daily in tepid water.
   B. use makeup to cover the wrinkles.
   C. avoid prolonged use of sunscreens.
   *D. use a lubricating cream daily.

Rationale: Clients with dry skin should be instructed to us a lubricating cream daily, avoid prolonged exposure to the sun, bathe only 1 to 2 times per week, and maintain a safe indoor temperature.

Reference: p. 152

Descriptors:

1. 11	2. 04	3. Application
4. IV–3	5. Self-Care	6. Moderate

9. A nurse is caring for a female client who has been diagnosed with bladder distention and urinary frequency. The nurse should instruct the client to
   A. reduce fluid intake.
   B. drink plenty of iced tea.
   *C. reduce sugar intake.
   D. avoid citrus juices.

Rationale: The client should use good hygiene practices and avoid caffeinated products such as teas and colas. Maintenance of adequate fluid intake is recommended along with acidic juices such as cranberry juice. The client should avoid sugars and sweeteners because they can contribute to bacterial growth in the bladder.

Reference: p. 152

Descriptors:
1. 11 2. 03 3. Application
4. IV–3 5. Self-Care 6. Difficult

10. A nurse is planning a presentation on the topic of the normal signs of aging to a group of senior citizens. Which of the following should be included in the nurse's teaching plan?
*A. Female reproductive changes include vaginal dryness.
B. Male reproductive changes include increased androgen levels.
C. Disappearance of sexual desire for both males and females.
D. Increased sebaceous and sweat glands for both males and females.

Rationale: Normal signs of aging are female reproductive changes that include vaginal dryness and loss of elasticity, decreased androgen levels in males, decline but not disappearance of sexual desire, and decreased sebaceous and sweat glands for both males and females.

Reference: p. 153

Descriptors:
1. 11 2. 03 3. Application
4. IV–3 5. Self-Care 6. Difficult

11. A nurse is caring for a female client who has been diagnosed with kyphosis. The nurse should explain to the client that this term means
*A. increased convex curvature of the spine.
B. calcification of the sternum.
C. loss of bone density.
D. difficulty turning the head due to calcification.

Rationale: Kyphosis is an increased convex curvature of the spine and can lead to impaired gas exchange due to decreased mobility of the ribs. Osteoporosis is a loss of bone density.

Reference: p. 153

Descriptors:
1. 11 2. 03 3. Application
4. IV–3 5. Self-Care 6. Moderate

12. An elderly male client tells the nurse that he has frequent constipation. The nurse should assess the client for
A. nutritional intake of calcium rich foods.
*B. frequent use of laxatives and antacids.
C. excessive fluid intake.
D. adequate protein intake.

Rationale: Constipation is a common problem in aged people. The nurse should assess the client for frequent laxative and antacid use, which is associated with constipation. The client should eat high-fiber foods, drink 8 to 10 glasses of water daily, and establish regular bowel habits.

Reference: p. 154

Descriptors:
1. 11 2. 03 3. Analysis
4. IV–3 5. Self-Care 6. Moderate

13. An 80-year-old female client has been diagnosed with osteoporosis. The nurse should instruct the client to
*A. eat dairy products and dark, green vegetables.
B. exercise for only short periods of time.
C. eat red meats and foods high in phosphorus.
D. drink at least 8 glasses of fluids per day.

Rationale: Osteoporosis can be arrested through exercise, estrogens, and adequate calcium intake. The client should reduce phosphorus intake by decreasing the amounts of red meats and processed foods. Drinking 8 glasses of fluid is helpful for constipation, but not osteoporosis.

Reference: p. 154

Descriptors:
1. 11 2. 04 3. Comprehension
4. IV–3 5. Self-Care 6. Easy

14. A nurse is caring for a 76-year-old client who has been admitted to the hospital with a diagnosis of severe depression. The nurse should instruct the client's family that depression
A. can be a late sign of a chronic illness.
B. is rarely seen in clients after the age of 50 years.
C. is rarely associated with a physical illness.
*D. is the most common affective mood disorder of old age.

Rationale: Depression can be an early sign of a chronic illness and is the most common affective mood disorder of old age. Depression can result from a physical illness. It is self-perpetuating and often goes undiagnosed.

Reference: p. 156

Descriptors:
1. 11 2. 05 3. Application
4. III–1 5. Nursing Process 6. Moderate

15. An 84-year-old client is admitted to the hospital with a diagnosis of delirium. The nurse should explain to the client's family that delirium
A. usually remains until the client's death.
B. involves a progressive decline in memory loss.
*C. has symptoms that can be reversible.
D. is usually diagnosed only in male clients.

Rationale: Delirium differs from other types of dementia in that delirium begins with confusion and progresses to disorientation. It affects males and females equally, has symptoms that are reversible with treatment, and lasts from 1 day to 1 month. Progressive memory loss is seen in Alzheimer's disease.

Reference: p. 158

Descriptors:
1. 11 2. 05 3. Application
4. I–1 5. Nursing Process 6. Difficult

16. A nurse makes a home visit to a 90-year-old client who has cardiovascular disease. The nurse observes that the client is exhibiting symptoms of sudden confusion and hallucinations. The nurse contacts the client's physician because these symptoms are associated with
A. early Alzheimer's disease.
B. late Alzheimer's disease.
*C. multi-infarct dementia.
D. delirium.

Rationale: In more than half of the cases, sudden confusion and hallucinations are evident in multi-infarct dementia. This condition is also associated with cardiovascular disease.

Reference: p. 159

Descriptors:
1. 11 2. 05 3. Application
4. I–1 5. Nursing Process 6. Moderate

17. A client with early stage Alzheimer's disease has been prescribed tacrine hydrochloride. The nurse should explain to the client and his family that this medication enhances the body's production of
*A. acetylcholine.
B. prostaglandins.
C. norepinephrine.
D. adrenalin.

Rationale: Tacrine hydrochloride enhances the body's production of acetylcholine, which can decrease the symptoms of Alzheimer's disease.

Reference: p. 160

Descriptors:
1. 11 2. 06 3. Application
4. IV–2 5. Nursing Process 6. Difficult

18. A nurse is caring for an 86-year-old frail female client. The nurse has instructed the client to remove any hazardous rugs in her home to prevent falls because the most common fracture resulting from a fall is a fractured
*A. hip.
B. ankle.
C. wrist.
D. knee.

Rationale: The most common fracture resulting from a fall is a fractured hip, resulting from osteoporosis and the condition or situation that produced the fall. Falls have been associated with increased institutionalization of elderly clients.

Reference: p. 163

Descriptors:
1. 11 2. 06 3. Application
4. IV–3 5. Nursing Process 6. Moderate

19. The nurse makes a home visit to a 76-year-old widow who is taking multiple medications. The nurse should advise the client that
A. medications have a short action in older clients.
B. she should rely on her memory for taking daily medications.
C. high fiber diets can enhance absorption of medications.
*D. she should avoid over-the-counter medication use.

Rationale: Over-the-counter medication use and prescribed medications can lead to interactions that may be toxic. The client may need a pill reminder for taking her medications, and high fiber diets can decrease the rate of absorption with some medications.

Reference: pp. 164–165

Descriptors:
1. 11 2. 07 3. Application
4. IV–3 5. Nursing Process 6. Moderate

20. A nurse is caring for a 78-year-old widower in his home following bowel surgery. To encourage greater safety in the client's home, the nurse should advise the client to
*A. mark the edges of stairs with contrasting colors.
B. use only direct lighting in his rooms.
C. keep surfaces shiny rather than dull.
D. avoid the use of curtains to diffuse sunlight.

Rationale: Adequate lighting with minimal glare can be achieved through the use of small area lamps, indirect lighting, and sheer curtains to diffuse sunlight. Contrasting colors to mark the edges of the stairs can be useful for better discrimination.

Reference: p. 166

Descriptors:
1. 11 2. 08 3. Application
4. I–2 5. Nursing Process 6. Moderate

21. An elderly client asks the nurse how she can name someone to make decisions for her if she becomes incapacitated. The nurse should suggest that the client contact an attorney and draw up a
*A. durable power of attorney.
B. living trust.
C. guardian of the court.
D. power of attorney.

Rationale: A durable power of attorney allows another individual to make decisions for the client when the client is incapacitated. Power of attorney is a legal agreement that is invalidated if the client becomes incapacitated.

Reference: p. 167

Descriptors:
1. 11 2. 09 3. Application
4. I–1 5. Nursing Process 6. Moderate

UNIT 3 CONCEPTS AND CHALLENGES IN PATIENT MANAGEMENT

CHAPTER 12 Pain Management

1. An adult client is admitted to the hospital with a diagnosis of chronic back pain. The nurse should explain to the client that chronic pain
   A. lasts longer than 12 months.
   B. is an uncommon form of pain.
   C. is usually associated with an identifiable cause.
   *D. is often difficult to treat.

Rationale: Chronic pain persists for 6 months or longer and is a common form of pain.
Chronic pain is often difficult to treat because the etiology may not be clear.

Reference: p. 177

Descriptors:
1. 12 2. 01 3. Application
4. IV–1 5. Nursing Process 6. Moderate

2. A terminally ill client is being cared for in a hospice unit and is suffering from severe cancer pain. The nurse should explain to the client's family that clients with cancer have pain that is
   *A. a direct result of tumor involvement.
   B. not related to the cancer.
   C. due to the surgical interventions.
   D. due to the radiation therapies.

Rationale: Clients with cancer have pain that is usually a direct result of tumor involvement and nerve compression. However, some cancer victims suffer pain as a direct result of surgery or radiation, and some have pain that is not related to the cancer.

Reference: p. 177

Descriptors:
1. 12 2. 01 3. Application
4. IV–1 5. Nursing Process 6. Moderate

3. A client is seen in the clinic and complains of chronic pain, fatigue, stiffness, generalized muscle pain, and sleep disturbances. The nurse determines that the client is most likely experiencing a type of pain termed
   A. reflex sympathetic dystrophy.
   B. posttraumatic headache.
   C. AIDS-related pain.
   *D. fibromyalgia.

Rationale: Chronic pain, fatigue, stiffness, generalized muscle pain, and sleep disturbances are characteristic symptoms of fibromyalgia. RSD is characterized by weakness and skin color changes of the extremity. Posttraumatic headache results from head trauma. AIDS-related pain involves neuropathy, esophagitis, abdominal, and joint pain.

Reference: p. 178

Descriptors:
1. 12 2. 01 3. Analysis
4. IV–1 5. Nursing Process 6. Difficult

4. A 77-year-old postoperative client tells the nurse that she cannot sleep because of her pain. The nurse plans to administer a pain medication to the client to decrease the stress response that includes
   A. decreased mobility.
   B. decreased heart rate.
   *C. increased metabolic rate.
   D. decreased retention of fluids.

Rationale: Pain can produce the stress response, which includes increased metabolic rate, increased cardiac output, impaired insulin response, increased cortisol levels, and increased retention of fluids. The stress response may increase the client's risk for physiologic disorders.

Reference: p. 177

Descriptors:
1. 12 2. 02 3. Application
4. IV–2 5. Nursing Process 6. Moderate

5. An adult client is experiencing pain following abdominal surgery. During the pain response
   A. blood vessels constrict near the site.
   B. gastrointestinal peristalsis increases.
   *C. nocioreceptors in the brain are stimulated.
   D. endorphins are produced in response to the pain.

Rationale: During a pain response, nocioreceptors in the brain are stimulated, gastrointestinal peristalsis decreases or stops, and inflammation occurs. Prostaglandins are thought to increase the sensitivity of pain, while endorphins reduce or inhibit the perception of pain.

Reference: pp. 177–180

Descriptors:
1. 12 2. 03 3. Comprehension
4. IV–1 5. Nursing Process 6. Moderate

6. A nurse is caring for a client in severe pain following an automobile accident. One of the most common myths about pain and analgesia that many clients have is that
   *A. pain medication should be saved until the pain is severe.
   B. clients should inform the nurse when they have pain.
   C. pain is not good for you and can cause other physiologic changes.
   D. people rarely get addicted to pain medications.

Rationale: Common myths about pain and analgesia include pain medication should be saved until the pain is severe, clients shouldn't complain about their pain to the nurse, pain builds character, and people get addicted to pain medication easily.

Reference: p. 181

Descriptors:

1. 12	2. 04	3. Comprehension
4. IV–1	5. Nursing Process	6. Moderate

7. An essential aspect of pain management for all hospitalized clients is
   A. use of FACES pain rating scale.
   B. administration of pain medications.
   *C. a systematic pain assessment plan.
   D. use of relaxation techniques.

Rationale: Documentation of the client's pain level as rated on a pain scale is an essential component of care for all hospitalized clients. FACES is a pain scale that is used for children and low-literacy clients. Not all clients will require pain medication or relaxation techniques.

Reference: p. 181

Descriptors:

1. 12	2. 06	3. Comprehension
4. IV–1	5. Nursing Process	6. Moderate

8. To validate a client's pain level the nurse should
   *A. ask the client to rate the pain intensity.
   B. rely on physiologic responses to pain.
   C. observe the client's facial expressions.
   D. determine if the client appears angry.

Rationale: The nurse should ask the client to report the level of pain intensity unless the client is comatose. The nurse should not rely on physiologic or behavioral responses because these are unreliable.

Reference: p. 183

Descriptors:

1. 12	2. 06	3. Application
4. IV–1	5. Nursing Process	6. Moderate

9. A nurse is caring for an adult client with chronic fatigue and back pain that is unrelieved by medication. The nurse should assess the client for
   A. anxiety.
   B. the need for a placebo.
   *C. depression.
   D. pain tolerance.

Rationale: Depression is associated with chronic pain, and often, treatment of the pain may help relieve the depression. The client does not need a placebo. It is not necessarily true that anxiety is associated with pain.

Reference: p. 184

Descriptors:

1. 12	2. 07	3. Application
4. IV–1	5. Nursing Process	6. Moderate

10. A nurse is caring for a client with chronic pain following an automobile accident. In order to determine the goals for pain management, the nurse should first consider the
    A. anticipated harmful effects of pain.
    B. anticipated duration of the pain.
    C. client's pain tolerance level.
    *D. severity of the pain.

Rationale: A number of factors need to be considered to determine the goal of pain management. The first factor that should be considered is the severity of the pain as judged by the client. Next is anticipated harmful effects, and then anticipated duration.

Reference: p. 185

Descriptors:

1. 12	2. 11	3. Application
4. III–1	5. Nursing Process	6. Moderate

11. A nurse is preparing to administer morphine sulfate for the first time to a postoperative client. Before administering the medication, the nurse should
    *A. ask the client about allergies to the medication.
    B. determine if the client is in severe pain.
    C. ask the client if he is taking any over-the-counter medications.
    D. document the client's previous side effects to the medication.

Rationale: Before administering a medication such as morphine for the first time, the nurse should ask the client if he has ever experienced any allergies to the medication. Allergies, such as anaphylactic shock, are different from side effects such as rashes. Pain medication should be given before the client experiences severe pain.

Reference: p. 187

Descriptors:

1. 12	2. 11	3. Application
4. IV–2	5. Nursing Process	6. Moderate

12. When a nurse administers a narcotic analgesic and a nonsteroidal anti-inflammatory drug

together, the nurse should explain to the client that the medications are given together to
A. prevent respiratory depression from the narcotic.
B. eliminate the need for additional medication during the night.
*C. more effectively relieve the client's pain with less narcotic.
D. wean the client from the narcotic medications.

Rationale: When one agent is used alone, it must be used in a higher dose to be effective. Using the narcotic with the NSAID requires less narcotic to relieve the client's pain. This method also reduces but does not eliminate the potential for toxic effects of the narcotic.

Reference: p. 187

Descriptors:
1. 12 2. 09 3. Application
4. IV–2 5. Nursing Process 6. Difficult

13. A nurse is caring for a postoperative client who is receiving an opioid pain medication through a PCA pump. After the client has administered a bolus of the medication, the nurse should
A. document the amount the client has received.
B. assess the client for sedation.
*C. monitor the client for respiratory depression.
D. allow the client undisturbed rest for 4 hours.

Rationale: Whenever clients are receiving an opioid analgesic, the nurse should continue to monitor the client for respiratory depression, which is a toxic effect of the drug. The amount received is calculated by the PCA pump. The nurse should assess the client for pain relief, which may or may not include sedation.

Reference: p. 189

Descriptors:
1. 12 2. 10 3. Application
4. IV–2 5. Nursing Process 6. Moderate

14. A client with cancer is taking an opioid for chronic, unrelieved pain. Over time, the client is likely to become
*A. more tolerant of the dosage.
B. psychologically dependent on the drug.
C. immune to the drug's effects.
D. addicted to the medication.

Rationale: Over time, the client is likely to become more tolerant of the dosage. There is little evidence that clients with cancer become addicted to the opioid medications.

Reference: p. 191

Descriptors:
1. 12 2. 08 3. Application
4. IV–2 5. Nursing Process 6. Moderate

15. A client with rheumatoid arthritis is prescribed a nonsteroidal anti-inflammatory medication for pain. The nurse should explain to the client that these medications are thought to
A. prevent pain reception sites from receiving stimuli.
B. promote the release of endorphins.
C. reduce anxiety and decrease sensations.
*D. inhibit the production of prostaglandins.

Rationale: Nonsteroidal anti-inflammatory drugs are thought to inhibit the production of prostaglandins from traumatized or inflamed tissues. Endorphins are thought to decrease pain. These medications do not relieve anxiety.

Reference: p. 191

Descriptors:
1. 12 2. 09 3. Application
4. IV–2 5. Nursing Process 6. Moderate

16. A nurse is caring for a 79-year-old client with cancer and chronic pain and fatigue. The client is prescribed an opioid medication for pain relief. The nurse should explain to the client that for elderly clients
A. meperidine is usually the drug of choice.
B. intervals between doses are the same as for younger clients.
*C. absorption and metabolism of medications may be slower.
D. larger doses of medication are required for pain relief.

Rationale: For elderly clients meperidine should be avoided because of toxic effects, intervals between doses are usually longer than for younger clients, absorption and metabolism of medications may be slower because of decreased liver and GI function, and most elderly clients need less medication for pain relief.

Reference: p. 192

Descriptors:
1. 12 2. 05 3. Application
4. IV–2 5. Nursing Process 6. Moderate

17. A client is receiving transcutaneous electrical nerve stimulation following a total hip replacement. The nurse should explain to the client that the TENS unit works by
*A. stimulating the nonpain receptors.
B. providing distraction from the pain.
C. reducing the tissue damage that occurs with pain.
D. providing an electrical current to alter cell permeability.

Rationale: TENS is believed to work by stimulating the nonpain receptors in the same area as the fibers that transmit the pain. It does not provide a distraction, reduce tissue damage, or alter cell permeability.

Reference: p. 195

Descriptors:
1. 12 2. 11 3. Application
4. IV–2 5. Nursing Process 6. Moderate

CHAPTER 13
Fluid and Electrolytes: Balances and Disturbances

1. The term osmosis is best defined as a
   A. natural tendency of a substance to move from an area of higher concentration to one of lower concentration.
   B. ability of solutes to cause a driving force that promotes water movement.
   *C. fluid shifts through the membrane from a low concentration to a high concentration until the solutions are of equal concentration.
   D. energy expended for movement of a solution to occur against a concentration gradient.

Rationale: Osmosis occurs when two different solutions are separated by a membrane impermeable to the dissolved substances, fluid shifts through the membrane from the region of the low solute concentration to the region of high solute concentration until the solutions are of equal concentration. Active transport is the energy expenditure for movement of a solution to occur against a concentration gradient.

Reference: p. 203

Descriptors:
1. 13 2. 01 3. Comprehension
4. IV–4 5. Nursing Process 6. Moderate

2. The statement that best describes electrolytes in intracellular and extracellular fluid is that there is
   *A. a greater concentration of sodium in extracellular fluid and potassium in intracellular fluid.
   B. equal concentration of sodium and potassium in extracellular fluid.
   C. greater concentration of potassium in extracellular fluid and sodium in intracellular fluid.
   D. equal concentration of sodium and potassium between intracellular and extracellular fluid.

Rationale: There is a greater concentration of sodium in extracellular fluid and potassium in intracellular fluid.

Reference: pp. 203–204

Descriptors:
1. 13 2. 01 3. Comprehension
4. IV–4 5. Nursing Process 6. Moderate

3. A nurse is caring for a client with an elevated urine osmolarity. The nurse should assess the client for
   A. fluid volume excess.
   B. hyperkalemia.
   C. hypercalcemia.
   *D. fluid volume deficit.

Rationale: For a client with an elevated urine osmolarity, the nurse should assess the client for fluid volume deficit.

Reference: p. 204

Descriptors:
1. 13 2. 02 3. Application
4. IV–4 5. Nursing Process 6. Moderate

4. A physician orders a serum creatinine for a hospitalized client. The nurse should explain to the client and his family that this test
   A. is normal if the level is 4.0 to 5.5 mg/dl.
   B. can be elevated with increased protein intake.
   *C. is a better indicator of renal function than the BUN.
   D. reflects the fluid volume status of a person.

Rationale: A serum creatinine level should be 0.7 to 1.5 mg/dl and it does not vary with increased protein intake, thus it is a better indicator of renal function than the BUN.

Reference: p. 205

Descriptors:
1. 13 2. 02 3. Application
4. IV–4 5. Nursing Process 6. Moderate

5. One of the major functions of the kidneys in maintaining normal fluid balance is
   A. manufacturing of antidiuretic hormone.
   B. regulating calcium and phosphate balance.
   *C. regulating the pH of the extracellular fluid.
   D. controlling the levels of aldosterone.

Rationale: Major functions of the kidneys in maintaining normal fluid balance include regulation of extracellular fluid and osmolality by selective retention and excretion of fluids, regulation of pH of the extracellular fluid by retention of hydrogen ions, and excretion of metabolic wastes and toxic substances. ADH is manufactured by the pituitary, and the parathyroid regulates calcium and phosphate balance.

Reference: p. 205

Descriptors:
1. 13 2. 02 3. Comprehension
4. IV–4 5. Nursing Process 6. Moderate

6. A nurse is caring for a client with an elevated cortisol level. The nurse anticipates that the client will exhibit symptoms of
   A. urinary excess.
   B. hyperpituitarism.

*C. urinary deficit.
D. hyperthyroidism.

Rationale: High levels of cortisol can produce sodium and fluid retention and potassium deficit, thus creating urinary deficit.

Reference: p. 205

Descriptors:
1. 13 2. 02 3. Analysis
4. IV–4 5. Nursing Process 6. Difficult

7. A nurse is caring for a 76-year-old client following surgery. The client has a fluid volume deficit and a serum sodium level of 130 mEq/L. The nurse should monitor the client for symptoms of
*A. confusion.
B. thirst.
C. cardiac failure.
D. fatigue.

Rationale: Normal serum sodium levels should be 135 to 145 mEq/L, so this client has hyponatremia, which can lead to confusion in an elderly client. Thirst is more common in younger clients.

Reference: p. 207

Descriptors:
1. 13 2. 03 3. Application
4. IV–4 5. Nursing Process 6. Moderate

8. A nurse is caring for a 66-year-old client diagnosed with renal insufficiency. The nurse should monitor the client for symptoms of
A. fluid volume excess.
*B. fluid volume deficit.
C. potassium excess.
D. sodium excess.

Rationale: Clients diagnosed with renal insufficiency can exhibit symptoms of hyperkalemia and fluid volume deficit.

Reference: p. 208

Descriptors:
1. 13 2. 04 3. Application
4. IV–4 5. Nursing Process 6. Moderate

9. The nurse is caring for a 90-year-old client with fluid volume deficit. The nurse should assess the client's skin turgor over the
A. arms.
B. hands.
C. feet.
*D. forehead.

Rationale: In an elderly client, skin turgor is best assessed over the forehead or the sternum because alterations in elasticity are less marked in these areas.

Reference: p. 208

Descriptors:
1. 13 2. 04 3. Application
4. IV–1 5. Nursing Process 6. Moderate

10. A nurse is caring for a client with congestive heart failure and fluid volume excess. A priority assessment for the nurse to make for this client is assessment of
*A. breath sounds.
B. skin color.
C. skin turgor.
D. pedal pulses.

Rationale: Shortness of breath and wheezing are common symptoms of clients with congestive heart failure and fluid volume excess, therefore the priority assessment is assessment of breath sounds.

Reference: p. 211

Descriptors:
1. 13 2. 04 3. Application
4. IV–1 5. Nursing Process 6. Moderate

11. A client with severe hypervolemia due to renal failure is hospitalized. The nurse should plan to administer
A. hydrochlorthiazide.
B. trichlormethiazide.
C. methychlorothiazide.
*D. furosemide.

Rationale: Furosemide (Lasix) is a loop diuretic and indicated for clients with severe hypervolemia. Hydrochlorthiazide, trichlormethiazide, and methychlorothiazide are thiazide diuretics and are usually indicated for mild or moderate hypervolemia.

Reference: p. 211

Descriptors:
1. 13 2. 04 3. Application
4. IV–1 5. Nursing Process 6. Moderate

12. A nurse is caring for a hospitalized adult client who has a serum sodium level of 145 mEq/L and a serum potassium level of 4.0 mEq/L. The nurse should monitor this client for signs of
*A. thirst.
B. fatigue.
C. nausea.
D. anorexia.

Rationale: The client is experiencing hypernatremia. Signs of this condition include thirst, flushed skin, dry tongue, and increased muscle tone. Fatigue, nausea, and anorexia are symptoms of hyperkalemia; however, this client's potassium level is within a normal range.

Reference: p. 216

Descriptors:
1. 13 2. 05 3. Application
4. IV–4 5. Nursing Process 6. Moderate

13. A nurse is caring for a client who is taking diuretic medications. The nurse should instruct the client to eat foods that are high in potassium such as
A. frozen yogurt.
*B. bananas.

C. figs.
D. peanuts.

Rationale: Foods that are high in potassium include raisins, fruits such as bananas and oranges, milk, whole grains, and meat.

Reference: p. 218

Descriptors:
1. 13 2. 05 3. Application
4. IV–4 5. Nursing Process 6. Moderate

14. A nurse is preparing to administer a potassium supplement intravenously to a hospitalized client. The nurse should plan to
A. administer the potassium only with a normal saline solution.
B. stop the potassium administration if polyuria occurs.
C. administer the potassium only through a central venous line.
*D. administer the potassium using an infusion pump.

Rationale: IV potassium must be administered using an infusion pump to avoid replacing the potassium too quickly, which can result in life-threatening dysrhythmias.

Reference: p. 219

Descriptors:
1. 13 2. 05 3. Application
4. IV–1 5. Nursing Process 6. Difficult

15. A nurse is caring for a client who is hospitalized and diagnosed with Addison's disease. The nurse should monitor the client for symptoms of
A. hypocalcemia.
B. hypernatremia.
C. hypokalemia.
*D. hyperkalemia.

Rationale: A client with Addison's disease is at risk for hyperkalemia because this condition is characterized by deficient adrenal hormones, leading to sodium loss and potassium retention.

Reference: p. 219

Descriptors:
1. 13 2. 05 3. Application
4. IV–4 5. Nursing Process 6. Moderate

16. A nurse is caring for a hospitalized client diagnosed with renal failure and hypocalcemia. The nurse should monitor the client for symptoms of
*A. tetany.
B. muscle weakness.
C. constipation.
D. anorexia.

Rationale: The most characteristic manifestation of hypocalcemia is tetany. Other symptoms include seizures and mental changes such as confusion. Muscle weakness, constipation, and anorexia are symptoms of hypercalcemia.

Reference: p. 221

Descriptors:
1. 13 2. 05 3. Application
4. IV–3 5. Nursing Process 6. Moderate

17. A nurse is caring for a hospitalized adult client with a serum magnesium level of 1.3 mEq/L and a serum phosphorus level of 4.2 mEq/L. The nurse should monitor the client for symptoms of
*A. athetoid movements.
B. facial flushing.
C. dysarthria.
D. drowsiness.

Rationale: A serum magnesium level of 1.3 mEq/L is indicative of hypomagnesemia. The nurse should monitor the client for athetoid movements, tetany, and muscle weakness. Facial flushing, dysarthria, and drowsiness are symptoms of hypermagnesemia.

Reference: p. 223

Descriptors:
1. 13 2. 05 3. Application
4. IV–1 5. Nursing Process 6. Moderate

18. The bicarbonate levels of the extracellular fluid are regulated by the
A. lungs.
B. liver.
C. thalamus.
*D. kidneys.

Rationale: The kidneys are responsible for regulating the bicarbonate levels of the extracellular fluid, while the lungs control the CO_2 and carbonic acid content of the extracellular fluid.

Reference: p. 228

Descriptors:
1. 13 2. 06 3. Comprehension
4. IV–4 5. Nursing Process 6. Moderate

19. A nurse is caring for a hospitalized adult client with chronic renal failure. The nurse should monitor the client for symptoms of
A. respiratory acidosis.
*B. metabolic acidosis.
C. respiratory alkalosis.
D. metabolic alkalosis.

Rationale: Clients with chronic renal failure usually have chronic metabolic acidosis. Vomiting is associated with metabolic alkalosis.

Reference: p. 229

Descriptors:
1. 13 2. 10 3. Application
4. IV–1 5. Nursing Process 6. Moderate

20. A nurse is caring for an elderly client diagnosed with chronic obstructive pulmonary disease. The nurse should monitor the client for symptoms of
   A. lightheadedness.
   B. inability to concentrate.
   *C. papilledema.
   D. tinnitus.

   Rationale: Clients with chronic obstructive pulmonary disease often experience respiratory acidosis. The nurse should monitor the client for symptoms of hypercapnia, mental cloudiness, papilledema, and dilated conjunctival blood vessels. Lightheadedness, inability to concentrate, and tinnitus are symptoms associated with respiratory alkalosis.

   Reference: p. 230

   Descriptors:
   1. 13 2. 07 3. Application
   4. IV–3 5. Nursing Process 6. Moderate

21. A client is hospitalized with a diagnosis of chronic hepatic insufficiency and has a $PaCO_2$ level of 35 mmHg. The nurse determines that this client is most likely experiencing
   A. respiratory acidosis.
   *B. respiratory alkalosis.
   C. metabolic acidosis.
   D. metabolic alkalosis.

   Rationale: A client with a $PaCO_2$ level of 35 mmHg is experiencing respiratory alkalosis, since the $PaCO_2$ level is below 40 mmHg.

   Reference: p. 230

   Descriptors:
   1. 13 2. 10 3. Application
   4. IV–3 5. Nursing Process 6. Moderate

22. The physician has ordered intravenous fluids for a hospitalized client. Before choosing an IV site for peripheral administration of the fluids, the nurse should consider the
   A. client's level of consciousness.
   B. reason for the intravenous fluids.
   *C. type of fluid to be administered.
   D. client's preferences.

   Rationale: Factors to consider before administering intravenous fluids include the type of fluid to be administered, the duration of the therapy, the condition of the vein, client's age and size, and whether the client is right- or left-handed.

   Reference: p. 233

   Descriptors:
   1. 13 2. 11 3. Application
   4. IV–4 5. Nursing Process 6. Moderate

23. The nurse assesses a hospitalized client and determines that the intravenous infusion has just become infiltrated at the peripheral site. After discontinuing the infusion, the nurse should
   A. place a clean dressing on the site.
   *B. place a cold compress on the site.
   C. keep the site lower than the client's head.
   D. apply a hot pack to the site for 24 hours.

   Rationale: The IV infusion should be started in a new site. For recent infiltration, a cold compress is recommended. The site should be elevated to promote reabsorption of fluid. A sterile dressing should be placed on the site.

   Reference: p. 240

   Descriptors:
   1. 13 2. 12 3. Application
   4. IV–4 5. Nursing Process 6. Moderate

CHAPTER 14
Shock and Multisystem Failure

1. Shock is most accurately defined as a/an
   A. decreased circulating blood volume.
   B. inability of the heart to pump blood.
   *C. inadequate oxygen supply to vital organs.
   D. hemorrhage as a result of trauma.

   Rationale: Shock is a life-threatening condition with a variety of underlying causes. The term shock is best defined as an inadequate oxygen supply to vital organs through the systemic blood pressure.

   Reference: p. 243

   Descriptors:
   1. 14 2. 01 3. Comprehension
   4. IV–4 5. Nursing Process 6. Moderate

2. Cellular derangements that occur in shock and lead to pathophysiologic alterations include
   *A. increased cellular permeability.
   B. aerobic metabolism of glucose.
   C. increased activity of the sodium-potassium pump.
   D. an alkalotic intracellular environment.

   Rationale: In shock, the cells lack adequate blood supply and are deprived of oxygen and nutrients, therefore they must produce energy through anaerobic metabolism. This results in low energy fields and an acidotic intracellular environment. The cell membrane becomes more permeable.

   Reference: p. 244

   Descriptors:
   1. 14 2. 01 3. Comprehension
   4. IV–4 5. Nursing Process 6. Moderate

3. A nurse is caring for a client in the compensatory stage of shock. The nurse should assess the client for
   A. hypotension.

B. bradycardia.
*C. mental status changes.
D. increased urine output.

Rationale: During the compensatory stage of shock, the blood pressure remains normal; however, the client exhibits a "fight or flight" response. The alkalotic state causes mental status changes such as confusion. Urine output would be decreased and tachycardia would be present.

Reference: p. 246

Descriptors:
1. 14 2. 02 3. Application
4. IV–4 5. Nursing Process 6. Moderate

4. A nurse is caring for a client in the progressive stage of shock. A priority goal for this client is to
   A. reduce anxiety.
   B. promote adequate rest.
   C. improve nutritional status.
   *D. restore tissue perfusion.

Rationale: A priority goal for a client in the progressive stage of shock is to restore tissue perfusion to prevent organ systems from decompensation. Reducting anxiety, rest, and nutrition are not immediate goals.

Reference: p. 247

Descriptors:
1. 14 2. 02 3. Application
4. IV–4 5. Nursing Process 6. Moderate

5. A nurse is caring for a client who has had a progressive stage of shock. To assess the client for complications from shock, the nurse should assess the client's
   *A. urine output.
   B. serum glucose.
   C. serum sodium.
   D. weight.

Rationale: Acute renal failure can occur as a result of shock. The nurse should assess the client's urinary output, which should be greater than 30 ml/hour.

Reference: p. 247

Descriptors:
1. 14 2. 03 3. Application
4. IV–4 5. Nursing Process 6. Moderate

6. A nurse is caring for a client in shock when the physician orders an intravenous infusion of lactated Ringer's solution. The nurse determines that the client will be receiving an intravenous solution termed
   A. colloid.
   B. plasma.
   *C. crystalloid.
   D. synthetic colloid.

Rationale: Crystalloids are electrolyte solutions used for resuscitation in hypovolemic shock and include lactated Ringer's solution and sodium chloride solutions. Colloids contain large molecules. Albumin is a plasma solution, and Dextran is a synthetic colloid preparation.

Reference: pp. 249–250

Descriptors:
1. 14 2. 05 3. Comprehension
4. IV–4 5. Nursing Process 6. Difficult

7. A nurse is caring for a client in progressive shock. The nurse should
   A. turn the client every 4 to 8 hours.
   B. provide a high caloric diet to replace nutritional losses.
   *C. keep the client warm and comfortable.
   D. provide stimulation to maintain level of consciousness.

Rationale: To conserve the client's energy, the nurse should protect the client from temperature extremes by keeping the client warm and comfortable. Turning the client, high caloric diets, and stimulation are not a priority at this time.

Reference: p. 248

Descriptors:
1. 14 2. 02 3. Application
4. IV–4 5. Nursing Process 6. Moderate

8. During the irreversible stage of shock, the nurse should monitor the client for
   A. irritability or confusion.
   B. warm, flushed skin.
   *C. severe metabolic acidosis.
   D. severe metabolic alkalosis.

Rationale: During the irreversible stage of shock, complete renal and liver failure, compounded by the release of necrotic tissue toxins, results in severe metabolic acidosis. The client's skin will be cool and clammy. Irritability or confusion is not a symptom in irreversible shock.

Reference: p. 248

Descriptors:
1. 14 2. 02 3. Application
4. IV–4 5. Nursing Process 6. Moderate

9. For a client in hypovolemic shock, the nurse should explain to the client's family that this type of shock
   A. is a rare form of shock.
   B. is marked by inadequate pumping of the heart.
   *C. is marked by a drop in the client's blood pressure.
   D. is usually due to an infectious agent.

Rationale: Hypovolemic shock occurs when there are external fluid losses resulting in a decrease in cardiac output and a subsequent drop in the blood pressure. Septic shock occurs as a result of an infectious agent.

Reference: p. 251

Descriptors:
1. 14 2. 04 3. Application
4. IV–4 5. Nursing Process 6. Moderate

10. A nurse is caring for a client who is receiving large volumes of intravenous solution as a result of shock. The nurse should monitor the client for symptoms of
 A. hyperthermia.
 B. bradycardia.
 *C. pulmonary edema.
 D. pain.

Rationale: The nurse should monitor the client for cardiovascular overload and pulmonary edema when large volumes of intravenous solution are administered. Hypothermia may occur as well as tachycardia. Pain is related to cardiogenic shock.

Reference: p. 253

Descriptors:
1. 14 2. 04 3. Application
4. IV–1 5. Nursing Process 6. Moderate

11. Cardiogenic shock occurs when
 *A. the heart's ability to pump blood is impaired.
 B. there is inadequate blood flow to the cells.
 C. there is an excessive fluid loss.
 D. blood volume is abnormally displaced in the vasculature.

Rationale: Cardiogenic shock occurs when the heart's ability to pump blood is impaired and the supply of oxygen is inadequate for the heart and tissues. Excessive fluid loss is associated with hypovolemic shock and distributive shock occurs when blood volume is abnormally displaced in the vasculature.

Reference: p. 253

Descriptors:
1. 14 2. 04 3. Comprehension
4. IV–4 5. Nursing Process 6. Moderate

12. A nurse is monitoring a client for symptoms of cardiogenic shock. The nurse should report which of these findings immediately?
 A. Increased urine output.
 *B. Angina pain.
 C. Elevated temperature.
 D. Diarrhea.

Rationale: Symptoms of cardiogenic shock include angina pain and dysrhythmias. Increased or decreased urine output, elevated temperature, and diarrhea are associated with septic shock.

Reference: p. 254

Descriptors:
1. 14 2. 04 3. Application
4. IV–3 5. Nursing Process 6. Moderate

13. A nurse is caring for a client with chest pain and potential cardiogenic shock. To relieve the client's anxiety and pain, the nurse can anticipate administering intravenous
 A. nubain.
 B. demerol.
 C. valium.
 *D. morphine.

Rationale: For clients experiencing chest pain, morphine is the drug of choice as it dilates the blood vessels and controls the client's anxiety.

Reference: p. 254

Descriptors:
1. 14 2. 04 3. Application
4. IV–4 5. Nursing Process 6. Moderate

14. A client is receiving low doses of dopamine following cardiogenic shock. The nurse should explain to the client that this medication
 *A. increases renal and mesentary blood flow.
 B. improves cardiac output.
 C. acts as a venous vasodilator.
 D. reduces fluid accumulation.

Rationale: Low doses of dopamine following cardiogenic shock are administered to increase renal and mesentary blood flow and prevent ischemia to these organs. Low doses of dopamine do not improve cardiac output, act as a venous vasodilator, or reduce fluid accumulation.

Reference: p. 253

Descriptors:
1. 14 2. 06 3. Application
4. IV–2 5. Nursing Process 6. Moderate

15. A nurse is caring for a critically ill client following an automobile accident. To prevent septic shock in this client, the nurse should
 A. administer prophylactic antibiotics.
 B. continually monitor the client for constipation.
 C. obtain urine specimens using clean technique.
 *D. use meticulous aseptic technique for all procedures.

Rationale: The incidence of nosocomial infections in critically ill clients is 20 to 25%, and this percentage could be decreased by the use of sterile procedures and meticulous aseptic technique for all procedures. The temperature may be normal or abnormal, depending on the stage of septic shock.

Reference: p. 256

Descriptors:
1. 14 2. 04 3. Application
4. IV–4 5. Nursing Process 6. Moderate

16. A nurse is caring for a client diagnosed with septic shock. The nurse should explain to the client and his family that nutritional support is essential during septic shock because
 A. the absence of nutrition can lead to gastric ulceration.

B. antibiotics are administered through enteral feedings.
*C. malnutrition further impairs the client's resistence to infection.
D. nutritional feedings assist in maintaining an adequate blood pressure.

Rationale: Aggressive nutritional supplementation is critical in the management of septic shock because malnutrition further impairs the client's resistence to infection. Enteral feedings are preferred whenever possible.

Reference: p. 257

Descriptors:
1. 14 2. 07 3. Application
4. IV–4 5. Nursing Process 6. Moderate

17. A nurse is assessing a client for symptoms of neurogenic shock following a spinal cord injury. The nurse should monitor the client for symptoms of
*A. bradycardia.
B. tachycardia.
C. cool, moist skin.
D. absence of Homan's sign.

Rationale: Symptoms of neurogenic shock include bradycardia and warm, flushed skin. Absence of Homan's sign indicates no thrombosis.

Reference: p. 258

Descriptors:
1. 14 2. 04 3. Analysis
4. IV–4 5. Nursing Process 6. Difficult

18. A nurse is caring for a client in the emergency room who is experiencing progressive shock. The nurse can help to alleviate the anxiety of the client's family by
A. offering reassurance that the client will survive.
*B. keeping the family members informed frequently.
C. requesting that they limit visitation to promote rest.
D. informing the family that this type of shock has a high mortality rate.

Rationale: To alleviate the anxiety of the client's family, the nurse should keep the family members informed frequently and allow them to be with the client.

Reference: p. 249

Descriptors:
1. 14 2. 08 3. Application
4. III–1 5. Nursing Process 6. Moderate

19. A nurse is caring for a client who is experiencing multiple organ dysfunction syndrome. A priority goal for this client is to
A. eliminate the sepsis.
B. enhance overall well-being.
*C. promote perfusion of organs.
D. decrease loss of fluids.

Rationale: Measures to reverse multiple organ dysfunction syndrome are aimed at controlling the initiating event, promoting adequate organ perfusion, and maintaining nutritional support.

Reference: p. 259

Descriptors:
1. 14 2. 09 3. Application
4. IV–4 5. Nursing Process 6. Moderate

CHAPTER 15
Oncology: Nursing Management in Cancer Care

1. Dysplasia is a pattern of cell growth that can best be defined as
A. normal cell growth that occurs during skin regeneration.
*B. bizarre cell growth that results in different cell sizes and shapes.
C. increased number of cells of a tissue, which then become enlarged.
D. malignant and lacking in normal cellular characteristics.

Rationale: Dysplasia is a pattern of bizarre cell growth resulting in cells that differ in size, shape, or arrangement from other cells of the same type of tissue.

Reference: p. 262

Descriptors:
1. 15 2. 01 3. Knowledge
4. II–1 5. Nursing Process 6. Moderate

2. Malignant neoplasms differ from benign neoplasms in that with malignant neoplasms the
*A. tumor grows at the periphery and sends out processes that destroy surrounding tissue.
B. cells are well differentiated and resemble the tissue from which the tumor originated.
C. tumor is localized and does not cause generalized effects.
D. rate of tumor growth is typically slow.

Rationale: Malignant neoplasms differ from benign neoplasms in that with malignant neoplasms the tumor grows at the periphery and sends out processes that destroy surrounding tissue and the rate of growth is variable and often causes generalized effects.

Reference: p. 264

Descriptors:
1. 15 2. 02 3. Knowledge
4. II–2 5. Nursing Process 6. Moderate

3. A client is scheduled to have a carcinoembryonic antigen blood level drawn. The nurse should explain to the client that this test
   A. evaluates the status of the client's immune system.
   B. identifies the stage and grade of a malignancy.
   C. detects chromosomal anomalies of cells.
   *D. differentiates between malignant and benign tissue cell growth.

Rationale: The cell membrane of malignant cells contains proteins called tumor specific antigens. A carcinoembryonic antigen blood test can differentiate between malignant and benign tissue cell growth and can track the course of an illness.

Reference: p. 265

Descriptors:
1. 15 2. 02 3. Application
4. II–2 5. Nursing Process 6. Moderate

4. A client tells the nurse that he has heard that certain foods can decrease the incidence of cancer. The nurse should instruct the client to increase his intake of
   A. ham.
   B. grapes.
   *C. broccoli.
   D. bananas.

Rationale: High-fiber foods; cruciferous vegetables such as broccoli, cauliflower, and spinach; and carotenoids such as apricots and peaches appear to reduce cancer risk. Salt-cured foods such as ham and processed luncheon meats should be avoided.

Reference: p. 267

Descriptors:
1. 15 2. 03 3. Application
4. II–2 5. Nursing Process 6. Moderate

5. A hormonal agent that has been associated with an increase in vaginal carcinoma is
   A. progesterone.
   B. estrogen.
   C. lactoferrin.
   *D. diethylstilbesterol.

Rationale: Diethylstilbesterol has long been recognized as a hormonal agent that has been associated with an increase in vaginal carcinoma. Prolonged estrogen replacement therapy is associated with a slight risk of endometrial and breast cancers.

Reference: p. 267

Descriptors:
1. 15 2. 03 3. Application
4. II–2 5. Nursing Process 6. Moderate

6. A nurse is caring for a client with AIDS who is hospitalized. The nurse recognizes that clients with AIDS have an increased incidence of
   *A. Kaposi's sarcoma.
   B. pancreatic tumors.
   C. bladder tumors.
   D. brain tumors.

Rationale: Clients with AIDS have an increased incidence of Kaposi's sarcoma; lymphoma; rectal, head, and neck cancers.

Reference: p. 267

Descriptors:
1. 15 2. 03 3. Application
4. II–2 5. Nursing Process 6. Moderate

7. A nurse is planning a cancer prevention program for a group of high school seniors. The nurse should plan to include physical factors that should be avoided, including
   A. hepatitis B virus.
   B. lead-based paint.
   C. x-rays of teeth.
   *D. ultraviolet radiation.

Rationale: Excessive exposure to radiation can contribute to skin cancers, especially for fair-haired individuals.

Reference: p. 266

Descriptors:
1. 15 2. 04 3. Application
4. II–2 5. Nursing Process 6. Moderate

8. A nurse is caring for a client who has had a lumpectomy, and the cancer has been diagnosed in the same breast. One of the types of surgery that is an option for the client is
   *A. salvage surgery.
   B. palliative surgery.
   C. prophylactic surgery.
   D. reconstructive surgery.

Rationale: Salvage surgery is an additional treatment option that uses an extensive surgical approach to treat the local recurrence of the cancer after a less extensive primary approach is used. Palliative surgery is used when cure is not possible. Prophylactic surgery is used when there is an extensive family history and nonvital tissues are removed. Reconstructive surgery is an attempt to obtain a more desirable cosmetic effect.

Reference: p. 271

Descriptors:
1. 15 2. 05 3. Application
4. I–1 5. Nursing Process 6. Moderate

9. An adult client is scheduled to undergo surgery for the treatment of cancer. The nurse should
   A. reassure the client and family that the outcome will be favorable.
   *B. encourage the client and family to express their fears.
   C. provide distraction activities to keep the client from worrying about the surgery.
   D. tell the client not to worry about being apprehensive because most clients experience fears.

Rationale: The nurse who is caring for a client who will undergo surgery for cancer should provide emotional support and education. The nurse should explore with the client and family any fears or misconceptions they have about the surgery. Telling the client not to worry or offering false reassurance is not helpful.

Reference: p. 266

Descriptors:
1. 15 2. 06 3. Application
4. IV–3 5. Nursing Process 6. Moderate

10. An adult client is scheduled for a radioactive implant for treatment of cervical cancer. The nurse has instructed the client about care following the procedure. The nurse determines that the client has understood the instructions when she says,
   A. "I will not be able to have any visitors while the implant is in place."
   B. "I will need to use a bedside commode for bowel movements."
   *C. "I will have an indwelling urinary catheter while the implant is in place."
   D. "I will need to eat a high-fiber diet while I am on bed rest."

Rationale: The client has understood the instructions when she says, "I will have an indwelling urinary catheter while the implant is in place." The purpose of the catheter is to keep the bladder empty. The client will have a low-residue diet and Lomotil to prevent bowel movements. Visitors are allowed with precautions.

Reference: p. 273

Descriptors:
1. 15 2. 06 3. Application
4. IV–3 5. Nursing Process 6. Moderate

11. While a client is receiving intravenous dactinomycin, the nurse observes that there is an absence of blood return from the intravenous catheter. The nurse should
   *A. stop the administration of the drug immediately.
   B. notify the client's physician.
   C. continue to administer the drug and assess for edema.
   D. apply a warm compress to the site.

Rationale: Dactinomycin is a chemotherapeutic vesicant that can cause severe tissue damage. The nurse should stop the administration of the drug immediately and then notify the client's physician. Ice can be applied to the site once the drug therapy has stopped.

Reference: p. 275

Descriptors:
1. 15 2. 06 3. Application
4. IV–3 5. Nursing Process 6. Moderate

12. A client is scheduled to receive chemotherapy for cancer. The nurse should explain that one of the most common side effects of chemotherapy is
   A. thrombosis.
   B. infection.
   C. altered glucose metabolism.
   *D. nausea and vomiting.

Rationale: One of the most common side effects of chemotherapy is nausea and vomiting, and antiemetic drugs are frequently prescribed for these clients. Other side effects include bone marrow suppression, anorexia, vaginal dryness, and hair loss. Less common effects include altered glucose metabolism and jaundice.

Reference: p. 275

Descriptors:
1. 15 2. 07 3. Application
4. IV–1 5. Nursing Process 6. Moderate

13. An adult client is receiving intravenous cisplatin for cancer. To determine the effects of the chemotherapy on the client's renal system, the nurse should monitor the client's
   A. white blood count.
   *B. serum creatinine.
   C. hematocrit.
   D. urine culture and sensitivity.

Rationale: Cisplatin can result in renal damage. The nurse should monitor the client's serum creatinine, blood urea nitrogen, creatinine clearance, and serum electolyte levels.

Reference: p. 278

Descriptors:
1. 15 2. 07 3. Application
4. IV–3 5. Nursing Process 6. Moderate

14. When the nurse prepares to administer an antineoplastic agent to a hospitalized client, the nurse should
   A. administer only prepackaged agents from the manufacturer.
   B. wear short sleeves and wash the arms following administration.
   *C. use surgical gloves and disposable long-sleeved gowns.
   D. dispose of the antineoplastic wastes in the client's bedside trash.

Rationale: The nurse should use surgical gloves and disposable long-sleeved gowns when administering antineoplastic agents. The antineoplastic wastes are disposed of as hazardous materials.

Reference: p. 288

Descriptors:
1. 15 2. 06 3. Application
4. IV–3 5. Nursing Process 6. Difficult

15. An adult client has just received a bone marrow transplant. The nurse should monitor the client for signs of

A. cataract formation.
B. cardiac shock.
C. nausea and vomiting.
*D. infection.

Rationale: Through the period of bone marrow aplasia until engulfment of the new marrow occurs, clients are at high risk of dying from sepsis and bleeding. Cataract formation may occur as a late effect. Cardiac shock is rare. Nausea and vomiting are side effects of chemotherapy.

Reference: p. 289

Descriptors:

1. 15	2. 06	3. Application
4. IV–3	5. Nursing Process	6. Moderate

16. The leading cause of death in oncology clients is
*A. infection.
B. renal failure.
C. malnutrition.
D. hemorrhage.

Rationale: For oncology clients, infection is the leading cause of death. This is due to impaired skin integrity and the suppression of bone marrow caused by many treatments for cancer.

Reference: p. 294

Descriptors:

1. 15	2. 07	3. Application
4. IV–3	5. Nursing Process	6. Moderate

17. A nurse is caring for an adult client who develops mild stomatitis following chemotherapy. The nurse should encourage the client to
A. rinse the mouth with a mouthwash after each meal.
B. drink hot tea with honey with each meal.
C. avoid the use of dental floss until the stomatitis is resolved.
*D. brush the teeth with a soft toothbrush after meals.

Rationale: Stomatitis is an inflammation of the oral cavity. The client should be encouraged to brush the teeth with a soft toothbrush after meals, use dental floss every 24 hours, rinse with normal saline, and to use a lip lubricant. Mouthwashes and hot foods should be avoided.

Reference: pp. 282, 296

Descriptors:

1. 15	2. 08	3. Application
4. IV–3	5. Nursing Process	6. Moderate

18. A nurse is caring for a client with cancer who has been receiving chemotherapy and has experienced severe nausea and vomiting and loss of appetite. The client consumed a total of 650 calories in a 24-hour period and appears fatigued. A priority nursing diagnosis for this client is
A. Pain related to chemotherapy treatments.
*B. Altered nutrition: less than body requirements due to anorexia.
C. Fatigue related to side effects of chemotherapy and lack of rest.
D. Body image disturbance related to weight loss and anorexia.

Rationale: A priority nursing diagnosis for this client is Altered nutrition: less than body requirements due to anorexia. Pain and fatigue may be present, but the priority is the client's nutritional status.

Reference: p. 295

Descriptors:

1. 15	2. 09	3. Application
4. IV–3	5. Nursing Process	6. Moderate

19. A nurse is caring for an oncology client who develops leukopenia following radiation therapy. The nurse should instruct the client to
A. stay in a semiprivate room.
B. eat only fresh fruits and vegetables.
C. ask the physician for a flu vaccination.
*D. do coughing and deep breathing exercises frequently.

Rationale: Leukopenia is a decrease in white blood cells, therefore the client is at risk for infection. The nurse should instruct the client to do coughing and deep breathing exercises frequently to prevent atelectasis. A private room and strict aseptic technique is warranted. Low bacterial diets without fresh fruits and vegetables is warranted.

Reference: p. 300

Descriptors:

1. 15	2. 09	3. Application
4. IV–3	5. Nursing Process	6. Moderate

20. A client is referred to a hospice for care. The nurse should explain to the client and her family that the primary goal of hospice care is to
*A. provide support to the client and family.
B. assist in managing the technology required for the client's care.
C. offer bereavement programs to the client and family.
D. teach the client and family how to provide home care.

Rationale: The hospice movement began in Great Britain. The primary goal of hospice care is to provide support to the client and family. Clients who are referred to hospice care generally have less than 6 months to live. Although hospice nurses are skilled in bereavement counseling, this is not the primary purpose of a hospice.

Reference: p. 303

Descriptors:

1. 15	2. 10	3. Application
4. IV–1	5. Nursing Process	6. Moderate

21. An oncology client has been diagnosed with thrombocytopenia following chemotherapy and radiation. A priority goal for this client is to prevent

*A. trauma related to decreased platelet count.
B. pain related to spontaneous bleeding episodes.
C. tissue integrity loss due to decreased perfusion.
D. alterations in nutrition due to anorexia.

Rationale: Clients with thrombocytopenia are at risk for bleeding due to decreased platelet counts. A priority goal for this client is to prevent trauma related to decreased platelet count. A soft toothbrush or an electric razor can be used. No invasive procedures should be performed.

Reference: p. 301

Descriptors:
1. 15 2. 09 3. Application
4. IV–3 5. Nursing Process 6. Moderate

22. A client who has been diagnosed with lymphoma and complains to the nurse of increasing shortness of breath and difficulty swallowing. The nurse observes that the client has edema of the neck and distended jugular veins. The nurse determines that these findings are indicative of
A. pulmonary embolus.
B. cardiac tamponade.
C. spinal cord compression.
*D. superior vena cava syndrome.

Rationale: Increasing shortness of breath, difficulty swallowing, edema of the neck, and distended jugular veins are indicative of superior vena cava syndrome and may lead to anoxia and death. Spinal cord compression involves pain with movement. Cardiac tamponade involves tachycardia. Pulmonary embolus involves chest pain.

Reference: p. 304

Descriptors:
1. 15 2. 11 3. Analysis
4. IV–3 5. Nursing Process 6. Moderate

23. A nurse is caring for a client with metastatic bone disease. The client complains to the nurse of excessive thirst and frequent urination. The client's reflexes are hypoactive and there is some mental confusion. The nurse determines that the client is most likely experiencing
*A. hypercalcemia.
B. hyperkalemia.
C. hypernatremia.
D. hyperphosphotemia.

Rationale: Excessive thirst, frequent urination, reflexes that are hypoactive, and some mental confusion are symptoms of hypercalcemia. Serum calcium levels exceeding 11 mg/dL are indicative of hypercalcemia. Hyponatremia is associated with nausea, vomiting, and fatigue.

Reference: p. 305

Descriptors:
1. 15 2. 11 3. Analysis
4. IV–3 5. Nursing Process 6. Moderate

UNIT 4 PERIOPERATIVE CONCEPTS AND NURSING MANAGEMENT

CHAPTER 16 Preoperative Nursing Management

1. A hospitalized client tells the nurse that she is worried about her upcoming surgery. The best response by the nurse is to tell the client
A. "That's ok. Most people are afraid of surgery."
B. "Don't worry. There's nothing to be afraid of."
*C. "Tell me more about what you are worried about."
D. "Your doctor is a fine surgeon. Everything will be fine."

Rationale: The nurse should acknowledge the client's concerns and communicate in a therapeutic manner. To respond to the client's fears with unwarranted reassurance is not helpful. The best response by the nurse is to say, "Tell me more about what you are worried about," because this opens the communication.

Reference: p. 317

Descriptors:
1. 16 2. 01 3. Application
4. IV–1 5. Communication 6. Moderate

2. A nurse is preparing a client for surgery in one hour. The client has not yet signed the consent form, although the client's physician has explained the procedure and risks. The client tells the nurse that he needs more information before signing the consent form. The nurse should
*A. contact the client's physician.
B. answer the client's questions.
C. administer the client's preoperative medications.
D. cancel the scheduled surgery in the operating room.

Rationale: If the client needs additional information to make his decision, the nurse should contact the client's physician. The consent form should be signed before any preoperative medication is given.

Reference: p. 315

Descriptors:
1. 16 2. 03 3. Application
4. IV–1 5. Nursing Process 6. Moderate

3. A client is 16 years old, married, and lives with her husband and her parents. The client is scheduled for surgery in the morning. The informed consent form should be signed by the
   A. parents.
   B. husband.
   *C. client.
   D. legal guardian.

Rationale: An emancipated minor (married) can sign his or her own surgical consent. The parents, husband, or legal guardian do not need to sign the consent.

Reference: p. 316

Descriptors:
1. 16 2. 03 3. Application
4. IV–1 5. Documentation 6. Difficult

4. An adult client tells the nurse that he has never had surgery before and doesn't know what to expect following the surgery to remove his appendix. The priority nursing diagnosis for the client is
   A. Anxiety related to fear of the unknown.
   B. Ineffective individual coping related to knowledge deficit.
   C. Fear of surgery related to the uncertainty of the outcomes.
   *D. Knowledge deficit related to postoperative procedures related to lack of experience.

Rationale: The priority nursing diagnosis for the client is Knowledge deficit related to postoperative procedures related to lack of experience. There is no evidence of ineffective coping, fear, or anxiety. The nurse should explain the postoperative procedures.

Reference: p. 317

Descriptors:
1. 16 2. 01 3. Analysis
4. IV–3 5. Nursing Process 6. Moderate

5. During a preoperative assessment, a client tells the nurse that she has been taking long-term corticosteroid therapy. The nurse should notify the client's physician as sudden termination of steroids can lead to
   *A. cardiovascular collapse.
   B. a severe electrolyte imbalance.
   C. respiratory failure.
   D. thyrotoxicosis.

Rationale: Corticosteroids are not to be discontinued abruptly before surgery because sudden termination may lead to cardiovascular collapse. Sudden termination of corticosteroids does not contribute to severe electrolyte imbalance, respiratory failure, or thyrotoxicosis.

Reference: p. 320

Descriptors:
1. 16 2. 02 3. Application
4. IV–3 5. Nursing Process 6. Moderate

6. A preoperative client tells the nurse during the nursing history that he has been taking monoamine oxidase inhibitors for several years. The nurse should alert the client's surgeon as these medications can lead to
   *A. hypotension.
   B. seizures.
   C. cardiac tamponade.
   D. ketoacidosis.

Rationale: Monoamine oxidase inhibitors can increase the hypotensive effects of the anesthesia. They do not contribute to seizures, cardiac tamponade, or ketoacidosis.

Reference: p. 320

Descriptors:
1. 16 2. 02 3. Application
4. IV–3 5. Nursing Process 6. Moderate

7. A nurse is caring for a client who is scheduled for abdominal surgery. Ideally, the preoperative teaching should be done
   A. only when the client asks for information.
   B. when all of the family members are present.
   *C. over a period of time to allow for assimilation and questions.
   D. during the immediate preoperative period so the client doesn't become fearful.

Rationale: Ideally, the preoperative teaching should be done over a period of time to allow for assimilation and questions. Teaching sessions are often combined with various preparation procedures.

Reference: p. 321

Descriptors:
1. 16 2. 05 3. Application
4. IV–3 5. Teaching/Learning 6. Moderate

8. A nurse has instructed a preoperative client about deep breathing and coughing exercises during the postoperative period. The nurse determines that the client has understood the instructions when the client says,
   A. "Taking deep breaths will help to decrease my incisional pain."
   *B. "If I cough and deep breathe I will be less likely to develop pneumonia."
   C. "My coughing and deep breathing exercises will be most effective if I lie on my back."
   D. "It is important that I cough at least twice before taking a deep breath."

Rationale: The client has understood the instructions when the client says, "If I cough and deep breathe I will be less likely to develop pneumonia," because these exercises enhance expiration. The exercises will not decrease incisional pain, they are more effective if the client is sitting upright, and the client should deep breathe before coughing.

Reference: p. 321

Descriptors:
1. 16 2. 04 3. Application
4. IV–3 5. Teaching/Learning 6. Moderate

9. A nurse is caring for a preoperative client scheduled for surgery in the morning. The nurse should explain to the client that food and fluid will be withheld after midnight to
   A. reduce the potential for diarrhea after the surgery.
   B. promote the effectiveness of the anesthesia.
   C. inhibit bacterial growth in the intestinal tract.
   *D. reduce the risk of aspiration during surgery.

Rationale: Food and fluid will be withheld after midnight to reduce the risk of aspiration during surgery, which results in inadequate oxygen exchange. Keeping the client NPO after midnight does not reduce the potential for diarrhea after the surgery, promote the effectiveness of the anesthesia, or inhibit bacterial growth.

Reference: p. 323

Descriptors:
1. 16 2. 04 3. Application
4. IV–3 5. Teaching/Learning 6. Moderate

10. A nurse is caring for a preoperative client who will be transported to the operating room in 5 minutes for an appendectomy. At this time, the nurse should
    A. allow the client to wear his dentures to the operating room.
    B. catheterize the client before he is transported.
    *C. encourage the client to void.
    D. tape the client's rings to his finger.

Rationale: The client should be encouraged to void immediately before going to the operating room to promote continence during low abdominal surgery. Dentures should not be worn to the operating room. Catheterization is done in the operating room if necessary. Rings should have already been removed or taped.

Reference: p. 324

Descriptors:
1. 16 2. 06 3. Application
4. IV–3 5. Nursing Process 6. Moderate

11. A nurse is caring for a preoperative client following administration of the preoperative sedation. The client tells the nurse that he needs to void. The nurse should
    A. assist the client to the bathroom.
    *B. offer the client a urinal.
    C. call the physician for a catheterization order.
    D. tell the client he will be catheterized in the operating room.

Rationale: If a client needs to void following administration of a sedative, the nurse should offer the client a urinal. The client should not get out of bed because of the potential for lightheadedness.

Reference: p. 324

Descriptors:
1. 16 2. 07 3. Application
4. IV–3 5. Nursing Process 6. Moderate

CHAPTER 17 Intraoperative Nursing Management

1. The nurse is caring for an elderly client in the operating room. The nurse should monitor the client for a side effect of the surgery and anesthesia that is common in elderly clients:
   A. hyperthermia.
   B. pulmonary edema.
   C. cerebral ischemia.
   *D. agitation or disorientation.

Rationale: Agitation or disorientation are common side effects of surgery and anesthesia, particularly in the elderly. Hypothermia, cardiac arrythmias, and hypotension are other common side effects.

Reference: p. 328

Descriptors:
1. 17 2. 04 3. Application
4. IV–3 5. Nursing Process 6. Moderate

2. One of the primary functions of the scrub nurse in the operating room is to
   *A. assist the surgeon with necessary instruments.
   B. coordinate the operating team.
   C. maintain proper lighting.
   D. ensure the availability of supplies.

Rationale: One of the primary functions of the scrub nurse in the operating room is to assist the surgeon with necessary instruments. In addition, the scrub nurse monitors the time that the client is under anesthesia and keeps track of drains and sponges.

Reference: p. 329

Descriptors:
1. 17 2. 01 3. Knowledge
4. IV–1 5. Nursing Process 6. Moderate

3. During a surgical procedure under anesthesia, the anesthesiologist is responsible for
   A. estimating the client's blood loss.
   B. maintaining a record of the fluid intake.
   C. positioning the client on the operating table.
   *D. monitoring the client's electrocardiogram.

Rationale: The responsibilities of the anesthesiologist include monitoring the client's electrocardiogram, vital signs, oxygen saturation, and tidal volume.

Reference: p. 324

Descriptors:
1. 17 2. 03 3. Application
4. I 5. Nursing Process 6. Moderate

4. Elderly clients are at greater risk for surgical procedures because they
   A. are more anxious and get agitated.
   *B. have decreased cardiac reserve.
   C. have immobility problems due to arthritis.
   D. require greater amounts of anesthetic than younger clients.

   Rationale: Elderly clients are at greater risk for surgical procedures because they have decreased cardiac reserve and reduced cardiac output. They usually need less anesthesia than younger clients.

   Reference: p. 328

   Descriptors:

1. 17	2. 04	3. Application
4. IV–3	5. Nursing Process	6. Moderate

5. A nurse is working in the operating room during a surgical procedure. Which of the following actions would be considered a break in sterile technique?
   A. Placing a sterile drape in position from front to back.
   B. Discarding sterile supplies into a waste receptacle.
   *C. Keeping sterile gloved hands below waist level.
   D. Replacement of a drape when it has been punctured.

   Rationale: Sterile gloved hands must always remain above the waist to maintain sterility. Placing a sterile drape in position from front to back, discarding sterile supplies into a waste receptacle, and replacement of a drape when it has been punctured are all examples of appropriate sterile procedures.

   Reference: p. 331

   Descriptors:

1. 17	2. 02	3. Application
4. I–1	5. Nursing Process	6. Moderate

6. A nurse is working in an operating room that will be using lasers. The nurse should plan to
   A. wear clean gloves to scrub.
   *B. wear protective goggles.
   C. use only latex-based gloves.
   D. take several breaks during the procedure.

   Rationale: Protective goggles specific to the type of laser being used are necessary to avoid eye damage. Sterile gloves are always used by the scrub nurse. Latex-based gloves may result in an allergic reaction. Breaks should be limited to time between surgical cases to prevent potential breaks in sterile technique due to leaving the OR and re-entry.

   Reference: p. 331

   Descriptors:

1. 17	2. 04	3. Application
4. I–1	5. Nursing Process	6. Moderate

7. The most common general gas anesthetic used in operating rooms is
   *A. nitrous oxide.
   B. isoflurane.
   C. enflurane.
   D. sevoflurane.

   Rationale: Nitrous oxide is the most common gas anesthetic used in operating rooms. Isoflurane, enflurane, and sevoflurane are volatile anesthetics.

   Reference: p. 332

   Descriptors:

1. 17	2. 04	3. Application
4. I–1	5. Nursing Process	6. Moderate

8. A nurse is working in the operating room during a surgical procedure. The client has been administered general anesthesia. When the client reaches Stage III of anesthesia, the nurse can anticipate that the client will be
   A. dizzy.
   B. warm.
   C. excited.
   *D. unconscious.

   Rationale: In Stage III of anesthesia, the client is unconscious. In Stage I, the client may feel warm and dizzy. In Stage II, the client may talk or laugh and be excited.

   Reference: p. 333

   Descriptors:

1. 17	2. 04	3. Application
4. I–1	5. Nursing Process	6. Moderate

9. A client is scheduled for surgery and is to have an intravenous anesthetic. The nurse should explain to the client that one advantage of intravenous anesthesia is that
   A. there is a decreased potential for respiratory depression.
   B. the client will be able to remain awake during the surgery.
   *C. the duration of the drug's action is brief.
   D. the drug causes a potent skeletal muscle relaxation.

   Rationale: Advantages of intravenous anesthesia include the brief duration of the drug, less nausea and vomiting, and little equipment is required. The client is unconscious, and there is an increased potential for respiratory depression. There is no indication that the drugs cause a potent skeletal muscle relaxation.

   Reference: p. 334

   Descriptors:

1. 17	2. 06	3. Application
4. IV–3	5. Nursing Process	6. Difficult

10. A client is scheduled to receive conscious sedation. The nurse should explain to the client that one commonly used drug for this type of sedation is
    *A. diazepam.
    B. meperidine.

C. morphine.
D. chlordiazepoxide.

Rationale: Midazolam (Versad) and diazepam (Valium) are two of the most commonly used drugs for conscious sedation. Meperidine, morphine, and chlordiazepoxide are not commonly used for conscious sedation.

Reference: p. 334

Descriptors:
1. 17 2. 06 3. Application
4. IV–2 5. Nursing Process 6. Moderate

11. A client is receiving morphine as an intravenous anesthetic agent. The priority assessment for the nurse to make is the client's
A. blood pressure.
B. gastrointestinal status.
*C. respiratory rate.
D. hallucinations.

Rationale: Morphine as an intravenous anesthetic can result in respiratory depression; therefore, the client's respiratory rate is the priority assessment. Ketamine can cause hallucinations and decrease the blood pressure. Meperidine can cause nausea and vomiting.

Reference: p. 335

Descriptors:
1. 17 2. 06 3. Application
4. IV–2 5. Nursing Process 6. Moderate

12. A nurse is caring for a client in the recovery room following surgery under a spinal anesthetic. The nurse determines that the client has recovered from the effects of spinal anesthesia when the client exhibits
A. return of spontaneous breathing.
*B. complete return of sensation to the legs.
C. stabilization of the blood pressure.
D. warm and dry extremities.

Rationale: The client has recovered from the effects of spinal anesthesia when the client exhibits complete return of sensation to the legs. Spinal anesthesia should not affect the client's breathing, blood pressure, or temperature of the extremities.

Reference: p. 337

Descriptors:
1. 17 2. 06 3. Application
4. IV–4 5. Nursing Process 6. Moderate

13. A nurse is caring for a client who has developed a spinal headache following surgery under a spinal anesthetic. The nurse should
*A. keep the client well hydrated.
B. elevate the head of the bed 45 degrees.
C. keep the client on NPO status.
D. perform hourly neurological assessments.

Rationale: If a client develops a spinal headache, the nurse should keep the client in a flat position, a quiet environment, and maintain adequate hydration. Hourly neurological assessments are not necessary.

Reference: p. 337

Descriptors:
1. 17 2. 06 3. Application
4. IV–1 5. Nursing Process 6. Moderate

14. A client is scheduled for vaginal surgery. The nurse should place the client in the position termed
A. dorsal recumbent.
B. Sims.
C. Trendelenberg.
*D. lithotomy.

Rationale: The lithotomy position is used for vaginal, perineal, or rectal surgery. Dorsal recumbent position is used for most abdominal surgery. Sims position is used for renal surgery, and Trendelenberg position is used for surgery on the lower abdomen.

Reference: p. 340

Descriptors:
1. 17 2. 06 3. Application
4. IV–1 5. Nursing Process 6. Easy

15. An operating room nurse is caring for a 75-year-old client who is scheduled for abdominal surgery. While caring for older clients in the operating room, a priority assessment for the nurse to make is the client's
A. hallucinations.
*B. temperature status.
C. gastrointestinal status.
D. anxiety.

Rationale: Hypothermia is a common problem for older clients, therefore the nurse should assess the client for symptoms of heat loss and keep the client's head warm with a heat-retaining cap. Hallucinations, gastrointestinal status, and anxiety are common reactions to surgery and anesthesia for all clients.

Reference: p. 341

Descriptors:
1. 17 2. 05 3. Application
4. IV–1 5. Nursing Process 6. Moderate

16. An operating room nurse is caring for a client during surgery when the client exhibits tachycardia and tetany-like movements of the jaw. The nurse suspects that the client is exhibiting symptoms of
A. respiratory depression.
B. induced hypertension.
C. hypokalemia.
*D. malignant hyperthermia.

Rationale: Tachycardia, hypotension, and tetany-like movements of the jaw are indicative of malignant hyperthermia, which is an emergency situation.

These symptoms are not associated with respiratory depression, induced hypertension, or hypokalemia.

Reference: p. 342

Descriptors:

1. 17	2. 06	3. Analysis
4. IV–3	5. Nursing Process	6. Moderate

CHAPTER 18
Postoperative Nursing Management

1. A client has just been transferred to the postanesthesia care unit following abdominal surgery. The first priority for assessment by the nurse is the client's
   A. blood pressure.
   B. evidence of malignancy.
   C. abdominal dressing.
   *D. respirations.

Rationale: Patency of the airway and respiratory status should be evaluated first, followed by cardiovascular status, and the condition of the surgical site.

Reference: p. 347

Descriptors:

1. 18	2. 01	3. Application
4. IV–1	5. Nursing Process	6. Moderate

2. Unless contraindicated, the nurse in the postanesthesia care unit should plan to maintain an unconscious postsurgical client in which position during the recovery phase?
   *A. Side-lying position with chin extended.
   B. High Trendelenberg position.
   C. Dorsal recumbent position.
   D. Prone position.

Rationale: To maintain a patent airway and prevent choking if the client vomits, the client should be maintained in a side-lying position with chin extended. High Trendelenberg, dorsal recumbent, and prone positions are not recommended, because they can lead to airway obstruction or aspiration.

Reference: pp. 337–348

Descriptors:

1. 18	2. 01	3. Application
4. IV–1	5. Nursing Process	6. Moderate

3. Upon admission to the postanesthesia care unit, a client's blood pressure was 130/90 and the pulse was 68. After 30 minutes, the client's blood pressure is 120/65 and the pulse is 100. The client's skin is cold, moist, and pale. The nurse should
   A. increase the rate of the intravenous fluids.
   *B. notify the client's physician.
   C. increase the nasal oxygen flow from 2 liters to 3 liters.
   D. elevate the head of the bed and encourage deep breathing.

Rationale: The client is exhibiting symptoms of hemorrhage and shock, therefore the nurse should first notify the client's physician. The client may be ordered to have a blood transfusion or increased intravenous fluids. Increasing the nasal oxygen flow from 2 liters to 3 liters, elevating the head of the bed, and encouraging deep breathing are not helpful.

Reference: pp. 348–349

Descriptors:

1. 18	2. 01	3. Application
4. IV–3	5. Nursing Process	6. Moderate

4. While caring for an adult client in the postanesthesia care unit following chest surgery, the client complains of severe nausea. The nurse should first
   A. administer an antiemetic.
   B. apply a cool cloth to the client's forehead.
   C. offer the client a small amount of ice chips.
   *D. turn the client completely to one side.

Rationale: Turning the client completely to one side allows collected fluid to escape from the side of the mouth if the client vomits. Ice chips can increase feelings of nausea. After turning the client to the side, the nurse can offer a cool cloth to the client's forehead and administer an antiemetic if one is ordered.

Reference: p. 349

Descriptors:

1. 18	2. 03	3. Application
4. IV–3	5. Nursing Process	6. Moderate

5. A nurse is caring for a client after abdominal surgery in the postanesthesia care unit. The client begins to complain of incisional pain and requests pain medication. The nurse assesses the client for a common side effect of stimulation of the sympathetic nervous system:
   A. warmth.
   B. respiratory depression.
   *C. hypertension.
   D. nausea and vomiting.

Rationale: Hypertension is common in the immediate postoperative period secondary to sympathetic nervous system stimulation from pain or hypoxia. Hypothermia is more common than warmth. Respiratory depression and nausea and vomiting are not common as a result of sympathetic nervous stimulation.

Reference: p. 349

Descriptors:

1. 18	2. 03	3. Application
4. IV–1	5. Nursing Process	6. Moderate

6. While caring for a 90-year-old newly postoperative client, the nurse observes that the client now appears confused and agitated. The nurse should assess the client for
   *A. pain.
   B. senility.
   C. hypertension.
   D. hypothermia.

Rationale: Postoperative confusion in elderly clients is common. Unrelieved pain may increase the risk for delirium, therefore this should be assessed. Senility, hypertension, and hypothermia are not common causes of confusion.

Reference: p. 349

Descriptors:
1. 18 2. 04 3. Application
4. IV–1 5. Nursing Process 6. Moderate

7. A nurse is preparing to discharge a 60-year-old client following ambulatory surgery for cataract removal. One of the important differences between clients who are released from ambulatory surgery and hospitalized clients is the need for
   A. prescription medications.
   *B. teaching and reinforcement.
   C. pain control.
   D. detection of surgical complications.

Rationale: One of the important differences between clients who are released from ambulatory surgery and hospitalized clients is the need for teaching and reinforcement. Written and verbal instructions should be given both to the client and a family member, since the effects of anesthesia and analgesia can alter the client's thinking abilities.

Reference: p. 351

Descriptors:
1. 18 2. 02 3. Application
4. IV–3 5. Nursing Process 6. Moderate

8. A nurse is caring for a group of preoperative clients who will undergo surgery. The preoperative teaching related to coughing and deep breathing following surgery should be provided to the client who will undergo
   A. intracranial surgery.
   B. facial plastic surgery.
   *C. lung surgery.
   D. eye surgery.

Rationale: Coughing is contraindicated for clients who have undergone intracranial surgery or eye surgery because of the increase in pressure and plastic surgery because of strain on delicate tissues. The client who will undergo lung surgery should be instructed in deep breathing and coughing exercises.

Reference: p. 352

Descriptors:
1. 18 2. 03 3. Application
4. IV–3 5. Nursing Process 6. Moderate

9. While caring for a postoperative client on the first postoperative day following chest surgery, the nurse assesses the client for deep vein thrombosis. To prevent venous stasis, the nurse should
   *A. encourage frequent position changes.
   B. raise the knee gatch on the bed.
   C. place a pillow under the client's knees.
   D. dangle the legs on the side of the bed for prolonged periods.

Rationale: Raising the knee gatch on the bed, placing a pillow under the client's knees, and dangling the legs on the side of the bed for prolonged periods can affect venous return and should not be done. Frequent position changes, leg exercises, and antiembolism stockings can improve venous return.

Reference: p. 353

Descriptors:
1. 18 2. 01 3. Application
4. IV–3 5. Nursing Process 6. Moderate

10. A nurse is assessing a two-day postoperative client following chest surgery. The client is reluctant to ambulate, has a nonproductive cough, and has crackles at the base of the lung. The nurse determines that the client is most likely exhibiting symptoms of
   A. bronchopneumonia.
   B. pleurisy.
   *C. static pulmonary secretions.
   D. malignant hyperthermia.

Rationale: When the client is reluctant to ambulate, has a nonproductive cough, and has crackles at the base of the lung, the client is most likely exhibiting symptoms of static pulmonary secretions. The client should be encouraged to turn every two hours and take deep breaths to prevent pneumonia. These are not symptoms of bronchopneumonia, pleurisy, or malignant hyperthermia.

Reference: p. 352

Descriptors:
1. 18 2. 01 3. Application
4. IV–3 5. Nursing Process 6. Moderate

11. A nurse is caring for a one-day postoperative client with a nasogastric tube. The last hourly urine output for the client was 30 mL. A priority nursing goal for this client should include
   A. observing the intravenous insertion site.
   *B. maintaining the fluid and electrolyte balance.
   C. documenting the wound irrigation procedure.
   D. maintaining the client on complete bedrest.

Rationale: Postoperative clients are at risk for fluid imbalances, particularly if there is a nasogastric tube in place and a urine output of 30 mL or below in one hour. Observing the intravenous insertion site is common practice. There is no need to document the wound irrigation procedure or to maintain the client on complete bedrest at this time.

Reference: p. 353

Descriptors:
1. 18 2. 01 3. Application
4. IV–3 5. Nursing Process 6. Moderate

12. A nurse is preparing to ambulate a one-day postoperative client for the first time. In order to decrease the potential for orthostatic hypotension, the nurse should plan to have the client
 A. avoid taking any narcotics for 30 minutes before ambulation.
 B. transfer the client directly from the bed to a bedside chair.
 C. stand at the bedside for 5 minutes before ambulation.
 *D. position himself completely upright on the side of the bed.

13. A nurse is caring for an adult client on the first postoperative day following an appendectomy for a ruptured appendix. The nurse should plan the instructions for wound care for this client based on the wound class status called
 A. clean.
 *B. clean-contaminated.
 C. contaminated.
 D. dirty.

Rationale: Appendectomies due to a ruptured appendix are considered clean-contaminated wounds, so the teaching should include special emphasis on signs of infection. Clean wounds do not involve any contamination. Dirty wounds are due to trauma or foreign bodies, such as gunshot wounds.

Reference: p. 360

Descriptors:
1. 18 2. 05 3. Application
4. IV–3 5. Nursing Process 6. Moderate

14. A nurse has instructed a client about caring for her surgical wound and changing the dressing. The nurse determines that the client has understood the instructions when the client says,
 A. "I should change the dressing only if it has a foul odor."
 B. "I will probably have a temperature elevation until the wound heals."
 *C. "It is normal for the edges of the wound to be slightly raised."
 D. "Red streaks in the skin near the wound are normal and will disappear."

Rationale: The client has understood the instructions when the client says, "It is normal for the edges of the wound to be slightly raised," because this is a normal finding. A foul odor, temperature elevation, and red streaks near the wound are signs of infection.

Reference: p. 364

Descriptors:
1. 18 2. 07 3. Application
4. IV–3 5. Nursing Process 6. Moderate

15. A nurse is preparing to change the abdominal dressing of a one-day postoperative client. After explaining the procedure to the client, the nurse should
 A. place the old dressing in the client's bedside trash.
 B. cut several pieces of surgical tape.
 C. remove the old adhesive with baby oil.
 *D. wash his or her hands.

Rationale: To prevent contamination, the nurse should first wash his or her hands and then don clean gloves. Old dressings should be placed in hazardous waste containers. Adhesive can be removed with alcohol or nonirritating solvents. Cutting surgical tape is not the first step.

Reference: p. 362

Descriptors:
1. 18 2. 06 3. Application
4. IV–1 5. Nursing Process 6. Moderate

16. A nurse is caring for a two-day postoperative client following a cesarean section. The client tells the nurse that she thinks "my incision has ruptured." After determining that the wound exhibits dehiscence and evisceration, the nurse should
 A. ask the client to sit in a chair.
 B. apply an abdominal binder to support the wound.
 C. place the client in a supine position.
 *D. apply a sterile dressing moistened with sterile saline.

Rationale: When there is dehiscence and evisceration of the wound, the nurse should place the client in a quiet, low Fowler's position and apply a sterile dressing moistened with sterile saline to the wound. The physician should be notified. Abdominal binders will not help at this point.

Reference: p. 365

Descriptors:
1. 18 2. 07 3. Application
4. IV–1 5. Nursing Process 6. Moderate

UNIT 5
GAS EXCHANGE AND RESPIRATORY FUNCTION

CHAPTER 19
Assessment of Respiratory Function

1. Airway resistance and slight obstruction of air flow is determined by the
   *A. radius or size of the airway through which air flows.
   B. movement of the diaphragm on inspiration.
   C. elasticity of the lung tissue.
   D. surface tension of the alveoli.

Rationale: Resistance is determined chiefly by the radius or size of the airway through which air flows. Movement of the diaphragm on inspiration, elasticity of the lung tissue, and surface tension of the alveoli do not determine resistance.

Reference: p. 373

Descriptors:
1. 19 2. 01 3. Comprehension
4. IV–1 5. Nursing Process 6. Moderate

2. Which of the following statements best describes a low-flow ventilation–perfusion ratio?
   A. An absence of ventilation and perfusion exists in the lungs.
   *B. Blood bypasses the alveoli without gas exchange occurring.
   C. The alveoli have inadequate blood supply to allow gas exchange to occur.
   D. A given amount of blood passes an alveolus and is matched with an equal amount of gas.

Rationale: A low-flow ventilation–perfusion ratio exists when blood bypasses the alveoli without gas exchange occurring. This may be due to pneumonia or chronic obstructive lung disease.

Reference: p. 378

Descriptors:
1. 19 2. 02 3. Comprehension
4. IV–1 5. Nursing Process 6. Moderate

3. The normal value of PaO_2 in an adult client is
   A. 40–59 mmHg.
   B. 60–79 mmHg.
   *C. 80–100 mmHg.
   D. 101–120 mmHg.

Rationale: The normal value of PaO_2 in an adult client is 80–100 mmHg, which provides adequate oxygenation to the tissues.

Reference: p. 379

Descriptors:
1. 19 2. 02 3. Application
4. IV–1 5. Nursing Process 6. Moderate

4. The inspiratory and expiratory centers that control the rate and depth of ventilation are in the
   A. hypothalamus.
   B. thalamus.
   C. occipital lobe.
   *D. medulla oblongata.

Rationale: The inspiratory and expiratory centers that control the rate and depth of ventilation are in the medulla oblongata and the pons.

Reference: p. 380

Descriptors:
1. 19 2. 02 3. Comprehension
4. IV–1 5. Nursing Process 6. Moderate

5. A nurse is assessing the respiratory system of a 78-year-old client. The nurse can anticipate that because of the client's age, the client will have
   A. increased elasticity of the alveoli.
   *B. decreased vital capacity.
   C. functional residual capacity.
   D. increased respiratory volume.

Rationale: A decrease in vital capacity occurs with loss of chest wall movement, thus restricting air flow in older clients. At about age 50, alveoli begin to lose their elasticity.

Reference: p. 380

Descriptors:
1. 19 2. 02 3. Application
4. IV–1 5. Nursing Process 6. Moderate

6. A nurse is caring for a client who has chronic dyspnea and an expiratory wheeze. The nurse suspects that the client may be exhibiting symptoms of
   A. muscular dystrophy.
   B. pneumonia.
   C. pulmonary embolism.
   *D. chronic obstructive pulmonary disease.

Rationale: Dyspnea and an expiratory wheeze are associated with chronic obstructive pulmonary disease. Sudden dyspnea may be associated with pulmonary embolism.

Reference: p. 381

Descriptors:
1. 19 2. 03 3. Application
4. IV–3 5. Nursing Process 6. Moderate

7. A nurse is assessing a newly admitted client and observes that the client has a cough in the morning with excessive sputum production. The nurse suspects that the client has
   A. emphysema.
   B. laryngotracheitis.

*C. bronchitis.
D. pleurisy.

Rationale: A cough in the morning with sputum production is indicative of bronchitis. Pleurisy involves chest pain. Wheezing is associated with emphysema. Laryngotracheitis is associated with an irritated, high-pitched cough.

Reference: p. 381

Descriptors:
1. 19 2. 04 3. Analysis
4. IV–4 5. Nursing Process 6. Moderate

8. A nurse is caring for a hospitalized client who has profuse pink, frothy mucous. The nurse notifies the client's physician, because these symptoms are indicative of
A. bronchiectasis.
B. lung tumors.
C. infection.
*D. pulmonary edema.

Rationale: Profuse, pink, frothy sputum is a symptom of pulmonary edema. Foul-smelling sputum is associated with bronchiectasis. Pink-tinged mucoid sputum is associated with a lung tumor. Infections are associated with greenish or yellowish sputum.

Reference: p. 382

Descriptors:
1. 19 2. 04 3. Analysis
4. IV–4 5. Nursing Process 6. Moderate

9. A nurse is caring for a client diagnosed with pleurisy who has a foul-tasting sputum. To assist the client in cleansing the palate of the foul taste, the nurse should encourage the client to begin the meal with
A. applesauce.
B. salads.
C. bread.
*D. orange juice.

Rationale: The nurse should encourage the client to begin the meal with a citrus juice, such as orange juice, because these juices cleanse the palate of the foul taste. Applesauce, salads, and bread do not cleanse the palate.

Reference: p. 382

Descriptors:
1. 19 2. 04 3. Application
4. IV–1 5. Nursing Process 6. Moderate

10. A nurse is caring for a hospitalized adult client diagnosed with pleurisy. The client tells the nurse that she has a sharp pain on inspiration. The nurse should encourage the client to maintain which position?
*A. Side-lying on the affected side.
B. Dorsal recumbent.
C. Prone.
D. Upright in a chair.

Rationale: Lying on the affected side tends to splint the chest wall, limit expansion and contraction of the lung, and reduce friction. The dorsal recumbent, prone, or upright in a chair positions will not alleviate the sharp pain.

Reference: p. 382

Descriptors:
1. 19 2. 04 3. Application
4. IV–1 5. Nursing Process 6. Moderate

11. A client tells the nurse that he recently vomited and that the emesis resembled "coffee grounds." The nurse notifies the physician, because this symptom is associated with hemorrhage from the
*A. stomach.
B. lungs.
C. nose.
D. duodenum.

Rationale: "Coffee grounds"-colored emesis is associated with hemorrhage from the stomach. Blood from the lungs is bright red, frothy, and mixed with sputum.

Reference: p. 383

Descriptors:
1. 19 2. 04 3. Analysis
4. IV–4 5. Nursing Process 6. Moderate

12. A nurse is assessing the chest of a client with emphysema. The nurse observes that there is an increase in the anteriorposterior diameter of the client's thorax. The nurse should document the presence of
A. pidgeon chest.
*B. barrel chest.
C. kyphoscoliosis.
D. funnel chest.

Rationale: Barrel chest occurs with overinflation of the client's lungs, such as with a client who has emphysema. There is an increase in the anteriorposterior diameter of the client's thorax. Pidgeon chest has a displaced sternum. Funnel chest has a depressed sternum. Kyphoscoliosis involves an elevation of the scapula.

Reference: p. 384

Descriptors:
1. 19 2. 04 3. Application
4. IV–1 5. Documentation 6. Moderate

13. Which of the following respiratory pattern descriptions is characteristic of a client who is hyperventilating?
*A. An increase in the rate and depth with a lowered arterial PCO_2.
B. A rapid increase in the respiratory rate with no change in depth.
C. Alternating periods of deep breathing and apnea.
D. Increased depth of breathing resulting in alkalosis.

Rationale: Hyperventilation is associated with an increase in the rate and depth with a lowered arterial PCO_2. Severe acidosis and hyperventilation is called Kussmaul's respirations and usually have a renal or diabetic origin. Cheyne–Stokes is associated with deep breathing and periods of apnea.

Reference: p. 385

Descriptors:
1. 19 2. 04 3. Analysis
4. IV–4 5. Nursing Process 6. Moderate

14. A nurse is planning to auscultate the lungs of an adult client. To begin at the client's point of maximal impulse of the heart, the nurse should place the stethoscope at the
*A. midclavicular line.
B. midsternal line.
C. midaxillary line.
D. posterior axillary line.

Rationale: The point of maximal impulse of the heart normally lies along the midclavicular line on the left thorax.

Reference: p. 385

Descriptors:
1. 19 2. 04 3. Application
4. IV–1 5. Nursing Process 6. Moderate

15. A nurse is assessing a female client for fremitus. To detect fremitus, the nurse should place his or her hands on the client's
A. lower rib cage.
B. sternum.
*C. upper thorax.
D. midclavicular line.

Rationale: While the client repeats the words "ninety-nine," the nurse's hands should move down the client's upper anterior or posterior thorax. Fremitus is most pronounced near the large bronchi closest to the chest wall.

Reference: p. 386

Descriptors:
1. 19 2. 04 3. Application
4. IV–1 5. Nursing Process 6. Moderate

16. A nurse is planning to percuss the anterior chest of an adult client. The nurse should ask the client to position himself in a
A. side-lying position.
B. Sims position.
C. sitting position with head flexed forward.
*D. upright position with shoulders arched backward.

Rationale: Percussion over the anterior chest is performed with the client in an upright position with shoulders arched backward and arms at the side. Percussion of the posterior thorax is done with the client in a sitting position with head flexed forward.

Reference: p. 387

Descriptors:
1. 19 2. 03 3. Application
4. IV–1 5. Nursing Process 6. Difficult

17. While percussing the thorax of an adult client, the nurse detects dullness over the left lung. The nurse suspects the client may be exhibiting symptoms of
*A. pneumonia.
B. pneumothorax.
C. emphysema.
D. bronchitis.

Rationale: Dullness over the lung occurs when air-filled lung tissue is replaced by fluid or solid tissue. This occurs with lung tumors and lobar pneumonia. Pneumothorax is associated with a tympanic or drumlike sound. Emphysema is associated with hyperresonance.

Reference: p. 387

Descriptors:
1. 19 2. 04 3. Application
4. IV–4 5. Nursing Process 6. Moderate

18. A nurse is preparing to auscultate an adult client's lungs. To hear vesicular breath sounds, the nurse should place the stethoscope on the client's
*A. lungs.
B. manubrium.
C. first intercostal space.
D. scapulae.

Rationale: Vesicular breath sounds are best heard over most of both lungs. Broncho-vesicular sounds are heard in the first and second intercostal spaces and between the scapulae. Bronchial sounds are heard over the manubrium.

Reference: p. 389

Descriptors:
1. 19 2. 04 3. Application
4. IV–1 5. Nursing Process 6. Moderate

19. A nurse is assessing the pulmonary system of an adult client. The nurse notes a significant decrease in respiratory excursion on the left side of the client's chest. Percussion reveals a hyperresonant sound. The nurse suspects that the client is most likely exhibiting symptoms of
A. pulmonary edema.
B. bronchitis.
*C. pneumothorax.
D. pneumonia.

Rationale: A significant decrease in respiratory excursion on the left side of the client's chest and percussion that reveals a hyperresonant sound is associated with pneumothorax. Pulmonary edema is associated with crackles and resonant sounds. Bronchitis would be associated with normal-to-decreased breath sounds with resonant percussion sounds. Pneumonia would reveal crackles and dull percussion sounds.

Reference: p. 390

Descriptors:
1. 19 2. 04 3. Application
4. IV–4 5. Nursing Process 6. Moderate

20. A nurse is caring for a client on the pulmonary unit. The noninvasive method of monitoring oxygen saturation levels includes
A. positron emission tomography.
*B. pulse oximetry.
C. arterial blood gas studies.
D. lung scans.

Rationale: The noninvasive method of monitoring oxygen saturation levels includes pulse oximetry. Invasive tests include arterial blood gases and lung scans.

Reference: p. 393

Descriptors:
1. 19 2. 05 3. Application
4. IV–4 5. Nursing Process 6. Moderate

21. Following a fiberoptic bronchoscopy, the nurse will determine that the client can have clear liquids when the client has
*A. a cough and gag reflex.
B. indicated he knows the date and place.
C. normal blood pressure levels.
D. regular, nondyspneic breathing.

Rationale: The client can have clear liquids when the client has a cough and gag reflex. Preoperative sedation and local anesthesia can impair the swallowing reflex.

Reference: p. 395

Descriptors:
1. 19 2. 05 3. Application
4. IV–1 5. Nursing Process 6. Moderate

22. A client is scheduled for a thoracoscopy. The nurse should explain to the client that this procedure is used in the diagnostic evaluation of
A. bleeding sites.
B. atelectasis.
C. abnormal lung fluids.
*D. pleural effusions.

Rationale: This procedure is used in the diagnostic evaluation of pleural effusions, pleural disease, and tumor staging. Bronchoscopy is used to detect bleeding sites. Thoracentesis is the procedure that removes fluids for diagnostic purposes.

Reference: p. 395

Descriptors:
1. 19 2. 05 3. Application
4. IV–1 5. Nursing Process 6. Moderate

CHAPTER 20
Management of Patients with Upper Respiratory Tract Disorders

1. The nurse is caring for an elderly client with a severe head cold. The nurse should instruct the client that one of the most effective methods of preventing transmission of the organism is to
A. take prescribed antibiotics.
B. use warm salt water gargles.
C. use cough suppressants.
*D. wash the hands frequently.

Rationale: Hand washing remains the most effective preventive measure to reduce the transmission of organisms. Taking prescribed antibiotics, using warm salt water gargles, and using cough suppressants do not suppress transmission.

Reference: p. 401

Descriptors:
1. 20 2. 01 3. Application
4. IV–4 5. Self-Care 6. Moderate

2. A client visits the clinic and is diagnosed with acute sinusitis. The nurse should instruct the client that to promote sinus drainage, the client should
A. use a cold pack over the area.
*B. inhale steam from a hot shower.
C. perform postural drainage.
D. sleep with the head down.

Rationale: For a client diagnosed with acute sinusitis, the nurse should instruct the client that inhalation of steam from a hot shower will promote sinus drainage. Hot packs, decongestants, and brief use of nasal sprays can also promote drainage.

Reference: p. 402

Descriptors:
1. 20 2. 01 3. Application
4. IV–4 5. Nursing Process 6. Moderate

3. A nurse has explained the use of a topical nasal decongestant to a client with sinusitis. The nurse determines that the client has understood the instructions when the client says,
A. "I should hold my head down before using the spray."
B. "I should apply pressure to my nose for 3 minutes after using the spray."
C. "The tip of the nasal spray bottle should be kept sterile."
*D. "There is a possibility that using the sprays will cause a rebound effect."

Rationale: The use of topical decongestants is controversial because of the potential for a rebound effect. The client should hold his head back for maximum distribution of the spray. There is no need to apply pressure to the nose for 3 minutes after using the spray, nor does the tip of the nasal spray bottle need to be kept sterile, but only the client should use the bottle.

Reference: p. 402

Descriptors:

1. 20	2. 02	3. Application
4. IV–4	5. Self-Care	6. Moderate

4. A client with pharyngitis has been given a prescription for antibiotics for a streptococcal infection. After three days, the client tells the nurse she feels better and wonders if she can discontinue the antibiotic medications. The nurse should instruct the client to
   A. call her physician for further instructions.
   B. discontinue the medications if the fever is gone.
   C. discontinue the medications for now, but resume if symptoms reappear.
   *D. take the medication for the entire 10-day period.

Rationale: Antibiotics should be taken for the entire 10-day period to eliminate the streptococcal organisms. There is no need to contact the physician. Even if the fever or other symptoms are gone, the medications should be continued.

Reference: pp. 404–405

Descriptors:

1. 20	2. 02	3. Application
4. IV–4	5. Self-Care	6. Moderate

5. A client visits the clinic and is diagnosed with pharyngitis. The nurse should instruct the client that one of the potential complications of pharyngitis due to hemolytic streptococcus is
   *A. nephritis.
   B. scarlet fever.
   C. laryngitis.
   D. adenoiditis.

Rationale: Potential complications of pharyngitis due to hemolytic streptococcus are nephritis and rheumatic fever. Scarlet fever, laryngitis, and adenoiditis are not common complications of pharyngitis.

Reference: p. 405

Descriptors:

1. 20	2. 02	3. Application
4. IV–4	5. Nursing Process	6. Moderate

6. A client is scheduled for a tonsillectomy in the morning. Following the surgery, the priority assessment for this client includes assessing the client for
   A. hoarseness.
   *B. hemorrhage.
   C. infection.
   D. acute pain.

Rationale: Hemorrhage is a potential complication of a tonsillectomy. Hoarseness or a sore throat is common. While infection and acute pain may occur, hemorrhage is the priority assessment. Clients need to report any bleeding to the physician if they are discharged to home following the surgery.

Reference: p. 406

Descriptors:

1. 20	2. 02	3. Application
4. IV–1	5. Nursing Process	6. Moderate

7. A client visits the clinic and is diagnosed with peritonsillar abscess. The nurse should instruct the client that the treatment that is most effective in treating this condition is
   A. warm saline gargles.
   B. ice collars to the neck.
   C. nasal decongestants.
   *D. antibiotic therapy.

Rationale: The treatment that is most effective in treating peritonsillar abscess is antibiotic therapy. If this is not successful, the abscess must be drained. Warm saline gargles, ice collars to the neck, and nasal decongestants are not effective therapies to cure the infection.

Reference: p. 406

Descriptors:

1. 20	2. 02	3. Application
4. IV–4	5. Nursing Process	6. Moderate

8. A nurse is caring for an alert postoperative client following a tonsillectomy. When the client is ready to eat, the nurse should offer the client
   A. milkshakes.
   B. mashed potatoes.
   *C. gelatin.
   D. ice cream soda.

Rationale: The client's diet should be liquid or semiliquid. The nurse should offer the client gelatin or sherbet. Milk products should be avoided because they create more mucous in some people.

Reference: p. 406

Descriptors:

1. 20	2. 02	3. Application
4. IV–4	5. Nursing Process	6. Moderate

9. A client visits the clinic and is diagnosed with acute laryngitis. The nurse should instruct the client to
   A. place warm clothes on the throat.
   *B. inhale cool steam.
   C. gargle with a mouth wash.
   D. decrease fluid intake.

Rationale: Acute laryngitis is usually treated by resting the voice and inhaling cool steam or an aerosol. Bacterial infections are treated with antibiotics. Fluid intake should be increased. Gargling with a mouthwash is not useful.

Reference: p. 407

Descriptors:
1. 20 2. 03 3. Application
4. IV–1 5. Self-Care 6. Moderate

10. A client visits the clinic and is diagnosed with chronic laryngitis. The nurse should instruct the client that an effective therapy for chronic laryngitis is
*A. topical corticosteroids.
B. limiting fluid intake.
C. warm cloths to the throat.
D. saline mouth rinses.

Rationale: For clients with chronic laryngitis, useful therapies include resting the voice, no smoking, and topical corticosteroids. Limiting fluid intake is not recommended. Warm cloths to the throat and saline mouth rinses are not very effective with chronic laryngitis.

Reference: p. 407

Descriptors:
1. 20 2. 03 3. Application
4. IV–1 5. Nursing Process 6. Difficult

11. A client visits the clinic and is diagnosed with sinusitis. The priority nursing diagnosis for the client is
A. Obstruction of the nasal passages due to an infection.
B. Fluid volume excess related to accumulation of fluid in the sinuses.
C. Impaired verbal communication related to throat irritation.
*D. Ineffective airway clearance related to excessive secretions.

Rationale: The priority nursing diagnosis for the client is Ineffective airway clearance related to excessive secretions. There is no indication of Fluid volume excess related to accumulation of fluid in the sinuses or Impaired verbal communication related to throat irritation. Obstruction of the nasal passages due to an infection is not a nursing diagnosis.

Reference: p. 407

Descriptors:
1. 20 2. 03 3. Analysis
4. IV–1 5. Nursing Process 6. Moderate

12. A client visits the clinic and is diagnosed with sleep apnea. The nurse should explain to the client that one of the risk factors for sleep apnea is
A. being female.
B. renal disease.
*C. obesity.
D. anorexia.

Rationale: Males are more apt to have sleep apnea than females. Renal disease and anorexia are not risk factors. Smoking, obesity, and ingestion of alcohol are risk factors.

Reference: p. 409

Descriptors:
1. 20 2. 03 3. Application
4. IV–1 5. Nursing Process 6. Moderate

13. The nurse is caring for a client with epistaxis. The nurse should position the client in the
A. supine position with head to the side.
B. Trendelenberg position.
*C. upright position with head tilted forward.
D. side-lying with neck hyperextended.

Rationale: The client should be positioned in an upright position with the head tilted forward to prevent swallowing and aspiration of the blood. The supine position with head to the side, the Trendelenberg position, and the side-lying position with neck hyperextended will not prevent aspiration and swallowing of the blood.

Reference: p. 409

Descriptors:
1. 20 2. 04 3. Application
4. IV–1 5. Nursing Process 6. Moderate

14. A nurse is preparing to discharge a client with recurrent epistaxis from the clinic. The nurse should instruct the client to
A. blow his nose vigorously to prevent mucous accumulation.
*B. provide adequate humidification of the air.
C. sleep with head elevated on two or three pillows.
D. apply ice to the nose before retiring at night.

Rationale: Adequate humidification may prevent drying of the nasal passages. Blowing the nose vigorously to prevent mucus accumulation will aggravate the condition. Sleeping with head elevated on two or three pillows and applying ice to the nose before retiring at night are not helpful.

Reference: p. 410

Descriptors:
1. 20 2. 03 3. Application
4. IV–4 5. Nursing Process 6. Moderate

15. A client visits the clinic and is diagnosed with a fractured nose following a sports injury. The nurse should instruct the client to
*A. apply ice packs for 20 minutes at least four times per day.
B. make an appointment with a surgeon for the next day.
C. test the fluid from the nose twice daily with a dextrostix.
D. remove the packing from the nose in 12 hours.

Rationale: Cool compresses and application of ice packs for 20 minutes at least four times per day will reduce the swelling. Surgery is usually done at 7 to 10 days following the injury. The client does not need to test the fluid from the nose twice daily with a dextrostix and the packing should not be removed in 12 hours.

Reference: p. 411

Descriptors:
1. 20 2. 05 3. Application
4. IV–4 5. Nursing Process 6. Moderate

16. A nurse is caring for a client who is suspected of having laryngeal cancer. The nurse should assess the client for an early symptom of laryngeal cancer—
*A. hoarseness.
B. dyspnea.
C. dysphagia.
D. weight loss.

Rationale: Hoarseness is an early symptom of laryngeal cancer. Dyspnea, dysphagia, weight loss, and lumps are later signs of laryngeal cancer.

Reference: p. 411

Descriptors:
1. 20 2. 03 3. Application
4. IV–1 5. Nursing Process 6. Difficult

17. A nurse is caring for a client who has had a supraglottic laryngectomy. The nurse should explain to the client that a common postoperative complaint from this type of surgery is
A. inability to speak.
B. permanent tracheal stoma.
C. chronic pharyngitis.
*D. difficulty in swallowing.

Rationale: A common postoperative complaint from this type of surgery is difficulty in swallowing. There is also a potential for aspiration. Inability to speak, permanent tracheal stoma, and chronic pharyngitis are not common complaints.

Reference: p. 413

Descriptors:
1. 20 2. 05 3. Application
4. IV–1 5. Nursing Process 6. Moderate

18. A nurse is caring for a postoperative client following a total laryngectomy. The nurse is preparing to feed the client and the client communicates to the nurse that his sense of smell seems altered. The nurse should explain to the client that his sense of smell
A. will return after the stoma disappears.
B. will return once the oxygen is discontinued.
*C. has been altered due to breathing through the stoma.
D. has been altered because the client has been NPO.

Rationale: The client's sense of smell has been altered due to breathing through the stoma. The senses of taste and smell should return in time.

Reference: p. 416

Descriptors:
1. 20 2. 05 3. Application
4. IV–1 5. Nursing Process 6. Moderate

19. While caring for a postoperative client following a laryngectomy, the nurse observes that the client is restless and has a respiratory rate of 26 per minute. The nurse should
*A. suction the client.
B. contact the client's physician immediately.
C. apply oxygen by mask at 4 liters.
D. assess the client for bleeding.

Rationale: Restlessness, irritation, confusion, and a respiratory rate of 26 per minute are signs of an obstruction. The nurse should first suction the client and have the client cough and deep breathe. If these measures are not successful, the nurse should contact the client's physician immediately as this may be life threatening. Cold, clammy skin and increased pulse are symptoms of hemorrhage.

Reference: p. 417

Descriptors:
1. 20 2. 05 3. Application
4. IV–4 5. Nursing Process 6. Moderate

20. A nurse has instructed a client who has had a total laryngectomy about self-care at home. The nurse determines that the client has understood the instructions when the client says,
A. "I can go swimming if I stay in shallow water."
*B. "I should wear a protective covering if I am in the shower."
C. "I can continue to use hair spray when I am fixing my hair."
D. "I should stay in the air-conditioned rooms until the stoma is healed."

Rationale: Swimming is not recommended as the client can drown. The client should wear a protective bib or covering when taking a shower. Hair spray and powders should be avoided due to potential aspiration. Adequate humidity is required.

Reference: p. 417

Descriptors:
1. 20 2. 05 3. Application
4. IV–4 5. Self-Care 6. Difficult

CHAPTER 21
Management of Patients with Chest and Lower Respiratory Tract Disorders

1. A nurse is caring for a postoperative client following lung surgery. To prevent atelectasis, the nurse should encourage the client to

A. lie in a supine position.
B. ask for pain medications every 4 hours.
*C. cough and deep breathe every 2 hours.
D. lie in a semi-Fowler's position.

Rationale: Coughing and deep breathing every 2 hours enhance lung expansion and can help to prevent atelectasis. Suctioning and aerosol nebulizers can also help to prevent atelectasis. Lying in a supine position or in a semi-Fowler's position is not helpful. Pain medications will help reduce the discomfort, but not prevent atelectasis.

Reference: p. 423

Descriptors:
1. 21 2. 01 3. Application
4. IV–4 5. Nursing Process 6. Moderate

2. A nurse is caring for a 78-year-old client diagnosed with bacterial pneumonia. The client is receiving oxygen therapy and is on bedrest. A priority nursing diagnosis for this client is
*A. Ineffective airway clearance related to copious tracheobronchial secretions.
B. Fever and dyspnea related to ineffective airway clearance and pneumonia.
C. Altered nutrition: Potential for more than body requirements.
D. Activity intolerance related to age and immobility.

Rationale: The priority nursing diagnosis for this client is Ineffective airway clearance related to copious tracheobronchial secretions, which is the most common symptom of bacterial pneumonia. Fever and dyspnea are not nursing diagnoses. There is a potential for less than body requirements, since these clients have a decreased appetite. Activity intolerance is not a priority nursing diagnosis.

Reference: p. 433

Descriptors:
1. 21 2. 03 3. Analysis
4. IV–1 5. Nursing Process 6. Difficult

3. A nurse is caring for a client with bacterial pneumonia who is receiving oxygen. The nurse assesses the effectiveness of the client's oxygen therapy by the
A. presence or absence of cyanosis.
B. client's respiratory rate and depth.
*C. arterial blood gas analysis.
D. client's level of consciousness.

Rationale: The effectiveness of the client's oxygen therapy is assessed by the arterial blood gas analysis or pulse oximetry. Presence or absence of cyanosis, the client's respiratory rate, and depth or level of consciousness are not good indicators of oxygen effectiveness.

Reference: p. 433

Descriptors:
1. 21 2. 02 3. Application
4. IV–2 5. Nursing Process 6. Moderate

4. A nurse is assessing a client's Mantoux test and determines that the reaction is significant when the nurse observes
*A. induration of 10 mm with redness.
B. blisters around the area.
C. erythema and itching near the area.
D. painful induration of 3 mm without redness.

Rationale: A significant reaction is an induration of 10 mm with redness, although this does not necessarily mean that the client has TB. Blisters around the area, erythema and itching near the area, and painful induration of 3 mm without redness are not considered significant.

Reference: p. 437

Descriptors:
1. 21 2. 02 3. Application
4. IV–4 5. Nursing Process 6. Moderate

5. An adult client is at high risk for developing tuberculosis. The nurse should explain to the client that one of the drugs that is used as a prophylactic measure for clients at risk for tuberculosis is
*A. isoniazid (INH).
B. rifampin (RIF).
C. ethambutol (EMB).
D. pyrazinamide (PZA).

Rationale: One of the drugs that is used as a prophylactic measure for clients at risk for tuberculosis is isoniazid (INH). Rifampin (RIF), ethambutol (EMB), and pyrazinamide (PZA) are used to treat active tuberculosis.

Reference: p. 438

Descriptors:
1. 21 2. 02 3. Application
4. IV–2 5. Nursing Process 6. Moderate

6. A client at high risk for tuberculosis is started on prophylactic medication therapy with isoniazid (INH). The nurse should instruct the client to avoid eating
A. red meat.
*B. tuna.
C. ham.
D. potatoes.

Rationale: Clients who are taking INH should avoid tuna, aged cheese, red wine, soy sauce, and yeast extracts because of the potential for side effects such as headache, hypotension, and diaphoresis.

Reference: p. 439

Descriptors:
1. 21 2. 02 3. Application
4. IV–4 5. Nursing Process 6. Moderate

7. A nurse has admitted a client to the hospital with a diagnosis of pleurisy. The nurse should instruct the client that the client's pain is usually controlled by the use of
A. morphine sulfate.

B. meperidine sulfate.
C. ibuprofen.
*D. indomethiacin.

Rationale: The drug that is commonly used to control pain for clients with pleurisy is indomethiacin. Morphine sulfate and meperidine sulfate are generally not used. Ibuprofen may not provide enough relief for the pain.

Reference: p. 442

Descriptors:
1. 21 2. 04 3. Application
4. IV–2 5. Nursing Process 6. Moderate

8. A nurse encourages a client who is diagnosed with chronic obstructive pulmonary disease not to smoke because smoking
A. decreases the amount of mucus production.
B. the hemoglobin becomes highly oxygenated.
C. shrinks the alveoli in the lungs.
*D. damages the ciliary cleansing mechanism of the respiratory tract.

Rationale: Smoking damages the ciliary cleansing mechanism of the respiratory tract. Smoking also increases the amount of mucus production, reduces the oxygen carrying capacity of hemoglobin, and distends the alveoli in the lungs.

Reference: p. 444

Descriptors:
1. 21 2. 05 3. Application
4. IV–4 5. Self-Care 6. Moderate

9. A nurse is caring for a client with chronic obstructive pulmonary disease. The nurse should assess the client for a complication of COPD that includes
A. bronchitis.
B. pericarditis.
C. pulmonary embolus.
*D. pneumothorax.

Rationale: Complications of COPD include pneumothorax, atelectasis, pneumonia, and pulmonary hypertension (cor pulmonale). Bronchitis, pericarditis, and pulmonary embolus are not common complications.

Reference: p. 445

Descriptors:
1. 21 2. 08 3. Application
4. IV–4 5. Nursing Process 6. Moderate

10. A nurse is caring for a client who is diagnosed with chronic bronchitis. During the nursing history, the priority assessment for the nurse to make is the client's
*A. history of smoking.
B. occupation.
C. age.
D. weight.

Rationale: The priority assessment for the nurse to make is the client's history of smoking, which is the major risk factor for chronic bronchitis. Other risk factors include air pollution, exposure to hazardous airborne substances, and second-hand smoke.

Reference: p. 449

Descriptors:
1. 21 2. 06 3. Application
4. IV–4 5. Nursing Process 6. Moderate

11. A nurse is preparing to discharge an adult client with emphysema. The nurse should explain to the client that one of the primary symptoms of pulmonary hypertension is
*A. dyspnea.
B. chronic cough.
C. frothy mucus.
D. central cyanosis.

Rationale: One of the primary symptoms of pulmonary hypertension is dyspnea. Other symptoms include fatigue, angina, near syncope, and palpitations.

Reference: p. 457

Descriptors:
1. 21 2. 07 3. Application
4. IV–4 5. Nursing Process 6. Difficult

12. A parent visits the clinic with her 9-year-old child, and the child is diagnosed with mild asthma. The nurse should explain to the client and her mother that one of the medications used for children with mild asthma is
A. ipatropium bromide.
B. theophylline.
*C. cromolyn sodium.
D. leukotrine modifiers.

Rationale: Cromolyn sodium and nedocromil are mild to moderate anti-inflammatory agents that are used more commonly with children. Ipatropium bromide is used more frequently with COPD clients. Theophylline is used with older individuals and is helpful for night-time attacks. Leukotrine modifiers are a new class of medications.

Reference: p. 462

Descriptors:
1. 21 2. 06 3. Application
4. IV–2 5. Nursing Process 6. Moderate

13. A nurse is caring for a postoperative adult client when the client is diagnosed with acute respiratory failure. The nurse anticipates that the client will receive
A. a regular diet with supplements.
B. morphine sulfate for pain management.
C. heparin to prevent clot formation.
*D. mechanical ventilation.

Rationale: When a client is diagnosed with acute respiratory failure, the nurse should anticipate that the client will receive intubation and mechanical ventilation such as positive end-expiratory pressure (PEEP). The client may be placed on enteral feedings but not a regular diet. Morphine and heparin are not used.

Reference: p. 466

Descriptors:
1. 21 2. 09 3. Application
4. IV–4 5. Nursing Process 6. Moderate

14. A nurse is caring for a 77-year-old client following abdominal surgery. To reduce the client's risk of developing a pulmonary embolism, the nurse should
*A. encourage the client to perform active leg exercises.
B. ask the physician for an order for anticoagulant therapy.
C. provide the client with a high calorie diet.
D. administer oxygen by mask at 2 to 3 liters.

Rationale: For those at risk, the most effective approach in preventing pulmonary embolism is to prevent deep vein thrombosis. Active leg exercises, early ambulation, and anti-embolic stockings or pneumatic leg compression devices can all prevent the development of pulmonary embolism.

Reference: p. 471

Descriptors:
1. 21 2. 02 3. Application
4. IV–4 5. Nursing Process 6. Moderate

15. A nurse assesses an adult client following an automobile accident. The nurse observes that a portion of the client's chest is pulled inward while the rest of his chest expands. The nurse suspects that the client may be experiencing
A. pneumothorax.
*B. flail chest.
C. subcutaneous emphysema.
D. cardiac tamponade.

Rationale: When the nurse observes that a portion of the client's chest is pulled inward while the rest of his chest expands, this is usually a sign of a flail chest. Ventilary support is required. These symptoms are not indicative of pneumothorax, subcutaneous emphysema, or cardiac tamponade.

Reference: p. 481

Descriptors:
1. 21 2. 01 3. Application
4. IV–4 5. Nursing Process 6. Moderate

CHAPTER 22
Respiratory Care Modalities

1. A client with chronic obstructive pulmonary disease who has been receiving oxygen therapy for an extended time enters the emergency room. The client complains of dyspnea, substernal pain, and restlessness. The nurse suspects that the client is experiencing
*A. oxygen toxicity.
B. pneumothorax.
C. cardiac tamponade.
D. flail chest.

Rationale: Oxygen toxicity can occur when clients receive too high a concentration of oxygen for an extended period. Symptoms of oxygen toxicity include dyspnea, substernal pain, restlessness, fatigue, and progressive respiratory difficulty. These symptoms are not associated with pneumothorax, cardiac tamponade, or flail chest.

Reference: p. 491

Descriptors:
1. 22 2. 01 3. Analysis
4. IV–4 5. Nursing Process 6. Moderate

2. A nurse is preparing to administer oxygen to a client with respiratory disease. The nurse should explain to the client that the type of mask that provides the most accurate method of oxygen delivery is
A. nonrebreather air mask.
B. aerosol mask.
*C. Venturi mask.
D. simple mask.

Rationale: The Venturi mask provides the most accurate method of oxygen delivery. Other methods of oxygen delivery include the aerosol mask, tracheostomy collar, and face tents.

Reference: p. 492

Descriptors:
1. 22 2. 01 3. Application
4. IV–1 5. Nursing Process 6. Moderate

3. To assist a client to deep breathe and prevent stasis of the pulmonary secretions after abdominal surgery, the nurse should use
A. IPPB therapy.
B. nebulizer therapy.
*C. incentive spirometry.
D. aerosol treatments.

Rationale: Incentive spirometry is used after surgery to promote the expansion of the alveoli and to prevent atelectasis. It is more effective than IPPB therapy.

Reference: p. 495

Descriptors:
1. 22 2. 01 3. Application
4. IV–4 5. Nursing Process 6. Moderate

4. A client is scheduled to receive postural drainage therapy. Before beginning the postural drainage, the nurse should
A. offer the client clear fluids.
*B. auscultate breath sounds.
C. auscultate heart sounds.

D. perform chest percussion.

Rationale: Postural drainage is typically performed 2 to 4 times daily before meals. Before beginning the postural drainage, the nurse should auscultate breath sounds. Auscultation following the therapy can help assess the effectiveness of the therapy. Auscultating heart sounds and performing chest percussion are not necessary.

Reference: p. 496

Descriptors:

1. 22	2. 01	3. Application
4. IV–4	5. Nursing Process	6. Moderate

5. Immediately after an endotracheal intubation of an adult client, the nurse should assess for potential complications by
   A. auscultating bowel sounds.
   B. palpating the carotid artery.
   C. monitoring the level of consciousness.
   *D. auscultating breath sounds.

Rationale: The nurse should assess for potential complications by auscultating breath sounds to be certain that the tube is in the trachea. A chest x-ray will confirm placement. It is not necessary to auscultate bowel sounds, palpate the carotid artery, or monitor the level of consciousness because these do not provide information about tube placement.

Reference: p. 501

Descriptors:

1. 22	2. 02	3. Application
4. IV–4	5. Nursing Process	6. Moderate

6. A nurse is caring for a client who has just had a tracheostomy performed. The nurse should assess the client for symptoms of early complications, which include
   *A. bleeding.
   B. airway obstruction.
   C. infection.
   D. stenosis.

Rationale: Early complications include bleeding, pneumothorax, air embolism, aspiration, and recurrent laryngeal nerve damage. Late complications include airway obstruction, infection, and tracheal stenosis.

Reference: p. 500

Descriptors:

1. 22	2. 02	3. Application
4. IV–4	5. Nursing Process	6. Difficult

7. A nurse is preparing to suction the tracheostomy tube of an adult client for the first time. After washing the hands, the nurse should
   A. put on sterile gloves.
   B. turn on the suction machine.
   *C. explain the procedure to the client.
   D. open the suction catheter kit.

Rationale: The nurse should obtain all necessary equipment before beginning the procedure. After washing the hands, the nurse should explain the procedure to the client and family. Clean gloves are used to discard the old dressing. Sterile supplies are prepared after the soiled dressing is removed.

Reference: p. 502

Descriptors:

1. 22	2. 03	3. Application
4. IV–1	5. Nursing Process	6. Moderate

8. A nurse is planning to teach a newly discharged client with a tracheostomy about care of the tracheostomy. The nurse should instruct the client to
   *A. avoid the use of tissues around the tracheostomy.
   B. use only sterile equipment for cleaning.
   C. have a family member perform all tracheotomy care.
   D. remain on oxygen at all times.

Rationale: The client should be instructed to avoid the use of tissues or any dressings that shred around the tracheostomy to prevent lint or thread from getting into the tube. At home, clean technique may be used. It is not necessary for the client to have a family member perform all tracheotomy care or to remain on oxygen at all times.

Reference: p. 503

Descriptors:

1. 22	2. 02	3. Application
4. IV–4	5. Nursing Process	6. Moderate

9. A nurse is caring for a hospitalized client who has muscular dystrophy. The nurse determines that mechanical ventilation is needed when the client
   A. has a respiratory rate of 24 breaths per minute.
   *B. has a PaO_2 of 45 mm Hg and a FiO_2 of 0.65.
   C. exhibits symptoms of dyspnea.
   D. has a PaO_2 less than 50 mm Hg with a pH of 7.26.

Rationale: Mechanical ventilation is needed when the client has a respiratory rate of 35 breaths per minute and has a PaO_2 of 45 mm Hg and a FiO_2 of 0.65 or a PaO_2 greater than 50 mm Hg with a pH of less than 7.25. Symptoms of dyspnea may not be accurate.

Reference: p. 504

Descriptors:

1. 22	2. 04	3. Analysis
4. IV–4	5. Nursing Process	6. Difficult

10. An adult client is scheduled to be placed on mechanical ventilation. The nurse who is caring for the client should
    A. set the machine to deliver tidal volume between 15 and 20 mL/kg.
    B. record the client's peak expiratory pressure.

*C. measure carbon dioxide partial pressure after 20 minutes of ventilation.
D. adjust the machine to deliver the highest level of oxygen to maintain oxygenation.

Rationale: The nurse who is caring for this client should set the machine to deliver tidal volume between 10 and 15 mL/kg, record the client's peak inspiratory pressure, measure carbon dioxide partial pressure after 20 minutes of ventilation, and adjust the machine to deliver the lowest level of oxygen to maintain oxygenation (80 to 100 mm Hg).

Reference: p. 507

Descriptors:

1. 22	2. 04	3. Application
4. IV–4	5. Nursing Process	6. Moderate

11. A nurse is caring for an adult client who is on a ventilator. While caring for this client, the nurse should
A. offer the client antacids every 4 hours.
*B. perform tracheostomy care at least every 8 hours.
C. keep the client on bedrest continually.
D. monitor cuff pressure every 2 hours.

Rationale: It is important to perform tracheostomy care at least every 8 hours because of the risk of infection. The use of antacids can contribute to nosocomial infections. The client should be encouraged to ambulate if possible. The cuff pressure should be monitored every 8 hours.

Reference: p. 510

Descriptors:

1. 22	2. 04	3. Application
4. IV–4	5. Nursing Process	6. Moderate

12. A nurse is planning to provide preoperative teaching to a client who will be undergoing a thoracotomy. The nurse should instruct the client about
*A. incentive spirometry.
B. wound care.
C. endotracheal suctioning.
D. signs of respiratory distress.

Rationale: Preoperative teaching for a client who will undergo a thoracotomy includes the use of incentive spirometry, turning, coughing, and deep breathing, and splinting of the incision. Wound care, endotracheal suctioning, and signs of respiratory distress are not a part of the preoperative teaching.

Reference: p. 515

Descriptors:

1. 22	2. 05	3. Application
4. IV–4	5. Nursing Process	6. Moderate

13. A client has a water-sealed chest drainage system following thoracic surgery. The nurse should instruct the client and the family that this drainage system is used to maintain
A. positive chest wall pressure.
B. negative chest wall pressure.
C. positive intrathoracic pressure.
*D. negative intrathoracic pressure.

Rationale: Water-sealed chest drainage systems operate by maintaining a negative intrathoracic pressure.

Reference: p. 516

Descriptors:

1. 22	2. 06	3. Application
4. IV–1	5. Nursing Process	6. Moderate

14. A nurse is caring for a client in the postanesthesia care unit immediately following a thoracotomy and insertion of a water-sealed drainage system. The priority nursing diagnosis for this client is
A. Pain related to surgical incision.
B. Fluid volume deficit related to thoracic surgery.
*C. Impaired gas exchange related to lung impairment and surgery.
D. Nutrition, less than body requirements related to dyspnea.

Rationale: In the immediate postoperative period, the priority nursing diagnosis for this client is Impaired gas exchange related to lung impairment and surgery. Since the client is most likely still under the effects of anethesia, pain and nutrition are not priorities at this time. Fluid volume deficit related to thoracic surgery may occur at a later time.

Reference: p. 516

Descriptors:

1. 22	2. 07	3. Application
4. IV–1	5. Nursing Process	6. Moderate

15. A client is to be discharged 5 days after having a thoracotomy. The nurse should instruct the client to notify the physician if the client has
A. constipation.
B. fatigue.
C. decreased respiratory rate.
*D. increased shortness of breath.

Rationale: The client's physician should be notified if the client experiences an increased shortness of breath, chest pain, bleeding, change in sputum color, restlessness, and an increased respiratory rate because these signs are symptomatic of complications.

Reference: p. 521

Descriptors:

1. 22	2. 07	3. Application
4. IV–4	5. Nursing Process	6. Moderate

UNIT 6 CARDIOVASCULAR, CIRCULATORY, AND HEMATOLOGIC FUNCTION

CHAPTER 23 Assessment of Cardiovascular Function

1. In the human cardiac system, the chamber that is responsible for the apex beat or point of maximal impulse is the
   A. right atrium.
   B. right ventricle.
   C. left atrium.
   *D. left ventricle.

Rationale: The chamber that is responsible for the apex beat or point of maximal impulse is the left ventricle. The right atrium receives blood, while the left atrium and left ventricle distribute oxygenated blood.

Reference: p. 533

Descriptors:
1. 23 2. 01 3. Knowledge
4. IV–1 5. Nursing Process 6. Moderate

2. Which of the following sequences correctly shows the electrical conduction through the heart?
   *A. SA node to the AV node to the bundle of His to the Purkinje fibers.
   B. AV node to the bundle of His to the SA node to the Purkinje fibers.
   C. Purkinje fibers to the SA node to the AV node to the bundle of His.
   D. Bundle of His to the AV node to the SA node to the Purkinje fibers.

Rationale: The correct sequence of electrical conduction is SA node to the AV node to the bundle of His to the Purkinje fibers.

Reference: p. 534

Descriptors:
1. 23 2. 01 3. Knowledge
4. IV–1 5. Nursing Process 6. Moderate

3. During the cardiac cycle of diastole
   A. pressure inside the ventricles rises.
   B. the pulmonic and aortic valves open.
   C. blood is ejected into the pulmonary aorta.
   *D. blood returning from the veins flows into the atria.

Rationale: During the cardiac cycle of diastole blood returning from the veins flows into the atria and then into the ventricles. During systole, pressure inside the ventricles rises, the pulmonic and aortic valves open, and blood is ejected into the pulmonary aorta.

Reference: p. 535

Descriptors:
1. 23 2. 01 3. Knowledge
4. IV–1 5. Nursing Process 6. Moderate

4. A nurse is caring for a client who has experienced a myocardial infarction. The nurse should instruct the client to avoid constipation and straining to have a bowel movement because
   A. this can lead to disease progression.
   *B. a vagal response can be triggered.
   C. straining can increase palpitations.
   D. shortness of breath can occur.

Rationale: Straining to have a bowel movement should be avoided because it can trigger a vagal response and cause a decrease in heart rate or syncope. Disease progression, shortness of breath, and palpitations are not associated with straining.

Reference: p. 539

Descriptors:
1. 23 2. 02 3. Application
4. IV–4 5. Nursing Process 6. Moderate

5. A nurse is caring for a 65-year-old client who has experienced a myocardial infarction. During the first 24 to 48 hours, the nurse can anticipate that the client will express a typical emotional response of
   *A. shock.
   B. aggression.
   C. adaptation.
   D. depression.

Rationale: During the first 24 to 48 hours, a typical emotional response is shock and disbelief. Aggression, adaptation, and depression are later responses.

Reference: p. 543

Descriptors:
1. 23 2. 02 3. Application
4. III–1 5. Nursing Process 6. Moderate

6. A nurse is assessing an adult client for peripheral cyanosis. The nurse should assess the client's
   A. chest.
   B. groin.
   *C. nails.
   D. sclera.

Rationale: Peripheral cyanosis is best detected in the nails, skin of the nose, extremities, and earlobes. Peripheral cyanosis suggests a decreased flow of blood to the area.

Reference: p. 545

Descriptors:
1. 23 2. 02 3. Application
4. IV–1 5. Nursing Process 6. Moderate

7. A nurse is assessing an adult client's pulse pressure. To obtain the client's pulse pressure, the nurse should
*A. subtract the diastolic blood pressure from the systolic blood pressure.
B. subtract the apical pulse rate from the radial pulse rate.
C. assess bilateral radial pulses for 1 minute and find the difference.
D. subtracting the radial pulse rate from the apical pulse rate.

Rationale: The difference between the diastolic blood pressure and the systolic blood pressure is called the pulse pressure. Normal pulse pressure is 30 to 40 mm Hg.

Reference: p. 545

Descriptors:
1. 23 2. 03 3. Application
4. IV–1 5. Nursing Process 6. Moderate

8. A nurse is caring for an adult client following a myocardial infarction. To assess the client for intravascular volume depletion, the nurse should evaluate the client for
A. widening pulse pressure.
B. apical-radial pulse deficit.
C. decreased capillary refill time.
*D. orthostatic hypotension.

Rationale: One of the causes of orthostatic hypotension is intravascular volume depletion. Other causes include inadequate vasoconstriction and insufficient autonomic effect on vascular constriction.

Reference: p. 545

Descriptors:
1. 23 2. 03 3. Application
4. IV–1 5. Nursing Process 6. Moderate

9. A nurse is planning to auscultate the heart sounds of an adult client. To auscultate the aortic area, the nurse should place the stethoscope at the
*A. second intercostal space to the right of the sternum.
B. second intercostal space to the left of the sternum.
C. third intercostal space to the left of the sternum.
D. fourth intercostal space to the right of the sternum.

Rationale: To auscultate the aortic area, the nurse should place the stethoscope at the second intercostal space to the right of the sternum. To determine the correct intercostal space, start at the angle of Louis by locating the bony ridge near the top of the sternum at the junction of the body and the manubrium.

Reference: p. 547

Descriptors:
1. 23 2. 03 3. Application
4. IV–1 5. Nursing Process 6. Moderate

10. While auscultating the heart sounds of an adult client, the nurse detects a murmur. The nurse realizes that murmurs are frequently due to
A. fluid volume overload.
*B. turbulent flow of blood across a valve.
C. pericardial surfaces rubbing together.
D. accumulation of fluid in the alveoli.

Rationale: Murmurs are created when there is a turbulent flow of blood across a valve. A friction rub occurs when there is an abrasion of the pericardial surfaces during the cardiac cycle.

Reference: p. 549

Descriptors:
1. 23 2. 03 3. Application
4. IV–4 5. Nursing Process 6. Moderate

11. An adult client has just had a lipid profile drawn. The nurse should explain to the client that
A. a total serum cholesterol greater than 100 mg/dL places a person at increased risk for heart diseases.
B. low density lipoproteins transfer cholesterol to the liver for excretion.
*C. high density lipoproteins transfer cholesterol to the liver for excretion.
D. triglycerides have a direct correlation with high density lipoproteins.

Rationale: High density lipoproteins transfer cholesterol to the liver for excretion, while low density lipoproteins transport cholesterol and triglycerides to the cell. Triglycerides have a direct correlation with low density lipoproteins.

Reference: p. 552

Descriptors:
1. 23 2. 04 3. Application
4. IV–4 5. Nursing Process 6. Moderate

12. An adult client who has been taking theophylline for several days is scheduled for a dipyridamole pharmacologic stress test. The nurse should instruct the client to
*A. avoid any ingestion of products with caffeine.
B. fast for 12 hours before the test.
C. continue taking the theophylline medication as prescribed.
D. ignore symptoms of chills during the test as these are transient.

Rationale: The nurse should instruct the client to avoid any ingestion of products with caffeine. If the client ingests any caffeine prior to a dipyridamole pharmacologic stress test, the test will need to be rescheduled. The client should fast 4 hours before the test. Transient flushing or nausea may occur during the test.

Reference: p. 555

Descriptors:
1. 23 2. 04 3. Application
4. IV–4 5. Nursing Process 6. Moderate

13. A nurse is caring for a client during the immediate recovery period following a cardiac catheterization. The nurse should
A. keep the client on bedrest for 12 hours.
B. monitor peripheral pulses every hour.
*C. monitor the puncture site for bleeding every 15 minutes for 1 hour.
D. keep the client NPO for 4 hours.

Rationale: During the immediate recovery period following a cardiac catheterization, the nurse should monitor peripheral pulses and the puncture site for bleeding every 15 minutes. Fluids should be encouraged to flush out the dye. If the procedure was performed through the femoral artery, the nurse should keep the client on bedrest for 4 to 6 hours.

Reference: p. 558

Descriptors:
1. 23 2. 04 3. Application
4. IV–4 5. Nursing Process 6. Moderate

14. A client is scheduled to have her pulmonary artery pressure monitored. The nurse should explain to the client that pulmonary artery pressure is a diagnostic test to assess for
A. dysrhythmias.
*B. left ventricular pressure.
C. right ventricular filling pressure.
D. cardiac isoenzymes.

Rationale: Pulmonary artery pressure is a diagnostic test to assess for left ventricular pressure. Right ventricular filling pressure is assessed through central venous pressure monitoring.

Reference: p. 560

Descriptors:
1. 23 2. 05 3. Application
4. IV–1 5. Nursing Process 6. Moderate

15. While caring for a client with a pulmonary artery catheter, the nurse should assess the client for a potential complication of
*A. pulmonary artery rupture.
B. congestive heart failure.
C. transient flushing of the skin.
D. pneumonia.

Rationale: Potential complications of pulmonary artery catheters include pulmonary artery rupture, pulmonary embolism, infection, and dysrhythmias. Congestive heart failure, transient flushing of the skin, and pneumonia are not complications of pulmonary artery catheters.

Reference: p. 561

Descriptors:
1. 23 2. 05 3. Application
4. IV–4 5. Nursing Process 6. Moderate

16. While caring for a client with systemic arterial pressure monitoring, the nurse should assess the client for a potential complication of
A. dysrhythmias.
*B. hemorrhage.
C. hypokalemia.
D. fluid volume deficit.

Rationale: Complications of systemic arterial pressure monitoring include hemorrhage, distal ischemia, massive eccymosis, and air embolism. Dysrhythmias, hypokalemia, and fluid volume deficit are not complications of systemic arterial pressure monitoring.

Reference: p. 562

Descriptors:
1. 23 2. 05 3. Application
4. IV–4 5. Nursing Process 6. Moderate

CHAPTER 24
Management of Patients with Dysrhythmias and Conduction Problems

1. The QRS complex of the electrocardiogram represents the
A. firing of the SA node.
B. atrial muscle depolarization.
*C. ventricular muscle depolarization.
D. Purkinje fiber repolarization.

Rationale: The QRS complex of the electrocardiogram represents the conduction of the impulses from the AV node through the ventricles, or ventricular muscle depolarization. A U wave represents Purkinje fiber repolarization and is usually due to low potassium.

Reference: p. 567

Descriptors:
1. 24 2. 01 3. Knowledge
4. IV–1 5. Nursing Process 6. Moderate

2. A nurse is caring for a client diagnosed with sinus bradycardia. During the client's electrocardiogram, the nurse anticipates that the electrocardiogram will be the same as for a normal sinus rhythm except for the
*A. rate.
B. P wave.
C. ventricular rhythm.
D. atrial rhythm.

Rationale: For a client diagnosed with sinus bradycardia, the electrocardiogram will be the same as for a normal sinus rhythm except for the rate, which will be decreased.

Reference: p. 569

Descriptors:
1. 24 2. 02 3. Application
4. IV–1 5. Nursing Process 6. Moderate

3. During an electrocardiogram, the P wave represents
*A. atrial muscle depolarization.
B. repolarization of the ventricles.
C. ventricular muscle depolarization.
D. Purkinje fiber repolarization.

Rationale: The P wave represents conduction of an electrical impulse through the atrium or atrial muscle depolarization. The T wave represents repolarization of the ventricles.

Reference: p. 567

Descriptors:
1. 24 2. 03 3. Knowledge
4. IV–1 5. Nursing Process 6. Moderate

4. While caring for a client with sinus bradycardia, the physician orders atropine 0.5 mg to be given intravenously. The nurse should explain to the client that atropine
A. is a calcium channel blocker.
B. improves myocardial contractility.
*C. blocks the vagal stimulation.
D. facilitates parasympathetic nervous system activity.

Rationale: Atropine blocks the vagal stimulation, thus allowing a normal rate to occur. It is not a calcium channel blocker, nor does it improve myocardial contractility.

Reference: p. 570

Descriptors:
1. 24 2. 04 3. Application
4. IV–4 5. Nursing Process 6. Moderate

5. An adult client is diagnosed with atrial flutter. The nurse should explain to the client that with this condition
A. an electrical impulse starts in the atrium before the next normal impulse.
B. there is a slowing of the SA node and the AV node automatically discharges.
C. the impulse is routed back over and over again at a fast rate.
*D. not all impulses are conducted through the ventricle, causing a therapeutic block.

Rationale: Atrial flutter creates impulses at an atrial rate between 250 and 400 times per minute. In a client diagnosed with atrial flutter, not all impulses are conducted through the ventricle, causing a therapeutic block.

Reference: p. 571

Descriptors:
1. 24 2. 09 3. Application
4. IV–4 5. Nursing Process 6. Difficult

6. The nurse is caring for a client with atrial fibrillation. The nurse should assess the client for
A. pericardial friction rub.
B. decreased pulse rate.
*C. apical-radial pulse deficit.
D. increased cardiac output.

Rationale: For a client with atrial fibrillation, the nurse should assess the client for apical-radial pulse deficit. There is a shorter time for diastole. Decreased pulse rate is a sign of sinus bradycardia.

Reference: p. 573

Descriptors:
1. 24 2. 04 3. Application
4. IV–1 5. Nursing Process 6. Moderate

7. A nurse is caring for a client with cardiovascular disease who has a continuous cardiac monitor in place. The nurse should assess the client for symptoms of ventricular tachycardia, which includes
A. rate greater than 100 beats per minute.
B. tall, peaked P waves.
C. fewer QRS complexes than P waves.
*D. bizarre, abnormal QRS complexes.

Rationale: Symptoms of ventricular tachycardia include no pulse, difficult-to-detect P waves, more QRS complexes than P waves, and bizarre, abnormal QRS complexes.

Reference: p. 575

Descriptors:
1. 24 2. 09 3. Application
4. IV–4 5. Nursing Process 6. Moderate

8. A nurse is caring for a client with cardiovascular disease on a continuous cardiac monitor. To assess the client for a third degree AV block, the nurse should examine the EKG strip for
*A. more P waves than QRS complexes.
B. a ventricular rate greater than 100 beats per minute.
C. lengthening of the PR intervals.
D. PP interval equal to the RR interval.

Rationale: To assess the client for a third degree AV block, the nurse should examine the EKG strip for more P waves than QRS complexes. The PR interval is very irregular and the PP interval is not equal to the RR interval.

Reference: p. 578

Descriptors:
1. 24 2. 04 3. Application
4. IV–4 5. Nursing Process 6. Moderate

9. When defibrillating an adult client, the nurse should
   *A. apply a conducting agent between the skin and the paddles.
   B. place the paddles near the client's medication patches.
   C. medicate the client to prevent pain from the shock.
   D. call "all clear" after discharging the machine.

Rationale: When defibrillating an adult client, the nurse should apply a conducting agent between the skin and the paddles and place the paddles away from the client's medication patches and linens. There is no need to medicate the client to prevent pain from the shock. "All clear" should be said before discharging the paddles.

Reference: p. 582

Descriptors:
1. 24 2. 05 3. Application
4. IV–4 5. Nursing Process 6. Moderate

10. A client has just had a temporary pacemaker implanted. The nurse should assess the client for potential complications following implantation, which include
   A. clotting defects.
   B. bradycardia.
   *C. bleeding.
   D. decreased respiratory rate.

Rationale: Complications of pacemaker implantations include bleeding, hematomas, local infections, perforation of the myocardium, and tachycardia.

Reference: p. 584

Descriptors:
1. 24 2. 08 3. Application
4. IV–4 5. Nursing Process 6. Moderate

11. A priority nursing goal for a client who has had a permanent pacemaker implanted is that the client will
   A. be able to read the EKG monitor.
   *B. have a white blood count of 5,000 to 10,000 mm^3.
   C. avoid strenuous activities.
   D. expect periodic palpitations.

Rationale: A priority nursing goal for a client who has had a permanent pacemaker implanted is that the client will have a white blood count of 5,000 to 10,000 mm^3 and remain free from infection. The client should also know when to contact the physician. Periodic palpitations are not normal.

Reference: p. 587

Descriptors:
1. 24 2. 10 3. Application
4. IV–4 5. Nursing Process 6. Moderate

12. A nurse is caring for a client with a temporary pacemaker. To prevent electrical hazards associated with pacemakers, the nurse should
   A. unplug all monitors in the client's room.
   *B. cover any exposed wires with nonconductive materials.
   C. remove all electrical equipment from the client's room.
   D. wear nonconductive shoes when caring for this client.

Rationale: All electrical equipment in the vicinity of the client should be grounded. The nurse should cover any exposed wires with nonconductive materials. It is not necessary to wear nonconductive shoes when caring for this client or to remove all electrical equipment from the client's room.

Reference: p. 586

Descriptors:
1. 24 2. 08 3. Application
4. IV–4 5. Nursing Process 6. Moderate

13. A client is scheduled for an electrophysiology study to evaluate his dysrhythmia. The nurse should explain to the client that an electrophysiology study is used to
   *A. assess the function or dysfunction of the SA and AV nodes.
   B. locate the source of arterial blockage in the heart.
   C. treat ventricular fibrillation in through electrical activity.
   D. deliver a timed current to terminate the dysrhythmia.

Rationale: An electrophysiology study is used to assess the function or dysfunction of the SA and AV nodes, identify impulse formation and propagation through the cardiac electrical conduction system, and assess the effectiveness of antidysrhythmic medications. Cardioversion delivers a timed current to terminate the dysrhythmia. Cardiac catheterization can be used to locate the source of arterial blockage in the heart.

Reference: p. 587

Descriptors:
1. 24 2. 06 3. Application
4. IV–1 5. Nursing Process 6. Difficult

14. A client is scheduled to have an implantable cardioverter defibrillator. The nurse should explain to the client that this device (ICD) detects and terminates
   A. sinus bradycardia.
   B. atrial fibrillation.
   *C. ventricular fibrillation.
   D. atrial flutter.

Rationale: The implantable cardioverter defibrillator (ICD) is a device that detects and terminates life-threatening episodes of ventricular tachycardia and ventricular fibrillation.

Reference: p. 589

Descriptors:
1. 24 2. 07 3. Application
4. IV–1 5. Nursing Process 6. Moderate

15. A client is scheduled to have radiofrequency ablation therapy. The nurse should instruct the client that this therapy is done to
A. resect the myocardium after removal of necrotic tissue.
B. pace a specific area of the myocardium.
C. facilitate pacemaker insertion.
*D. destroy myocardial tissue that causes a dysrhythmia.

Rationale: Catheter ablation therapy and radiofrequency ablation therapy destroy specific cells that have been identified as the cause or central conduction method of a tachydysrhythmia.

Reference: p. 590

Descriptors:
1. 24 2. 06 3. Application
4. IV–1 5. Nursing Process 6. Moderate

CHAPTER 25
Management of Patients with Coronary Vascular Disorders

1. A 66-year-old client visits the clinic and complains of chest pain after physical exertion. The nurse should explain to the client that, in most cases, angina pectoris is due to
A. hypertension.
*B. atherosclerosis.
C. overexertion of the heart.
D. dysrhythmias.

Rationale: In most cases, angina pectoris is due to atherosclerosis, particularly in older clients. Smoking, hypertension, high cholesterol levels, and diabetes mellitus are all associated with coronary atherosclerosis.

Reference: p. 595

Descriptors:
1. 25 2. 01 3. Application
4. II–2 5. Nursing Process 6. Moderate

2. A client is diagnosed with unstable angina pectoris. The nurse should explain to the client that with this condition
*A. symptoms occur at rest.
B. symptoms are relieved by rest.
C. pain is due to a coronary artery vasospasm.
D. there is severe incapacitating chest pain.

Rationale: With the condition of unstable angina pectoris, symptoms occur at rest and the pain threshold is lower. Severe incapacitating chest pain is associated with intractable angina. Symptoms that are relieved at rest occur with stable angina.

Reference: p. 597

Descriptors:
1. 25 2. 02 3. Application
4. II –2 5. Nursing Process 6. Moderate

3. An adult client is started on a beta-adrenergic blocker for treatment of angina. The nurse should instruct the client to
*A. never stop taking the medication abruptly.
B. take the medication only when there is chest pain.
C. crush the tablet between the teeth to hasten absorption.
D. have his blood sugar checked frequently.

Rationale: When beta-adrenergic blockers are prescribed for treatment of angina, the nurse should instruct the client to never stop taking the medication abruptly because the angina may worsen. Only clients who are diabetic need to check their blood sugars frequently due to potential hypoglycemia.

Reference: p. 598

Descriptors:
1. 25 2. 03 3. Application
4. IV–3 5. Nursing Process 6. Moderate

4. A client has been prescribed nitroglycerin to treat his angina pain. The nurse should explain to the client that this medication
A. constricts the veins and arteries.
B. increases the blood pressure.
C. improves the myocardial contractility.
*D. relieves pain in about 3 minutes.

Rationale: Nitroglycerin relieves pain in about 3 minutes, should be taken by the buccal route or topical patches, dilates the veins and arteries, and lowers blood pressure. It does not improve the myocardial contractility.

Reference: p. 598

Descriptors:
1. 25 2. 03 3. Application
4. IV–3 5. Self-Care 6. Moderate

5. Following a percutaneous transluminal coronary angioplasty (PTCA) procedure on an adult client, the nurse should monitor the client for a possible complication of
A. congestive heart failure
*B. abrupt closure of the artery.
C. hyperkalemia.
D. perforation of the artery.

Rationale: Complications of PTCA include abrupt closure of the artery, vascular complications, bleeding at the insertion site, retroperitoneal bleeding, and arterial thrombosis. Perforation of the artery may occur during the PTCA procedure.

Reference: p. 602

Descriptors:
1. 25 2. 05 3. Application
4. IV–3 5. Nursing Process 6. Moderate

6. A nurse is caring for a client who is undergoing cardiopulmonary bypass surgery. When the client is disconnnected from the cardiopulmonary bypass machine, the nurse should plan to administer
   A. morphine sulfate.
   B. digoxin.
   *C. protamine sulfate.
   D. sodium bicarbonate.

   Rationale: A client undergoing cardiac bypass surgery is given heparin to reduce the potential for clotting. When the client is disconnected from the bypass machine, the nurse should plan to administer protamine sulfate to reverse the effects of heparin. Morphine sulfate and digoxin may be administered later.

   Reference: p. 605

   Descriptors:
   1. 25 2. 05 3. Application
   4. IV–2 5. Nursing Process 6. Moderate

7. A nurse is caring for a client who has undergone cardiac bypass surgery. At 8 hours after the surgery, the client appears nauseated, restless, and weak. The nurse suspects that the client may be experiencing symptoms of
   *A. hyperkalemia.
   B. hypomagnesia.
   C. hypercalcemia.
   D. hypernatremia.

   Rationale: Mental confusion, nausea, restlessness, and weakness are symptomatic of hyperkalemia. Tetany, tremors, and muscle cramps are associated with hypomagnesia. Digitalis toxicity and asystole are associated with hypercalcemia. Weakness, convulsions, and coma are associated with hypernatremia.

   Reference: p. 609

   Descriptors:
   1. 25 2. 06 3. Application
   4. IV–3 5. Nursing Process 6. Moderate

8. A client returns to the clinic following cardiac bypass surgery one week ago. The client tells the nurse that he has had a fever, pleural pain, dyspnea, and arthralgia. The nurse suspects that the client may be experiencing
   A. pulmonary edema.
   B. congestive heart failure.
   C. pulmonary embolus.
   *D. postpericardiotomy syndrome.

   Rationale: Postpericardiotomy syndrome occurs in 10 to 40 % of clients following surgery. Fever, pericardial pain, pleural pain, dyspnea, and arthralgia may all be present. Bedrest and anti-inflammatory drugs can relieve the symptoms.

   Reference: p. 618

   Descriptors:
   1. 25 2. 07 3. Analysis
   4. IV–3 5. Nursing Process 6. Moderate

9. A client enters the emergency room and tells the nurse that he "thinks he is having a heart attack." The most common symptom of a myocardial infarction is
   A. left arm and shoulder pain.
   B. nausea unrelieved by antacids.
   *C. sudden chest pain that continues despite rest.
   D. bradycardia and warm moist skin.

   Rationale: The most common symptoms of an MI include sudden chest pain that continues despite rest. There may be tachycardia and cool moist skin.

   Reference: p. 619

   Descriptors:
   1. 25 2. 01 3. Application
   4. IV–1 5. Nursing Process 6. Moderate

10. A nurse is caring for a client during the immediate postoperative period following cardiac surgery. The nurse should notify the client's physician when the nurse observes that the client has
   A. serum sodium levels of 140 mEq/L.
   *B. urinary output of 20 ml in one hour.
   C. serum calcium level of 8.9 mg/100 ml
   D. pulse rate of 80 beats per minute.

   Rationale: The nurse should notify the client's physician when the nurse observes that the client has a urinary output of 20 ml in one hour as this is indicative of renal failure. Sodium serum levels of 140 mEq/L, serum calcium levels of 8.9 mg/100 ml, and a pulse rate of 80 beats per minute are all within normal limits.

   Reference: p. 617

   Descriptors:
   1. 25 2. 08 3. Application
   4. IV–3 5. Nursing Process 6. Moderate

11. A nurse is caring for a client who is mechanically ventilated during the immediate postoperative period following cardiac surgery. The nurse should monitor the client for symptoms of impaired gas exchange, which include
   *A. tachycardia.
   B. bradycardia.
   C. constricted pupil size.
   D. warm moist skin.

   Rationale: Symptoms of impaired gas exchange include tachycardia, restlessness, altered arterial blood gases, cyanosis of the tissues, and fighting the ventilator.

   Reference: p. 616

   Descriptors:
   1. 25 2. 01 3. Application
   4. IV–3 5. Nursing Process 6. Moderate

12. A nurse is monitoring a client during the first 8 hours following cardiac surgery. The nurse observes the client's cardiac monitor for a common dysrhythmia that can occur during the postoperative period that includes
    A. ventricular fibrillation.
    B. atrial fibrillation.
    *C. bradycardia.
    D. ventricular asystole.

    Rationale: Common dysrhythmias that can occur following cardiac surgery include bradycardia, tachycardia, and extra beats. Ventricular fibrillation, atrial fibrillation, and ventricular asystole are not common.

    Reference: p. 616

    Descriptors:
    1. 25 2. 06 3. Application
    4. IV–3 5. Nursing Process 6. Moderate

13. A client experienced a myocardial infarction at 0900. At what time would the nurse anticipate that the client's myoglobin analysis would show an increase?
    A. 0930
    *B. 1000.
    C. 1300.
    D. 1500.

    Rationale: Myoglobin is a heme protein that helps to transport oxygen. The test can be run more quickly than a creatinine kinase and an increase would appear in 1 to 3 hours or around 1000.

    Reference: p. 626

    Descriptors:
    1. 25 2. 01 3. Application
    4. IV–1 5. Nursing Process 6. Moderate

14. A client who has experienced a myocardial infarction is ordered to have tissue type plasminogen activator. Following administration, the nurse should monitor the client for
    A. shortness of breath.
    B. hypermagnesia.
    C. decreased respiratory rate.
    *D. internal bleeding.

    Rationale: Following administration of tissue type plasminogen activator, which is usually given with heparin, the nurse should monitor the client for internal bleeding.

    Reference: p. 628

    Descriptors:
    1. 25 2. 08 3. Application
    4. IV–2 5. Nursing Process 6. Moderate

15. Following a myocardial infarction, a client is referred to a cardiac rehabilitation center. The nurse should instruct the client that during cardiac rehabilitation, the client should
    *A. increase his activity gradually.
    B. perform strenuous activity daily.
    C. eat 6 small meals per day.
    D. begin a weight lifting program.

    Rationale: The client should be instructed to increase activities gradually, avoid activity if chest pain occurs, and to modify the diet and lose weight if indicated. Six small meals per day are not necessary. Exercises that require tensing of the muscles, or sudden bursts of energy, such as weight lifting, should be avoided.

    Reference: p. 631

    Descriptors:
    1. 25 2. 08 3. Application
    4. IV–3 5. Nursing Process 6. Moderate

CHAPTER 26
Management of Patients with Structural, Infectious, and Inflammatory Cardiac Disorders

1. While assessing an adult female's heart sounds, the nurse hears an extra heart sound. The client tells the nurse that she has had anxiety, fatigue, and shortness of breath. The nurse refers the client to a physician as these symptoms are indicative of
    A. aortic stenosis.
    *B. mitral valve prolapse.
    C. aortic regurgitation.
    D. myocarditis.

    Rationale: An extra heart sound, known as a mitral click, plus anxiety, fatigue, shortness of breath, lightheadedness, chest pain, and palpitations are symptoms of mitral valve prolapse. Aortic stenosis and aortic regurgitation are often asymptomatic. Myocarditis is an infection of the myocardium and depends on the infectious agent.

    Reference: p. 637

    Descriptors:
    1. 26 2. 01 3. Application
    4. II–2 5. Nursing Process 6. Moderate

2. A nurse is caring for a client diagnosed with mitral valve stenosis. The nurse should assess the client for one of the most common symptoms of this disorder—
    *A. fatigue.
    B. palpitations.
    C. angina.
    D. forceful heartbeat in the head.

    Rationale: Common symptoms of mitral valve prolapse include fatigue, hemoptysis, and dyspnea on exertion. Palpitations are common symptoms of mitral valve regurgitation. A forceful heartbeat in the head is associated with aortic regurgitation.

Reference: p. 638

Descriptors:
1. 26 2. 01 3. Application
4. IV–1 5. Nursing Process 6. Moderate

3. Incomplete closure of the mitral valve during systole is termed
A. myocarditis.
B. mitral valve stenosis.
C. mitral valve prolapse.
*D. mitral valve regurgitation.

Rationale: Mitral valve regurgitation is the incomplete closure of the mitral valve during systole. It may be asymptomatic or present as heart failure. Mitral valve stenosis is a narrowing of the valve. Mitral valve prolapse is the prolapse of the valve.

Reference: p. 638

Descriptors:
1. 26 2. 01 3. Application
4. IV–1 5. Nursing Process 6. Easy

4. Which of the following adult clients would be a candidate for a balloon valvuloplasty? The client who is diagnosed with
*A. mitral stenosis.
B. mitral regurgitation.
C. rotation of the great vessels.
D. thoracolumbar scoliosis.

Rationale: Balloon valvuloplasty is used for clients diagnosed with mitral stenosis or aortic valve stenosis in elderly clients. Balloon valvuloplasty is contraindicated for clients with mitral regurgitation, rotation of the great vessels, and thoracolumbar scoliosis.

Reference: p. 640

Descriptors:
1. 26 2. 02 3. Application
4. IV–3 5. Nursing Process 6. Moderate

5. A nurse is caring for a client following a cardiac valve replacement. The nurse should assess the client for a complication which includes
A. hypotension.
B. myocardial infarction.
C. pericarditis.
*D. congestive heart failure.

Rationale: Complications following valve replacement surgery include hypertension, congestive heart failure, dysrhythmias, bleeding, and thromboembolism. Hypotension, myocardial infarction, and pericarditis are usually not complications of valve replacement surgery.

Reference: p. 643

Descriptors:
1. 26 2. 02 3. Application
4. IV–3 5. Nursing Process 6. Moderate

6. An adult client is diagnosed with dilated cardiomyopathy. The nurse should explain to the client that this condition is usually due to
A. amyloidosis.
*B. infection.
C. valve prolapse.
D. congestive heart failure.

Rationale: Dilated cardiomyopathy is usually due to infection. Other causes include pregnancy and heavy alcohol intake. Amyloidosis is associated with restrictive cardiomyopathy.

Reference: p. 643

Descriptors:
1. 26 2. 03 3. Application
4. IV–3 5. Nursing Process 6. Moderate

7. A client is ready to be discharged from the hospital following a valve replacement. The nurse should instruct the client that before any dental surgery is performed, the client should
A. check with her physician.
B. be NPO for 12 hours.
C. take a prescribed course of heparin.
*D. take a prescribed course of antibiotics.

Rationale: To prevent bacterial endocarditis, the client should be instructed to take a prescribed course of antibiotics before any surgical procedure. The client does not need to be NPO for 12 hours or check with the physician. Usually these clients are on long-term anticoagulant therapy.

Reference: p. 643

Descriptors:
1. 26 2. 05 3. Application
4. IV–3 5. Nursing Process 6. Moderate

8. A nurse is caring for a client with dilated cardiomyopathy. During the assessment of the client, the nurse can anticipate
A. a nonpalpable liver.
B. chest tenderness.
*C. jugular vein distention.
D. a weak, slow pulse.

Rationale: Assessment findings for a client with dilated cardiomyopathy include jugular vein distention, pulmonary crackles, dysrhythmias, enlarged liver, and pitting edema. Chest tenderness and a weak, slow pulse are not typical with dilated cardiomyopathy.

Reference: p. 644

Descriptors:
1. 26 2. 03 3. Application
4. IV–1 5. Nursing Process 6. Moderate

9. A nurse is caring for a 67-year-old client diagnosed with dilated cardiomyopathy. The client is easily fatigued and has a dysrhythmia and a poor appetite. A priority nursing diagnosis for the client is
*A. Activity intolerance related to decreased cardiac output.
B. Poor appetite related to cardiac strain.

C. Noncompliance related to no desire for low fat diet.
D. Anxiety related to fear of outcome of hospitalization.

Rationale: A priority nursing diagnosis for the client is Activity intolerance related to decreased cardiac output. Poor appetite is not a diagnosis. There is no evidence of noncompliance or anxiety.

Reference: p. 645

Descriptors:
1. 26 2. 03 3. Analysis
4. IV–1 5. Nursing Process 6. Moderate

10. A nurse is preparing to discharge a client who has been hospitalized with a diagnosis of cardiomyopathy. The expected outcomes for this client should include
A. maintains bedrest while at home.
*B. adheres to prescribed medication schedule.
C. maintains a high protein diet.
D. increases walking activities daily.

Rationale: The expected outcomes for this client should include that the client adheres to prescribed medication schedule, modifies diet for fluid and sodium restriction, modifies lifestyle to accommodate activity limitations, and identifies signs and symptoms to report to the health care professional.

Reference: p. 646

Descriptors:
1. 26 2. 04 3. Application
4. IV–3 5. Nursing Process 6. Moderate

11. Prevention of rheumatic heart disease includes
A. avoidance of cigarette smoking.
B. limited intake of alcohol.
*C. prompt treatment of streptococcal infections.
D. adequate control of hypertension.

Rationale: Rheumatic endocarditis results directly from rheumatic heart fever caused by a group A streptococcal infection. It is not associated with cigarette smoking, intake of alcohol, or hypertension.

Reference: p. 648

Descriptors:
1. 26 2. 04 3. Application
4. IV–3 5. Nursing Process 6. Moderate

12. Clinical manifestations of rheumatic endocarditis include
*A. small vegetations on the valve leaflets.
B. coronary artery disease.
C. mitral valve prolapse.
D. cardiac enlargement.

Rationale: Clinical manifestations of rheumatic endocarditis include small vegetations on the valve leaflets. These tiny beads thicken the leaflets and prevent them from closing completely, resulting in mitral valve regurgitation.

Reference: p. 648

Descriptors:
1. 26 2. 04 3. Application
4. IV–1 5. Nursing Process 6. Moderate

13. A client visits the emergency room 2 months after a mitral valve replacement and complains of malaise, anorexia, weight loss, cough, and joint pain. The nurse observes splinter hemorrhages under the fingernails. The nurse suspects that the client may be experiencing
A. rheumatic fever.
B. myocarditis.
C. mitral regurgitation.
*D. infective endocarditis.

Rationale: Infective endocarditis is a risk for clients who have had valve replacement surgery. Symptoms include malaise, anorexia, weight loss, cough, splinter hemorrhages under the fingernails, and joint pain. Treatment consists of antibiotic therapy.

Reference: pp. 649–650

Descriptors:
1. 26 2. 04 3. Application
4. IV–1 5. Nursing Process 6. Difficult

14. A nurse is caring for a client with pericarditis. The nurse should notify the physician immediately when the nurse observes that the client has
A. a fever.
*B. falling arterial pressures.
C. decreased diastolic pressure.
D. severe pain.

Rationale: The client is at risk for cardiac tamponade. One of the earliest signs of cardiac tamponade is falling arterial pressure. Usually the systolic pressure falls, while the diastolic pressure remains stable. Neck vein distention may be present. Pain is the primary symptom of pericarditis.

Reference: p. 652

Descriptors:
1. 26 2. 04 3. Application
4. IV–4 5. Nursing Process 6. Moderate

CHAPTER 27
Management of Patients with Complications from Heart Disease

1. The nurse is caring for a client following a myocardial infarction. The nurse notifies the physician when the nurse observes that the client is fatigued and has a dry, hacking cough. These symptoms are associated with
A. cardiac failure.
B. congestive heart failure.
C. pericarditis.
*D. pulmonary edema.

Rationale: Pulmonary congestion, fatigue, an increase in weight, activity intolerance, and a dry hacking cough are associated with pulmonary edema. Bradycardia is associated with cardiac failure. Pericarditis is associated with pain and infection.

Reference: p. 656

Descriptors:

1. 27	2. 01	3. Application
4. IV–3	5. Nursing Process	6. Moderate

2. Following cardiac surgery, a client is diagnosed with early signs of pulmonary edema. The nurse should anticipate that the physician will order
   *A. elevation of the client's feet and legs.
   B. administration of protamine sulfate.
   C. digitalis therapy.
   D. intravenous sodium solutions.

Rationale: For a client is diagnosed with early signs of pulmonary edema, the nurse should anticipate that the physician will order placing the client in an upright position and elevation of the client's feet and legs. Morphine sulfate, oxygen, and diuretics will also be ordered. Digitalis therapy is used for clients with congestive heart failure. No sodium solutions should be given.

Reference: p. 656

Descriptors:

1. 27	2. 01	3. Application
4. IV–1	5. Nursing Process	6. Moderate

3. A nurse is caring for a client diagnosed with left-sided heart failure. The nurse can anticipate that one of the client's primary symptoms will be
   *A. dyspnea on exertion.
   B. edema of the legs and feet.
   C. anorexia.
   D. hepatomegaly.

Rationale: Orthopnea and dyspnea on exertion are common symptoms of left-sided heart failure. Edema of the legs and feet, nocturia, anorexia, and hepatomegaly are associated with right-sided heart failure.

Reference: pp. 662–663

Descriptors:

1. 27	2. 02	3. Application
4. IV–1	5. Nursing Process	6. Moderate

4. A client with heart failure is receiving diuretics and benazepril, an ACE inhibitor. The nurse should monitor the client for
   A. hypertension.
   B. excess serum creatinine.
   C. hypernatremia.
   *D. hypotension.

Rationale: Clients who are receiving diuretics and ACE inhibitors should be monitored for hypotension, hypovolemia, hyperkalemia, and hyponatremia as these can be side effects when ACE inhibitors are used with diuretics.

Reference: p. 664

Descriptors:

1. 27	2. 02	3. Application
4. IV–3	5. Nursing Process	6. Moderate

5. A nurse is caring for an adult client with congestive heart failure when the client is prescribed digoxin. The nurse should explain to the client that digoxin
   *A. increases the force of the myocardial contraction.
   B. quickens cardiac conduction through the AV node.
   C. promotes fluid retention to prevent excessive diuresis.
   D. slows cardiac output by enhancing the force of the contraction.

Rationale: The medication digoxin increases the force of the myocardial contraction, slows cardiac conduction through the AV node, increases cardiac output by enhancing the force of the contraction, and promotes diuresis by increasing cardiac output.

Reference: p. 665

Descriptors:

1. 27	2. 03	3. Application
4. IV–2	5. Nursing Process	6. Moderate

6. An adult client has been receiving digitalis therapy for congestive heart failure. The nurse observes the client for symptoms of digitalis toxicity, which include
   A. hyperkalemia.
   B. vasodilitation.
   *C. bradycardia.
   D. hypernatremia.

Rationale: Symptoms of digitalis toxicity include fatigue, malaise, bradycardia, or other irregular rhythms, nausea, and vomiting. Hyperkalemia, vasodilitation, and hypernatremia are not symptoms of digitalis toxicity.

Reference: p. 665

Descriptors:

1. 27	2. 02	3. Application
4. IV–2	5. Nursing Process	6. Difficult

7. A nurse is preparing to administer digitalis for the third time to a client with heart failure. The nurse should
   A. assess pedal pulses.
   B. withhold the dose if the heart rate is 70 bpm.
   C. give the dose with only sips of water.
   *D. assess the client's apical heart rate.

Rationale: Before administering digitalis, the nurse should assess the client's apical heart rate. If the heart rate is greater than 60 bpm or the rhythm is regular, the dose should be given. Water intake is not restricted, but sodium intake is restricted. Assessing pedal pulses is not necessary. Observing for symptoms of toxicity is necessary.

Reference: p. 665

Descriptors:
1. 27 2. 03 3. Application
4. IV–2 5. Nursing Process 6. Moderate

8. An adult client with congestive heart failure has been prescribed milrinone (Primacor). The nurse should assess the client for a primary side effect of this medication, which is
*A. hypotension.
B. excessive diuresis.
C. increased platelets.
D. fluid retention.

Rationale: Side effects of milrinone (Primacor) include hypotension, decreased platelets, GI dysfunction, and an increase in ventricular dysrhythmias. Excessive diuresis, increased platelets, and fluid retention are not typical side effects of the drug.

Reference: p. 666

Descriptors:
1. 27 2. 03 3. Application
4. IV–2 5. Nursing Process 6. Moderate

9. A client with congestive heart failure has been ordered a 2 gram sodium diet. The nurse should explain to the client that the primary purpose of a low sodium diet is to
A. improve mortality.
*B. decrease circulatory volume.
C. help the client lose weight.
D. decrease the incidence of arrythmias.

Rationale: The primary purpose of a low sodium diet is to decrease circulatory volume and reduce the amount pumped by the heart. It does not improve mortality, nor is it to help the client lose weight or decrease arrythmias.

Reference: p. 666

Descriptors:
1. 27 2. 03 3. Application
4. IV–3 5. Nursing Process 6. Moderate

10. To assess his fluid balance at home, the nurse should instruct the client diagnosed with congestive heart failure to
*A. weigh himself daily.
B. assess radial pulses.
C. monitor his blood pressure.
D. monitor output amounts.

Rationale: A daily weight at the same time every day can be a good indicator of the client's fluid balance once he is at home. Assessing radial pulses, monitoring the blood pressure, and output amounts may be done, but do not provide information about fluid balance.

Reference: p. 666

Descriptors:
1. 27 2. 03 3. Application
4. IV–3 5. Nursing Process 6. Moderate

11. An elderly client is brought to the emergency room and presents with periorbital edema, oliguria, orthopnea, and edema of the feet and hands. The nurse suspects that the client may be experiencing
A. cardiomyopathy. pulmonary edema
B. ventricular tachycardia.
C. essential hypertension.
*D. cardiac failure.

Rationale: Periorbital edema, sleep disturbances, oliguria, orthopnea, and edema of the feet and hands are symptoms of cardiac failure. Cardiomyopathy is associated with an infection. These are not symptoms of essential hypertension or ventricular tachycardia.

Reference: p. 667

Descriptors:
1. 27 2. 03 3. Analysis
4. IV–3 5. Nursing Process 6. Difficult

12. A nurse is preparing to discharge a client who was diagnosed with cardiac failure to home. The nurse should instruct the client to
A. sleep in a supine position.
*B. rest with the head elevated.
C. maintain bedrest as much as possible.
D. eat only three meals per day.

Rationale: For a client who was diagnosed with cardiac failure, the goal is to encourage the client to maintain as much activity as can be tolerated. The client should be taught to rest with the head elevated to reduce preload on the heart and pulmonary congestion. Six smaller meals may provide the client with more energy than three meals.

Reference: p. 668

Descriptors:
1. 27 2. 03 3. Application
4. IV–3 5. Nursing Process 6. Moderate

13. A nurse is caring for a client in the acute care setting when the client is diagnosed with cardiogenic shock and transferred to the intensive care unit. On admission to the unit, the ICU nurse can anticipate
A. administration of vasoconstrictor medications.
*B. arterial blood gas analysis.
C. daily intake and output evaluations.
D. pericardial fluid aspiration therapy.

Rationale: The ICU nurse can anticipate arterial blood gas analysis, pulse oximetry, frequent intake and output measurements, intravenous fluids, diuretic and vasopressor medications, and continuous cardiac monitoring. Pericardial fluid aspiration therapy is used for clients with pericardial effusion.

Reference: p. 671

Descriptors:
1. 27 2. 04 3. Application
4. IV–3 5. Nursing Process 6. Moderate

14. A nurse is caring for a client who has just been diagnosed with myocardial rupture. The nurse monitoring the client can anticipate
A. pericardial aspiration.
B. administration of vasoconstrictors.
*C. immediate cardiac surgery.
D. administration of digitalis.

Rationale: Death will occur unless there is immediate cardiac surgery. Pericardial aspiration, administration of vasoconstrictors, and administration of digitalis are not warranted with cardiac rupture.

Reference: p. 674

Descriptors:
1. 27 2. 05 3. Application
4. IV–3 5. Nursing Process 6. Moderate

15. While caring for a client with congestive heart failure who is on a continuous cardiac monitor, the client develops signs of cardiac arrest. The nurse should first
A. take the client's blood pressure.
B. start decompression at 80 times per minute.
*C. activate the emergency code team.
D. get the emergency cart with the defibrillator.

Rationale: Airway, breathing, circulation, and defibrillation are the steps taken in a cardiac arrest. The nurse should first activate the emergency code team. Next is ventilation, then compression and defibrillation. Checking the carotid pulse is necessary but not the blood pressure.

Reference: p. 674

Descriptors:
1. 27 2. 06 3. Application
4. IV–3 5. Nursing Process 6. Moderate

CHAPTER 28
Assessment and Management of Patients with Vascular Disorders and Problems of Peripheral Circulation

1. The outer layer of the artery is termed the
A. endothelial cell.
*B. adventitia.
C. media.
D. intima.

Rationale: The walls of the arteries are composed of three layers: the intima, which is the inner endothelial layer; the media, which is the middle layer; and the adventitia, which is the outer layer.

Reference: p. 680

Descriptors:
1. 28 2. 01 3. Knowledge
4. IV–1 5. Nursing Process 6. Easy

2. Arterial vessel diameter is controlled by contraction and relaxation of which type of muscle?
A. Cardiac.
B. Striated.
*C. Smooth.
D. Skeletal.

Rationale: Smooth muscle controls the diameter of the vessels by contracting and relaxing. Because of the large amount of muscle, the walls of the arteries are relatively thick. Cardiac muscle is part of the heart.

Reference: p. 680

Descriptors:
1. 28 2. 01 3. Knowledge
4. IV–1 5. Nursing Process 6. Easy

3. The neurotransmitter responsible for sympathetic vasoconstriction is
*A. norepinephrine.
B. histamine.
C. bradykinin.
D. prostaglandin.

Rationale: Sympathetic activation occurs in response to physiologic and psychologic stressors. The neurotransmitter responsible for sympathetic vasoconstriction is norepinephrine. Histamine, bradykinin, and prostaglandin are vasodilators.

Reference: p. 683

Descriptors:
1. 28 2. 01 3. Knowledge
4. IV–1 5. Nursing Process 6. Easy

4. When the nurse assesses the vascular system of an elderly client, the nurse can anticipate that the
A. media layer of the vessels softens with age.
B. collagen decreases within the vessels.
*C. intima layer of the vessels thickens.
D. peripheral vascular resistence weakens.

Rationale: As one ages, the intima layer of the vessels thickens. Elastin fibers of the media become calcified. Peripheral vascular resistence is greater.

Reference: p. 683

Descriptors:
1. 28 2. 01 3. Application
4. IV–1 5. Nursing Process 6. Moderate

5. When the nurse assesses a client with peripheral vascular disease, the nurse anticipates signs and symptoms of ischemia, including
*A. intermittant claudication.
B. increased pulse pressure.
C. increased hair production on affected extremity.
D. warm, pink extremities.

Rationale: Clients with peripheral vascular disease often have intermittant claudication, which causes pain to the affected extremity. There is decreased pulse pressure, decreased hair production, and extremities may be pale or cyanotic.

Reference: p. 684

Descriptors:
1. 28 2. 02 3. Application
4. IV–3 5. Nursing Process 6. Moderate

6. A nurse is preparing to assess the ankle brachial index of an elderly client. The nurse should plan to
   A. use a cuff that is 40% greater than the client's limb.
   *B. allow the client to rest in a supine position for 5 minutes.
   C. deflate the pressure cuff rapidly after reading the blood pressure.
   D. inflate the cuff 10 mmHg beyond the point where the arterial signal is heard.

Rationale: The nurse should allow the client to rest in a supine position for at least 5 minutes before checking the ABI. The nurse should use a cuff that is 20 to 30% greater than the client's limb. Do not deflate the pressure cuff rapidly after reading the blood pressure. The cuff should be inflated 20 to 30 mmHg beyond the point where the arterial signal is heard.

Reference: p. 686

Descriptors:
1. 28 2. 03 3. Application
4. IV–3 5. Nursing Process 6. Moderate

7. Following an arteriogram produced by angiography, the adult client complains of nausea, sweating, and numbness of both extremities. The nurse should first
   A. apply warmth to the extremities.
   B. administer an ordered antiemetic.
   C. check the site for bleeding.
   *D. contact the client's physician.

Rationale: Allergic reactions to the iodine in the dye include nausea, sweating, dyspnea, and numbness of both extremities. The nurse should first contact the client's physician for a medication order such as corticosteroids, antihistamines, or adrenalin. Applying warmth to the extremities, administering an ordered antiemetic, and checking the site for bleeding are not helpful.

Reference: p. 687

Descriptors:
1. 28 2. 03 3. Application
4. IV–3 5. Nursing Process 6. Moderate

8. The layer of the artery that is most affected by the disease arteriosclerosis is the
   A. connective tissue.
   B. adventitia.
   C. media.
   *D. intima.

Rationale: Arteriosclerosis affects the intima of the large and medium-sized arteries. There is an accumulation of lipids, calcium, blood components, carbohydrates, and fibrous tissue on the intimal layer of the artery. These are referred to as plaques.

Reference: p. 688

Descriptors:
1. 28 2. 04 3. Knowledge
4. IV–3 5. Nursing Process 6. Easy

9. An adult client tells the nurse that her mother has been diagnosed with arteriosclerosis. The nurse should instruct the client that one of the strongest risk factors for this condition is
   A. genetic predisposition.
   B. high protein intake.
   C. malnutrition.
   *D. smoking.

Rationale: One of the strongest risk factors for this condition is smoking. Other factors include high fat diets, diabetes mellitus, hypertension, and a sedentary lifestyle.

Reference: pp. 689–690

Descriptors:
1. 28 2. 04 3. Application
4. IV–3 5. Nursing Process 6. Moderate

10. When instructing an adult client how to perform Buerger–Allen exercises to promote circulation, the nurse should instruct the client to first
   *A. lie flat with both feet elevated above the heart for 2 to 3 minutes.
   B. sit in an upright position with feet lower than the heart for 3 minutes.
   C. lie in a straight supine position for 10 minutes before beginning the exercise.
   D. stand for 8 to 10 minutes in one position without moving.

Rationale: To perform Buerger–Allen exercises to promote circulation, the nurse should instruct the client to first lie flat with both feet elevated above the heart for 2 to 3 minutes. Next the legs are in a dependent position for about 3 minutes, and finally the client lies flat with legs at the same level as the heart.

Reference: p. 693

Descriptors:
1. 28 2. 06 3. Application
4. IV–1 5. Teaching-Learning 6. Moderate

11. The nurse is caring for a client with intermittant claudication. Evidence that the outcome of increased arterial circulation to the extremity has been met includes
   *A. reduced muscle pain.
   B. reduced sensation to touch.

C. increased coolness of the extremity.
D. decreased hair production on the extremity.

Rationale: For a client with intermittant claudication, evidence that the outcome of increased arterial circulation to the extremity has been met includes reduced muscle pain, increased sensation, increased warmth, and increased hair production.

Reference: p. 694

Descriptors:
1. 28 2. 06 3. Application
4. IV–3 5. Nursing Process 6. Moderate

12. A nurse is caring for a postoperative client following vascular grafting in the leg due to intermittant claudication. During the next 24 hours, the nurse should plan to assess the
*A pulse every hour for 24 hours.
B. color of the leg every 4 hours.
C. blood pressure every 2 hours.
D. ankle–arm indices every 8 hours.

Rationale: Following a vascular grafting, the nurse should plan to assess the pulse, color, capillary refill, and temperature of the extremity every hour for the first 24 hours. Disappearance of a pulse warrants immediate notification of the physician as this may indicate thrombotic occlusion.

Reference: p. 698

Descriptors:
1. 28 2. 05 3. Application
4. IV–3 5. Nursing Process 6. Moderate

13. A 69-year-old client visits the clinic and tells the nurse that she has constant pain when she is supine, dyspnea, a brassy cough, and slight dysphagia. The nurse suspects that the client may be experiencing
A. an aortoiliac disease.
B. an arterial embolism.
*C. a thoracic aortic aneurysm.
D. Raynaud's disease.

Rationale: Although often asymptomatic, clients experiencing a thoracic aortic aneurysm may experience constant, boring pain when lying supine, dyspnea, a brassy cough, and slight dysphagia. Back pain, impotence, and decreased femoral pulses are symptoms of aortoiliac disease. Cessation of distal blood flow is associated with arterial embolism. Cold hands are associated with Raynaud's disease.

Reference: p. 701

Descriptors:
1. 28 2. 04 3. Analysis
4. IV–3 5. Nursing Process 6. Moderate

14. A nurse is caring for a client who will be undergoing surgery for an arterial embolism in his left leg. The nurse should plan to
A. provide heat to the affected leg.
B. provide ice to the affected leg.
C. elevate the affected leg 30 degrees.
*D. use a sheepskin under the affected leg.

Rationale: Sheepskins or foot cradles should be used to protect the affected leg from trauma. Heat and ice is contraindicated as this may cause further damage. The affected leg should be level or slightly dependent.

Reference: p. 704

Descriptors:
1. 28 2. 04 3. Application
4. IV–3 5. Nursing Process 6. Difficult

15. A client visits the clinic and complains of burning and numbness of the hands. The nurse determines that the client is most likely experiencing symptoms of
A. venous thrombosis.
*B. Raynaud's phenomenon.
C. arterial occlusion.
D. intermittant claudication.

Rationale: Burning and numbness of the hands or toes is a symptom of Raynaud's phenomenon. Symptoms of venous thrombosis include redness, coolness, and pain at the thrombosed site. Arterial occlusion is associated with absence of a pulse. Intermittant claudication is associated with rubor and pain.

Reference: pp. 704–705

Descriptors:
1. 28 2. 04 3. Analysis
4. IV–3 5. Nursing Process 6. Moderate

16. When assessing a client for the presence of deep vein thrombosis, the nurse anticipates which of the following clinical manifestations?
A. Absence of a peripheral pulse in the affected extremity.
*B. Swelling of the affected extremity.
C. Localized swelling around the site of the clot.
D. Absence of Homan's sign in the extremity.

Rationale: Clinical manifestations of a client with deep vein thrombosis include swelling of the affected extremity, which is also painful and cool to the touch. Absence of a peripheral pulse in the affected extremity is associated with arterial occlusion. Localized swelling around the site of the clot is associated with superficial thrombosis. Absence of Homan's sign in the extremity is a normal finding in clients.

Reference: p. 706

Descriptors:
1. 28 2. 05 3. Application
4. IV–3 5. Nursing Process 6. Moderate

17. A client has been prescribed warfarin sodium (Coumadin) to be taken daily.The nurse should instruct the client to
A. monitor his blood pressure weekly.
B. observe for signs and symptoms of infection.

C. discontinue the medication if there is pain at the site.
*D. avoid using products that contain aspirin.

Rationale: Medications that potentiate oral anticoagulants include salicylates (aspirin), anabolic steroids, chloral hydrate, and neomycin. The client should be instructed to avoid taking aspirin because bleeding can occur. Blood pressure, infection, and discontinuation of the medication if there is pain at the site are not necessary.

Reference: p. 708

Descriptors:
1. 28 2. 06 3. Application
4. IV–3 5. Nursing Process 6. Moderate

18. To promote a moist environment for granulation and healing of a leg ulcer that is not deep or infected, the nurse should apply a
*A. Tegapore dressing.
B. sterile dressing.
C. gauze dressing.
D. hydrogen peroxide dressing.

Rationale: A Tegapore dressing maintains a moist environment and can be left in place for several days. Hydrocolloids are also good choices to promote granulation, but should not be used if the ulcer is infected. Sterile, gauze, or hydrogen peroxide dressings do not provide a moist environment.

Reference: p. 711

Descriptors:
1. 28 2. 07 3. Application
4. IV–4 5. Nursing Process 6. Moderate

19. Evidence that the outcome of "restore skin integrity" for a client with a leg ulcer has been met when the nurse observes
A. absence of bleeding.
B. no requests for pain medication.
C. an increase in the client's activity.
*D. an absence of inflammation.

Rationale: Evidence that the outcome of "restore skin integrity" in a client with a leg ulcer has been met is present when the nurse observes an absence of inflammation. Absence of bleeding, pain medication, and increased activity do not relate to skin integrity outcomes.

Reference: p. 712

Descriptors:
1. 28 2. 07 3. Application
4. IV–3 5. Nursing Process 6. Moderate

20. A nurse is caring for a client diagnosed with lymphangitis. The nurse uses strict aseptic technique with this client since the disorder is usually caused by
*A. hemolytic streptococcus.
B. staphylococcus aureus.
C. streptococcus thermophilus.
D. staphylococcus epidermidis.

Rationale: Lymphangitis is most often caused by the organism hemolytic streptococcus and is typically treated with antibiotic therapy. There are characteristic red streaks that extend from the infected wound area.

Reference: p. 714

Descriptors:
1. 28 2. 08 3. Application
4. IV–3 5. Nursing Process 6. Moderate

CHAPTER 29
Assessment and Management of Patients with Hypertension

1. Hypertension often accompanies risk factors for
*A. atherosclerosis.
B. gallstones.
C. renal calculi.
D. emphysema.

Rationale: Hypertension often accompanies risk factors for atherosclerotic heart disease, such as dyslipidemia and diabetes mellitus. The incidence of gallstones, renal calculi, or emphysema are not increased with hypertension.

Reference: p. 715

Descriptors:
1. 29 2. 01 3. Knowledge
4. IV–1 5. Nursing Process 6. Easy

2. A client visits the clinic and the nurse observes that the client's blood pressure is 138/88. The nurse should instruct the client that his blood pressure should be reevaluated in
A. one week.
B. one month.
*C. one year.
D. two years.

Rationale: A client who exhibits a blood pressure of 138/88 should be reevaluated in one year. A blood pressure of 140–159 / 90–99 should be reevaluated in 2 months. A blood pressure of <130/<85 should be rechecked in 2 years.

Reference: p. 716

Descriptors:
1. 29 2. 02 3. Application
4. IV–3 5. Nursing Process 6. Moderate

3. A nurse is caring for a client who is noncompliant about taking his anti–hypertensive medications. The nurse should instruct the client that prolonged uncontrolled hypertension can result in
A. pulmonary embolism.
B. polycythemia.
C. glaucoma.
*D. myocardial infarction.

Rationale: Prolonged uncontrolled hypertension can result in myocardial infarction, cardiac failure, renal failure, strokes, and impaired vision. Hypertension is not associated with pulmonary embolism, polycythemia, or glaucoma.

Reference: p. 716

Descriptors:
1. 29 2. 02 3. Application
4. IV–3 5. Nursing Process 6. Moderate

4. A nurse is caring for an adult client who has been diagnosed with primary hypertension. The nurse should instruct the client that lifestyle modification should include
   A. reduction of sodium intake to 4 grams per day.
   *B. weight loss if overweight.
   C. limitation of whiskey intake to no more than 4 ounces per day.
   D. increase anaerobic physical activity to 30 minutes per day.

Rationale: Lifestyle modifications should include weight loss if overweight, reduction of sodium intake to 2.4 grams per day, limitation of whiskey intake to no more than 2 ounces per day, and increasing aerobic physical activity to 30 to 45 minutes per day.

Reference: p. 719

Descriptors:
1. 29 2. 03 3. Application
4. IV–3 5. Nursing Process 6. Moderate

5. A nurse is caring for an adult client who has been diagnosed with primary hypertension. To assist the client with hypertension to adhere to the medication treatment, the nurse should
   A. explain that with medication therapy other risk factors are not important.
   B. discuss the side effects of the medication and ways to relieve them.
   C. provide the client and family with pamphlets about low fat diets.
   *D. involve the client's family members to support the client's efforts.

Rationale: Although the therapeutic regimen is the responsibility of the client, involving the client's family members to support the client's efforts can assist the client to adhere to the treatment regimen. Other risk factors are still important. Discussing the side effects of the medication should be done, but this will not necessarily increase compliance and may decrease compliance. Poviding the client and family with pamphlets about low fat diets will not necessarily increase compliance.

Reference: p. 723

Descriptors:
1. 29 2. 04 3. Application
4. IV–3 5. Nursing Process 6. Moderate

6. A client is rescheduled to visit the clinic in two months to have his blood pressure reevaluated. The nurse should instruct the client that prior to the next clinic visit the client should
   A. be NPO for at least 4 hours.
   B. refrain from smoking for at least 8 hours.
   *C. try to rest quietly for 5 minutes before the reading is taken.
   D. avoid drinking herbal teas for 24 hours before the visit.

Rationale: Prior to the next clinic visit the client should try to rest quietly for 5 minutes before the reading is taken. The forearm should be positioned at heart level. The client does not need to be NPO for at least 4 hours, refrain from smoking for at least 8 hours, or avoid drinking herbal teas for 24 hours before the visit. Caffeine products should be avoided for at least 30 minutes prior to the visit.

Reference: p. 723

Descriptors:
1. 29 2. 04 3. Application
4. IV–3 5. Nursing Process 6. Moderate

7. A client with hypertension has been prescribed chlorothiazide (Diuril) as part of his treatment regimen. The nurse should explain to the client that one of the side effects of this medication is
   *A. postural hypotension.
   B. hyperkalemia.
   C. depression.
   D. nasal stuffiness.

Rationale: Side effects of this medication are postural hypotension, hypokalemia, and hyponatremia. Depression and nasal stuffiness are associated with peripheral agents such as reserpine (Serpasil).

Reference: p. 720

Descriptors:
1. 29 2. 04 3. Application
4. IV–2 5. Nursing Process 6. Moderate

8. A client with hypertension has been prescribed methydopa (Aldomet) for part of his medication regimen. The nurse should instruct the client that one of the side effects of this medication is
   A. anorexia.
   *B. drowsiness.
   C. diarrhea.
   D. anemia.

Rationale: Some of the side effects of methyldopa include drowsiness, dry mouth, and dizziness. Anorexia is associated with clonodine hydrochloride (Catapres). Diarrhea is associated with prazosin hydrochloride. Anemia is not associated with methyldopa.

Reference: p. 721

Descriptors:
1. 29 2. 04 3. Application
4. IV–2 5. Self-Care 6. Difficult

9. A client diagnosed with hypertension has been prescribed verapamil (Calan SR) as part of his medication regimen. The nurse should instruct the client to
   A. monitor his potassium intake.
   B. have regular dental checkups.
   C. report any excessive hair growth.
   *D. take the medication on an empty stomach.

Rationale: The nurse should instruct a client who has been prescribed verapamil (Calan SR), to take the medication on an empty stomach and not to discontinue the medication suddenly. Hypokalemia is associated with diuretics. Gingivitis may be caused by diltiazem hydrochloride (Cardizem). Excessive hair growth (hirsutism) is associated with Minoxodil.

Reference: p. 722

Descriptors:

1. 29	2. 03	3. Application
4. IV–2	5. Self-Care	6. Difficult

10. A client visits the emergency room and is diagnosed with a hypertensive crisis. The nurse anticipates that the physician will order
   *A. sodium nitroprusside.
   B. minoxodil.
   C. hydralazine hydrochloride.
   D. captopril.

Rationale: Medication treatment for a hypertensive crisis includes intravenous vasodilators such as sodium nitroprusside, nicardipine hydrochloride, and nitroglycerin, which have an immediate reaction that is short lived. Minoxodil, hydralazine hydrochloride, and captopril are used for blood pressure control.

Reference: p. 724

Descriptors:

1. 29	2. 05	3. Application
4. IV–2	5. Nursing Process	6. Difficult

CHAPTER 30
Assessment and Management of Patients with Hematologic Disorders

1. In humans, the primary site for hematopoiesis is the
   A. liver.
   B. spleen.
   C. heart.
   *D. bone marrow.

Rationale: The primary site for hematopoiesis is the bone marrow. During embryonic development, the liver and spleen may be involved. The heart is not involved in hematopoiesis.

Reference: p. 729

Descriptors:

1. 30	2. 01	3. Knowledge
4. IV–1	5. Nursing Process	6. Easy

2. Dietary intake of essential vitamins and iron have important effects on erythropoiesis. The vitamin that has the greatest effect on erythropoiesis is vitamin
   A. A.
   *B. B_{12}.
   C. C.
   D. D.

Rationale: Vitamin B_{12} and folic acid have the greatest effect on erythropoiesis. Vitamins A, C, and D are also important to maintain health, but they do not have the same effect as B_{12} and folic acid.

Reference: p. 732

Descriptors:

1. 30	2. 01	3. Comprehension
4. IV–1	5. Nursing Process	6. Moderate

3. When a human being's tissue is injured, a series of reactions occurs. Which of the following occurs during the reaction cascade that forms fibrin?
   *A. Prothrombin is converted to thrombin.
   B. Plasmin activates plasminogen.
   C. Fibrinogen digests the plasmin.
   D. Plasmin forms the clotting factors.

Rationale: During the reaction cascade that forms fibrin, prothrombin is converted to thrombin. Plasminogen activates plasmin and plasmin digests the fibrinogen. Clotting factors are activated and form fibrin.

Reference: p. 735

Descriptors:

1. 30	2. 02	3. Knowledge
4. IV–1	5. Nursing Process	6. Difficult

4. A client is being evaluated for anemia. Diagnostic evaluation reveals a low serum iron level and a low ferritin level. The client is most likely experiencing an anemia termed
   A. aplastic.
   B. pernicious.
   *C. iron deficient.
   D. hemolytic.

Rationale: A low serum iron level and a low ferritin level are associated with iron deficiency anemia. TIBC may also be elevated. Neutropenia and thrombocytopenia are associated with aplastic anemia.

Reference: p. 741

Descriptors:

1. 30	2. 03	3. Analysis
4. IV–1	5. Nursing Process	6. Moderate

5. A nurse is caring for a client who is diagnosed with aplastic anemia. The nurse anticipates that the medical treatment for this client will be
   *A. bone marrow transplantation.
   B. antibiotics.
   C. administration of folic acid daily.
   D. blood transfusions.

Rationale: Medical management of aplastic anemia consists of bone marrow–peripheral stem cell transplant. Other treatments include immunosuppressive therapy with cyclosporine. Folic acid is used for megaloblastic anemias, and blood transfusions may be used for sickle cell anemia.

Reference: p. 744

Descriptors:
1. 30 2. 03 3. Application
4. IV–2 5. Nursing Process 6. Moderate

6. A nurse is caring for an adult client who is hospitalized with sickle cell crisis. When assessing this client, the nurse can anticipate
   A. bradycardia.
   B. below normal temperature.
   *C. tachycardia.
   D. small skull bones.

Rationale: Sickle cell anemia is associated with tachycardia, cardiac murmurs, and an enlarged heart. Often the bones of the skull and face are enlarged. Fever is associated with sickle cell crisis.

Reference: p. 747

Descriptors:
1. 30 2. 04 3. Application
4. IV–1 5. Nursing Process 6. Moderate

7. A nurse is caring for a 6-year-old child who is diagnosed with thalassemia major. The nurse should explain to the child and the parents that treatment for this condition includes
   A. immunosuppressive therapy.
   B. administration of folic acid.
   C. administration of vitamin B_{12}.
   *D. RBC transfusions.

Rationale: For a child with thalassemia major (Cooley's anemia), regular transfusion therapy facilitates growth and development. Bone marrow transplantation is also used. Immunosuppressive therapy is used for aplastic anemia. Folic acid and vitamin B_{12} are used for megaloblastic anemia.

Reference: p. 751

Descriptors:
1. 30 2. 04 3. Application
4. IV–2 5. Nursing Process 6. Difficult

8. An adult client visits the clinic complaining of headache, fatigue, dizziness, and tinnitus. The client has a very ruddy complexion and splenomegaly with an elevation in red blood cells. The nurse determines that the client most likely is exhibiting symptoms of
   *A. polycythemia vera.
   B. megaloblastic anemia.
   C. sickle cell anemia.
   D. hereditary spherocytosis.

Rationale: Symptoms of headache, fatigue, dizziness, tinnitus, a very ruddy complexion, splenomegaly, and an elevation in red blood cells is associated with polycythemia vera. Megaloblastic anemia is associated with abnormally large RBCs. Sickle cell anemia is associated with pain, tachycardia, and sickled cells. Hereditary spherocytosis is associated with spherical RBCs.

Reference: p. 753

Descriptors:
1. 30 2. 04 3. Analysis
4. IV–1 5. Nursing Process 6. Difficult

9. A nurse is caring for a client diagnosed with leukemia. The nurse should explain to the client that the common feature of leukemia is
   A. unregulated proliferation of red blood cells.
   B. depressed production of red blood cells.
   C. depressed production of white blood cells.
   *D. unregulated proliferation of white blood cells.

Rationale: The common feature of leukemia is unregulated proliferation of white blood cells. Depressed production of red blood cells is associated with anemias. Depressed production of white blood cells is associated with leukopenia.

Reference: p. 755

Descriptors:
1. 30 2. 05 3. Application
4. IV–3 5. Nursing Process 6. Moderate

10. A nurse is caring for an adult client who is diagnosed with acute myeloid leukemia. The nurse anticipates that medical management of the client will include
   *A. chemotherapy.
   B. fibrinogen transfusions.
   C. antibiotic therapy.
   D. interferon injections.

Rationale: For a client with AML, medical management includes chemotherapy and transfusions of RBCs and platelets. Antibiotic therapy is not used. Interferon injections are used with chronic myeloid leukemias.

Reference: p. 757

Descriptors:
1. 30 2. 06 3. Application
4. IV–1 5. Nursing Process 6. Moderate

11. An adult client is hospitalized for treatment of acute myeloid leukemia. One of the potential complications of the therapy that the nurse should assess for is
   A. increased appetite.
   B. splenomegaly.

C. pruritis.
*D. renal stone formation.

Rationale: Common complications of chemotherapy used to treat AML include renal stone formation, anorexia, nausea, vomiting, and mucositis. Splenomegaly is associated with sickle cell disease. Pruritis is not a typical complication.

Reference: p. 758

Descriptors:
1. 30 2. 06 3. Application
4. IV–3 5. Nursing Process 6. Difficult

12. A nurse is caring for a client who is being discharged after treatment for acute leukemia. The nurse should instruct the client to increase his nutritional intake of
*A. soft meats such as meatloaf.
B. fresh fruits such as apples.
C. fresh vegetables such as eggplant.
D. high fat foods such as cheddar cheese.

Rationale: One complication of therapy for acute leukemia is mucositis and sore mucous membranes. The nurse should encourage the client to eat soft meats that are high in protein, and nutritional supplements. Fresh fruits and vegetables should be avoided because there is a potential for infection. High fat foods should be avoided.

Reference: p. 762

Descriptors:
1. 30 2. 06 3. Application
4. IV–3 5. Nursing Process 6. Moderate

13. A nurse is preparing to discharge a client who has been hospitalized and treated for Hodgkin's disease. The priority teaching item for this client is
A. nutritional intake.
*B. prevention of infection.
C. coping with fatigue.
D. need for daily exercise.

Rationale: The priority teaching item for clients who have received immunosuppressive therapy for treatment of Hodgkin's disease is prevention of infection. Treatment related myelosuppression occurs and the defective immune response that results from the disease itself make these clients highly susceptible to infections. Nutrition, fatigue, and exercise are not the priority at this time.

Reference: p. 765

Descriptors:
1. 30 2. 06 3. Application
4. IV–3 5. Self-Care 6. Moderate

14. A nurse is caring for a client diagnosed with primary thrombocytopenia. The nurse should explain to the client that with this condition there is
A. an attack on the platelets by the antibodies.
B. decreased production of clotting factors.
*C. elevated platelet production.
D. decreased white blood cell production.

Rationale: With primary thrombocytopenia there is an elevated platelet production. Decreased production of clotting factors is associated with hemophilia, and decreased white blood cell production is associated with leukopenia.

Reference: p. 767

Descriptors:
1. 30 2. 07 3. Application
4. IV–1 5. Nursing Process 6. Moderate

15. A nurse preparing to discharge an adolescent client who has been hospitalized and treated for complications related to hemophilia. The nurse should instruct the client to
A. use a nasal packing if a nosebleed occurs.
B. apply heat to an injured wound with bleeding.
*C. avoid medications such as aspirin.
D. take any prescribed medications by injection if possible.

Rationale: For a client with hemophilia, the nurse should instruct the client to avoid medications such as aspirin because they can interfere with platelet aggregation. A nasal packing should not be used if a nosebleed occurs because this can increase bleeding. Application of cold to an injured wound with bleeding is effective. Injections should always be avoided.

Reference: p. 771

Descriptors:
1. 30 2. 06 3. Application
4. IV–3 5. Nursing Process 6. Moderate

16. A nurse is caring for a group of hospitalized clients on a surgical unit of the hospital. The client who is at particular risk of developing disseminated intravascular coagulation is the client diagnosed with
A. cardiac disease.
B. renal calculi.
C. gallstones.
*D. cancer.

Rationale: The client who is at particular risk of developing disseminated intravascular coagulation (DIC) is the client diagnosed with cancer because of the side effects of chemotherapy. Other risk factors for DIC include sepsis, viremia, trauma, acute hemolysis, and extensive burns.

Reference: p. 773

Descriptors:
1. 30 2. 07 3. Application
4. IV–3 5. Nursing Process 6. Moderate

17. A nurse is caring for a client who is receiving an infusion of packed RBCs. Fifteen minutes after the infusion has begun, the client complains of difficulty breathing. The nurse should first

A. notify the client's physician.
B. assess the client's vital signs.
C. obtain a blood specimen from the client.
*D. stop the transfusion immediately.

Rationale: Allergic reactions can often be controlled by antihistamines. However, bronchospasm, laryngeal edema, shock, fever, chills, and jugular vein distention are severe reactions. The nurse should stop the transfusion immediately, monitor the client's vital signs, notify the physician, and send the blood container and tubing to the blood bank. A blood specimen may be needed if a transfusion reaction or a bacterial infection is suspected.

Reference: p. 784

Descriptors:
1. 30 2. 09 3. Application
4. IV–3 5. Nursing Process 6. Moderate

18. A client is ordered to receive fresh plasma intravenously. Fresh plasma is indicated for clients who have
*A. coagulation factor deficiencies.
B. hypoproteinemia.
C. symptomatic anemia.
D. significant blood loss.

Rationale: Fresh plasma is indicated for clients who have coagulation factor deficiencies. Albumin is administered to clients with hypoproteinemia. Red blood cells are administered when there is symptomatic anemia. Whole blood is administered when there is significant blood loss.

Reference: p. 779

Descriptors:
1. 30 2. 10 3. Application
4. IV–4 5. Nursing Process 6. Moderate

UNIT 7 DIGESTIVE AND GASTROINTESTINAL FUNCTION

CHAPTER 31 Assessment of Digestive and Gastrointestinal Function

1. Which is most accurate regarding the anatomy and physiology of the gastrointestinal tract?
*A. Pancreatic secretions empty into the duodenum and neutralize stomach acid.
B. Sympathetic nerves generally increase gastric secretions and motility.
C. The common bile duct empties into the jejunum in the small intestine.
D. The ileocecal valve prevents reflux of gastric contents into the esophagus.

Rationale: Pancreatic secretions empty into the duodenum and neutralize stomach acid. Parasympathetic nerves generally increase gastric secretions and motility. The common bile duct empties into the duodenum at the ampulla of Vater. The lower esophageal sphincter prevents reflux of gastric contents into the esophagus.

Reference: p. 795

Descriptors:
1. 31 2. 01 3. Knowledge
4. I–1 5. Nursing Process 6. Moderate

2. Which of the following statements is true regarding digestive processes?
A. Carbohydrates are broken down into amino acids and peptides.
B. Gastric secretions contain pepsin, which helps to digest fats.
C. Pancreatic secretions include trypsin, which helps digest starches.
*D. Salivary amylase begins the breakdown of starches.

Rationale: Salivary amylase begins the breakdown of starches. Carbohydrates are broken down into disaccharides. Gastric secretions contain pepsin, which helps to digest proteins. Pancreatic secretions include trypsin, which helps digest proteins, while amylase aids in digesting starches.

Reference: p. 793

Descriptors:
1. 31 2. 01 3. Comprehension
4. I–1 5. Nursing Process 6. Easy

3. A tarry black-colored stool is termed
A. acholia.
*B. melena.
C. scybala.
D. steatorrhea.

Rationale: A tarry black-colored stool is termed melena. Scybala are small, dry rock-hard masses. Steatorrhea are greasy stools and often are associated with cystic fibrosis.

Reference: p. 797

Descriptors:
1. 31 2. 01 3. Comprehension
4. I–1 5. Nursing Process 6. Easy

4. The enzyme that aids in the digestion of emulsified fats is
*A. bile.
B. trypsin.
C. amylase.
D. gastrin.

Rationale: The enzyme that aids in the digestion of emulsified fats is bile. Trypsin aids in the digestion of protein, amylase aids in the digestion of starch, and gastrin is produced when the stomach distends with food.

Reference: p. 794

Descriptors:
1. 31 2. 02 3. Knowledge
4. I–1 5. Nursing Process 6. Moderate

5. An adult client visits the clinic and tells the nurse that he "feels bloated all of the time and has a lot of intestinal gas." The nurse suspects that the client may be exhibiting symptoms of
*A. gallbladder disease.
B. pancreatic disease.
C. liver disease.
D. stomach ulcers.

Rationale: Symptoms of feeling bloated all of the time and a lot of intestinal gas are usually associated with gallbladder disease or food intolerance. Pancreatic disease is associated with diabetes mellitus. Liver disease causes jaundice, and stomach ulcers are associated with epigastric pain.

Reference: p. 796

Descriptors:
1. 31 2. 03 3. Analysis
4. IV–3 5. Nursing Process 6. Moderate

6. A nurse is planning to teach an adult client about an upper gastrointestinal series. The nurse should instruct the client that he will
A. need to drink only clear liquids the evening before the test.
B. be given a cleansing enema the morning of the test.
*C. pass clay-colored stools following the test.
D. receive a sedative prior to the test.

Rationale: The nurse should instruct the client that he will pass clay-colored stools following the test. The client should remain NPO after midnight before the morning of the test. The client will not be given a cleansing enema the morning of the test. nor will he receive a sedative prior to the test.

Reference: p. 799

Descriptors:
1. 31 2. 04 3. Application
4. IV–3 5. Nursing Process 6. Moderate

7. An adult client is scheduled for a lower GI series that will use Gastrografin as the contrast media. The nurse should instruct the client that
A. laxatives will be necessary following the procedure.
B. some clients have complained of constipation following the procedure.
*C. clients who are sensitive to iodine should alert the physician.
D. the procedure takes about 2 hours to complete.

Rationale: Clients who are sensitive to iodine should alert the physician because an allergic reaction may occur. Some clients have complained of diarrhea following the procedure and laxatives are generally not necessary. The procedure takes about 15 to 30 minutes to complete.

Reference: p. 799

Descriptors:
1. 31 2. 04 3. Application
4. IV–3 5. Nursing Process 6. Moderate

8. A client is scheduled for a gastric acid stimulation test in the morning. The nurse should explain to the client that he will
A. not be allowed to drink any fluids for an hour or two after the test.
*B. most likely experience a flushed feeling when the medication is injected.
C. receive a laxative the evening before to cleanse the bowel.
D. take all of his prescribed morning medications as usual.

Rationale: The client is NPO for 8 to 12 hours before the test. He will most likely experience a flushed feeling when the medication is injected. The test does not require a laxative the evening before to cleanse the bowel. Any medications affecting gastric secretions are withheld before the test.

Reference: p. 799

Descriptors:
1. 31 2. 04 3. Application
4. IV–3 5. Nursing Process 6. Moderate

9. An adult client tells the nurse that he is scheduled for an upper GI fiberoscopy in the morning. The nurse determines that the client is having this procedure for
A. evaluation of rectal bleeding.
B. evaluation of diarrhea of unknown origin.
C. removal of rectal polyps.
*D. removal of common bile duct stones.

Rationale: An upper GI fiberoscopy is used for removal of common bile duct stones, to dilate strictures, and to treat gastric bleeding and esophageal varices. Fiberoptic colonoscopy is used for evaluation of rectal bleeding, evaluation of diarrhea of unknown origin, and removal of rectal polyps.

Reference: p. 800

Descriptors:
1. 31 2. 04 3. Application
4. IV–1 5. Nursing Process 6. Moderate

10. An adult client is preparing to have a sigmoidoscopy with a biopsy using a flexible scope. The nurse should position the client
A. in a knee–chest position.
*B. lying on the left side with legs drawn toward the chest.

C. lying on the right side with the left leg bent.
D. in a prone position with two pillows elevating the legs.

Rationale: For best visualization during the procedure, the nurse should position the client lying on the left side with legs drawn toward the chest. A knee–chest position, lying on the right side with the left leg bent, or a prone position with two pillows elevating the legs does not allow for the best visualization.

Reference: p. 802

Descriptors:

1. 31	2. 04	3. Application
4. IV–3	5. Nursing Process	6. Moderate

11. A client is scheduled for a fiberoptic colonoscopy in the morning. He has an order for Golytely solution to be given today. The nurse should
A. continue to administer the prescribed medications.
*B. offer to put ice in the Golytely lavage solution.
C. offer a low residue diet for the rest of the day.
D. keep the client NPO after administration of the Golytely.

Rationale: When clients are to receive Golytely solutions to cleanse the bowel, the nurse should offer to put ice in the Golytely lavage solution. After the solution is administered, no prescribed medications should be taken. The client should be placed on a clear liquid diet starting at the noon meal. The client should continue to take oral fluids throughout the day administration of the Golytely to prevent fluid imbalances.

Reference: p. 802

Descriptors:

1. 31	2. 04	3. Application
4. IV–3	5. Nursing Process	6. Moderate

12. A client is scheduled to have a Hematest. Before the test, the nurse should instruct the client to avoid taking
*A. aspirin.
B. benadryl.
C. penicillin.
D. vitamin D.

Rationale: A false positive Hematest can result from medications such as iron, salicylates (aspirin), corticosteriods, and vitamin C.

Reference: p. 805

Descriptors:

1. 31	2. 04	3. Application
4. IV–3	5. Nursing Process	6. Moderate

CHAPTER 32
Management of Patients with Oral and Esophageal Disorders

1. A client visits the clinic with a painful canker sore on his mouth. The nurse should instruct the client to
A. brush the teeth several times per day.
B. drink an adequate amount of fruit juices.
C. use sun block on the lips daily.
*D. rinse the mouth with warm saline solutions.

Rationale: The nurse should instruct the client with a painful canker sore to rinse the mouth frequently with warm saline solutions and eat a soft bland diet. Brushing the teeth, drinking fruit juices which are acid, and using sun blocks on the lips are not helpful.

Reference: p. 809

Descriptors:

1. 32	2. 01	3. Application
4. IV–3	5. Nursing Process	6. Moderate

2. The nurse is planning to provide oral hygiene to a hospitalized client. The nurse should explain to the client that the most effective method of cleansing the teeth is the use of
A. lemon glycerin swabs.
B. mouthwash and peroxide.
*C. a soft-bristled toothbrush.
D. a moistened sponge stick.

Rationale: The most effective method of cleansing the teeth is the use of a soft-bristled toothbrush. Lemon glycerin swabs should not be used because they dry out the mucosa. The use of mouthwash and peroxide or moistened sponge sticks are not as effective as a toothbrush.

Reference: p. 810

Descriptors:

1. 32	2. 01	3. Application
4. IV–3	5. Nursing Process	6. Moderate

3. An adult client with an abscessed tooth had an incision made to provide drainage. The nurse should instruct the client to
A. massage the gumline to increase drainage.
B. pack the gums with gauze if bleeding occurs.
*C. rinse the mouth with warm saline to keep it clean.
D. eat a regular diet that is high in fiber.

Rationale: The nurse should instruct the client with an abscessed tooth and an incision made to provide drainage to rinse the mouth with warm saline to keep it clean. Antibiotics may be prescribed for infection. Massaging the gumline to increase drainage and packing the gums with gauze if bleeding occurs are not recommended. The client should advance from a liquid to a soft diet as tolerated.

Reference: p. 811

Descriptors:
1. 32 2. 03 3. Application
4. IV–3 5. Nursing Process 6. Moderate

4. An adult client had a fractured jaw repaired with a rigid plate fixation. To reduce the risk of aspiration for this client, the nurse should
*A. administer the prescribed antiemetics to prevent vomiting.
B. irrigate the nasogastric tube every 3 hours.
C. monitor the client for symptoms of nausea.
D. clear any secretions in the mouth with a bulb syringe.

Rationale: To reduce the risk of aspiration for this client, the nurse should administer the prescribed antiemetics to prevent vomiting and keep the client in a side-lying position. The client will have continuous nasogastric suctioning. Monitoring the client for symptoms of nausea will not help. Secretions in the mouth should be cleared with a small suction catheter.

Reference: p. 812

Descriptors:
1. 32 2. 03 3. Application
4. IV–3 5. Nursing Process 6. Difficult

5. An adult client is admitted to the hospital with sialadenitis. The nurse can anticipate that the physician will order
A. warm, moist packs.
*B. antibiotics.
C. lithotripsy.
D. room isolation.

Rationale: Sialadenitis is an inflammation of the salivary glands due to poor oral hygiene, S. aureus, or pneumococcus. The nurse can anticipate that the physician will order corticosteriods and antibiotics. Lithotripsy is used for calculi in the salivary glands. The client does not need room isolation or warm, moist packs.

Reference: p. 812

Descriptors:
1. 32 2. 03 3. Application
4. IV–1 5. Nursing Process 6. Moderate

6. The most common symptom the nurse should expect to note in a client in the early stages of oral cancer is
*A. a painless sore that does not heal.
B. a swollen, hard nodule in the mouth.
C. oral drainage of pus and blood.
D. difficulty in swallowing foods.

Rationale: Often oral cancer is asymptomatic. An early symptom is a painless sore that does not heal. Later there is tenderness, difficulty swallowing, and tenderness.

Reference: p. 813

Descriptors:
1. 32 2. 04 3. Application
4. IV–1 5. Nursing Process 6. Moderate

7. Clients with oral cancer frequently experience dryness of the mouth, which is termed
A. gingivitis.
B. leukoplakia.
C. stomatitis.
*D. xerostomia.

Rationale: Dryness of the mouth in oral cancer clients is termed xerostomia. Gingivitis is an inflammation of the gums. Leukoplakia are white patches of the mouth. Stomatitis is an inflammation of the oral mucosa.

Reference: p. 815

Descriptors:
1. 32 2. 04 3. Application
4. IV–1 5. Nursing Process 6. Moderate

8. A nurse is caring for a client following neck dissection surgery. The nurse should
A. place the client in a side-lying position.
B. monitor the continuous nasogastric suctioning equipment.
*C. notify the physician if the client develops stridor.
D. perform oral hygiene with hydrogen peroxide.

Rationale: While caring for a client following neck dissection surgery, the nurse should place the client in a high Fowler's position to assist the expansion of lungs. The client should be suctioned intermittantly with a soft catheter. The physician should be notified if the client develops stridor because this indicates an obstructed airway.

Reference: p. 819

Descriptors:
1. 32 2. 05 3. Application
4. IV–3 5. Nursing Process 6. Moderate

9. A nurse is caring for a client who had a radical neck dissection 12 hours ago. The nurse observes that the client has 300 ml in his surgical suction drainage device in the last 8 hours. The nurse should
A. culture the drainage.
B. increase the client's fluid intake.
*C. notify the physician.
D. take the client's temperature.

Rationale: When the nurse observes that the client has 300 ml in his surgical suction drainage device in the last 8 hours, the nurse should notify the physician as this may be indicative of hemorrhage. 80 to 120 ml of drainage in 24 hours is normal.

Reference: p. 819

Descriptors:
1. 32 2. 05 3. Application
4. IV–3 5. Nursing Process 6. Moderate

10. When a client has a neck dissection with a graft, the nurse anticipates that the normal graft will appear
 A. slightly bluish and cool.
 *B. pale pink and warm.
 C. white and cool.
 D. purplish and warm.

Rationale: The normal graft will appear pale pink and warm, which indicates adequate blood perfusion. Bluish or purplish colors indicate cyanosis.

Reference: p. 819

Descriptors:
1. 32 2. 06 3. Application
4. IV–3 5. Nursing Process 6. Moderate

11. The nurse is caring for a client who is diagnosed with achalasia. The nurse determines that the primary symptom of this disorder is
 *A. difficulty in swallowing.
 B. burning sensation in the esophagus.
 C. epigastric pain after eating.
 D. diarrhea after eating.

Rationale: The primary symptom of achalasia is difficulty in swallowing. Pain may or may not be associated with eating. Epigastric pain after eating may be indicative of an ulcer. A burning sensation in the esophagus is associated with hiatal hernias.

Reference: p. 824

Descriptors:
1. 32 2. 07 3. Application
4. IV–1 5. Nursing Process 6. Moderate

12. A nurse is caring for a client diagnosed with esophageal reflux disorder. The nurse should instruct the client to
 *A. keep the head of the bed elevated.
 B. drink a cup of hot tea before bedtime.
 C. avoid high fiber foods.
 D. drink a carbonated drink after meals.

Rationale: For a client diagnosed with esophageal reflux disorder, the nurse should instruct the client to keep the head of the bed elevated. Carbonated drinks, caffeine, and tobacco should be avoided. A high-fiber low-fat diet should be eaten daily.

Reference: p. 826

Descriptors:
1. 32 2. 08 3. Application
4. IV–3 5. Nursing Process 6. Moderate

13. A client visits the clinic and tells the nurse that he has difficulty swallowing; a feeling of fullness in the neck; belching, gurgling noises after eating; and halitosis. The nurse determines that the client is most likely experiencing
 A. hiatal hernia.
 B. cancer of the esophagus.
 *C. a diverticulum.
 D. aphthous stomatitis.

Rationale: Difficulty swallowing; a feeling of fullness in the neck; belching, gurgling noises after eating; and halitosis are associated with a diverticulum, usually termed Zenker's diverticulum. Aphthous stomatitis is a canker sore. Lesions are associated with cancer of the esophagus. Hiatal hernia is associated with burning sensations.

Reference: p. 827

Descriptors:
1. 32 2. 08 3. Application
4. IV–3 5. Nursing Process 6. Difficult

CHAPTER 33
Gastrointestinal Intubation and Special Nutritional Modalities

1. A client has been ordered a nasoenteric tube to administer tube feedings. The nurse should plan to anchor which type of tube?
 *A. Dubhoff.
 B. Miller Abbott.
 C. Salem pump.
 D. Sengstaken–Blakemore.

Rationale: The nurse should plan to anchor a Dubhoff or Keofeed II. Salem pump and Sengstaken–Blakemore are nasogastric tubes for lavage, while the Miller Abbott tube is for nasogastric decompression.

Reference: p. 837

Descriptors:
1. 33 2. 01 3. Application
4. IV–1 5. Nursing Process 6. Moderate

2. A client is ordered to have a tube anchored to control bleeding from esophageal varices. The nurse should plan to anchor a
 A. Salem pump.
 B. Baker tube.
 C. Harris tube.
 *D. Sengstaken–Blakemore tube.

Rationale: Sengstaken–Blakemore tubes are used to control bleeding from esophageal varices. Salem pumps, Baker tubes, and Harris tubes are nasogastric tubes.

Reference: p. 834

Descriptors:
1. 33 2. 01 3. Application
4. IV–1 5. Nursing Process 6. Moderate

3. After the insertion of a feeding tube into an adult client, the nurse should
 A. test the pH of the gastric aspirate.
 *B. ask the client to lie on the right side.

C. maintain the client in a high Fowler's position.
D. flush the tubing with sterile water.

Rationale: After the insertion of a feeding tube into an adult client, the nurse should ask the client to lie on the right side to help move the tube into the duodenum. X-ray not aspirate should confirm placement of the tube. Flushing should only be done with normal saline.

Reference: p. 838

Descriptors:

1. 33	2. 02	3. Application
4. IV–3	5. Nursing Process	6. Moderate

4. The nurse is preparing to insert a Cantor tube into an adult client. Once the tube has reached the client's nasopharynx, the nurse should
*A. offer the client sips of water.
B. ask the client to hold his breath.
C. have the client tilt the head backward.
D. tell the client to breathe slowly.

Rationale: Once the Cantor tube has reached the client's nasopharynx, the nurse should offer the client sips of water because swallowing will aid in the insertion of the tube. The client's head should be tilted upward.

Reference: p. 838

Descriptors:

1. 33	2. 01	3. Application
4. IV–1	5. Nursing Process	6. Moderate

5. The nurse is caring for a client who has had a nasogastric tube in place for two days. The nurse determines that the client's aspirate is from the gastric area when the nurse observes that the color of the aspirate is
A. clear.
B. tan mucous.
C. pale yellow.
*D. green.

Rationale: The client's aspirate is from the gastric area when the nurse observes that the color of the aspirate is green. Clear, yellow, and bile-colored are associated with intestinal aspirate. Tan mucus is associated with tracheobronchial secretions and pleural secretions are pale yellow.

Reference: p. 838

Descriptors:

1. 33	2. 02	3. Analysis
4. IV–1	5. Nursing Process	6. Moderate

6. The nurse is caring for a client who has had a nasogastric tube in place for 24 hours. The pH of the aspirate is 3.0, which most liikely indicates
*A. gastric aspirate.
B. intestinal aspirate.
C. pleural aspirate.
D. tracheoesophageal aspirate.

Rationale: Normal gastric aspirate has a pH of 0–4, while intestinal aspirate is 6 or greater and respiratory aspirate is 7 or greater.

Reference: p. 838

Descriptors:

1. 33	2. 02	3. Application
4. IV–3	5. Nursing Process	6. Moderate

7. While caring for a client with a nasogastric tube, the nurse should irrigate the tubing every 8 hours with normal saline to prevent
A. dehydration.
B. fluid overload.
*C. electrolyte imbalance.
D. gastric irritation.

Rationale: The nurse should irrigate the tubing every 8 hours with normal saline to prevent electrolyte imbalance. Gastric irritation, dehydration, and fluid overload are not prevented by the use of normal saline.

Reference: p. 839

Descriptors:

1. 33	2. 02	3. Application
4. IV–3	5. Nursing Process	6. Moderate

8. While caring for a client with a nasogastric tube, the client appears lethargic and has a decreased body temperature. The nurse should assess the client for fluid volume deficit by evaluating the client's laboratory values for
A. hematocrit.
*B. blood urea nitrogen.
C. white blood cell count.
D. serum amylase.

Rationale: To assess the client for fluid volume deficit, the nurse should evaluate the client's laboratory values for the blood urea nitrogen and creatinine, which will be low. Hematocrit, white blood cell count, and serum amylase will not give an accurate picture of fluid volume deficit.

Reference: p. 839

Descriptors:

1. 33	2. 02	3. Application
4. IV–3	5. Nursing Process	6. Moderate

9. A nurse is caring for a client who has been receiving nasogastric tube feedings for 12 hours. The nurse should monitor the client for symptoms of the dumping syndrome, which includes
A. constipation.
B. bradycardia.
C. hypertension.
*D. diarrhea.

Rationale: The symptoms of dumping syndrome include diarrhea, feelings of fullness, nausea, hypotension, and dehydration. Constipation, bradycardia, and hypertension are not associated with the dumping syndrome.

Reference: p. 840

Descriptors:
1. 33 2. 02 3. Application
4. IV–3 5. Nursing Process 6. Moderate

10. Jevity or Ultracal may be prescribed for clients with nasogastric tube feedings to provide
 A. easy-to-absorb nutrients.
 B. high fats and low carbohydrates.
 *C. fiber to minimize diarrhea.
 D. high calories for wound healing.

Rationale: Jevity or Ultracal may be prescribed for clients with nasogastric tube feedings to provide fiber to minimize diarrhea. Isocal has easy-to-absorb nutrients. Nepro is high in calories.

Reference: p. 841

Descriptors:
1. 33 2. 02 3. Application
4. IV–3 5. Nursing Process 6. Moderate

11. A client has just had a gastrostomy performed. The nurse should monitor the client for a postoperative complication of the procedure that includes
 *A. bleeding.
 B. dehydration.
 C. diarrhea.
 D. electrolyte imbalance.

Rationale: A postoperative complication of a gastrostomy is GI bleeding. Other complications include wound infection and premature removal of the tube. Dehydration, diarrhea, and electrolyte imbalances are not typical complications.

Reference: p. 848

Descriptors:
1. 33 2. 03 3. Application
4. IV–3 5. Nursing Process 6. Moderate

12. A nurse makes a home visit to a client who has had a gastrostomy tube feeding in place for two weeks. Nursing interventions for routine site care should include
 A. applying an antibiotic ointment twice daily.
 B. changing the dressing daily using sterile technique.
 *C. cleansing the site daily with soap and water.
 D. washing the site every other day with iodine and alcohol.

Rationale: Routine site care should include cleansing the site daily with soap and water. Applying an antibiotic ointment twice daily is not necessary. Clean dressing changes are acceptable. Washing the site every other day with iodine and alcohol can damage the skin.

Reference: p. 847

Descriptors:
1. 33 2. 04 3. Application
4. IV–3 5. Nursing Process 6. Moderate

13. A nurse is caring for a client who is receiving total parenteral nutrition (TPN) through the subclavian site and his feeding bag is empty. While waiting for the next bag to be delivered, the nurse should
 *A. hang a bag of D10W until the new bag arrives.
 B. mix a new bag of supplement from emergency supplies.
 C. notify the physician immediately.
 D. turn off the TPN solution until the new bag arrives.

Rationale: While waiting for the next bag to be delivered, the nurse should hang a bag of D10W until the new bag arrives. The nurse should not mix a new bag of supplement from emergency supplies. Notifying the physician immediately is not helpful. The TPN should not be turned off until the new bag arrives.

Reference: p. 854

Descriptors:
1. 33 2. 07 3. Application
4. IV–3 5. Nursing Process 6. Moderate

CHAPTER 34
Management of Patients with Gastric and Duodenal Disorders

1. Which of the following terms refers to tarry or black stools?
 A. Dumping syndrome
 B. Hematemesis
 *C. Melena
 D. Pyrosis

Rationale: Melena is indicative of blood in stools. Hematemesis refers to vomiting blood, pyrosis refers to heartburn, and dumping syndrome refers to rapid emptying of gastric contents into the jejunum.

Reference: p. 858

Descriptors:
1. 34 2. 01 3. Knowledge
4. IV–4 5. Nursing Process 6. Easy

2. Characteristics of gastric ulcer, as compared with duodenal ulcer, include
 *A. increased incidence in patients 50 and older.
 B. uncommon vomiting.
 C. hemorrhage less likely.
 D. pain occurs 2–3 hours after a meal.

Rationale: Gastric ulcers occur in individuals usually 50 and over, cause vomiting, are more likely to hemorrhage, and cause pain within 1/2 to 1 hour after eating.

Reference: p. 861

Descriptors:
1. 34 2. 01 3. Comprehension
4. IV–4 5. Nursing Process 6. Moderate

3. A nurse teaches that the patient who has been diagnosed with peptic ulcer and has demonstrated the presence of Helicobacter pylori should
*A. take antibiotics until entire prescription is consumed.
B. expect that reinfection with H. pylori will likely recur.
C. take antibiotics with antacids.
D. expect to take antibiotics prophylactically when having dental work performed.

Rationale: Peptic ulcers treated with antibiotics to eradicate H. pylori have a 10% recurrence rate; those not treated have a 95% recurrence. Treatment requires completion of prescribed antibiotics. Antacids are known to affect absorption of medications.

Reference: p. 862

Descriptors:
1. 34 2. 03 3. Application
4. IV–3 5. Teaching/Learning 6. Difficult

4. Which of the following medications is categorized as a Histamine 2 (H2) receptor antagonist?
*A. Nizantidine (Axid).
B. Omperazole (Prilosec).
C. Misoprostol (Cytotec).
D. Sucralfate (Carafate).

Rationale: Nizantidine is a H2 receptor antagonist or H2 blocker that inhibits gastric acid secretion. Prilosec is a proton pump inhibitor. Cytotec and Carafate are cytoprotective agents.

Reference: p. 863

Descriptors:
1. 34 2. 04 3. Comprehension
4. IV–2 5. Nursing Process 6. Difficult

5. Which of the following categories of drugs used for peptic ulcer disease acts by coating the gastric mucosa?
A. Bismuth salts.
B. Histamine 2 (H2) receptor antagonists.
C. Proton pump inhibitors.
*D. Cytoprotective drugs.

Rationale: Bismuth salts suppress H. pylori in the gastric mucosa, and H2 blockers inhibit acid secretion. Proton pump inhibitors decrease gastric acid secretion. Cytoprotective agents protect the gastric mucosa by increasing mucus or creating a viscous protective layer at the site of the ulcer.

Reference: pp. 863, 862–863

Descriptors:
1. 34 2. 04 3. Comprehension
4. IV–2 5. Nursing Process 6. Difficult

6. Which of the following terms refers to the surgical procedure that results in removal of the distal third of the stomach and anastomosis of the remaining stomach to the duodenum?
A. Vagotomy.
B. Pyloroplasty.
*C. Subtotal gastrectomy.
D. Antrectomy.

Rationale: Vagotomy refers to severing of the vagal nerve, while pyloroplasty is a surgical procedure involving the pylorus. An antrectomy involves removal of the antral portion of the stomach. A subtotal gastrectomy results in removal of the gastrin-producing cells in the antrum and part of the parietal cells.

Reference: p. 865

Descriptors:
1. 34 2. 04 3. Comprehension
4. IV–4 5. Nursing Process 6. Moderate

7. The nurse anticipates which of the following signs that may indicate perforation in the patient diagnosed and hospitalized with peptic ulcer?
A. Bradycardia.
B. Anorexia.
*C. Right shoulder pain.
D. Soft abdomen.

Rationale: Pain accompanying ulcer perforation may be referred to the shoulders, especially the right shoulder, because of irritation of the phrenic nerve in the diaphragm. Other symptoms include hypotension and tachycardia; tender, rigid abdomen; vomiting and collapse.

Reference: p. 867

Descriptors:
1. 34 2. 04 3. Analysis
4. IV–4 5. Nursing Process 6. Moderate

8. A nurse evaluates the patient education provided to the patient with peptic ulcer disease as successful when the patient describes symptoms of complication of his disease, including
*A. distended abdomen.
B. warm, moist skin.
C. subnormal temperature.
D. anorexia.

Rationale: Indicators of hemorrhage include cool skin, confusion, tachycardia, and labored breathing. Indications of perforation include severe abdominal pain; rigid, tender abdomen; vomiting, fever, and increased heart rate. Indicators of pyloric obstruction include nausea and vomiting, abdominal distention, and abdominal pain.

Reference: p. 867

Descriptors:
1. 34 2. 04 3. Comprehension
4. II–2 5. Teaching/Learning 6. Moderate

9. Which of the following signs or symptoms may indicate an early symptom of gastric cancer?

*A. Stomach pain relieved with antacids.
B. Indigestion.
C. Anorexia.
D. Anemia.

Rationale: The early symptoms of gastric cancer and are often not definite. Some studies have shown that early symptoms, such as pain relieved with antacids, resemble those of benign ulcers. Symptoms of progressive disease include indigestion, anorexia, weight loss, abdominal pain, constipation, anemia, and nausea and vomiting.

Reference: p. 868

Descriptors:
1. 34 2. 06 3. Comprehension
4. II–2 5. Nursing Process 6. Moderate

10. During the early postoperative period, the nurse closely observes the morbidly obese patient who has undergone vertical banded gastroplasty for which of the following indicator of complications?
A. Pain.
B. Weight loss.
*C. Rigid, tender abdomen.
D. Increased urine output.

Rationale: Pain is an expected postoperative occurrence. Weight loss is anticipated postoperatively. Increased urine output is not problematic. A rigid, tender abdomen may indicate peritonitis and must be evaluated by the surgeon.

Reference: p. 868

Descriptors:
1. 34 2. 05 3. Analysis
4. II–2 5. Nursing Process 6. Moderate

11. When the patient who has undergone gastric surgery has some bloody drainage during the first 8 hours postoperatively, the nurse advises the family that
A. he or she will contact the physician immediately
*B. some bloody drainage is expected for the first 12 hours post surgery
C. bleeding can be expected to continue for 24 hours
D. hemorrhage is a common complication after gastric surgery

Rationale: Hemorrhage is occasionally a complication gastric surgery, and some bloody drainage is expected from the nasogastric tube for the first 12 hours post surgery. However, excessive bleeding will be reported to the physician immediately, and the patient will be monitored closely for signs of shock.

Reference: p. 867

Descriptors:
1. 34 2. 07 3. Analysis
4. I–1 5. Nursing Process 6. Difficult

12. A nurse teaches the patient post gastric surgery dietary self-management guidlines, including:
A. meals should contain more liquid items than dry.
B. carbohydrate intake should be high.
*C. sucrose and glucose are to be avoided.
D. 3 balanced meals per day are recommended.

Rationale: Because of complications such as dysphagia, gastric retention, bile reflux, and dumping syndrome that may occur in the post gastric surgery patient, the nurse teaches the patient that meals should contain more dry than liquid items; smaller but more frequent meals should be eaten; fat may be taken to tolerance, but carbohydrate intake should be kept low. Sucrose and glucose are to be avoided because of fluid imbalances that may be caused during digestion in the jejunum.

Reference: p. 872

Descriptors:
1. 34 2. 07 3. Analysis
4. IV–4 5. Teaching/Learning 6. Difficult

13. A nurse provides guidelines to the patient diagnosed with ulcer disease and being treated with a histamine receptor antagonist (H2 blocker), including:
A. take the medication until the symptoms disappear, and then as needed.
B. medication alone will cure the disease.
*C. small, frequent feedings are unnecessary as long as the patient is taking the H2 blocker.
D. smoking has no relationship to ulcer disease.

Rationale: Because most patients become symptom-free in a week, it is important to stress following the prescribed regimen so healing can continue uninterrupted and the return of chronic ulcer symptoms can be prevented. Medication, stress reduction and rest, smoking cessation, and dietary modification all contribute to management of the disease.

Reference: p. 864

Descriptors:
1. 34 2. 04 3. Analysis
4. IV–2 5. Teaching/learning 6. Moderate

14. A nurse instructs the patient who has been prescribed tetracycline therapy for eradication of Helicobacter pylori to avoid which of the following food groups when taking the medication?
A. Green, leafy vegetables.
*B. Milk and dairy products.
C. Whole grains.
D. Legumes.

Rationale: When taken with milk or dairy products, the effectiveness of tetracyclines may be reduced.

Reference: p. 863

Descriptors:
1. 34 2. 04 3. Knowledge
4. IV–2 5. Nursing Process 6. Moderate

15. Which of the following medications used to treat peptic ulcer disease is administered as a preventive medication in patients using NSAIDs?
   A. Bismuth salicylate.
   B. Cimetidine (Tagamet).
   *C. Misoprostol (Cytotec).
   D. Famotidine (Pepcid).

Rationale: Because cytoprotective agents such as Cytotec protect the gastric mucosa from ulcerogenic agents, such as NSAIDs, it is often used as a preventive method for treating peptic ulcer disease.

Reference: p. 863

Descriptors:
1. 34 2. 04 3. Comprehension
4. IV–2 5. Nursing Process 6. Difficult

CHAPTER 35
Management of Patients with Intestinal and Rectal Disorders

1. Which of the following terms refers to inflammation of the lining of the abdominal cavity?
   A. Appendicitis.
   B. Diverticulitis.
   C. Irritable bowel syndrome.
   *D. Peritonitis.

Rationale: Peritonitis occurs usually as a result of a bacterial infection of an area of the GI system with related leakage of contents into the abdominal cavity.

Reference: p. 876

Descriptors:
1. 35 2. 08 3. Knowledge
4. IV–4 5. Nursing Process 6. Easy

2. To prevent constipation, the nurse teaches the patient to
   *A. establish a bowel routine by knowing that the best time for defecation is after breakfast.
   B. limit fluid intake.
   C. consume low-residue, low-fiber foods.
   D. resist the urge to defecate until the scheduled time.

Rationale: Identifying a regular time, such as after stimulation of the GI tract by breakfast intake, may aid in initiating the reflex. The urge to defecate should be heeded. Fluid intake should be increased unless contraindicated, and intake of high-residue, high-fiber foods is suggested.

Reference: p. 879

Descriptors:
1. 35 2. 01 3. Analysis
4. IV–4 5. Teaching/Learning 6. Moderate

3. The main aim of intervention for the patient suffering malabsorption syndrome is to
   *A. avoid dietary substances that aggravate malabsorption
   B. eradicate the syndrome with antibiotics
   C. prevent diarrhea
   D. induce weight gain

Rationale: Intervention is aimed at avoiding dietary substances that aggravate malabsorption as well as supplementing nutrients that have been lost. Antibiotics are used to treat disease of bacterial overgrowth. Diarrhea is a consequence of dietary aggravation of the GI system. Weight gain may or may not be indicated.

Reference: p. 881

Descriptors:
1. 35 2. 02 3. Analysis
4. I–1 5. Nursing Process 6. Moderate

4. A nurse teaches the patient who demonstrates lactose intolerance which of the following guidelines in order to manage the disorder?
   A. Avoid "active culture" yogurts.
   *B. Decreased milk intake without supplements can lead to osteoporosis.
   C. Processed foods do not contain lactose.
   D. Products, such as Lactaid drops, should be taken immediately after eating.

Rationale: Lactase activity of yogurt with "active cultures" helps digestion of lactose in the intestine better than lactase preparations. While elimination of milk and milk substances can abolish symptoms, vitamin D and calcium deficiencies can lead to osteoporosis. Processed foods may contain fillers such as dried milk, and foods should be pretreated with Lactaid before ingestion to reduce symptoms.

Reference: p. 883

Descriptors:
1. 35 2. 02 3. Analysis
4. IV–1 5. Teaching/Learning 6. Difficult

5. The nurse caring for the patient with acute diverticulitis observes the patient and her laboratory data closely for indicators of perforation, specifically
   A. decreased sedimentation rate.
   B. bradycardia.
   C. hypertension.
   *D. increased abdominal pain and tenderness.

Rationale: If a diverticulum ruptures, it leaks intestinal contents into the peritoneum with resulting signs of peritonitis. Other signs of diverticular perforation include elevated WBC, elevated sedimentation rate, increased temperature, tachycardia, and hypotension.

Reference: p. 885

Descriptors:
1. 35 2. 03 3. Comprehension
4. IV–4 5. Nursing Process 6. Moderate

6. When comparing the pathophysiology and clinical manifestation of regional enteritis with ulcerative colitis, the nurse is aware that ulcerative colitis
   *A. is a disease of remissions and exacerbations.
   B. affects the ileum and right colon.
   C. usually does not involve bleeding.
   D. is commonly associated with fistula development.

Rationale: Regional enteritis is a prolonged and variable disease. Ulcerative colitis, a disease of exacerbations and remissions, affects the rectum and left colon, commonly results in severe bleeding, and is rarely associated with development of fistula.

Reference: p. 890

Descriptors:
1. 35 2. 04 3. Knowledge
4. I–1 5. Nursing Process 6. Moderate

7. Diagnostic findings of regional enteritis anticipated by the nurse include
   A. no narrowing of the colon.
   B. diffuse tissue involvement.
   C. no mucosal edema.
   *D. multiple areas of stenosis.

Rationale: In regional enteritis, the colon is narrowed; there are regional, discontinuous lesions; the bowel wall is thickened; and stenosis and fistulas are common findings.

Reference: p. 890

Descriptors:
1. 35 2. 04 3. Knowledge
4. I–1 5. Nursing Process 6. Moderate

8. The nurse teaches the patient diagnosed with inflammatory bowel disease which of the following dietary guidelines? The diet should include foods that are
   A. high-residue.
   B. low-protein.
   C. high-fiber.
   *D. bland.

Rationale: Nutritional management of inflammatory bowel disease requires ingestion of a diet that is bland, low-residue, high-protein, and high-vitamin.

Reference: p. 893

Descriptors:
1. 35 2. 05 3. Comprehension
4. IV–1 5. Teaching/Learning 6. Moderate

9. Which of the following terms is used to describe intestinal obstruction caused by the bowel twisting and turning on itself?
   A. intussusception
   *B. volvulus
   C. herniation
   D. adhesion

Rationale: Volvulus causes gas and fluid to accumulate in the tapped bowel. Intussusception refers to a telescoped shortening of the intestine, while herniation refers to protrusion of intestine through a weakened area in the abdominal muscle or wall. Adhesion is the adherence of loops of intestine to areas that heal slowly or scar after abdominal surgery.

Reference: p. 902

Descriptors:
1. 35 2. 08 3. Knowledge
4. IV–4 5. Nursing Process 6. Easy

10. Risk factors associated with colorectal cancer include
    A. age less than 40.
    B. history of bowel obstruction.
    *C. family history of familial polyposis.
    D. low-fat, low-protein, low-fiber diet.

Rationale: Risk factors include age older than 40; history of rectal or colon polyps; presence of adenomatous polyps or villous adenomas; family history of colon cancer or familial polyposis; history of inflammatory bowel disease; and high-fat, high-protein (with high intake of beef), low-fiber diet.

Reference: p. 903

Descriptors:
1. 35 2. 07 3. Knowledge
4. II–2 5. Nursing Process 6. Easy

11. When the patient with colon cancer asks the nurse why the physician stated that carcinoembryonic antigen (CEA) levels will be measured for the remainder of her life, the nurse informs the patient that
    A. CEA is secreted by colon cancers.
    B. CEA levels are used to diagnose colon cancer.
    *C. elevations of CEA at a later date may suggest recurrence.
    D. with complete resection of the colon tumor, CEA returns to normal immediately.

Rationale: CEA is not a highly reliable indicator for diagnosing colon cancer, because not all lesions secrete CEA. Studies show, however, that it is reliable in predicting prognosis, returns to normal within 48 hours of complete resection of the colon tumor, and may become elevated with recurrence of the tumor.

Reference: p. 904

Descriptors:
1. 35 2. 07 3. Comprehension
4. IV–4 5. Nursing Process 6. Difficult

12. A permanent sigmoid colostomy results in which type of discharge?
    *A. Solid feces.
    B. Semimushy feces.
    C. Mushy feces.
    D. Liquid feces.

Rationale: With a sigmoid colostomy, feces are solid. With a descending colostomy, feces are semimushy. With a transverse colostomy, feces are mushy. With an ascending colostomy, feces are fluid.

Reference: p. 907

Descriptors:

1. 35	2. 06	3. Comprehension
4. IV–1	5. Nursing Process	6. Moderate

13. Which of the following actions is appropriate when irrigating a colostomy?
*A. Allow some of the solution to flow through the tubing and catheter/cone prior to insertion into the stoma.
B. Do not lubricate catheter/cone.
C. Insert the catheter no more than 8 inches into the stoma.
D. Apply pressure, as necessary, to advance the catheter.

Rationale: Air bubbles in the setup must be released and should not be introduced into the colon because they will cause crampy pain. The catheter/cone should be lubricated, inserted no more than 3 inches, and should never be forced into the stoma.

Reference: p. 910

Descriptors:

1. 35	2. 06	3. Application
4. I–1	5. Nursing Process	6. Difficult

14. A permanent ascending colostomy results in which type of discharge?
A. Solid feces.
B. Semimushy feces.
C. Mushy feces.
*D. Liquid feces.

Rationale: With a sigmoid colostomy, feces are solid. With a descending colostomy, feces are semimushy. With a transverse colostomy, feces are mushy. With an ascending colostomy, feces are fluid.

Reference: p. 907

Descriptors:

1. 35	2. 06	3. Comprehension
4. IV–1	5. Nursing Process	6. Moderate

15. A permanent transverse colostomy results in which type of discharge?
A. Solid feces.
B. Semimushy feces.
*C. Mushy feces.
D. Liquid feces.

Rationale: With a sigmoid colostomy, feces are solid. With a descending colostomy, feces are semimushy. With a transverse colostomy, feces are mushy. With an ascending colostomy, feces are fluid.

Reference: p. 907

Descriptors:

1. 35	2. 06	3. Comprehension
4. IV–1	5. Nursing Process	6. Moderate

16. A permanent descending colostomy results in which type of discharge?
A. Solid feces.
*B. Semimushy feces.
C. Mushy feces.
D. Liquid feces.

Rationale: With a sigmoid colostomy, feces are solid. With a descending colostomy, feces are semimushy. With a transverse colostomy, feces are mushy. With an ascending colostomy, feces are fluid.

Reference: p. 907

Descriptors:

1. 35	2. 06	3. Comprehension
4. IV–1	5. Nursing Process	6. Moderate

UNIT 8
METABOLIC AND ENDOCRINE FUNCTION

CHAPTER 36
Assessment and Management of Patients with Hepatic and Biliary Disorders

1. The liver uses amino acids from protein breakdown for the metabolic processes of
A. take up of glucose.
B. conversion glucose to glycogen.
C. release of glucose.
*D. synthesis of glucose.

Rationale: Additional glucose can be synthesized by the liver through a process called gluconeogenesis. For this process, the liver uses amino acids from protein breakdown or lactate produced by exercising muscles.

Reference: pp. 920–921

Descriptors:

1. 36	2. 01	3. Comprehension
4. IV–4	5. Nursing Process	6. Moderate

2. Which of the following metabolic functions does the liver fulfill?
A. Conversion of urea into ammonia.
B. Synthesis of gamma globulin.
*C. Breakdown of fatty acids into ketones.
D. Storage of vitamin K.

Rationale: The liver converts metabolically generated ammonia and urea and synthesizes almost all of the plasma proteins *except* gamma globulin. The liver requires Vitamin K for the synthesis of prothrombin and some of the other clotting factors. Breakdown of fatty acids into ketone bodies occurs primarily when the availability of metabolism is limited, as during starvation or in uncontrolled diabetes. Vitamins stored in the liver include A, B_{12}, D, and several of the B-complex vitamins.

Reference: p. 921

Descriptors:
1. 36 2. 02 3. Analysis
4. IV–4 5. Nursing Process 6. Difficult

3. Which of the following statements accurately describes drug metabolism by the liver?
   A. When oral medications absorbed from the GI tract are metabolized to a large extent in the liver, a greater amount of the drug will actually reach the systemic circulation.
   B. The first-pass effect of a drug may indicate that the administration of a drug must be limited to oral administration in small amounts.
   C. All drugs undergo the first-pass effect of the liver.
   *D. Liver metabolism of drugs generally results in loss of activity of the medication.

Rationale: If an oral medication that is absorbed from the GI tract is metabolized by the liver to a great extent before it reaches the systemic circulation (first-pass effect), the amount of drug actually reaching the systemic circulation (oral bioavailability) will be decreased. Some medications have such a large first-pass effect that their use is essentially limited to the parenteral route or oral doses are substantially larger than parenteral doses. Metabolism generally results in loss of activity of the medication, although in some cases activation of the medication may occur.

Reference: p. 921

Descriptors:
1. 36 2. 01 3. Analysis
4. IV–4 5. Nursing Process 6. Difficult

4. Which of the following substances is a pigment derived from the breakdown of hemoglobin?
   A. bile.
   *B. bilirubin.
   C. taurine.
   D. bile salts.

Rationale: Bilirubin is a pigment derived from the breakdown of hemoglobin by cells of the reticuloendothelial system, including the Kupffer cells of the liver. Bile is composed mainly of water and electrolytes. Bile salts are synthesized by the hepatocytes from cholesterol. Taurine is an amino acid.

Reference: p. 922

Descriptors:
1. 36 2. 02 3. Knowledge
4. IV–4 5. Nursing Process 6. Easy

5. The function of the gallbladder is the
   A. synthesis of bile salts.
   *B. storage of bile.
   C. formation of bile.
   D. reabsorption of bile salts.

Rationale: Bile and bile salts are formed in the liver. Bile salts are reabsorbed primarily in the distal ileum. The gallbladder functions as a storage depot for bile.

Reference: p. 923

Descriptors:
1. 36 2. 02 3. Knowledge
4. IV–4 5. Nursing Process 6. Easy

6. Liver function is generally measured in terms of serum
   A. electrolytes
   B. creatinine and BUN
   *C. proteins
   D. antibodies

Rationale: Generally, liver function is measured in terms of serum enzyme activity, serum proteins, bilirubin, ammonia, clotting factors, and lipids.

Reference: p. 923

Descriptors:
1. 36 2. 02 3. Knowledge
4. IV–4 5. Nursing Process 6. Easy

7. When the nurse notes that the patient is demonstrating jaundice, he or she reviews which of the following liver function tests, in particular, as associated clinically with jaundice? Serum
   A. ammonia.
   B. alkaline phosphatase.
   C. albumin/globulin ratio.
   *D. bilirubin.

Rationale: Serum bilirubin (direct and indirect) measures the ability of the liver to conjugate and excrete bilirubin. Results are abnormal in liver and biliary tract disease and are associated clinically with jaundice.

Reference: p. 924

Descriptors:
1. 36 2. 02 3. Comprehension
4. IV–4 5. Nursing Process 6. Moderate

8. The nurse assists the patient to which of the following positions immediately after undergoing a liver biopsy?
   A. On the left side with the head of the bed flat.
   *B. On the right side with a pillow under the costal margin.
   C. On the left side with a pillow under the costal margin.
   D. On the right side with the head of the bed flat.

Rationale: Immediately after the biopsy, the nurse assists the patient to turn onto the right side and places a pillow under the costal margin. In this position, the liver capsule at the site of penetration is compressed against the chest wall, and the escape of blood or bile through the perforation is impeded.

Reference: p. 926

Descriptors:
1. 36 2. 05 3. Application
4. IV–3 5. Nursing Process 6. Difficult

9. Which of the following consequences of liver disease result in marked sodium and fluid retention?
   A. Jaundice.
   B. Nutritional deficiencies.
   *C. Portal hypertension.
   D. Hepatic encephalopathy.

Rationale: Portal hypertension and ascites, resulting from circulatory changes within the disease liver produce severe GI hemorrhages and marked sodium and fluid retention.

Reference: p. 924

Descriptors:
1. 36 2. 03 3. Comprehension
4. IV–4 5. Nursing Process 6. Difficult

10. Which of the following guidelines is indicated when the patient with an impaired liver demonstrates altered nutrition, less than body requirements related to abdominal distention, discomfort, nausea, and anorexia? The nurse instructs the patient to:
   A. eat three, balanced meals per day with supplements
   B. decrease alcohol intake
   C. consume a high protein diet
   *D. apply an ice collar for nausea.

Rationale: In general, patients with impaired liver function become malnourished and are instructed to eat small, more frequent meals (6 per day), eliminate alcohol, restrict protein intake consistent with liver function, and use an ice collar for nausea (may reduce incidence of nausea).

Reference: p. 927

Descriptors:
1. 36 2. 05 3. Application
4. IV–1 5. Teaching/Learning 6. Difficult

11. Which type of hepatitis results in the largest number of deaths among health care workers?
   A. A.
   *B. B.
   C. Drug-induced.
   D. Toxic.

Rationale: Hepatitis B, transmitted through contaminated body fluids, is responsible for the largest numbers of deaths of health care workers annually.

Reference: pp. 942–943

Descriptors:
1. 36 2. 04 3. Knowledge
4. IV–3 5. Nursing Process 6. Easy

12. Of the following clinical manifestations, which will indicate to the nurse that the patient is demonstrating compensated cirrhosis?
   A. Muscle wasting.
   *B. Continuous mild fever.
   C. Purpura.
   D. Clubbing of fingers.

Rationale: In compensated cirrhosis, the patient demonstrates intermittent mild fever, while in decompensated disease the fever is continuous. The decompensated cirrhosis also demonstrates purpura, clubbing of fingers, and muscle wasting.

Reference: p. 947

Descriptors:
1. 36 2. 05 3. Application
4. IV–4 5. Nursing Process 6. Difficult

13. The nurse recognizes which of the following symptoms, in addition to pain, as an early manifestation of liver malignancy?
   A. Continuous dull ache in the left upper quadrant, epigastrium, or back.
   B. Weight gain.
   *C. Anemia.
   D. Jaundice.

Rationale: The early manifestations of malignancy of the liver include pain, a continuous dull ache in the right upper quadrant epigastrium, or back. Weight loss, anorexia, and anemia may occur. Jaundice is present only if the larger bile ducts are occluded by the pressure of malignant nodules in the hilum of the liver.

Reference: p. 957

Descriptors:
1. 36 2. 07 3. Analysis
4. IV–4 5. Nursing Process 6. Moderate

14. The nurse anticipates that which of the following therapies will most likely be the initial mode of therapy for the nonsurgical treatment of the patient with bleeding esophageal varices?
   *A. Pharmacologic.
   B. Balloon tamponade.
   C. Endoscopic sclerotherapy.
   D. Esophageal banding.

Rationale: Pharmacologic therapy with vasopressin (Pitressin) may be the initial mode of nonsurgical therapy in the patient with bleeding esophageal varices because it produces constriction of the splanchnic arterial bed and a resulting decrease in portal pressure.

Reference: p. 952

Descriptors:
1. 36 2. 06 3. Application
4. I–1 5. Nursing Process 6. Moderate

15. Of the following instructions given to the patient who has undergone liver transplant, the nurse recognizes that the MOST important is

A. the measurement of drainage from the T-tube.
B. the need for follow-up blood work.
*C. to ensure an adequate supply of medication at all times.
D. to monitor for signs of liver dysfunction.

Rationale: The patient is given written as well as verbal instructions about how and when to take the medications and is instructed to take steps to be sure that an adequate supply of medication is available so that there is NO CHANCE of running out of the medication or skipping a dose. Failure to take medications as instructed may precipitate rejection.

Reference: p. 961

Descriptors:

1. 36	2. 08	3. Analysis
4. IV–3	5. Teaching/Learning	6. Difficult

CHAPTER 37
Assessment and Management of Patients with Diabetes Mellitus

1. In Type 1 Insulin-dependent diabetes mellitus (IDDM), the patient demonstrates
   *A. need for insulin for life.
   B. obesity at diagnosis.
   C. no islet cell antibodies.
   D. rare ketosis.

Rationale: Individuals with IDDM demonstrate the following characteristics: onset at any age, but usually young (< 30 years); thin at diagnosis with recent weight loss; islet cell antibodies (often); little or no endogenous insulin; need insulin to preserve life; ketosis-prone when insulin is absent.

Reference: pp. 976–977

Descriptors:

1. 37	2. 01	3. Comprehension
4. IV–1	5. Nursing Process	6. Moderate

2. Which of the following characteristics is associated with development Type 2 diabetes mellitus (NIDDM)?
   *A. Obesity.
   B. Immunologic factors.
   C. Viral diseases.
   D. Pancreatic disease.

Rationale: Obesity is the characteristic associated with Type 2 (NIDDM) along with heredity or environmental factors. Type 1 (IDDM) is associated with immunologic, genetic, and environmental (viral) factors. Secondary diabetes is associated with pancreatic disease.

Reference: p. 976

Descriptors:

1. 37	2. 02	3. Knowledge
4. IV–4	5. Nursing Process	6. Moderate

3. Of the following clinical manifestations of diabetes mellitus, which results from the catabolic state induced by insulin deficiency?
   A. Polydipsia.
   B. Polyurea.
   *C. Polyphagia.
   D. Sudden vision changes.

Rationale: Polyuria and polydipsia occur as a result of the excess loss of fluid associated with osmotic diuresis. Polyphagia results from the catabolic state induced by insulin deficiency and the breakdown of proteins and fats. Sudden vision changes result from the elevated level of glucose in the blood.

Reference: p. 979

Descriptors:

1. 37	2. 03	3. Analysis
4. IV–4	5. Nursing Process	6. Difficult

4. A diagnosis of diabetes mellitus is made in the evaluation of the patient who demonstrates which of the following criteria?
   *A. Fasting plasma glucose greater than or equal to 126 mg/dL.
   B. 2-hour postload glucose greater than 126 mg/dL.
   C. Fasting plasma glucose greater than 200 mg/dL.
   D. Casual plasma glucose greater than 126 mg/dL.

Rationale: Criteria for the diagnosis of diabetes mellitus include symptoms of diabetes plus casual plasma glucose greater than or equal to 200 mg/dL, fasting plasma glucose greater than or equal to 126 mg/dL, or 2-hour postload glucose greater than or equal to 200 mg/dL.

Reference: p. 979

Descriptors:

1. 37	2. 04	3. Analysis
4. I–1	5. Nursing Process	6. Difficult

5. The nurse teaches the newly diagnosed, diet-controlled patient with diabetes mellitus which of the following general guidelines?
   A. The calorie distribution is usually higher in protein than in carbohydrates and fats.
   B. Complex carbohydrates must be eaten in moderation.
   *C. Once converted during digestion, approximately 50% of protein foods are converted to glucose.
   D. Dietary cholesterol should be limited to 500 mg/day.

Rationale: In general, calorie distribution recommended is higher in carbohydrates than in fat and protein, and all carbohydrates should be eaten in moderation to avoid high postprandial blood glucose levels. While 100% of carbohydrates are converted to blood glucose during digestion, 50% of proteins (meat, fish, and poultry) are also converted to glucose. Dietary cholesterol should be limited to 300 mg/day.

Reference: pp. 981–982

Descriptors:
1. 37 2. 05 3. Application
4. IV–3 5. Teaching/Learning 6. Difficult

6. The nurse teaches the newly diagnosed patient with diabetes mellitus which of the following general guidelines regarding exercise? Exercise
   A. increases blood glucose.
   B. decreases levels of high-density lipoproteins.
   *C. decreases the body's need for insulin.
   D. increases total cholesterol and triglyceride levels.

Rationale: Exercise lowers blood glucose, increases levels of HDLs, and decreases total cholesterol and triglyceride levels. The physiologic decrease in circulating insulin that normally occurs with exercise cannot occur in patients treated with insulin, and hypoglycemia many hours after exercise can occur. In addition, it may be necessary to have the patient reduce the dosage of insulin that peaks at the time of exercise.

Reference: p. 984

Descriptors:
1. 37 2. 06 3. Application
4. IV–4 5. Teaching/Learning 6. Difficult

7. Which of the following types of insulins is the MOST rapidly acting?
   *A. Humalog.
   B. Regular.
   C. NPH.
   D. Ultralente.

Rationale: Humalog's onset of action is 10–15 minutes, while regular insulin acts in 1/2 to 1 hour. NPH acts in 3–4 hours, and ultralente acts in 6–8 hours.

Reference: p. 987

Descriptors:
1. 37 2. 07 3. Knowledge
4. IV–2 5. Nursing Process 6. Moderate

8. The nurse teaches and practices which of the following general guidelines related to care of insulin?
   A. Insulin may be stored in the freezer until needed.
   *B. If a vial of insulin will be used up in 1 month, it may be kept at room temperature.
   C. Longer-acting insulins should be shaken vigorously before use.
   D. A frosted, whitish coating inside the bottle of intermediate- or longer-acting insulins is common and acceptable.

Rationale: Extremes of temperature are to be avoided when storing insulin. If a vial will be used up in one month, it may be stored at room temperature. Longer-acting insulins must be gently inverted or rolled in the hands before use. If the patient notes a frosted, adherent coating in the vial, some of the insulin is bound and should not be used.

Reference: p. 999

Descriptors:
1. 37 2. 07 3. Application
4. IV–2 5. Nursing Process 6. Moderate

9. Which of the following categories of oral antidiabetic agents exert their primary action by directly stimulating the pancreas to secrete insulin?
   *A. Sulfonylureas.
   B. Biguanides.
   C. Thiazolidinediones.
   D. Alpha glucosidase inhibitors.

Rationale: Sulfonylureas exert their primary action by directly stimulating the pancreas to secrete insulin and therefore require a functioning pancreas to be effective. Biguanides facilitate insulin's action on peripheral receptor sites. Thiazolidinediones enhance insulin action at the receptor site without increasing insulin secretion from the beta cells of the pancreas. Alpha glucosidase inhibitors work by delaying the absorption of glucose in the intestinal system, resulting in a lower postprandial blood glucose level.

Reference: p. 993

Descriptors:
1. 37 2. 08 3. Comprehension
4. IV–2 5. Nursing Process 6. Difficult

10. Which of the following categories of oral antidiabetic agents exert their primary action by facilitating insulin's action on peripheral receptor sites?
   A. Sulfonylureas.
   *B. Biguanides.
   C. Meglitinides.
   D. Alpha glucosidase inhibitors.

Rationale: Sulfonylureas exert their primary action by directly stimulating the pancreas to secrete insulin and therefore require a functioning pancreas to be effective. Biguanides facilitate insulin's action on peripheral receptor sites. Meglitinides lower the blood glucose by stimulating the release of insulin from the beta cells of the pancreas. Alpha glucosidase inhibitors work by delaying the absorption of glucose in the intestinal system, resulting in a lower postprandial blood glucose level.

Reference: pp. 993–994

Descriptors:
1. 37 2. 08 3. Comprehension
4. IV–2 5. Nursing Process 6. Difficult

11. Which of the following categories of oral antidiabetic agents exert their primary action by delaying the absorption of glucose in the intestinal system?
    A. Sulfonylureas.
    B. Biguanides.
    C. Thiazolidinediones.
    *D. Alpha glucosidase inhibitors.

Rationale: Sulfonylureas exert their primary action by directly stimulating the pancreas to secrete insulin and therefore require a functioning pancreas to be effective. Biguanides facilitate insulin's action on peripheral receptor sites. Thiazolidinediones enhance insulin action at the receptor site without increasing insulin secretion from the beta cells of the pancreas. Alpha glucosidase inhibitors work by delaying the absorption of glucose in the intestinal system, resulting in a lower postprandial blood glucose level.

Reference: p. 994

Descriptors:
1. 37 2. 08 3. Comprehension
4. IV–2 5. Nursing Process 6. Difficult

12. When the patient informs the nurse that he is experiencing hypoglycemia, the nurse provides immediate treatment by providing
    A. one (1) commercially prepared glucose tablet.
    B. two (2) hard candies (e.g., Life Savers).
    C. 4 to 6 ounces of fruit juice with (1) teaspoon of sugar added.
    *D. 2 to 3 teaspoons of honey.

Rationale: The usual recommendation for treatment of hypoglycemia is for 10 to 15 grams of a fast-acting, simple carbohydrate orally, such as 3 or 4 commercially prepared glucose tablets; 4 to 6 oz of fruit juice or regular soda; 6 to 10 Life Savers or other hard candies; or 2 to 3 teaspoons of sugar or honey. It is unnecessary to add sugar to juice, even it if is labeled as unsweetened juice, because the fruit sugar in juice contains enough simple carbohydrate to raise the blood glucose level and addition of sugar may result in a sharp rise in blood sugar that will last for several hours.

Reference: p. 1004

Descriptors:
1. 37 2. 09 3. Application
4. IV–4 5. Nursing Process 6. Difficult

13. The nurse teaches the person with diabetes which of the following guidelines to follow during periods of illness ("sick day rules")?
    A. Do not take oral antidiabetic agent or insulin while sick.
    B. Report elevated glucose levels greater than 126 mg/dL
    *C. If vomiting, diarrhea, or fever persists, take 1/2 cup regular cola or orange juice every 1/2 to 1 hour.
    D. If nauseated, do not eat solid foods.

Rationale: The most important issue to teach patients with diabetes who become ill is NOT to eliminate insulin doses when nausea and vomiting occur. Rather, they should take their usual insulin or oral hypoglycemic agent dose, and then attempt to consume frequent small portions of food. In general, blood sugar levels will rise but should be reported if they are greater than 300 mg/dL.

Reference: p. 1006

Descriptors:
1. 37 2. 10
3. Application/Analysis 4. IV–1
5. Teaching/Learning 6. Difficult

14. Which of the following complications of diabetes is termed "microvascular"?
    A. Myocardial infarction (MI).
    B. Cerebral vascular accident (CVA).
    *C. Retinopathy.
    D. Peripheral neuropathy.

Rationale: MI and CVA are considered macrovascular complications of diabetes mellitus, while peripheral neuropathy is related the effects of elevated blood glucose levels over a period of years directly affecting the nerves. Microvascular complications include diabetic retinopathy and nephropathy.

Reference: p. 1012

Descriptors:
1. 37 2. 11 3. Analysis
4. IV–4 5. Nursing Process 6. Moderate

15. The nurse teaches the patient which of the following general guidelines regarding foot care?
    A. Wash your feet in hot water every day.
    B. Rub a thin coat of lotion between your toes.
    C. Walk barefoot only at the beach.
    *D. Feel the inside of your shoes with your hands before putting your feet into the shoes.

Rationale: Feet should be washed in warm water, and lotion should be applied to the tops and bottoms of the feet, but not between the toes. The patient should NEVER walk barefoot. Because of decreased sensation associated with peripheral neuropathy, the patient must be certain that the lining is smooth and that there are not objects in the shoes prior to wearing.

Reference: p. 1018

Descriptors:
1. 37 2. 13 3. Application
4. IV–1 5. Teaching/Learning 6. Moderate

CHAPTER 38
Assessment and Management of Patients with Endocrine Disorders

1. Which of the following hormones is secreted by the POSTERIOR pituitary gland?
   A. Growth hormone.
   B. Thyroid stimulating hormone.
   *C. Antidiuretic hormone.
   D. Adrenocorticotropic hormone.

Rationale: Antidiuretic hormone (vasopressin) and oxytocin are the only two hormones secreted by the posterior pituitary. The anterior pituitary secretes growth hormone, TSH, ACTH, FSH, LH, prolactin, melanocyte-stimulating hormone, and beta lipotropin.

Reference: p. 1030

Descriptors:
1. 38 2. 01 3. Knowledge
4. IV–2 5. Nursing Process 6. Easy

2. The nurse explains to the patient undergoing a hormone stimulation test that
   A. if the endocrine gland responds to the stimulation, endocrine problems are ruled out.
   B. if the endocrine gland fails to respond to the stimulation, problems with the particular endocrine gland stimulated are ruled out.
   *C. stimulation tests may be used to determine how an endocrine gland responds to the administration of stimulating hormones that are normally produced by the pituitary gland.
   D. stimulation tests are used to evaluate negative feedback mechanisms.

Rationale: If the endocrine gland responds to the stimulation, the specific disorder may be in the hypothalamus or pituitary (still endocrine-related problem), while if the gland fails to response, it may indicate the problem as being in the gland itself. Stimulation tests may be used to determine how an endocrine gland responds to pituitary- or hypothalamus-secreted hormones. Suppression tests are used to evaluate negative feedback mechanisms.

Reference: p. 1031

Descriptors:
1. 38 2. 02
3. Application/Analysis 4. IV–4
5. Teaching/Learning 6. Difficult

3. The nurse assesses the patient with Hashimoto's thyroiditis for which of the following clinical manifestations, typical of hypothyroidism?
   *A. Extreme fatigue.
   B. Emotional hyperexcitability.
   C. Palpitations.
   D. Flushed skin.

Rationale: Symptoms of hypothyroidism include extreme fatigue; reports of hair loss, brittle nails, dry skin; voice huskiness or hoarseness; menstrual disturbance; and numbness and tingling of the fingers.

Reference: p. 1038

Descriptors:
1. 38 2. 03 3. Comprehension
4. IV–4 5. Nursing Process 6. Easy

4. Which of the following terms is used to refer to a form of hyperthyroidism characterized by a diffuse goiter and exophthalmos?
   A. Addison's disease.
   B. Cushing's syndrome.
   *C. Graves' disease.
   D. Myxedema.

Rationale: Addisons's disease is characterized by chronic adrenocortical insufficiency secondary to destruction of the adrenal glands, while Cushing's syndrome is a group of symptoms produced by an excess of free circulating cortisol from the adrenal cortex. Grave's disease is a form of hyperthyroidism characterized by a diffuse goiter and exophthalmos and is also called Basedow's or Parry's disease. Myxedema is a severe form of hypothyroidism.

Reference: p. 1027–1028

Descriptors:
1. 38 2. 03 3. Comprehension
4. IV–4 5. Nursing Process 6. Moderate

5. Which of the following positions is the most comfortable for the patient post thyroidectomy?
   A. Side-lying (lateral) with one pillow under the head.
   B. Head of the bed elevated 30 degrees and no pillows placed under the head.
   *C. Semi-Fowler's with the head supported on two pillows.
   D. High-Fowler's with no pillows placed under the head.

Rationale: Semi-Fowler's position with head elevated and supported by pillows is believed to provide the most comfort and least tension on the suture line.

Reference: p. 1051

Descriptors:
1. 38 2. 04
3. Application/Analysis 4. IV–1
5. Nursing Process 6. Difficult

6. Increased secretion of parathormone results in
   A. increase of blood phosphorus level.
   B. decrease of blood calcium level.
   C. decreased calcium absorption from the kidney.
   *D. increased calcium absorption from the bones.

Rationale: Increased secretion of parathormone results in increased calcium absorption from the kidney, the intestines, and bones, thereby raising the blood calcium level. Parathormone also tends to lower the blood phosphorus level.

Reference: p. 1052

Descriptors:
1. 38 2. 05 3. Comprehension
4. IV–4 5. Nursing Process 6. Moderate

7. The nurse anticipates acute hypoparathyroidism in the care of the postoperative care of the patient who has undergone
*A. thyroidectomy.
B. fractured hip plating and nailing.
C. gastric resection.
D. pelvic surgery.

Rationale: Care of postoperative patients having thyroidectomy, parathyroidectomy, and radical neck dissection is directed toward detecting early signs of hypoparathyroidsm and subsequent hypocalcemia and anticipating signs of tetany, seizures, and respiratory difficulties.

Reference: p. 1054

Descriptors:
1. 38 2. 05
3. Application/Analysis 4. IV–3
5. Nursing Process 6. Difficult

8. The patient with Addison's disease likely will demonstrate:
A. truncal obesity
B. hypertension
*C. dark pigmentation of the skin
D. abdominal striae

Rationale: Patient's with Addison's disease demonstrate muscular weakness, anorexia, gastrointestinal symptoms, fatigue, emaciation and dark pigmentation of the skin, and hypotension. Patient's with Cushing's syndrome demonstrate truncal obesity, "moon" face, acne, abdominal striae, and hypertension.

Reference: p. 1058

Descriptors:
1. 38 2. 06 3. Comprehension
4. IV–4 5. Nursing Process 6. Moderate

9. When teaching the patient with Addison's disease about hormone replacement, the nurse instructs that TOO HIGH a dose may be indicated by
*A. weight gain.
B. dizziness on standing.
C. increase in systolic blood pressure.
D. lightheadedness.

Rationale: The development of edema or weight gain may signify too high a dose of hormone; postural hypotension (decrease in systolic blood pressure, lightheadedness, dizziness on standing) and weight loss may indicate too low a dose.

Reference: p. 1059

Descriptors:
1. 38 2. 07 3. Application
4. IV–3 5. Teaching/Learning 6. Easy

10. The nurse teaches the patient who is prescribed corticosteroid therapy that
A. her diet should be low protein with ample fat.
B. her changes in appearance are permanent.
C. she is resistant to infection.
*D. she is at risk for development of thrombophlebitis and thromboembolism.

Rationale: The cardiovascular effects of corticosteroid therapy may result in development of thrombophlebitis or thromboembolism. Diet should be high protein with limited fat. Changes in appearance usually disappear when therapy is no longer necessary. The patient is at increased risk of infection and masking of signs of infection.

Reference: p. 1066

Descriptors:
1. 38 2. 09 3. Application
4. IV–3 5. Teaching/Learning 6. Moderate

11. The major symptom of pancreatitis that brings the patient to medical care is
A. jaundice.
B. extreme fatigue.
*C. severe abdominal pain.
D. hypoglycemia.

Rationale: Severe abdominal pain is the major symptom of pancreatitis that brings the patient to medical care. Abdominal pain and tenderness and back pain result from irritation and edema of the inflamed pancreas that stimulate nerve endings.

Reference: p. 1068

Descriptors:
1. 38 2. 10 3. Comprehension
4. IV–4 5. Nursing Process 6. Moderate

12. When the physician prescribes morphine sulfate injections for the relief of pain associated with acute pancreatitis, the nurse's FIRST action is to
A. assess the patient for allergy.
B. assess the patient's pain level and respiratory rate.
C. administer the medication prior to report of severe pain.
*D. verify the order with the physician.

Rationale: Meperidine (Demerol) is the medication of choice to treat the pain of the patient with acute pancreatitis. Morphine sulfate is avoided because it causes spasms of the sphincter of Oddi.

Reference: p. 1070

Descriptors:
1. 38 2. 10 3. Application
4. IV–2 5. Nursing Process 6. Moderate

13. Which of the following statements, if made by the patient (post acute pancreatitis) to the nurse, would indicate to the nurse that expected outcomes of teaching have been met? "I will:
   A. limit my intake of alcohol."
   B. include high-protein foods in my diet."
   *C. measure my waist daily."
   D. eat three, full meals a day."

Rationale: In general, the patient should report that he will eliminate alcohol intake, eat high-carbohydrate, low-protein foods, and avoid heavy meals. The patient learns to measure his girth to quickly detect signs of complications.

Reference: p. 1071

Descriptors:
1. 38 2. 10 3. Analysis
4. IV–1 5. Nursing Process 6. Moderate

14. To reduce the stimulation of the pancreas in the patient with acute pancreatitis, the nurse plans which of the following interventions?
   A. Administration of meperidine (Demerol).
   B. Providing ice chips.
   C. Ambulating the patient each shift.
   *D. Using continuous nasogastric drainage.

Rationale: Anticholinergic drugs are used to reduce gastric and pancreatic secetion, while Demerol is used to treat the pain associated with acute pancreatitis. ALL oral intake is withheld, and the paint is maintained on bedrest. Nasogastric suction removes gastric contents and prevents gastric secretions from entering the duodenum and stimulating the secreting mechanism.

Reference: p. 1072

Descriptors:
1. 38 2. 10 3. Analysis
4. IV–1 5. Nursing Process 6. Difficult

15. The nurse instructs the patient who is undergoing diagnostic testing for chronic pancreatitis that the most useful study is the
   A. computerized tomography (CT) scan.
   B. ultrasound.
   *C. endoscopic retrograde cholepancreatography (ERCP).
   D. glucose tolerance test.

Rationale: ERCP is the most useful study in the diagnosis of chronic pancreatitis because it provides detail about the anatomy of the pancreas and of the pancreatic and biliary ducts. CT scan or ultrasound is helpful to detect the presence of pancreatic cysts. A glucose tolerance test evaluates pancreatic islet cell function, information necessary for making decisions about surgical resection of the pancreas.

Reference: p. 1074

Descriptors:
1. 38 2. 10 3. Application
4. IV–4 5. Teaching/Learning 6. Moderate

UNIT 9
URINARY AND RENAL FUNCTION

CHAPTER 39
Assessment of Urinary and Renal Function

1. When the kidneys are functioning normally, which of the statements accurately reflects the kidneys' regulation of electrolyte excretion? The volume of
   A. sodium chloride excreted will exceed the volume of potassium chloride excreted.
   B. potassium chloride excreted will exceed the volume of sodium chloride excreted.
   *C. electrolytes excreted per day is exactly equal to the amount ingested.
   D. potassium chloride and sodium chloride excreted will be less than the amount ingested.

Rationale: When the kidneys are functioning normally, the volume of electrolytes excreted per day is exactly equal to the amount ingested.

Reference: p. 1087

Descriptors:
1. 39 2. 01 3. Comprehension
4. IV–4 5. Nursing Process 6. Moderate

2. Which of the following substances is released from specialized cells in the kidney?
   A. Aldosterone.
   B. Angiotensin I.
   C. Angiotensin II.
   *D. Renin.

Rationale: Release of aldosterone from the adrenal cortex is largely under the control of angiotensin II. Angiotensin II levels are in turn controlled by renin, an enzyme that is released from special cells in the kidneys.

Reference: p. 1088

Descriptors:
1. 39 2. 01 3. Knowledge
4. IV–4 5. Nursing Process 6. Easy

3. Which of the following changes results in activation of the renin-angiotensin system?
   *A. Fall in renal arteriole blood pressure below normal.
   B. Increased sodium chloride delivery to the tubules.
   C. Retention of water.
   D. Expansion of intravascular volume.

Rationale: The renin-angiotensin system is activated when pressure in the renal arterioles falls below normal levels, as occurs with shock and dehydration, or when there is decreased sodium chloride delivery to the tubules. Activation of this system increases the retention of water and expansion of intravascular volume.

Reference: p. 1088

Descriptors:
1. 39 2. 01 3. Analysis
4. IV–4 5. Nursing Process 6. Moderate

4. The nurse recognizes that a urine specific gravity of 1.030 indicates
   A. a normal value.
   *B. an abnormal–high value.
   C. an abnormal–low value.
   D. dilute urine.

Rationale: Normal urine specific gravity is 1.010 to 1.025 when fluid intake is normal. The specific gravity of water is 1.000. Therefore, the closer the urine specific gravity to 1.000, the more dilute the urine.

Reference: p. 1088

Descriptors:
1. 39 2. 02 3. Knowledge
4. IV–1 5. Nursing Process 6. Moderate

5. Which of the following terms is used to indicate total urine output of less than 50 mL in 24 hours?
   *A. Anuria.
   B. Oliguria.
   C. Dysuria.
   D. Polyuria.

Rationale: Anuria refers to total urine output less than 50 mL in 24 hours, while oliguria refers to total urine output less than 400 mL in 24 hours. Dysuria refers to painful urination, and polyuria refers to frequent urination.

Reference: p. 1091

Descriptors:
1. 39 2. 02 3. Comprehension
4. IV–4 5. Nursing Process 6. Easy

6. Which of the following terms is used to indicate total urine output of less than 400 mL in 24 hours?
   A. Anuria.
   *B. Oliguria.
   C. Dysuria.
   D. Polyuria.

Rationale: Anuria refers to total urine output less than 50 mL in 24 hours, while oliguria refers to total urine output less than 400 mL in 24 hours. Dysuria refers to painful urination and polyuria refers to frequent urination.

Reference: p. 1091

Descriptors:
1. 39 2. 02 3. Comprehension
4. IV–4 5. Nursing Process 6. Easy

7. When the patient who is collecting a 24-hour urine specimen asks the nurse what the test will show, the nurse informs that patient the test
   A. evaluates the ability of the kidneys to concentrate solutes in urine.
   B. evaluates hydration status.
   *C. detects and evaluates progression of renal disease.
   D. serves as an index of renal function.

Rationale: The urine specific gravity evaluates concentration abilities of the kidneys, while the BUN-to-creatinine ratio evaluates hydration status. The 24-hour creatinine clearance test measures volume of blood cleared of endogenous creatinine in 1 minute, which provides an approximation of the glomerular filtration rate and is a sensitive indicator of renal disease. The blood urea nitrogen value serves as an index of renal function.

Reference: p. 1094

Descriptors:
1. 39 2. 02 3. Application
4. IV–4 5. Nursing Process 6. Difficult

8. Which of the following statements reflects accurate instruction regarding nursing care of the patient post kidney biopsy? The patient will be
   A. kept in a supine position immediately after biopsy.
   B. ambulated 4 hours after biopsy.
   C. observed closely for signs of infection.
   *D. asked to save his urine for comparison to prebiopsy specimens.

Rationale: All urine voided by the patient post kidney biopsy is inspected for evidence of bleeding and compared with the prebiopsy specimen and subsequent voiding specimens. The patient is kept in a prone position, on bedrest for 6 to 8 hours to minimize the risk of hemorrhage.

Reference: p. 1097

Descriptors:
1. 39 2. 04 3. Application
4. IV–3 5. Nursing Process 6. Moderate

9. A nurse instructs the patient preparing to undergo urodynamic testing that
   A. "Only one catheter will be placed at a time for measurement."
   *B. "You may have electrodes placed in the perianal area for electromyography."
   C. "Your bladder will be filled only at the beginning of the procedure."
   D. "You must not cough during the procedure."

Rationale: During the procedure, several catheters may be placed at one time; electrodes may be used to assess perianal muscle functioning; the patient may be asked to cough or perform a Valsalva maneuver. The bladder will be filled through the urethral catheter one or more times during the procedure.

Reference: p. 1098

Descriptors:
1. 39 2. 04 3. Application
4. IV–1 5. Nursing Process 6. Difficult

10. A nurse teaches the patient who has undergone urodynamic testing to report which of the following signs or symptoms to the physician immediately?
 A. Slight hematuria.
 B. Urinary frequency.
 C. Urgency.
 *D. Chills.

Rationale: Hematuria, urinary frequency, urgency, and dysuria are expected abnormals. Chills, fever, lower back pain, or continued dysuria or hematuria should be reported to the physician because they may indicate onset of a urinary tract infection.

Reference: p. 1098

Descriptors:
1. 39 2. 04 3. Application
4. IV–1 5. Teaching/Learning 6. Moderate

11. When the kidneys sense a decrease in the oxygen tension in the blood flow, they release which of the following hormones?
 A. Antidiuretic.
 *B. Erythropoietin.
 C. Renin.
 D. Angiotensin.

Rationale: When the kidneys sense a decrease in the oxygen tension in renal blood flow, they release erythropoietin. Erythropoietin stimulates the bone marrow to produce red blood cells, thereby increasing the amount of hemoglobin available to carry oxygen.

Reference: p. 1089

Descriptors:
1. 39 2. 01 3. Knowledge
4. IV–4 5. Nursing Process 6. Moderate

12. Normally, residual urine amounts to no more than
 A. 30 cc.
 *B. 50 cc.
 C. 100 cc.
 D. 150 cc.

Rationale: Normally, residual urine (urine left in the bladder after voiding) amounts to no more than 50 mL.

Reference: p. 1089

Descriptors:
1. 39 2. 02 3. Knowledge
4. IV–4 5. Nursing Process 6. Easy

13. A nurse advises the patient that he or she may experience which of the following sensations as an expected abnormal reaction when the contrast agent is injected during the patient's planned intravenous pyelogram. "You may
 A. begin to breathe faster."
 B. feel your heart racing."
 *C. experience an unusual seafood taste sensation in the mouth."
 D. become very drowsy."

Rationale: Expected abnormal experiences for the patient during urologic testing with contrast agents include a temporary feeling of warmth, flushing of the face, and an unusual taste (seafood) sensation in the mouth when the contrast agent is infused. Any other untoward symptoms must be considered a potential anaphylactoid reaction to the contrast agent.

Reference: p. 1095

Descriptors:
1. 39 2. 04 3. Application
4. IV–3 5. Nursing Process 6. Moderate

14. A nurse anticipates that a laxative may be prescribed for the patient undergoing which of the following urologic diagnostic tests?
 A. Magnetic resonance imaging.
 B. Computerized tomography scanning.
 C. Cytoscopy.
 *D. Renal angiography.

Rationale: Before the procedure, a laxative may be prescribed to evacuate the colon so that unobstructed radiographs may be obtained by renal angiography.

Reference: p. 1096

Descriptors:
1. 39 2. 04 3. Comprehension
4. IV–1 5. Nursing Process 6. Moderate

15. In 24 hours, the average person voids how many mL of urine?
 A. 1000 mL.
 *B. 1200–1500 mL.
 C. 1800–2000 mL.
 D. 2500–3000 mL.

Rationale: The average person voids 1200–1500 mL of urine in 24 hours, although this varies depending on fluid intake, sweating, environmental temperature, vomiting, or diarrhea.

Reference: p. 1090

Descriptors:
1. 39 2. 02 3. Knowledge
4. IV–4 5. Nursing Process 6. Easy

CHAPTER 40
Management of Patients with Urinary and Renal Dysfunction

1. The most accurate indicator of fluid loss or gain in an acutely ill patient is
   A. intake and output measurements.
   B. hematocrit.
   *C. weight.
   D. blood pressure.

   Rationale: The most accurate indicator of fluid loss or gain in an acutely ill patient is weight. An accurate daily weight must be obtained and recorded. A one (1) kilogram weight gain is equal to 1,000 mL of retained fluid.

   Reference: p. 1102

   Descriptors:
   1. 40 2. 07 3. Analysis
   4. IV–4 5. Nursing Process 6. Difficult

2. Which of the following terms refers to incontinence that results from cognitive or physical impairments that make it difficult or impossible for the patient to reach the toilet in time for voiding?
   A. Stress incontinence.
   B. Reflex incontinence.
   C. Overflow incontinence.
   *D. Functional incontinence.

   Rationale: Stress incontinence is the involuntary loss of urine through an intact urethra as a result of sudden increase in intra-abdominal pressure. Reflex incontinence is loss of urine due to hyperreflexia or involuntary urethral relaxation in the absence of normal sensations usually associated with voiding. Overflow incontinence is an involuntary urine loss associated with overdistension of the bladder. Functional incontinence refers to those instances in which the function of the lower urinary tract is intact, but other factors (outside the urinary system) make it difficult or impossible for the patient to reach the toilet in time for voiding).

   Reference: p. 1105

   Descriptors:
   1. 40 2. 03 3. Comprehension
   4. IV–4 5. Nursing Process 6. Moderate

3. Which of the following terms refers to incontinence that results from a sudden increase in intra-abdominal pressure?
   *A. Stress incontinence.
   B. Reflex incontinence.
   C. Overflow incontinence.
   D. Functional incontinence.

   Rationale: Stress incontinence is the involuntary loss of urine through an intact urethra as a result of sudden increase in intra-abdominal pressure. Reflex incontinence is loss of urine due to hyperreflexia or involuntary urethral relaxation in the absence of normal sensations usually associated with voiding. Overflow incontinence is an involuntary urine loss associated with overdistension of the bladder. Functional incontinence refers to those instances in which the function of the lower urinary tract is intact, but other factors (outside the urinary system) make it difficult or impossible for the patient to reach the toilet in time for voiding).

   Reference: p. 1105

   Descriptors:
   1. 40 2. 03 3. Comprehension
   4. IV–4 5. Nursing Process 6. Moderate

4. The nurse teaches the patient which of the following general strategies to manage urinary incontinence?
   A. Void hourly.
   B. Use Nutrasweet (aspartame) in place of sugar.
   C. Restrict fluid intake.
   *D. Avoid taking diuretics after 4 pm.

   Rationale: The patient should be taught to void regularly (about every 2 to 3 hours); avoid bladder irritants, such as caffeine, alcohol, or aspartame; drink adequate fluids; and avoid taking diuretics after 4 pm.

   Reference: p. 1107

   Descriptors:
   1. 40 2. 03 3. Application
   4. IV–1 5. Teaching/Learning 6. Easy

5. Which of the following actions is appropriate to prevent urinary infection in the patient with a closed urinary drainage system?
   A. Vigorously clean the meatus daily.
   B. Rotate the taped placement of the catheter bag daily.
   C. Disconnect the tubing using aseptic technique.
   *D. Empty the collection bag at least every 8 hours.

   Rationale: Vigorous cleaning of the meatus while the catheter is in place is discouraged because the cleaning action can move the catheter to and fro, increasing the risk of infection. The catheter is anchored as securely as possible to prevent it from moving in the urethra. The tubing should NEVER be disconnected. The collection bag should be emptied at least every 8 hours or more frequently, if indicated.

   Reference: p. 1110

   Descriptors:
   1. 40 2. 02 3. Application
   4. IV–3 5. Nursing Process 6. Moderate

6. Which of the following actions are appropriate to prevent urinary infection in the patient with a closed urinary drainage system?
   *A. Gently clean the meatus daily.
   B. Rotate the taped placement of the catheter bag daily.

C. Disconnect the tubing using aseptic technique.
D. Empty the collection bag at least every 4 hours.

Rationale: Vigorous cleaning of the meatus while the catheter is in place is discouraged because the cleaning action can move the catheter to and fro, increasing the risk of infection. The catheter is anchored as securely as possible to prevent it from moving in the urethra. The tubing should NEVER be disconnected. The collection bag should be emptied at least every 8 hours or more frequently, if indicated.

Reference: p. 1108

Descriptors:

1. 40	2. 02	3. Application
4. IV–3	5. Nursing Process	6. Moderate

7. The most common cause of incontinence in patients who self-catheterize is a mismatch between
*A. high fluid intake and infrequent catheterization.
B. high fluid intake and frequent catheterization.
C. low fluid intake and infrequent catheterization.
D. low fluid intake and frequent catheterization.

Rationale: The most common cause of incontinence in patients who self-catheterize is a mismatch between high fluid intake and infrequent catheterization.

Reference: p. 1110

Descriptors:

1. 40	2. 04	3. Knowledge
4. IV–4	5. Nursing Process	6. Easy

8. The nurse teaches the male patient to use which penile position for self-catheterization?
A. Hold the penis parallel to the body, with the glans penis directed downward.
*B. Hold the penis at a right angle to the body.
C. Hold the penis parallel to the body, with the glans penis directed upward.
D. Hold the penis at a 45-degree angle to the body.

Rationale: The male patient should be taught to hold the penis at a right angle to the body since this maneuver straightens the urethra and makes it easier to insert the catheter.

Reference: p. 1111

Descriptors:

1. 40	2. 04	3. Application
4. IV–1	5. Nursing Process	6. Moderate

9. Which method of dialysis is the most commonly used?
*A. Hemodialysis.
B. Continuous renal replacement therapy.
C. Continuous arteriovenous hemofiltration.
D. Continuous ambulatory peritoneal dialysis.

Rationale: Hemodialysis is the most commonly used method of dialysis.

Reference: p. 1112

Descriptors:

1. 40	2. 05	3. Knowledge
4. IV–9	5. Nursing Process	6. Easy

10. A nurse teaches the patient preparing to undergo peritoneal dialysis that the entire exchange will take from
*A. 1–4 hours.
B. 6–10 hours.
C. 12–16 hours.
D. at least 24 hours.

Rationale: The entire exchange (infusion, dwell time, and drainage) takes from 1 to 4 hours, depending on the prescribed dwell time.

Reference: p. 1120

Descriptors:

1. 40	2. 05	3. Knowledge
4. IV–1	5. Nursing Process	6. Easy

11. A nurse teaches the patient with end stage renal disease who is preparing for hemodialysis which of the following statements regarding a fistula?
*A. The fistula connects the arterial and venous systems.
B. The fistula is ready to use immediately after it is created.
C. The patient should limit the movement of the arm used to create the fistula.
D. The nurse should always obtain a blood pressure in the arm with the fistula prior to beginning hemodialysis.

Rationale: The fistula joins an artery and a vein, either side to side or end to end. The fistula requires 4 to 5 weeks to mature, and the patient is encouraged to perform exercises to increase the size of the affected vessels (e.g., squeezing a rubber ball for forearm fistulas). A blood pressure should NEVER be taken in an extremity containing a fistula since it may damage the structure.

Reference: p. 1113

Descriptors:

1. 40	2. 05	3. Application
4. IV–4	5. Teaching/Learning	6. Moderate

12. Which of the following nursing interventions is appropriate in the care of the patient with a nephrostomy tube?
A. Clamp a nephrostomy tube when ambulating the patient.
B. If the tube dislodges, cover the opening with a moist, sterile dressing.

C. Irrigate the nephrostomy tube to maintain clear drainage.
*D. Measure the output from each kidney's tube separately.

Rationale: The activity of each kidney is carefully assessed. The nephrostomy tube is never clamped and should never be irrigated without specific order. If the tube dislodges, the surgeon must be notified so that he or she may replace the tube immediately to prevent the opening from contracting.

Reference: p. 1126

Descriptors:
1. 40 2. 07 3. Application
4. IV–3 5. Nursing Process 6. Moderate

13. When the patient who has undergone ureteral surgery asks the nurse how long the stent must remain in place, the nurse responds that stents are usually removed
A. 24 hours after surgery.
B. prior to discharge.
C. two weeks after surgery.
*D. four to six weeks after surgery.

Rationale: Stents are used to maintain urine flow in patients with ureteral obstruction, to divert urine, to promote healing, and to maintain the caliber and patency of the ureter after surgery. They are usually removed 4 to 6 weeks after surgery in an outpatient setting without the need for general anesthesia.

Reference: p. 1127

Descriptors:
1. 40 2. 07 3. Application
4. IV–1 5. Nursing Process 6. Moderate

14. When the nurse observes bloody drainage during the first peritoneal dialysis procedure performed on the patient, the nurse's MOST APPROPRIATE response is to
*A. document the observation.
B. contact the physician immediately.
C. monitor the patient for signs of shock.
D. monitor the patient for signs of infection.

Rationale: Bloody drainage may be seen in the first few exchanges after insertion of a new catheter but should not occur after that time.

Reference: pp. 1120–1121

Descriptors:
1. 40 2. 06 3. Application
4. IV–4 5. Nursing Process 6. Moderate

15. When the patient has experienced an episode of peritonitis following peritoneal dialysis, the nurse recognizes that:
A. the catheter must be removed immediately.
*B. the catheter must be removed if the peritonitis is unresolved after 4 days of appropriate therapy.
C. the catheter may be used as long as the dialysate solution contains antibiotics.
D. the patient must begin hemodialysis.

Rationale: Peritonitis that is unresolved after 4 days of appropriate therapy necessitates catheter removal. The patient is maintained on hemodialysis for about 1 month before a new catheter is inserted.

Reference: p. 1121

Descriptors:
1. 40 2. 05 3. Analysis
4. IV–4 5. Nursing Process 6. Difficult

CHAPTER 41
Management of Patients with Urinary and Renal Disorders

1. Which of the following factors contributes to the development of urinary tract infections?
A. Diabetes insipidus.
B. Cardiovascular disease.
*C. Immunosuppression.
D. Cirrhosis.

Rationale: Risk factors for urinary tract infection include inability or failure to empty the bladder completely, obstructed urinary flow, immunosuppression, instrumentation of the urinary tract, inflammation or abrasion of the urethral mucosa, and systemic conditions such as diabetes mellitus.

Reference: p. 1137

Descriptors:
1. 41 2. 01 3. Comprehension
4. IV–4 5. Nursing Process 6. Moderate

2. Which of the following routes of infection is most commonly associated with the development of urinary tract infections (UTIs)?
*A. Transurethral.
B. Hematogenous.
C. Direct extension.
D. Transfusion reactions.

Rationale: The most common route of infection is transurethral, in which bacteria colonize the periurethral area and subsequently enter the bladder. Bacteria may also enter the urinary tract by means of the blood (hemtaogenous) from a distant site of infection or through direct extension by way of a fistula from the gut.

Reference: p. 1137

Descriptors:
1. 41 2. 01 3. Comprehension
4. IV–4 5. Nursing Process 6. Easy

3. A nurse teaches the patient with a urinary tract infection (UTI) that
   A. pain associated with UTIs is controlled with narcotics.
   B. application of cold compresses to the pubic area will relieve bladder spams.
   C. liberal intake of fluids such as coffee, tea, and colas is recommended.
   *D. frequent voiding (every 2 to 3 hours) is encouraged.

Rationale: Pain associated with UTI is quickly relieved once effective antimicrobial therapy is initiated, and heat to the perineum may relieve spasm. The patient should avoid urinary tract irritants (e.g., coffee, tea, spices, colas, citrus, and alcohol). Frequent voiding to empty the bladder completely can significantly lower urine bacterial counts, reduce urinary stasis, and prevent reinfection.

Reference: p. 1140

Descriptors:
1. 41 2. 02 3. Application
4. IV–1 5. Teaching/Learning 6. Moderate

4. Which of the following terms refers to a disorder characterized by proteinuria, edema, hypoalbuminuria, and hyperlipidemia?
   A. Pyelonephritis.
   B. Interstitial cystitis.
   *C. Nephrotic syndrome.
   D. Glomerulonephritis.

Rationale: Nephrotic syndrome, characterized by the aforementioned signs and symptoms, is apparent in any condition that seriously damages the glomerular capillary membrane and results in increased glomerular capillary permeability.

Reference: p. 1136

Descriptors:
1. 41 2. 03 3. Comprehension
4. IV–4 5. Nursing Process 6. Moderate

5. Which of the following renal disorders is associated with a recent infection with group A beta-hemolytic streptococcus?
   A. Pyelonephritis.
   *B. Acute glomerulonephritis.
   C. Nephrotic syndrome.
   D. Nephrosis.

Rationale: In most cases of acute glomerulonephritis, there is a history of a group A beta-hemolytic streptococcal infection of the throat preceding the onset of glomerulonephritis by 2 to 3 weeks.

Reference: p. 1143

Descriptors:
1. 41 2. 03 3. Comprehension
4. IV–4 5. Nursing Process 6. Moderate

6. Which of the following clinical problems are known causes of chronic renal failure?
   *A. Diabetes mellitus.
   B. Myocardial infarction.
   C. Anaphylaxis.
   D. Hemorrhage.

Rationale: Causes of chronic renal failure include diabetes mellitus (leading cause), hypertension, chronic glomerulonephritis, pyelonephritis, obstruction of the urinary tract, hereditary lesions, vascular disorders, infections, medications, or toxic agents.

Reference: p. 1151

Descriptors:
1. 41 2. 04 3. Knowledge
4. IV–4 5. Nursing Process 6. Moderate

7. Which of the following problems is categorized as an INTRARENAL cause of acute renal failure?
   A. Calculi (stones).
   B. Sepsis.
   C. Congestive heart failure.
   *D. Nonsteroidal anti-inflammatory drugs.

Rationale: NSAIDs are known nephrotoxic agents that may precipitate acute renal failure.

Reference: p. 1147

Descriptors:
1. 41 2. 04 3. Knowledge
4. IV–4 5. Nursing Process 6. Easy

8. Which of the fluid and electrolyte disturbances that occur in acute renal failure is most life threatening?
   *B. Hyperkalemia.
   B. Fluid excess.
   C. Hypoproteinemia.
   D. Anemia.

Rationale: Because hyperkalemia is the most life threatening of the fluid and electrolyte disturbances in the patient in acute renal failure, the patient is monitored through serum electrolyte levels, electrocardiogram, and change in clinical status.

Reference: p. 1150

Descriptors:
1. 41 2. 05 3. Analysis
4. IV–4 5. Nursing Process 6. Difficult

9. A nurse anticipates use of which of the following agents to drive potassium into the cell in an acute renal failure patient who demonstrates hyperkalemia?
   A. Kayexelate.
   *B. Glucose and insulin.
   C. Calcium gluconate.
   D. Low dose dopamine.

Rationale: Glucose and insulin drive potassium into the cells, thereby lowering serum potassium levels temporarily. Calcium gluconate helps protect the heart from the effects of hyperkalemia. Kayexelate is an ion-exchange resin introduced orally or by retention enema. Low dose dopamine is not used to treat hyperkalemia.

Reference: p. 1150

Descriptors:
1. 41 2. 05 3. Application
4. IV–2 5. Nursing Process 6. Difficult

10. The nurse recognizes that the decreased erythropoietin, decreased red blood cell life span, bleeding in the gastrointestinal tract from irritating toxins, and blood loss during hemodialysis of the patient with end stage renal disease causes which of the following complications?
A. Hyperkalemia.
B. Hypertension.
C. Pericarditis.
*D. Anemia.

Rationale: Anemia is due to the aforementioned problems. Hypertension and hyperkalemia are due to the fluid and electrolyte disturbances that occur with ESRD. Pericarditis is due to retention of uremic waste products and inadequate dialysis.

Reference: p. 1153

Descriptors:
1. 41 2. 06 3. Comprehension
4. IV–4 5. Nursing Process 6. Moderate

11. Which of the following signs and symptoms does the nurse teach the postoperative kidney transplant patient most likely indicates infection?
A. Elevated serum creatinine.
B. Elevated blood urea nitrogen.
C. Fever.
*D. Leukocytosis.

Rationale: Impaired renal function and fever are evidence of both infection and rejection. Leukocytosis, however, is associated with infection. Any of these signs or symptoms should be reported to the physician.

Reference: p. 1161

Descriptors:
1. 41 2. 07 3. Application
4. IV–3 5. Teaching/Learning 6. Moderate

12. The nurse teaches the patient who has been diagnosed with oxalate renal calculi which of the following nutritional guidelines?
A. Restrict protein intake to 20 grams per day.
B. Restrict sodium intake to ½ gram per day.
C. Follow a low-calcium diet.
*D. Restrict intake of oxalates (peanuts, wheat bran, strawberries, rhubarb, tea, and spinach).

Rationale: Protein is restricted to 60 g/day, while sodium is restricted to 3–4 g/day. Low-calcium diets are generally not recommended except for true absorptive hypercalciuria.

Reference: p. 1164

Descriptors:
1. 41 2. 08 3. Application
4. IV–3 5. Teaching/Learning 6. Difficult

13. The nurse teaches the patient which of the following general guidelines to avoid recurrent renal stones?
*B. Drink two glasses of water at bedtime and an additional glass at each nighttime awakening.
B. Incorporate vigorous exercise into his or her daily routine.
C. Increase intake of vitamins and minerals.
D. Increase intake of milk.

Rationale: The patient is taught to drink two glasses of water at bedtime and an additional glass at each nighttime awakening to prevent urine from becoming too concentrated during the night.

Reference: p. 1167

Descriptors:
1. 41 2. 09 3. Application
4. IV–3 5. Teaching/Learning 6. Moderate

14. The nurse evaluates the expected outcome that the patient who has undergone creation of urinary diversion will verbalize characteristics of a healthy stoma when the patient reports that a healthy stoma appears
A. slightly pink.
*B. beefy red.
C. dark purplish.
D. brown.

Rationale: A healthy stoma is beefy red. A change from this normal color to a dark purplish color suggests that the vascular supply may be compromised.

Reference: p. 1172

Descriptors:
1. 41 2. 10 3. Analysis
4. IV–4 5. Nursing Process 6. Difficult

15. Which of the following terms refers to inflammation of the bladder wall?
*B. Interstitial cystitis.
B. Interstitial nephritis.
C. Urethritis.
D. Pyelonephritis.

Rationale: Interstitial cystitis refers to inflammation of the bladder wall that eventually causes disintegration of the lining and the loss of bladder elasticity. Patients with interstitial cystitis have to void more than 60 times per day.

Reference: p. 1136

Descriptors:
1. 41 2. 11 3. Knowledge
4. IV–4 5. Nursing Process 6. Easy

UNIT 10 REPRODUCTIVE FUNCTION

CHAPTER 42 Assessment and Management: Problems Related to Female Physiologic Processes

1. Which of the following hormones is the most important hormone for conditioning the endometrium for implantation?
   A. Estrogen.
   *B. Progesterone.
   C. Androgens.
   D. Follicle-stimulating hormone.

Rationale: Progesterone is the most important hormone for conditioning the endometrium in preparation for implantation of the fertilized ovum. Estrogens are responsible for developing and maintaining the female reproductive organs. Androgens, secreted by the ovaries in small amounts, are involved in the early development of the follicle and affect the female libido. Follicle-stimulating hormone is responsible for stimulating the ovaries to secrete estrogen.

Reference: p. 1194

Descriptors:

1. 42	2. 02	3. Comprehension
4. IV–4	5. Nursing Process	6. Moderate

2. Which of the following statements, if made by the nurse, demonstrates an appropriate approach to effective sexual assessment?
   *A. "Are you involved in an intimate relationship at this time?"
   B. "How many sexual partners have you had?"
   C. "Are you single, married, widowed, divorced, or separated?"
   D. "Have you ever been diagnosed with a sexually transmitted disease?"

Rationale: Asking about a partner or about current meaningful relationships may be a less offensive way to initiate a sexual history.

Reference: p. 1196

Descriptors:

1. 42	2. 02	3. Application
4. I–1	5. Communication	6. Moderate

3. The Abuse Assessment Screen includes which of the following questions?
   A. Did your husband hit you?
   *B. In the past year, have you been hit, slapped, kicked, or otherwise physically hurt by someone?
   C. Do you make your husband angry?
   D. Is this the first time you have been hit, slapped, kicked, or otherwise physically hurt by someone?

Rationale: The Abuse Assessment Screen consists of three questions: (1) In the past year, have you been hit, slapped, kicked, or otherwise physically hurt by someone? (2) If pregnant, since you have been pregnant, have you been hit, slapped, kicked, or otherwise physically hurt by someone? (3) Have you ever been forced into sexual activity?

Reference: p. 1196

Descriptors:

1. 42	2. 03	3. Knowledge
4. I–2	5. Nursing Process	6. Moderate

4. Which of the following guidelines directs the nurse in providing appropriate care to the victim of domestic abuse?
   A. If the woman chooses to go to a shelter, seek a social work consult for transfer.
   B. If the woman chooses to return to the abuser, contact protective services.
   *C. Assist the woman to set up a safety plan in case she decides to return home.
   D. If the husband appears at the emergency room, contact the police immediately.

Rationale: The nurse should assist the woman to set up a safety plan (an organized departure with packed bags and important papers hidden in a safe spot). However, the woman should make any contact with a shelter. If the woman chooses to return home, the nurse should remain nonjudgmental and provide information that will make her safer than she was before disclosing her information. The information disclosed to the nurse is confidential, and any contact with authorities must be based on the consent and desire of the woman.

Reference: p. 1197

Descriptors:

1. 42	2. 03	3. Application
4. I–2	5. Self-Care	6. Moderate

5. A nurse teaches the patient who is to undergo a pelvic examination that, during the examination, it is NOT normal to feel
   A. apprehensive.
   B. uncomfortable.
   C. pressure.
   *D. pain.

Rationale: A pelvic examination should never hurt. Women often describe a feeling of fullness or pressure. Feelings of apprehension and discomfort are normal. Relaxation is important because women who are very tense tend to feel discomfort.

Reference: p. 1198

Descriptors:
1. 42 2. 04 3. Application
4. IV–1 5. Teaching/Learning 6. Easy

6. When the patient asks the nurse the meaning of white discharge from the vagina, in the absence of symptoms or odor, the nurse responds that the
*A. drainage is physiologic and normal.
B. patient may have a Candida species infection.
C. drainage is caused by vaginal dryness.
D. patient may have a Trichomonas species infection.

Rationale: Mucus or white discharge from the vagina is physiologic and normal. Drainage caused by Candida is curd-like and white in color, while infection with Trichomonas is often frothy/yellow green in color. Vaginal dryness causes scant and mucoid drainage that may be blood-tinged.

Reference: p. 1199

Descriptors:
1. 42 2. 04 3. Application
4. I–2 5. Teaching/Learning 6. Moderate

7. The nurse teaches the young female patient who inquires about the need for Pap smear that
A. the test may be performed at any time during the patient's menstrual cycle.
B. the patient should douche before the examination.
C. the test detects uterine cancer.
*D. false-negative Pap smear results occur mostly from sampling errors.

Rationale: The test should be performed when the patient is not menstruating, and douching washes away cellular material. The test detects cervical cancer, and false-negative Pap smear results occur mostly from sampling errors or improper technique.

Reference: pp. 1200–1201

Descriptors:
1. 42 2. 04 3. Application
4. IV–3 5. Teaching/Learning 6. Moderate

8. A nurse understands that a Class V Pap smear is considered
A. normal.
B. probably negative.
C. suspicious.
*D. malignant.

Rationale: A Class 1 result is negative (normal); Class 2 is probably negative; Class 3 is suspicious; Class 4 is more suspicious; and Class 5 is malignant.

Reference: p. 1202

Descriptors:
1. 42 2. 04 3. Knowledge
4. IV–4 5. Nursing Process 6. Easy

9. Which of the following statements is an accurate point regarding sexual activity in the woman approaching menopause?
*A. Frequent sexual activity helps to maintain the elasticity of the vagina.
B. Contraception is no longer necessary when menses stop.
C. Safe sex practices are no longer necessary when menses stop.
D. Disinterest in sexual activity is common.

Rationale: The nurse should state the following points about sexual activity: frequent sexual activity helps to maintain the elasticity of the vagina; contraception is advised until 1 year passes without menses; safe sex is important at any age; and sexual functioning may be enhanced at midlife.

Reference: p. 1208

Descriptors:
1. 42 2. 07 3. Application
4. IV–1 5. Teaching/Learning 6. Moderate

10. The nurse teaches the patient who experiences premenstrual syndrome which of the following treatment guidelines?
A. Decrease water intake.
B. Limit exercise.
*C. Limit intake of caffeine, salt, sweets, and alcohol.
D. Decrease intake of fruits and vegetables.

Rationale: In general, the patient is encouraged to follow a nutritious diet consisting of whole grains, fruit, and vegetables; increase water intake; decrease intake of caffeine, salt, sweets, and alcohol; and increase or initiate an exercise program.

Reference: p. 1209

Descriptors:
1. 42 2. 06 3. Application
4. IV–3 5. Teaching/Learning 6. Moderate

11. Which of the following terms refers to prolonged or excessive bleeding at the time of the regular menstrual flow?
A. Amenorrhea.
B. Dysmenorrhea.
*C. Menorrhagia.
D. Metrorrhagia.

Rationale: Amenorrhea refers to absence of menstrual flow, while dysmenorrhea is painful menstruation. Menorrhagia is also called hypermenorrhea and is defined as prolonged or excessive bleeding at the time of the regular menstrual flow. Metrorrhagia refers to vaginal bleeding between regular menstrual periods.

Reference: p. 1210

Descriptors:
1. 42 2. 05 3. Knowledge
4. IV–4 5. Nursing Process 6. Easy

12. A nurse teaches the patient who is inquiring about an intrauterine device (IUD) as a form of birth control which of the following guidelines?
 A. The IUD destroys fertilized eggs.
 *B. Pregnancy can occur with the IUD in place.
 C. An IUD method is recommended in women who have not had children.
 D. An IUD is easily expelled during menstruation.

Rationale: The IUD does not destroy fertilized eggs, and pregnancy can occur. An IUD method is not recommended in the nulliparous patient because uterine size may be too small to tolerate it. An IUD remains in place over time and must be removed by the health care provider.

Reference: p. 1213

Descriptors:
1. 42 2. 08 3. Application
4. IV–3 5. Teaching/Learning 6. Moderate

13. Administration of which of the following agents is used in elective abortions and terminates the pregnancy <u>because it is toxic to the fetus?</u>
 A. Prostaglandins.
 B. Mifepristone.
 *C. Methotrexate.
 D. Misoprostol.

Rationale: Methotrexate is a teratosen that is lethal to the fetus. Prostaglandins precipitate strong uterine contractions that result in abortion, while Mifepristone prevents implantation of the ovum. Misoprostol is a synthetic prostaglandin analog that produces cervical effacement and uterine contractions.

Reference: p. 1217

Descriptors:
1. 42 2. 09 3. Analysis
4. IV–4 5. Nursing Process 6. Difficult

14. Which of the following categories of females should NOT take oral contraceptives?
 A. Nonsmokers under age 35.
 B. Nonsmokers age 35 and over.
 C. Smokers under age 35.
 *D. Smokers age 35 and over.

Rationale: Women who smoke and who are age 35 years or older should not take oral contraceptives because of an increased risk for heart problems.

Reference: p. 1212

Descriptors:
1. 42 2. 07 3. Knowledge
4. IV–3 5. Nursing Process 6. Easy

15. A nurse teaches the patient who is undergoing a vasectomy that
 A. the procedure is easily and successfully reversed.
 B. he no longer requires contraceptive protection.
 *C. the procedure is highly effective.
 D. he will never experience serious long-term effects.

Rationale: A vasectomy is potentially reversible, but results cannot be guaranteed. Contraception must be used until the sperm count is zero. Once the sperm remaining in the reproductive system are ejaculated, the procedure is highly effective. Serious long-term side effects are suspected but unproven.

Reference: p. 1211

Descriptors:
1. 42 2. 08 3. Application
4. IV–3 5. Teaching/Learning 6. Moderate

CHAPTER 43
Management of Women with Reproductive Disorders

1. Of the following attributes, which is classified as a risk factor for vulvovaginal infection?
 A. Menopause.
 B. Infrequent douching.
 C. High estrogen levels.
 *D. Tight undergarments.

Rationale: Risk factors for vulvovaginal infections include premenarche, perimenopause, and pregnancy; frequent douching; low estrogen levels; and tight undergarments.

Reference: p. 1227

Descriptors:
1. 43 2. 01 3. Knowledge
4. IV–3 5. Nursing Process 6. Moderate

2. Which of the following terms is used to describe inflammation causing pain with intercourse?
 A. Vaginitis.
 *B. Vestibulitis.
 C. Vulvitis.
 D. Vulvodynia.

Rationale: Vaginitis is inflammation of the vagina, usually secondary to infection, while vulvitis is inflammation of the vulva, usually secondary to infection or irritation. Vestibulitis is refers to inflammation causing dyspareunia, and vulvodynia refers to a painful condition that affects the vulva.

Reference: p. 1226

Descriptors:
1. 43 2. 01 3. Knowledge
4. IV–4 5. Nursing Process 6. Easy

3. When the patient informs the nurse that she has noted inflammation of her vagina and a white, cheese-like discharge, the nurse recognizes that the clinical manifestations described are typical of which of the following vaginal infections?

A. Trichomonas vaginalis.
*B. Candidiasis.
C. Gardnerella.
D. Chlamydia.

Rationale: The clinical manifestations indicate candidiasis, which is treated with an antifungal agent in the form of vaginal suppositories or cream.

Reference: p. 1227

Descriptors:
1. 43 2. 01 3. Comprehension
4. IV–4 5. Nursing Process 6. Moderate

4. The nurse would include which of the following general guidelines regarding prevention in an educational program for the patient who has experienced a vaginal infection?
A. Repeated douching after sexual intercourse is encouraged.
B. Tub bathing is recommended.
C. Feminine hygiene products (sprays) decrease the likelihood of vaginal infection.
*D. Loose-fitting cotton underwear is recommended.

Rationale: Instead of tight-fitting synthetic, nonabsorbent, heat-retaining underwear, cotton underwear is recommended to prevent vaginal infections. Douching is generally discouraged, as is the use of feminine hygiene products. Type of daily bathing is not restricted.

Reference: pp. 1229–1230

Descriptors:
1. 43 2. 02 3. Application
4. IV–1 5. Teaching/Learning 6. Moderate

5. When the nurse assesses the female patient at an outpatient clinic and learns that the patient has experienced clear, thin, nonfrothy discharge, the nurse's BEST response is to:
A. advise the patient that she may have a sexually transmitted disease (STD).
B. obtain a specimen for vaginal smear (wet mount).
*C. describe the vaginal discharge in documentation as normal.
D. contact the physician or nurse practitioner directing the clinic.

Rationale: Normal vaginal discharge is thin, clear, and nonfrothy.

Reference: p. 1230

Descriptors:
1. 43 2. 03 3. Analysis
4. IV–4 5. Nursing Process 6. Moderate

6. When the nurse reviews the Emergency Department physician notes for the newly admitted patient and reads that the patient has a history of HSV–2 or herpes simplex 2 viral infection, the nurse recognizes that the
A. virus causes "cold sores" of the lips.
*B. patient may experience a recurrence during hospitalization.
C. patient may develop shingles during hospitalization.
D. virus does not remain in the body after initial infection.

Rationale: HSV-2 causes genital herpes and is known to ascend the peripheral sensory nerves and remain inactive after infection, becoming active in times of stress. HSV–1 causes "cold sores," and varicella zoster causes shingles.

Reference: p. 1230

Descriptors:
1. 43 2. 04 3. Analysis
4. IV–4 5. Nursing Process 6. Difficult

7. A nurse teaches the patient who has been diagnosed with genital herpes which of the following general guidelines?
A. Intercourse with the use of a condom is allowed during treatment.
B. Sun bathing assists in eradicating the virus.
C. Occlusive ointments should be used on lesions.
*D. Self-infection can occur from touching lesions during a breakout.

Rationale: Intercourse during treatment is avoided, and exposure to the sun may precipitate recurrence. The lesions should be allowed to dry. Touching of lesions during an outbreak should be avoided, and, if touched, appropriate hygiene practices must be followed.

Reference: pp. 1230–1231

Descriptors:
1. 43 2. 04
3. Application/Analysis 4. IV–3
5. Teaching/Learning 6. Difficult

8. The nurse teaches the patient who has experienced toxic shock syndrome (TSS) which of the following general guidelines?
A. Use of superabsorbent tampons is recommended.
B. Tampons may be left in place up to 4 hours.
C. A diaphragm or cervical cap may be used during menses.
*D. TSS is associated with postpartal bleeding as well as menses.

Rationale: Use of superabsorbent tampons is not recommended. Tampons should NOT be used by women who have had TSS. Use of a diaphragm or cervical cap during menses or the first 3 months postpartum is discouraged. The risk of development of TSS increases anytime a woman bleeds vaginally.

Reference: p. 1231

Descriptors:

1. 43	2. 05
3. Application/Analysis	4. IV–3
5. Teaching/Learning	6. Difficult

9. Which of the following terms is used to refer to a benign ovarian tumor of undefined origin that consists of embryonal cells?
   A. Bartholin's cyst.
   *B. Dermoid cyst.
   C. Hydatidiform mole.
   D. Leiomyoma.

Rationale: A Bartholin's cyst is a cyst in a paired vestibular bland in the vulva, while a dermoid cyst is a benign tumor that is thought to arise from parts of the ovum and normally disappears with maturation. A hydatidiform mole is a type of gestational neoplasm, and a leiomyoma is a usually benign tumor of the uterus, commonly referred to as a "fibroid."

Reference: p. 1241

Descriptors:

1. 43	2. 07	3. Comprehension
4. IV–4	5. Nursing Process	6. Moderate

10. Because the incidence of deep vein thrombosis (DVT) increases when the patient has any type of pelvic surgery, the nurse teaches the patient undergoing hysterectomy which of the following guidelines intended to prevent the development of DVT?
   A. When sitting, position body so that one's back rests against the chair back, and one's knees press against the chair seat.
   B. Limit the amount of walking during the first weeks postoperatively.
   C. Stop drinking fluids 3 hours before bedtime.
   *D. Change positions frequently.

Rationale: Crossing legs and pressure against knees is to be avoided. Exercising the legs and ankles is recommended as well as adequate hydrate to avoid hemoconcentration. Changing positions promotes venous return and decreases pooling in the extremities.

Reference: p. 1249

Descriptors:

1. 43	2. 08
3. Application/Analysis	4. IV–3
5. Teaching/Learning	6. Moderate

11. When planning a patient education for woman diagnosed with ovarian cancer, the nurse recognizes that the patient has a three to fourfold increased risk for developing
   *B. breast cancer.
   B. cervical cancer.
   C. vulvar cancer.
   D. bowel cancer.

Rationale: A woman with ovarian cancer has a threefold to fourfold increased risk for breast cancer, and women with breast cancer have an increased risk for ovarian cancer.

Reference: p. 1250

Descriptors:

1. 43	2. 07	3. Knowledge
4. IV–3	5. Nursing Process	6. Easy

12. When the female patient undergoes intracavitary brachytherapy, the patient should be be instructed to
   A. ambulate in the patient's room only.
   B. refrain from coughing.
   C. consume a high-fiber diet.
   *D. keep the head of the bed no higher than 15 degrees.

Rationale: A patient receiving intracavitary radiation must stay on absolute bed rest, but may move from side to side with the head of the bed raised to 15 degrees. Diet should be low residue to prevent frequent bowel movements. The patient should be encouraged to deep breathe, cough, and flex and extend feet to reduce incidence of complications of immobility.

Reference: p. 1255

Descriptors:

1. 43	2. 07
3. Application/Analysis	4. I–2
5. Nursing Process	6. Difficult

13. Which of the following instructions are typically provided when the patient undergoes internal irradiation?
   A. Visitors must wear film badges or pocket ion chambers to monitor exposure.
   B. Rubber gloves provide protection from sealed radiation sources.
   C. The patient is allowed no visitors.
   *D. Specific laundry and housekeeping procedures are required.

Rationale: Generally, health care providers are required to monitor exposure while visitors are not. Rubber gloves are needed to dispose of any soiled matter that may be contaminated, but they do NOT provide protection from sealed radiation sources. The patient is restricted to her room and allowed no visitors who are or may be pregnant or who are younger than 18 years of age. Specific laundry and housekeeping procedures are required.

Reference: p. 1256

Descriptors:

1. 43	2. 07	3. Analysis
4. I–2	5. Nursing Process	6. Moderate

14. In providing postoperative care to the patient who has undergone vulvectomy, which of the following nursing interventions is indicated?

*A. Administration of analgesics around the clock at designated times.
B. Ambulation on the evening of the operative day.
C. Placement of two pillows under the knees.
D. High Fowler's positioning.

Rationale: Because of the wide excision, the patient may experience severe pain even with minimal movement. Therefore, analgesics are administered preventively. Immobility is prolonged to promote healing. No more than one pillow should be placed under the knees (DVT prevention), and a low Fowler's position is recommended.

Reference: p. 1248

Descriptors:
1. 43 2. 09, 10 3. Application
4. IV–1 5. Nursing Process 6. Difficult

15. In which of the following surgical procedures is laser energy always used to remove tissue?
A. Brachytherapy.
B. Cryotherapy.
*C. Loop electrocautery excision procedure (LEEP).
D. Laparoscopy.

Rationale: Cryotherapy involves freezing of tissue and brachytherapy involves radiating tissue. LEEP is a procedure in which laser energy is used to remove a portion of cervical tissue after abnormal biopsy.

Reference: p. 1244

Descriptors:
1. 43 2. 07 3. Comprehension
4. I–1 5. Nursing Process 6. Moderate

CHAPTER 44
Assessment and Management of Patients with Breast Disorders

1. The nurse teaches the patient that breast self-examination (BSE) may be performed
A. any time during the month.
B. on the first day of every month.
C. on the first day of menstruation.
*D. five to seven days after menses, counting the first day of menses as day 1.

Rationale: Because most women notice increased tenderness and lumpiness before their menstrual period, BSE is best performed after menses when less fluid is retained.

Reference: pp. 1263–1264

Descriptors:
1. 44 2. 01
3. Application 4. IV–3
5. Teaching/Learning; Self-Care 6. Easy

2. Which of the following general guidelines, based upon recent research, should be explained to the daughters of a patient diagnosed with breast cancer at age 58 whose mother was diagnosed with breast cancer at age 68? The daughters should begin screening activities at age
A. 28.
B. 38.
*C. 48.
D. 58.

Rationale: Several studies suggest that screening for high-risk women should begin about 10 years before the diagnosis of the family member with breast cancer. In families with a history of breast cancer, a downward shift in age of diagnosis of about 10 years is seen.

Reference: p. 1264

Descriptors:
1. 44 2. 02 3. Comprehension
4. IV–3 5. Teaching/Learning 6. Moderate

3. The nurse teaches the female patient that American Cancer Society (ACS) recommends that a baseline mammogram should be obtained by the age of
A. 20 years.
B. 30 years.
*C. 40 years.
D. 50 years.

Rationale: The ACS recommends that a baseline mammogram be obtained after the age of 35 years and by the age of 40 years.

Reference: p. 1264

Descriptors:
1. 44 2. 02 3. Knowledge
4. IV–3 5. Nursing Process 6. Easy

4. The nurse teaches the patient that mammography
A. seldom fails to detect breast cancer.
*B. may detect a breast tumor before it is clinically palpable.
C. uses radiation that may cause skin cancer.
D. should never be uncomfortable.

Rationale: Generally, a tumor smaller than 1 cm is not detected clinically but may be detected through mammography. Mammography has a false-negative rate ranging between 5% and 10%. The radiation exposure of mammogram is equivalent to about 1 hour of exposure to sunlight. Women may experience some fleeting discomfort because maximum compression is necessary for proper visualization.

Reference: p. 1264

Descriptors:
1. 44 2. 02
3. Application/Analysis 4. IV–3
5. Teaching/Learning 6. Moderate

5. To prepare the patient for a breast ultrasound, the nurse informs the patient that
   A. a needle will be inserted to draw tissue and fluid from her breast.
   B. a radiopaque material will be injected into her breast.
   C. her breast will be mechanically compressed while X-ray films are taken.
   *D. a transducer will be passed over the breast and echo waves will be viewed on a screen.

Rationale: Ultrasonography is used to distinguish fluid-filled cysts from other lesions. High-frequency sound waves are transmitted through the breast and echo signals are measured.

Reference: pp. 1264, 1266

Descriptors:
1. 44 2. 02 3. Application
4. IV–3 5. Teaching/Learning 6. Moderate

6. When explaining how to perform breast self-examination, the nurse instructs the learner to use which of the following measures?
   A. Use 1 or 2 fingers to feel the breast.
   B. Use the hand on the same side as the breast to complete the examination.
   C. Place a pillow or folded towel under the shoulder of the breast you are NOT examining.
   *D. Pay special attention to the area between the breast and the underarm, including the underarm itself.

Rationale: Many breast tumors occur in the upper outer quadrant of the breast, and enlarged lymph nodes may indicate a breast cancer.

Reference: p. 1265

Descriptors:
1. 44 2. 01 3. Application
4. IV–3 5. Teaching/Learning 6. Moderate

7. A breast cancer mass that indicates a malignant tumor usually is characterized by
   A. tenderness.
   B. a regular shape.
   *C. firmness and hardness.
   D. being easily moved.

Rationale: A malignant breast tumor usually occurs as a single mass in one breast; is usually nontender; has an irregular shape; is firm, hard, and embedded in surrounding tissue (not easily mobile).

Reference: pp. 1262, 1268

Descriptors:
1. 44 2. 01 3. Comprehension
4. IV–3 5. Nursing Process 6. Moderate

8. When the nurse examines the patient and notes an inverted nipple, which of the following questions is MOST appropriate?
   A. When was your last mammogram?
   B. Do you perform monthly breast self-examination?
   *C. How long has your nipple been inverted?
   D. Do you have a family history of breast cancer?

Rationale: Nipple inversion is considered normal if long-standing, but is associated with fibrosis and malignancy if recently developed.

Reference: p. 1262

Descriptors:
1. 44 2. 03 3. Application
4. IV–3 5. Nursing Process 6. Difficult

9. A nurse recognizes that the most common type of invasive breast cancer is
   A. medullary carcinoma.
   B. mucinous cancer.
   *C. infiltrating ductal carcinoma.
   D. infiltrating lobular carcinoma.

Rationale: Infiltrating ductal carcinoma accounts for 75% of all breast cancers, while infiltrating lobular carcinoma accounts for 5 to 10%. Mucinous and medullary carcinomas of the breast are rare, accounting for 3% and 6%, respectively, of breast cancers.

Reference: p. 1269

Descriptors:
1. 44 2. 03 3. Comprehension
4. IV–3 5. Nursing Process 6. Moderate

10. Which of the following attributes are known risk factors related to hormones as an etiology for breast cancer?
   A. Multiparity.
   B. Childbirth during adolescence.
   *C. Late menopause.
   D. Early menarche.

Rationale: Early menarche, nulliparity, childbirth after 30 years of age, and late menopause are known but minor risk factors and are associated with prolonged exposure to estrogen because of menstruation.

Reference: p. 1270

Descriptors:
1. 44 2. 03 3. Analysis
4. IV–3 5. Nursing Process 6. Moderate

11. A breast tumor of any size with direct extension to the breast wall, any regional lymph node involvement, and no signs of metastasis would be categorized as
   A. Stage IIA.
   B. Stage IIB.
   C. Stage IIIA.
   *D. Stage IIIB.

Rationale: Stage IIB is characterized by any size tumor with direct extension to the chest wall or skin, any regional lymph node involvement, and no metastasis.

Reference: p. 1274

Descriptors:
1. 44 2. 03 3. Comprehension
4. IV–4 5. Nursing Process 6. Difficult

12. A nurse teaches the patient who has undergone total mastectomy and axillary dissection to report which of the following signs or symptoms to the physician immediately?
    A. Collection of fluid at the incision site.
    B. Sensations of burning and tingling along the chest wall and in the axilla.
    *C. Temperature of 100.4 or greater.
    D. Swelling in the arm on the side of the mastectomy.

Rationale: Seroma formation, development of paresthesias, and lymphedema are anticipated abnormals following total mastectomy and axillary dissection. Elevated temperature may indicate infection, known to follow breast surgery in about 1 in 100 patients.

Reference: pp. 1284–1286

Descriptors:
1. 44 2. 05
3. Application/Analysis 4. IV–3
5. Teaching/Learning 6. Moderate

13. A nurse teaches the patient who has undergone total mastectomy and axillary dissection to report which of the following signs or symptoms to the physician immediately?
    *A. Gross swelling at the surgical site.
    B. Sensations of burning and tingling along the chest wall and in the axilla.
    C. Temperature of 100.2.
    D. Swelling in the arm on the side of the mastectomy.

Rationale: Development of paresthesias and lymphedema are anticipated abnormals following total mastectomy and axillary dissection. Elevated temperature above 100.4 may indicate infection and is known to follow breast surgery in about 1 in 100 patients. Hematoma formation is indicated by gross swelling at the surgical site.

Reference: pp. 1284–1286

Descriptors:
1. 44 2. 05
3. Application/Analysis 4. IV–3
5. Teaching/Learning 6. Moderate

14. When the patient asks the nurse about reconstructive surgery after mastectomy, the nurse explains to the patient that:
    A. a permanent implant provides the most natural-looking breast.
    B. nipple and areola reconstruction are performed at the same time the breast is reconstructed.
    *C. the transrectus abdominal myocutaneous (TRAM) flap uses the patient's own tissue.
    D. recovery is shortest when tissue transfer procedures are used.

Rationale: Tissue transfer methods provide the most natural-looking breast. Breast reconstruction is staged, with nipple and areolar reconstruction occurring after the breast mound has been created and healed. The transrectus abdominal muscle, gluteal muscle, and latissimus dorsi muscle are used for flap surgeries. Flap surgeries require a greater recovery period than tissue expansion with permanent implant.

Reference: pp. 1291–1292

Descriptors:
1. 44 2. 05 3. Application
4. IV–1 5. Teaching/Learning 6. Moderate

15. When the patient asks the nurse about reconstructive surgery after mastectomy, the nurse explains to the patient that:
    *A. tissue transfer procedures provide the most natural-looking breast.
    B. nipple and areola reconstruction are performed at the same time the breast is reconstructed.
    C. a tissue expander is usually in place for 4 to 6 weeks, at which time a permanent implant is placed.
    D. recovery is shortest when tissue transfer procedures are used.

Rationale: Tissue transfer methods provide the most natural-looking breast. Breast reconstruction is staged, with nipple and areolar reconstruction occurring after the breast mound has been created and healed. The transrectus abdominal muscle, gluteal muscle, and latissimus dorsi muscle are used for flap surgeries. Flap surgeries require a greater recovery period than tissue expansion with permanent implant. The patient generally has a tissue expander in place for 4 to 6 months before it is exchanged for a permanent implant.

Reference: pp. 1291–1292

Descriptors:
1. 44 2. 05 3. Application
4. IV–1 5. Teaching/Learning 6. Moderate

CHAPTER 45
Assessment and Management: Problems Related to Male Reproductive Processes

1. Which of the following terms refers to failure of the testes to descend into the scrotum?
    *A. Cryptorchidism.
    B. Orchitis.

C. Hydrocele.
D. Prostatism.

Rationale: Cryptorchidism, or failure of the testes to descend into the scrotum, is the most common congenital defect of the male reproductive system.

Reference: p. 1298

Descriptors:
1. 45 2. 01 3. Knowledge
4. IV–1 5. Nursing Process 6. Moderate

2. Which of the following terms is used to describe the buildup of fibrous plaques in the sheath of the corpus cavernosum, causing curvature of the penis when it is erect?
A. Bowen's disease.
*B. Peyronie's disease.
C. Phimosis.
D. Priapism.

Rationale: Peyronie's disease results in painful and difficult intercourse. Surgical removal of the plaques may be necessary.

Reference: pp. 1298, 1322

Descriptors:
1. 45 2. 07 3. Knowledge
4. IV–1 5. Nursing Process 6. Moderate

3. The purpose of the prostate gland is to
A. produce spermatozoa from germinal cells.
*B. produce a secretion that is suitable to the needs of spermatozoa.
C. lubricate the urethra at the time of ejaculation.
D. induce and preserve male sex characteristics.

Rationale: Testes produce spermatozoa, and Cowper's gland provides lubrication at ejaculation. Testosterone, produced by the testes, is responsible for inducing and preserving male sex characteristics. The prostate gland produces a secretion that is chemically and physiologically suitable to the needs of the spermatozoa in their passage from the testes.

Reference: p. 1299

Descriptors:
1. 45 2. 01 3. Comprehension
4. IV–1 5. Nursing Process 6. Difficult

4. The digital rectal examination (DRE) is recommended as part of the regular health checkup for every man
A. who has begun sexual activity.
B. over age 18.
C. over age 30.
*D. over age 40.

Rationale: The DRE is recommended for every man over age 40 as an invaluable screening test for cancer of the prostate.

Reference: p. 1300

Descriptors:
1. 45 2. 02 3. Comprehension
4. IV–3 5. Nursing Process 6. Moderate

5. Nocturnal penile tumescence test is performed when the patient demonstrates
A. prostatism.
B. priapism.
*C. erectile dysfunction.
D. premature ejaculation.

Rationale: In healthy men, nocturnal penile erections closely parallel rapid-eye movement sleep in occurrence and duration. The nocturnal penile tumescence test can help to determine whether erectile impotence has an organic or psychological cause.

Reference: p. 1301

Descriptors:
1. 45 2. 02 3. Analysis
4. IV–1 5. Nursing Process 6. Moderate

6. A nurse teaches the patient who has been prescribed Viagra that
A. the drug will cause erection to occur.
B. the drug should be taken early in the day of planned intercourse.
C. facial flushing or indigestion should be reported to the physician immediately.
*D. a dose of more than 100 mg will result in a change of vision, making everything appear blue.

Rationale: The patient must have sexual stimulation to create the erection, and the drug should be taken 1 hour before intercourse. Facial flushing, mild headache, indigestion, and running nose are common side effects of Viagra. The "blue haze" that occurs with 100 mg dosage is transient and will last for about one hour.

Reference: p. 1304

Descriptors:
1. 45 2. 03 3. Application
4. IV–3 5. Nursing Process 6. Moderate

7. A nurse teaches the patient who has been prescribed Viagra that
*A. the patient must have sexual stimulation to create the erection.
B. the drug should be taken early in the day of planned intercourse.
C. any vision change that occurs when the drug is taken must be reported to the physician immediately.
D. Viagra may be used with penile injections.

Rationale: The patient must have sexual stimulation to create the erection, and the drug should be taken 1 hour before intercourse. Facial flushing, mild headache, indigestion, and running nose are common side effects of Viagra. The "blue haze" that occurs with 100 mg dosage is transient and will last for about one hour. Use of Viagra with other forms of therapy has not been tested and should be avoided.

Reference: p. 1304

Descriptors:
1. 45 2. 03 3. Application
4. IV–3 5. Nursing Process 6. Moderate

8. A nurse assesses the patient older than 50 years for signs of benign prostatic hyperplasia (BPH), specifically,
*A. nocturia.
B. anemia.
C. hematuria.
D. backache.

Rationale: The obstructive and irritative symptoms complex (prostatism) found in BPH patients include increased frequency of urination, nocturia, urgency, hesitancy in starting urination, abdominal straining with urination, decrease in force and volume of stream, interruption of stream, and dribbling.

Reference: p. 1305

Descriptors:
1. 45 2. 05 3. Comprehension
4. IV–4 5. Nursing Process 6. Moderate

9. When the progress notes reflect that digital rectal examination (DRE) revealed a nodule within the substance of the prostate gland, the nurse recognizes that the observation typically indicates
A. a normal finding.
*B. a sign of early prostate cancer.
C. evidence of a more advanced lesion.
D. metastatic disease.

Rationale: Routine repeated DRE is important because early cancer may be felt as a nodule within the substance of the gland or as an extensive hardening in the posterior lobe.

Reference: p. 1307

Descriptors:
1. 45 2. 05 3. Comprehension
4. IV–3 5. Nursing Process 6. Moderate

10. Which of the following surgical approaches to prostatectomy offers direct anatomic approach?
A. Transurethral resection.
B. Suprapubic approach.
C. Retropubic approach.
*D. Perineal approach.

Rationale: The perineal approach offers direct anatomic contact but carries higher postoperative incidence of impotence and urinary incontinence.

Reference: p. 1313

Descriptors:
1. 45 2. 04 3. Comprehension
4. IV–1 5. Nursing Process 6. Easy

11. Which of the following surgical approaches to prostatecomy requires incision through the bladder?
*A. Suprapubic.
B. Perineal.
C. Retropubic.
D. Perianal.

Rationale: The suprapubic approach requires surgical incision through the bladder, and urine may leak around the suprapubic tube.

Reference: p. 1313

Descriptors:
1. 45 2. 04 3. Comprehension
4. IV–1 5. Nursing Process 6. Easy

12. When the nurse notes that the urinary drainage of the patient post prostatectomy is reddish pink, his or her BEST response is to
A. increase frequency of measurement of vital signs.
B. notify the urologist.
*C. document the finding and continue to observe output.
D. apply traction to the catheter.

Rationale: The urinary drainage post prostatectomy begins as reddish pink and then clears to a light pink within 24 hours after surgery.

Reference: p. 1316

Descriptors:
1. 45 2. 05
3. Application/Analysis 4. IV–3
5. Nursing Process 6. Moderate

13. The nurse teaches the post-prostatectomy patient which of the following general guidelines regarding urination?
A. Resist the first urge to void.
B. Dribbling will continue for the remainder of his life.
C. Cloudy urine should be reported to the physician immediately.
*D. Avoid straining at stool.

Rationale: Straining at increases venous pressure and may produce hematuria. Dribbling should gradually diminish. Cloudy urine for several weeks after surgery may occur but should clear as the prostate area heals.

Reference: p. 1317

Descriptors:
1. 45 2. 05 3. Application
4. IV–1 5. Teaching/Learning 6. Moderate

14. The nurse recognizes that testicular cancer:
A. is most common among men over 65.
*B. is one of the most curable solid tumors.
C. generally produces a painful enlargement of the testis.
D. tend to metastasize late in the development of the disease.

Rationale: Testicular cancer is most common among men 15 to 35 years of age and produces a painless enlargement of the testicle. Testicular cancers metastasize early, but are one of the most curable solid tumors, being highly responsive to chemotherapy.

Reference: p. 1319

Descriptors:
1. 45 2. 06 3. Comprehension
4. IV–1 5. Nursing Process 6. Moderate

15. Which of the following conditions affecting the penis presents a urological emergency?
 A. Phimosis.
 B. Bowen's disease.
 *C. Priapism.
 D. Peyronie's disease.

Rationale: Priapism is an uncontrolled, persistent erection of the penis that causes the penis to become large, hard, and painful. Priapism is a urological emergency because the condition may result in gangrene and often results in impotence, whether treated or not.

Reference: p. 1322

Descriptors:
1. 45 2. 07 3. Analysis
4. IV–3 5. Nursing Process 6. Moderate

UNIT 11 IMMUNOLOGIC FUNCTION

CHAPTER 46 Assessment of Immune Function

1. Which of the following terms is used to describe the immune system's third line of defense?
 A. Agglutination.
 *B. Cellular immune response.
 C. Humoral response.
 D. Phagocytic immune response.

Rationale: Agglutination refers to the clumping effect occurring when an antibody acts as a cross-link between two antigens. Cellular immune response, the immune system's third line of defense, involves the attack of pathogens by T-cells. Humoral response is the immune system's second line of defense, often termed the antibody response. The phagocytic immune response, or immune response, is the system's first line of defense, involving white blood cells that have the ability to ingest foreign particles.

Reference: p. 1330

Descriptors:
1. 46 2. 01 3. Comprehension
4. IV–4 5. Nursing Process 6. Moderate

2. Which of the following terms is used to describe the immune system's first line of defense?
 A. Agglutination.
 B. Cellular immune response.
 C. Humoral response.
 *D. Phagocytic immune response.

Rationale: Agglutination refers to the clumping effect occurring when an antibody acts as a cross-link between two antigens. Cellular immune response, the immune system's third line of defense, involves the attack of pathogens by T-cells. Humoral response is the immune system's second line of defense, often termed the antibody response. The phagocytic immune response, or immune response, is the system's first line of defense, involving white blood cells that have the ability to ingest foreign particles.

Reference: p. 1330

Descriptors:
1. 46 2. 01 3. Comprehension
4. IV–4 5. Nursing Process 6. Moderate

3. Which of the following terms is used to describe the immune system's second line of defense?
 A. Agglutination.
 B. Cellular immune response.
 *C. Humoral response.
 D. Phagocytic immune response.

Rationale: Agglutination refers to the clumping effect occurring when an antibody acts as a cross-link between two antigens. Cellular immune response, the immune system's third line of defense, involves the attack of pathogens by T-cells. Humoral response is the immune system's second line of defense, often termed the antibody response. The phagocytic immune response, or immune response, is the system's first line of defense, involving white blood cells that have the ability to ingest foreign particles.

Reference: p. 1330

Descriptors:
1. 46 2. 01 3. Comprehension
4. IV–4 5. Nursing Process 6. Moderate

4. During which type of response to invasion to pathogens can the T-lymphocytes turn into killer T-cells?
 A. Antibody immune response.
 B. Phagocytic immune response.
 C. Humoral response.
 *D. Cellular immune response.

Rationale: During the third mechanism of defense, T-lymphocytes can turn into special cytotoxic (killer) T-cells that can attack the pathogens themselves.

Reference: pp. 1335–1336

Descriptors:
1. 46 2. 01 3. Analysis
4. IV–4 5. Nursing Process 6. Difficult

5. During which type of response to invasion of pathogens do white blood cells ingest foreign particles?
   A. Antibody immune response.
   *B. Immune response.
   C. Humoral response.
   D. Cellular immune response.

Rationale: During the first mechanism of defense, WBCs, which have the ability to ingest foreign particles, move to the point of attack, where they engulf and destroy the invading agents.

Reference: p. 1332

Descriptors:
1. 46 2. 01 3. Analysis
4. IV–4 5. Nursing Process 6. Difficult

6. B-lymphocyte response occurs during which of the following types of immune responses to invading pathogens?
   A. Preliminary immune.
   B. Phagocytic immune response.
   *C. Humoral response.
   D. Cellular immune response.

Rationale: The second protective response, the humoral response, begins with the B-lymphocytes, which can transform themselves into plasma cells that manufacture antibodies.

Reference: p. 1332

Descriptors:
1. 46 2. 03 3. Analysis
4. IV–4 5. Nursing Process 6. Difficult

7. During which stage of the immune response does the antibody or cytotoxic T-cell reach and couple with the antigen on the surface of the foreign invader?
   A. Recognition.
   B. Proliferation.
   C. Response.
   *D. Effector.

Rationale: In the effector stage, either the antibody of the humoral response or the cytotoxic (killer) T-cell of the cellular response reaches and couples with the antigen on the surface of the foreign invader. The coupling initiates a series of events that in most instances results in total destruction of the invading microbes or the complete neutralization of the toxin.

Reference: p. 1333

Descriptors:
1. 46 2. 02 3. Comprehension
4. IV–4 5. Nursing Process 6. Moderate

8. The B-lymphocytes are believed to have a specific role in
   A. transplant rejection.
   *B. allergic hay fever and asthma.
   C. graft-versus-host disease.
   D. intracellular infections.

Rationale: Some specific roles of B-lymphocytes (humoral responses) include bacterial phagocytosis and lysis, anaphylaxis, allergic hay fever and asthma, immune complex disease, bacterial and some viral infections. Some specific roles of T-lymphocytes (cellular response) include transplant rejection; delayed hypersensitivity (tuberculin reaction); graft-versus-host disease; tumor surveillance or destruction; intracellular infections; viral, fungal, and parasitic infections.

Reference: p. 1333

Descriptors:
1. 46 2. 03 3. Comprehension
4. IV–4 5. Nursing Process 6. Difficult

9. The cytotoxic (killer) T-lymphocytes are believed to have a specific role in:
   A. bacterial phagocytosis and lysis
   B. anaphylaxis
   C. immune complex disease
   *D. tumor surveillance and destruction

Rationale: Some specific roles of B-lymphocytes (humoral responses) include bacterial phagocytosis and lysis, anaphylaxis, allergic hay fever and asthma, immune complex disease, bacterial and some viral infections. Some specific roles of T-lymphocytes (cellular response) include transplant rejection; delayed hypersensitivity (tuberculin reaction); graft-versus-host disease; tumor surveillance or destruction; intracellular infections; viral, fungal, and parasitic infections.

Reference: p. 1333

Descriptors:
1. 46 2. 03 3. Comprehension
4. IV–4 5. Nursing Process 6. Difficult

10. When the patient is vaccinated against communicable diseases, the nurse anticipates that the healthy patient will develop
   A. natural immunity.
   *B. active acquired immunity.
   C. passive acquired immunity.
   D. hypersensitivity.

Rationale: Active acquired immunity usually develops as a result of vaccination or contracting a disease. Natural immunity is present at birth and provides a nonspecific response to any foreign invader. Passive acquired immunity is temporary immunity transmitted from another source that has developed immunity through previous disease or immunization.

Reference: p. 1332

Descriptors:
1. 46 2. 01 3. Comprehension
4. IV–4 5. Nursing Process 6. Difficult

11. Injection of which of the following substances will provide passive acquired immunity to the recipient?

*A. Gamma globulin.
B. Antibiotics.
C. Albumin.
D. Measles-mumps-rubella vaccine.

Rationale: Gamma globulin, obtained from the blood plasma of people with acquired immunity, is used in emergencies to provide immunity to diseases when the risk for contacting a specific disease is great and there is not enough time for a person to develop adequate active immunity.

Reference: p. 1332

Descriptors:
1. 46 2. 01 3. Analysis
4. IV–4 5. Nursing Process 6. Difficult

12. Which of the following categories of medications is known to inhibit prostaglandin synthesis or release?
A. Antibiotics (in large doses).
*B. Nonsteroidal anti-inflammatory drugs (in large doses).
C. Adrenal corticosteroids.
D. Antimetabolites.

Rationale: NSAIDs inhibit prostaglandin synthesis or release. Adrenalcortical steroids, antineoplastics, and antimetabolites cause immunosuppression. Antibiotics in large doses cause bone marrow suppression.

Reference: p. 1340

Descriptors:
1. 46 2. 04 3. Comprehension
4. IV–2 5. Nursing Process 6. Difficult

13. Which of the following assessment findings may indicate immune dysfunction?
*A. Rhinitis.
B. Hypertension.
C. Constipation.
D. Oliguria.

Rationale: Rhinitis may indicate immune dysfunction. Hypotension, vomiting, diarrhea, and hematuria are also indicators of immune dysfunction.

Reference: p. 1340

Descriptors:
1. 46 2. 05 3. Comprehension
4. IV–4 5. Nursing Process 6. Moderate

14. Which of the following organs, if removed, may place the patient at risk for impaired immune function?
A. Lung.
*B. Thymus.
C. Colon.
D. Gallbladder.

Rationale: A history of surgical removal of the spleen, lymph nodes, or thymus may place the patient at risk for impaired immune function.

Reference: p. 1339

Descriptors:
1. 46 2. 05 3. Comprehension
4. IV–3 5. Nursing Process 6. Easy

15. Depletion of which of the following nutrients results in atrophy of lymphoid tissue, depression of antibody response, and impaired phagocytic function?
A. Carbohydrates.
B. Fats.
*C. Proteins.
D. Vitamin C.

Rationale: Depletion of protein reserves results in atrophy of lymphoid tissues, depression of antibody response, reduction in the number of circulating T-cells, and impaired phagocytic function.

Reference: p. 1338

Descriptors:
1. 46 2. 05 3. Knowledge
4. IV–1 5. Nursing Process 6. Moderate

CHAPTER 47
Management of Patients with Immunodeficiency

1. Agammaglobulinemia is the term that refers to a
A. disorder involving a complete absence of humoral and cellular immunity resulting from an X-linked or autosomal genetic abnormality.
*B. disorder marked by an almost complete lack of immunoglobulins or antibodies.
C. lack of one or more of the five immunoglobulins.
D. T-cell deficiency that occurs when the thymus gland fails to develop normally during embryogenesis.

Rationale: Agammaglobulinemia (Bruton's disease) is an inherited B-cell deficiency in which plasma cells are lacking and the germinal centers of all lymphatic tissue disappear, leading to a complete lack of antibody production against invading bacteria, viruses, and other pathogens.

Reference: p. 1343

Descriptors:
1. 47 2. 01 3. Comprehension
4. IV–4 5. Nursing Process 6. Difficult

2. Hypogammaglobulinemia is the term that refers to a
A. disorder involving lack of a thymus gland and subsequent B-cell deficiencies in combination with increased, decreased, or normal immunoglobulins.
B. disorder marked by an almost complete lack of immunoglobulins or antibodies.

*C. lack of one or more of the five immunoglobulins.
D. T-cell deficiency that occurs when the thymus gland fails to develop normally during embryogenesis.

Rationale: Hypogammaglobulinemia is caused by B-cell deficiency.

Reference: p. 1343

Descriptors:
1. 47 2. 01 3. Comprehension
4. IV–4 5. Nursing Process 6. Difficult

3. Nezelof's syndrome is characterized as a
*A. disorder involving a complete absence of humoral and cellular immunity resulting from an X-linked or autosomal genetic abnormality.
B. disorder marked by an almost complete lack of immunoglobulins or antibodies.
C. lack of one or more of the five immunoglobulins.
D. T-cell deficiency that occurs when the thymus gland fails to develop normally during embryogenesis.

Rationale: Nezelhof's syndrome results in severe infections and malignancies.

Reference: p. 1343

Descriptors:
1. 47 2. 01 3. Comprehension
4. IV–4 5. Nursing Process 6. Difficult

4. DiGeorge's syndrome is characterized as a
A. disorder involving a complete absence of humoral and cellular immunity resulting from an X-linked or autosomal genetic abnormality.
B. disorder marked by an almost complete lack of immunoglobulins or antibodies.
C. lack of one or more of the five immunoglobulins.
*D. T-cell deficiency that occurs when the thymus gland fails to develop normally during embryogenesis.

Rationale: DiGeorge's syndrome, thymic hypoplasia, results in recurrent infections.

Reference: p. 1343

Descriptors:
1. 47 2. 01 3. Comprehension
4. IV–4 5. Nursing Process 6. Difficult

5. Angioneurotic edema is the term used to describe
A. a yeast infection of skin or mucous membranes.
B. uncoordinated muscle movement.
C. vascular lesions caused by dilated blood vessels.
*D. a condition marked by development of urticaria.

Rationale: Angioneurotic edema is a condition marked by development of urticaria and an edematous area of skin, mucous membranes, or viscera.

Reference: p. 1343

Descriptors:
1. 47 2. 01 3. Knowledge
4. IV–1 5. Nursing Process 6. Easy

6. Ataxia is the term used to refer to
A. a yeast infection of skin or mucous membranes.
*B. uncoordinated muscle movement.
C. vascular lesions caused by dilated blood vessels.
D. a condition marked by development of urticaria.

Rationale: Ataxia refers to uncoordinated muscle movement and is a clinical manifestation of combined B-cell and T-cell deficiencies.

Reference: p. 1343

Descriptors:
1. 47 2. 01 3. Knowledge
4. IV–1 5. Nursing Process 6. Moderate

7. Telangiectasia refers to
A. a yeast infection of skin or mucous membranes.
B. uncoordinated muscle movement.
*C. vascular lesions caused by dilated blood vessels.
D. a condition marked by development of urticaria.

Rationale: Telangiectasia refers to vascular lesions caused by dilated blood vessels and is a clinical manifestation of combined B-cell and T-cell deficiencies.

Reference: p. 1343

Descriptors:
1. 47 2. 01 3. Knowledge
4. IV–1 5. Nursing Process 6. Moderate

8. Patient teaching regarding infection prevention for the patient with an immunodeficiency includes which of the following guidelines?
A. Consume raw fruits daily.
B. Refrain from using creams or emollients on skin.
*C. Avoid people who have been vaccinated recently.
D. Report any diarrhea or vaginal discharge immediately.

Rationale: Individuals who have been vaccinated recently may be shedding an attenuated virus that would cause disease in an exposed immunocompromised host. All foods must be cooked, skin must be kept supple, and the patient should only report PERSISTENT diarrhea or vaginal discharge.

Reference: p. 1347

Descriptors:

1. 47	2. 04
3. Application/Analysis	4. IV–3
5. Teaching/Learning	6. Difficult

9. Patient teaching regarding infection prevention for the patient with an immunodeficiency includes which of the following guidelines?
   *A. Cook all foods.
   B. Refrain from using creams or emollients on skin.
   C. People who have been vaccinated recently may visit.
   D. Report any diarrhea or vaginal discharge immediately.

Rationale: Individuals who have been vaccinated recently may be shedding an attenuated virus that would cause disease in an exposed immunocompromised host. All foods must be cooked, skin must be kept supple, and the patient should only report PERSISTENT diarrhea or vaginal discharge.

Reference: p. 1347

Descriptors:

1. 47	2. 04
3. Application/Analysis	4. IV–3
5. Teaching/Learning	6. Difficult

10. Patient teaching regarding infection prevention for the patient with an immunodeficiency includes which of the following guidelines?
   A. Consume raw fruits daily.
   *B. Use creams or emollients on skin.
   C. People who have been vaccinated recently may visit.
   D. Report any diarrhea or vaginal discharge immediately.

Rationale: Individuals who have been vaccinated recently may be shedding an attenuated virus that would cause disease in an exposed immunocompromised host. All foods must be cooked, skin must be kept supple, and the patient should only report persistent diarrhea or vaginal discharge.

Reference: p. 1347

Descriptors:

1. 47	2. 04
3. Application/Analysis	4. IV–3
5. Teaching/Learning	6. Difficult

11. Patient teaching regarding infection prevention for the patient with an immunodeficiency includes which of the following guidelines?
   A. Consume raw fruits daily.
   B. Refrain from using creams or emollients on skin.
   C. People who have been vaccinated recently may visit.
   *D. Report persistent diarrhea or vaginal discharge immediately.

Rationale: Individuals who have been vaccinated recently may be shedding an attenuated virus that would cause disease in an exposed immunocompromised host. All foods must be cooked, skin must be kept supple, and the patient should report persistent diarrhea or vaginal discharge.

Reference: p. 1347

Descriptors:

1. 47	2. 04
3. Application/Analysis	4. IV–3
5. Teaching/Learning	6. Difficult

12. Which of the following medical problems is a cardinal symptom of immunodeficiency?
   *A. Recurrent severe infections.
   B. Skin rashes.
   C. Rhinitis.
   D. Joint pain.

Rationale: The cardinal symptoms of immunodeficiency include chronic or recurrent severe infections, infections caused by unusual organisms or organisms that are normal body flora, poor response to treatment of infections, and chronic diarrhea.

Reference: p. 1342

Descriptors:

1. 47	2. 01	3. Knowledge
4. IV–4	5. Nursing Process	6. Easy

13. Which of the following medical problems is a cardinal symptom of immunodeficiency?
   *A. Chronic severe infections.
   B. Skin rashes.
   C. Rhinitis.
   D. Joint pain.

Rationale: The cardinal symptoms of immunodeficiency include chronic or recurrent severe infections, infections caused by unusual organisms or organisms that are normal body flora, poor response to treatment of infections, and chronic diarrhea.

Reference: p. 1342

Descriptors:

1. 47	2. 01	3. Knowledge
4. IV–4	5. Nursing Process	6. Easy

14. Which of the following medical problems is a cardinal symptom of immunodeficiency?
   *A. Opportunistic infections.
   B. Skin rashes.
   C. Rhinitis.
   D. Joint pain.

Rationale: The cardinal symptoms of immunodeficiency include chronic or recurrent severe infections, infections caused by unusual organisms or organisms that are normal body flora, poor response to treatment of infections, and chronic diarrhea.

Reference: p. 1342

Descriptors:
1. 47 2. 01 3. Knowledge
4. IV–4 5. Nursing Process 6. Easy

15. Which of the following medical problems is a cardinal symptom of immunodeficiency?
*A. Chronic diarrhea.
B. Skin rashes.
C. Rhinitis.
D. Joint pain.

Rationale: The cardinal symptoms of immunodeficiency include chronic or recurrent severe infections, infections caused by unusual organisms or organisms that are normal body flora, poor response to treatment of infections, and chronic diarrhea.

Reference: p. 1342

Descriptors:
1. 47 2. 01 3. Knowledge
4. IV–4 5. Nursing Process 6. Easy

CHAPTER 48
Management of Patients with HIV and AIDS

1. Human immunodeficiency virus belongs to a group of viruses known as *retroviruses*, which indicates that the virus
*A. carries its genetic material in ribonuclei acid (RNA) rather than deoxyribonucleic acid (DNA).
B. has heightened virulence and infectious ability.
C. impairs the function of cytotoxic T-lymphocytes.
D. stimulates the immune system.

Rationale: HIV belongs to a group of viruses known as *retroviruses,* which indicates that the virus carries its genetic material in RNA rather than DNA. Some recent strains of HIV–1 have heightened virulence and infectious ability, but most strains of HIV–1 are relatively weak viruses. The HIV–1 virus impairs functioning of the helper T4 lymphocytes and "hides" from the immune system by way of its sugar "cloak."

Reference: pp. 1350–1351

Descriptors:
1. 48 2. 01 3. Comprehension
4. IV–4 5. Nursing Process 6. Difficult

2. Which of the following terms is used to refer to the substance used by HIV to reprogam the genetic materials of the infected lymphocyte?
A. Alpha-interferon.
B. Protease inhibitor.
C. p24 antigen.
*D. Reverse transcriptase.

Rationale: Reverse transcriptase is the enzyme that used by HIV that reprograms the single-stranded RNA into a double-stranded RNA within the infected T4 cell. Alpha-interferon is a protein substance that has antiviral and antitumor activity. Protease inhibitors are a category of medications that inhibit the function of protease, an enzyme needed for HIV replication. The p24 antigen is a blood test that measures viral core protein.

Reference: p. 1351

Descriptors:
1. 48 2. 01 3. Comprehension
4. IV–4 5. Nursing Process 6. Moderate

3. HIV–1 is transmitted by way of:
A. air.
B. droplet nuclei.
C. fomites.
*D. body fluids.

Rationale: HIV–1 is transmitted by way of body fluids that contain HIV–1 or CD4+ T-lymphocytes. These fluids include serum, seminal fluid, vaginal secretions, amniotic fluid, and breast milk.

Reference: p. 1351

Descriptors:
1. 48 2. 02 3. Knowledge
4. IV–3 5. Nursing Process 6. Easy

4. Which of the following time periods is recommended by the Centers for Disease Control (CDC) as the timeframe within which prophylaxis post exposure to HIV infection must be started in order to be of benefit?
A. 24 hours.
*B. 72 hours.
C. 3 months.
D. 6 months.

Rationale: Ideally, prophylaxis needs to start within hours of exposure. Therapy started more than 72 hours after exposure is thought to be of no benefit and therefore is not recommended.

Reference: p. 1352

Descriptors:
1. 48 2. 02 3. Knowledge
4. IV–3 5. Nursing Process 6. Easy

5. Which of the following statements accurately describes the emphasis that is recommended be given by health care workers to prevention of transmission of disease?
*A. Standard precautions must be applied to all hospitalized patients regardless of their diagnosis or presumed infectious status.
B. Standard precautions always incorporate airborne precautions.

C. Airborne, Droplet, and Contact precautions must be applied to all hospitalized patients regardless of their diagnosis or presumed infectious status.
D. Implementation of Airborne, Droplet, and Contact precautions eliminate the need for incorporation of standard precautions.

Rationale: Standard precautions incorporate the major features of universal precautions and Body Substance Isolation and applies to all patients receiving care in hospitals regardless of their diagnosis or presumed infectious status (Hospital Infection Control Practices Advisory Committee, 1996, p. 64). Transmission-based precautions (airborne, droplet, contact) were designed for use in addition to standard precautions for patients with documented or suspected infections involving highly transmissible pathogens.

Reference: p. 1352

Descriptors:
1. 48 2. 02 3. Analysis
4. IV–3 5. Nursing Process 6. Difficult

6. Of the following generalizations, which applies MOST APPROPRIATELY to the implementation of Standard Precautions?
A. Wear sterile gloves when touching blood or body fluids.
B. Use an antimicrobial soap for routine hand washing.
C. Carefully recap needles after administration of medication to the patient.
*D. Never manipulate used needles by hand.

Rationale: Gloves recommended for use for Standard Precautions should be clean and unsterile. Nonantimicrobial soap should be used for routine hand washing with an antimicrobial soap or waterless antiseptic agent used for special circumstances. Needles should NEVER be recapped or otherwise manipulated.

Reference: p. 1354

Descriptors:
1. 48 2. 02 3. Knowledge
4. IV–3 5. Nursing Process 6. Moderate

7. Which of the following statements accurately describes the physiology underlying the associated clinical manifestation of HIV infection?
A. GI symptoms directly result from the action of HIV on the cells lining the intestines.
B. Patients with AIDS have a higher than usual incidence of cancer because of the underlying immune deficiency caused by the virus.
*C. Neurologic dysfunction results from the direct effects of HIV on nervous tissue.
D. Endocrine manifestations of HIV infection result from the action of the HIV on the pituitary gland.

Rationale: GI symptoms *may* result from the action of HIV on the lining of the intestines, but opportunistic infections of the GI tract result in symptoms associated with the disorder. Patients with AIDS have a higher than usual incidence of cancer. Neurologic dysfunction results from the direct effects of HIV on nervous tissue. Endocrine manifestations are not completely understood.

Reference: p. 1356

Descriptors:
1. 48 2. 03 3. Analysis
4. IV–4 5. Nursing Process 6. Difficult

8. Of the following clinical manifestations of HIV infections, which is KNOWN to be the direct result of action of the viral infection?
A. Depression.
B. Endocrine disturbance.
C. Wasting syndrome.
*D. Neurologic dysfunction.

Rationale: Depression is multifactorial. Endocrine manifestations of the HIV infection are not completely understood. Wasting syndrome results from the *effects* of HIV as well as opportunistic infections. Neurologic dysfunction results from the direct effects of HIV on neurologic tissue.

Reference: p. 1356

Descriptors:
1. 48 2. 03 3. Comprehension
4. IV–4 5. Nursing Process 6. Moderate

9. A nurse teaches the patient undergoing HIV testing which of the following considerations? Positive test results
A. indicate that AIDS has been diagnosed.
B. do not indicate that AIDS is active in the body.
C. mean that the patient is immune to AIDS.
*D. mean that antibodies to the AIDS virus are present in the blood.

Rationale: Consideration of positive test results include the following: antibodies to the AIDS virus are present in the blood, HIV is probably active in the body, the patient does not necessarily have AIDS, the patient is not immune to AIDS, and the patient may not necessarily get AIDS in the future.

Reference: p. 1359

Descriptors:
1. 48 2. 04 3. Analysis
4. IV–3 5. Nursing Process 6. Difficult

10. A nurse teaches the patient undergoing HIV testing which of the following considerations? Positive test results
*A. indicate that the patient has been infected with HIV and produced antibodies.
B. do not indicate that AIDS is active in the body.

C. mean that the patient is immune to AIDS.
D. does not mean that the patient will get AIDS in the future.

Rationale: Consideration of positive test results include the following: antibodies to the AIDS virus are present in the blood, HIV is probably active in the body, the patient does not necessarily have AIDS, the patient is not immune to AIDS, and the patient may not necessarily get AIDS in the future.

Reference: p. 1359

Descriptors:
1. 48 2. 04 3. Analysis
4. IV–3 5. Nursing Process 6. Difficult

11. A nurse teaches the patient with AIDS which of the following guidelines related to the diarrhea experienced by the patient?
*A. Refrain from smoking.
B. Eat three balanced meals and a snack at bedtime.
C. Restrict fluid intake.
D. Include at least three servings of raw vegetables daily.

Rationale: Measures that will reduce hyperactivity of the bowel include no smoking, avoiding bowel irritants (fatty or fried foods, raw vegetables, and nuts), and eating small, frequent meals. Unless contraindicated, fluid intake of at least 3 liters/day is recommended to prevent hypovolemia.

Reference: p. 1367

Descriptors:
1. 48 2. 06
3. Application/Analysis 4. IV–1
5. Teaching/Learning 6. Moderate

12. Of the following antiretroviral agents, which is categorized as a protease inhibitor?
A. Zidovudine (Retrovir; formerly AZT).
B. Nevirapine (Viramune).
*C. Saquinavir (Infirase).
D. Didanosine (Videa).

Rationale: Saquinavir is a protease inhibitor, while Nevirapine is a non-nucleoside reverse transcriptase inhibitor. Zidovudine and Didanosine are nucleoside reverse transcriptase inhibitors.

Reference: pp. 1362–1363

Descriptors:
1. 48 2. 04 3. Knowledge
4. IV–2 5. Nursing Process 6. Moderate

13. Of the following antiretroviral agents, which is categorized as a non-nucleoside reverse transcriptase inhibitor?
A. Zidovudine (Retrovir; formerly AZT).
*B. Nevirapine (Viramune).
C. Saquinavir (Infirase).
D. Didanosine (Videx).

Rationale: Saquinavir is a protease inhibitor, while Nevirapine is a non-nucleoside reverse transcriptase inhibitor. Zidovudine and Didanosine are nucleoside reverse transcriptase inhibitors.

Reference: pp. 1362–1363

Descriptors:
1. 48 2. 04 3. Knowledge
4. IV–2 5. Nursing Process 6. Moderate

14. Of the following expected outcomes, which is REALISTIC regarding the AIDS patient?
A. Establishes normal bowel habits.
B. Demonstrates normal nutritional status.
*C. Maintains usual level of thought processes.
D. Increases level of self-care activities.

Rationale: Realistic expected outcomes for the AIDS patient include resuming usual bowel habits, maintaining adequate nutritional status, maintaining usual level of thought processes (neurological complications are irreversible), and participating in self-care activities as possible.

Reference: p. 1378

Descriptors:
1. 48 2. 07 3. Application
4. IV–4 5. Nursing Process 6. Moderate

15. Patient education regarding condom use would include which of the following guidelines?
A. Attach the condom prior to erection.
B. Hold the condom by the cuff for application.
C. Use skin lotion or petroleum jelly for lubrication.
*D. Hold the condom by the cuff upon withdrawal.

Rationale: The condom should be unrolled over the hard penis before any kind of sex. The condom should be held by the tip to squeeze out air. Skin lotions, baby oil, petroleum jelly, or cold cream should NOT be used with condoms (they cause latex deterioration/condom breakage). The condom should be held during withdrawal so it does not come off the penis.

Reference: p. 1377

Descriptors:
1. 48 2. 02 3. Application
4. IV–3 5. Nursing Process 6. Moderate

CHAPTER 49
Assessment and Management of Patients with Allergic Disorders

1. Antibodies formed by lymphocytes and plasma cells in response to an immunogenic stimulus constitute a group of serum substances called
A. haptens.
*B. immunoglobulins.

C. leukotrienes.
D. prostaglandins.

Rationale: Immunoglobulins are a family of closely related proteins capable of acting as antibodies formed by lymphocytes and plasma cells in response to an immunogenic stimulus. Haptens are incomplete antigens, while leukotrienes are a group of chemical mediators that initiate the inflammatory response. Prostaglandins are unsaturated fatty acids that have a wide assortment of biologic activity.

Reference: p. 1383

Descriptors:
1. 49 2. 01 3. Comprehension
4. IV–4 5. Nursing Process 6. Moderate

2. Which of the following analogies describe the way that antibodies combine with antigens?
*A. Keys fitting into a lock.
B. Paint coating a wall.
C. Sugar dissolving in water.
D. Glue sticking to paper.

Rationale: Antibodies combine with antigens in a special way, likened to keys fitting into a lock. Antigens (the keys) only fit certain antibodies (the locks).

Reference: p. 1383

Descriptors:
1. 49 2. 01 3. Knowledge
4. IV–4 5. Nursing Process 6. Easy

3. Which of the following properties of antibody molecules causes them to agglutinate?
*A. Bivalency.
B. Polarity.
C. Osmolarity.
D. Osmolality.

Rationale: Antibody molecules are bivalent; that is, they have two combining sites. Therefore, the antibody easily becomes a cross-link between two antigen groups, causing them to clump together (agglutination). By this action, foreign invaders are cleared from the bloodstream.

Reference: p. 1383

Descriptors:
1. 49 2. 01 3. Comprehension
4. IV–4 5. Nursing Process 6. Moderate

4. Which of the following chemical mediators initiates the inflammatory response?
A. Histamine.
*B. Leukotrienes.
C. Bradykinin.
D. Serotonin.

Rationale: Leukotrienes are chemical mediators that initiate the inflammatory response.

Reference: p. 1384

Descriptors:
1. 49 2. 01 3. Knowledge
4. IV–4 5. Nursing Process 6. Easy

5. Which type of hypersensitivity reaction is characterized by an immediate reaction beginning within minutes of exposure to an antigen?
*A. Type I.
B. Type II.
C. Type III.
D. Type IV.

Rationale: Anaphylactic (Type I) hypersensitivity is an immediate reaction mediated by IgE antibodies and requires previous exposure to the specific antigen. Type II reactions, or cytotoxic hypersensitivity, occur when the system mistakenly identifies a normal constituent of the body as foreign. Type III, or immune complex hypersensivity, occurs as the result of two factors, the increased amount of circulating complexes and the presence of vasoactive amines. Type IV, or delayed-type hypersensitivity, occurs 24 to 72 hours after exposure to an allergen and is mediated by sensitized T-cells and macrophages.

Reference: pp. 1385–1386

Descriptors:
1. 49 2. 02 3. Comprehension
4. IV–4 5. Nursing Process 6. Moderate

6. Which type of hypersensitivity reaction is characterized by the body mistakenly identifying its normal constituent as foreign?
A. Type I.
*B. Type II.
C. Type III.
D. Type IV.

Rationale: Anaphylactic (Type I) hypersensitivity is an immediate reaction mediated by IgE antibodies and requires previous exposure to the specific antigen. Type II reactions, or cytotoxic hypersensitivity, occurs when the system mistakenly identifies a normal constituent of the body as foreign. Type III, or immune complex hypersensivity, occurs as the result of two factors, the increased amount of circulating complexes and the presence of vasoactive amines. Type IV, or delayed-type hypersensitivity, occurs 24 to 72 hours after exposure to an allergen and is mediated by sensitized T-cells and macrophages.

Reference: pp. 1385–1386

Descriptors:
1. 49 2. 02 3. Comprehension
4. IV–4 5. Nursing Process 6. Moderate

7. Which type of hypersensitivity reaction is characterized by delayed reaction that occurs 24 to 72 hours after exposure to an antigen?
A. Type I.
B. Type II.
C. Type III.
*D. Type IV.

Rationale: Anaphylactic (Type I) hypersensitivity is an immediate reacation mediated by IgE antibodies and requires previous exposure to the specific antigen. Type II reactions, or cytotoxic hypersensitivity, occur when the system mistakenly identifies a normal constituent of the body as foreign. Type III, or immune complex hypersensivity, occurs as the result of two factors, the increased amount of circulating complexes and the presence of vasoactive amines. Type IV, or delayed-type hypersensitivity, occurs 24 to 72 hours after exposure to an allergen and is mediated by sensitized T-cells and macrophages.

Reference: pp. 1385–1386

Descriptors:
1. 49 2. 02 3. Comprehension
4. IV–4 5. Nursing Process 6. Moderate

8. When the patient asks the nurse to explain RAST testing for allergies, the nurse explains that the test involves
   A. simultaneous intradermal injection of several solutions at several sites to identify skin reactions.
   B. direct administration of a suspected allergen to the sensitive tissue, such as nasal or bronchial mucosa, with observation of target organ response.
   *C. exposing the patient's serum, obtained through a blood sample, to a variety of suspected radiolabeled allergen particle complexes.
   D. obtaining samples from the patient's nasal secretions during a symptomatic episode to determine the presence of eosinophils.

Rationale: RAST is a radioimmunoassay that measures allergen-specific IgE. A sample of the patient's serum is exposed to a variety of suspected allergen particle complexes. If antibodies are present, they will combine with radiolabeled allergens.

Reference: p. 1390

Descriptors:
1. 49 2. 03 3. Application
4. IV–1 5. Teaching/Learning 6. Moderate

9. When the nurse examines the patient's skin after interdermal skin testing, at the appropriate time for evaluating response, and determines that the area presents a wheal (7–10 mm) with associated erythema, the nurse records the result as
   A. 1+.
   *B. 2+.
   C. 3+.
   D. 4+.

Rationale: Interpretations of skin testing reactions: Negative = wheal soft with minimal erythema; 1+ = wheal present (5–8 mm) with associated erythema; 2+ = wheal (7–10 mm) with associated erythema; 3+ = wheal (9–15 mm), slight pseudopodia possible with associated erythema; 4+ = wheal (12 mm+) with pseudopodia and diffuse erythema.

Reference: p. 1391

Descriptors:
1. 49 2. 03 3. Comprehension
4. IV–4 5. Nursing Process 6. Moderate

10. Which of the following sites does the nurse teach the patient to use for self-administration of epinephrine in the event of an anaphylactic reaction?
   A. Forearm vein.
   *B. Thigh.
   C. Buttocks.
   D. Upper arm.

Rationale: The patient is taught to position the device at the middle portion of the thigh and push the device into the thigh as far as possible. The device will autoinject a premeasured dose of epinephrine into the subcutaneous tissue.

Reference: p. 1392

Descriptors:
1. 49 2. 04 3. Application
4 IV–3 5. Teaching/Learning 6. Easy

11. Of the following of chemical classes of H1 antihistamines, which is categorized as nonsedating?
   A. diphenhydramine (Benadryl).
   B. alkylamines (Chlor-trimeton).
   C. cetirizine (Zyrtec).
   *D. astemizole (Hismanal).

Rationale: Astemizole (Hismanal), loratadine (Claritin), and fexufenadine (Allegra) are nonsedating H1 antihistamines.

Reference: p. 1394

Descriptors:
1. 49 2. 03 3. Knowledge
4. IV–2 5. Nursing Process 6. Moderate

12. Which of the following types of contact dermatitis requires sun and a chemical in combination to damage the epidermis?
   A. Allergic.
   B. Irritant.
   *C. Phototoxic.
   D. Photoallergic.

Rationale: Phototoxic contact dermatitis resembles the irritant type but requires sun and a chemical in combination to damage the epidermis.

Reference: p. 1399

Descriptors:
1. 49 2. 02 3. Comprehension
4. IV–4 5. Nursing Process 6. Moderate

13. Which class of immunoglobulins are involved in allergic disorders and some parasitic infections?
   A. IgA.
   B. IgM.
   *C. IgE.
   D. IgG.

Rationale: Antibodies of the IgM, IgG, and IgA classes function to neutralize toxins and viruses and to precipitate, agglutinate, and lyze bacteria and other foreign cellular material. IgE class immunoglobulines are involved in allergic disorders, and IgE-producing cells are located in the respiratory and intestinal mucosa.

Reference: p. 1383

Descriptors:
1. 49 2. 01 3. Knowledge
4. IV–4 5. Nursing Process 6. Easy

14. Histamine produces which of the following effects?
A. Bronchial smooth muscle dilation.
B. Small venule contraction.
C. Decreased secretion of gastric and mucosal cells.
*D. Larger vessel constriction.

Rationale: Histamine plays an important role in regulating the immune response, causing contraction of bronchial smooth muscle, dilation of small venules and constriction of larger vessels, and increased secretion secretion of gastric and mucosal cells.

Reference: p. 1384

Descriptors:
1. 49 2. 01 3. Comprehension
4. IV–4 5. Nursing Process 6. Moderate

15. Regarding chemical mediators of hypersensitivity, which of the following are classified as secondary?
A. Histamine.
B. Prostaglandins.
C. Platelet-activating factor.
*D. Bradykinin.

Rationale: Bradykinin, a polypeptide, contracts smooth muscles of the bronchi and blood vessels. It causes increased permeability of the capillaries, resulting in edema. Bradykinin stimulates nerve cell fibers and produces pain.

Reference: p. 1384

Descriptors:
1. 49 2. 01 3. Knowledge
4. IV–4 5. Nursing Process 6. Moderate

CHAPTER 50
Assessment and Management of Patients with Rheumatic Disorders

1. Which of the following terms refers to newly formed synovial tissue infiltrated with inflammatory cells?
A. Cytokines.
*B. Pannus.
C. Leukotriene.
D. Tophi.

Rationale: Pannus is the newly formed synovial tissue infiltrated with inflammatory cells, the effects of which cause degeneration in human joints.

Reference: p. 1406

Descriptors:
1. 50 2. 01 3. Knowledge
4. IV–4 5. Nursing Process 6. Moderate

2. Of the following body components, which is the area most commonly affected by the inflammation and degeneration seen in rheumatic diseases? The
A. heart.
*B. joints.
C. skin.
D. blood vessels.

Rationale: The joint is the area most commonly affected by the inflammation and degeneration seen in rheumatic disease.

Reference: p. 1406

Descriptors:
1. 50 2. 01 3. Knowledge
4. IV–1 5. Nursing Process 6. Easy

3. When assessing the patient with a suspected diagnosis of rheumatic disease, the nurse anticipates which of the following manifestations?
A. Pigmented skin.
B. Scleral jaundice.
C. Normal grip strength.
*D. Alopecia.

Rationale: Skin may show rashes, lesions, increased bruising, erythema, thinning, warmth, and photosensivity. Hair may show alopecia. Conjunctiva may be inflamed, but not jaundiced. Grip strength usually is decreased due to joint debility.

Reference: pp. 1408–1409

Descriptors:
1. 50 2. 02 3. Application
4. IV–4 5. Nursing Process 6. Moderate

4. Of the following diagnostic tests, which would be used to assess the degree to which the crystal lattice of bone absorbs a bone-seeking radioactive isotope?
A. Radiographs.
B. Arthrography.
*C. Bone scan.
D. Serum studies.

Rationale: A bone scan can reflects the degree to which the crystal lattice of bone "takes up" a bone-seeking radioactive isotope. An area demonstrating increased uptake is considered abnormal. Bone scans are not the most cost-effective method for detecting early disease, and they are not done routinely at the time of diagnosis.

Reference: p. 1410

Descriptors:
1. 50 2. 02 3. Comprehension
4. IV–1 5. Nursing Process 6. Easy

5. An elevation in which of the following common serum studies for rheumatic disorders indicates inflammation?
   A. Hematocrit.
   B. Red blood cell count.
   C. Serum complement (C3, C4).
   *D. Antinuclear antibody level.

Rationale: Antinuclear antibody (ANA) measures serum antibodies that react with a variety of nuclear antigens. The higher the titre, the greater the inflammation.

Reference: p. 1411

Descriptors:
1. 50 2. 02 3. Knowledge
4. IV–1 5. Nursing Process 6. Easy

6. A decrease in which of the following common serum studies for rheumatic disorders indicates chronic inflammation?
   *A. Hematocrit.
   B. Creatinine.
   C. Erythrocyte sedimentation rate.
   D. Antinuclear antibody level.

Rationale: A decrease in hematocrit, RBC count, and WBC count may be seen with rheumatic disorders.

Reference: p. 1410

Descriptors:
1. 50 2. 02 3. Knowledge
4. IV–1 5. Nursing Process 6. Easy

7. Of the following medications used in rheumatic disease, which not only has anti-inflammatory effects but also inhibits lysosomal enzymes?
   A. Salicylates.
   B. Nonsteroidal anti-inflammatory drugs (NSAIDs).
   *C. Disease-modifying antirheumatic drugs (DMARDs).
   D. Corticosteroids.

Rationale: DMARDs are slow acting and administered concurrently with NSAIDs.

Reference: pp. 1413–1414

Descriptors:
1. 50 2. 03 3. Comprehension
4. IV–2 5. Nursing Process 6. Moderate

8. Of the following medications used in rheumatic disease, which not only has anti-inflammatory effects but also inhibits T-cell function?
   *A. Penicillamine.
   B. Nonsteroidal anti-inflammatory drugs (NSAIDs).
   C. Disease-modifying antirheumatic drugs (DMARDs).
   D. Corticosteroids.

Rationale: Penicillamine is a DMARD that acts as anti-inflammatory, inhibiting T-cell function, and impairing antigen presentation.

Reference: pp. 1413–1414

Descriptors:
1. 50 2. 03 3. Comprehension
4. IV–2 5. Nursing Process 6. Moderate

9. When the nurse learns that the patient with rheumatic disease is being prescribed an antimalarial agent for treatment, he or she teaches the patient to monitor himself or herself for
   A. tinnitus.
   *B. visual changes.
   C. stomatitis.
   D. hirsutism.

Rationale: The DMARD category of antimalarials may cause visual changes, GI upset, skin rash, headaches, photosensitivity, and bleaching of hair. Tinnitis is associated with salicylate therapy, stomatitis is associated with gold therapy, and hirsutism is associated with corticosteroid therapy.

Reference: pp. 1413–1414

Descriptors:
1. 50 2. 04 3. Application
4. IV–3 5. Teaching/Learning 6. Moderate

10. When the nurse learns that the patient with rheumatic disease is being prescribed salicylates for treatment, he or she teaches the patient to monitor himself or herself for
   *A. tinnitus.
   B. visual changes.
   C. stomatitis.
   D. hirsutism.

Rationale: The DMARD category of antimalarials may cause visual changes, GI upset, skin rash, headaches, photosensitivity, and bleaching of hair. Tinnitis is associated with salicylate therapy, stomatitis is associated with gold therapy, and hirsutism is associated with corticosteroid therapy.

Reference: pp. 1413–1414

Descriptors:
1. 50 2. 04 3. Application
4. IV–3 5. Teaching/Learning 6. Moderate

11. When the nurse learns that the patient with rheumatic disease is being prescribed gold-containing compounds for treatment, he or she teaches the patient to monitor himself or herself for
   A. tinnitus.
   B. visual changes.
   *C. stomatitis.
   D. hirsutism.

Rationale: The DMARD category of antimalarials may cause visual changes, GI upset, skin rash, headaches, photosensitivity, and bleaching of hair. Tinnitis is associated with salicylate therapy, stomatitis is associated with gold therapy, and hirsutism is associated with corticosteroid therapy.

Reference: pp. 1413–1414

Descriptors:
1. 50 2. 04 3. Application
4. IV–3 5. Teaching/Learning 6. Moderate

12. The nurse teaches the patient with rheumatic disease that it is acceptable to perform isometric exercises during which phase of the inflammatory process?
A. Acute exacerbation, severe pain.
B. Subacute exacerbation, moderate pain.
C. Subacute exacerbation, minimal pain.
*D. Remission.

Rationale: Active range of motion and isometric exercises are recommended for periods of inactive disease. Active assisted or active range of motion within pain tolerance is suggested for subacute inflammation. Passive range of motion is suggested during periods of acute exacerbation with severe pain.

Reference: p. 1414

Descriptors:
1. 50 2. 06 3. Application
4. IV–1 5. Teaching/Learning 6. Moderate

13. When the patient with rheumatic disease is experiencing an acute exacerbation with severe pain, the nurse suggests that the patient perform which type of exercise to promote mobility?
*A. Passive range of motion.
B. Active range of motion.
C. Active assisted range of motion.
D. Isometric.

Rationale: Active range of motion and isometric exercises are recommended for periods of inactive disease. Active assisted or active range of motion within pain tolerance is suggested for subacute inflammation. Passive range of motion is suggested during periods of acute exacerbation with severe pain.

Reference: p. 1414

Descriptors:
1. 50 2. 06 3. Application
4. IV–1 5. Teaching/Learning 6. Moderate

14. Which of the following diffuse connective tissue diseases (CTD) is the result of an autoimmune reaction that occurs primarily in the synovial fluid?
*A. Rheumatoid arthritis (RA).
B. Systemic lupus erythematosus (SLE).
C. Scleroderma.
D. Polymyositis.

Rationale: In RA, the autoimmune reaction results in phagocytosis producing enzymes within the joint that break down collagen, cause edema and proliferation of the synovial membrane, and ultimately form pannus. Pannus destroys cartilage and bone.

Reference: pp. 1422, 1424, 1426, 1427

Descriptors:
1. 50 2. 05 3. Comprehension
4. IV–4 5. Nursing Process 6. Moderate

15. Purine metabolism is altered in which of the following disorders?
A. Ankylosing spondylitis.
B. Reiter's syndrome.
C. Psoriatic arthritis.
*D. Gout.

Rationale: Gout is a heterogeneous group of conditions related to a generic defect of purine metabolism resulting in hyperuricemia. Then the urate crystals precipitate within a joint, an inflammatory response occurs, and an attack of gout begins.

Reference: p. 1430

Descriptors:
1. 50 2. 02 3. Knowledge
4. IV–4 5. Nursing Process 6. Moderate

UNIT 12 INTEGUMENTARY FUNCTION

CHAPTER 51
Assessment of Integumentary Function

1. Which of the following cells, common to the epidermis, are believed to play a significant role in cutaneous immune system reactions?
   A. Keratin cells.
   B. Melanocytes.
   C. Merkel cells.
   *D. Langerhans cells.

   Rationale: Dead cells of the epidermis contain keratin, an insoluble, fibrous protein that forms the outer barrier of the skin. Melanocytes are primarily involved in producing the pigment melanin. Merkel cells are the receptors that transmit stimuli to the axon via a chemical synapse. Langerhans cells are believed to play a significant role in cutaneous immune system reactions.

   Reference: p. 1439

   Descriptors:
   1. 51 2. 01 3. Knowledge
   4. IV–1 5. Nursing Process 6. Easy

2. Which of the following cells, common to the epidermis, are the receptors that transmit stimuli to the axon via a chemical synapse?
   A. Keratin cells.
   B. Melanocytes.
   *C. Merkel cells.
   D. Langerhans cells.

   Rationale: Dead cells of the epidermis contain keratin, an insoluble, fibrous protein that forms the outer barrier of the skin. Melanocytes are primarily involved in producing the pigment melanin. Merkel cells are the receptors that transmit stimuli to the axon via a chemical synapse. Langerhans cells are believed to play a significant role in cutaneous immune system reactions.

   Reference: p. 1439

   Descriptors:
   1. 51 2. 01 3. Knowledge
   4. IV–1 5. Nursing Process 6. Easy

3. Which of the following cells, common to the epidermis, are primarily involved in producing pigment?
   A. Keratin cells.
   *B. Melanocytes.
   C. Merkel cells.
   D. Langerhans cells.

   Rationale: Dead cells of the epidermis contain keratin, an insoluble, fibrous protein that forms the outer barrier of the skin. Melanocytes are primarily involved in producing the pigment melanin. Merkel cells are the receptors that transmit stimuli to the axon via a chemical synapse. Langerhans cells are believed to play a significant role in cutaneous immune system reactions.

   Reference: p. 1439

   Descriptors:
   1. 51 2. 01 3. Knowledge
   4. IV–1 5. Nursing Process 6. Easy

4. Which skin glands are confined to the axillae, anal region, scrotum, and labia majora?
   A. Sebaceous.
   B. Eccrine.
   *C. Apocrine.
   D. Papillary.

   Rationale: Sebaceous glands are associated with hair follicles, and for each hair there is a sebaceous gland. Eccrine glands are a type of sweat gland with ducts which open directly onto the skin surface. Apocrine glands are a type of sweat gland with ducts that generally open into hair follicles and are confined to the axillae, anal region, scrotum, and labia majora.

   Reference: p. 1441

   Descriptors:
   1. 51 2. 01 3. Knowledge
   4. IV–1 5. Nursing Process 6. Easy

5. Which skin layer provides the most effective barrier to both epidermal water loss and penetration of environmental factors? The stratum
   *A. corneum.
   B. lucidum.
   C. granulosum.
   D. germinativum.

   Rationale: The stratum corneum, the outer layer of the epidermis, provides the most effective barrier to both epidermal water loss and penetration of environmental factors, such as chemicals, microbes, insect bites, and other trauma.

   Reference: p. 1441

   Descriptors:
   1. 51 2. 02 3. Knowledge
   4. IV–1 5. Nursing Process 6. Easy

6. The "true skin" is the
   A. rete ridges.
   B. epidermis.
   *C. dermis.
   D. subcutaneous tissue.

   Rationale: The dermis is often referred to as the "true skin," because it makes up the largest portion of the skin, providing strength and structure.

   Reference: p. 1439

   Descriptors:
   1. 51 2. 02 3. Comprehension
   4. IV–1 5. Nursing Process 6. Moderate

7. Of the following terms, which is used to describe red marks on the skin caused by stretching of the superficial blood vessels?
   *A. Telangiectasias.
   B. Ecchymoses.
   C. Purpura.
   D. Urticaria.

   Rationale: Telangiectasias are red marks on the skin caused by stretching of superficial blood vessels. Ecchymoses are bruises, and purpura are pinpoint hemorrhages into the skin. Urticaria are wheals or hives.

   Reference: p. 1442

   Descriptors:
   1. 51 2. 03 3. Comprehension
   4. IV–4 5. Nursing Process 6. Easy

8. Benign changes in elderly skin that appear as yellowish waxy deposits on upper eyelids are termed
   A. cherry angiomas.
   B. solar lentigo.
   C. seborrheic keratoses.
   *D. xanthelasma.

   Rationale: Cherry angiomas appear as bright red "moles," while solar lentigo are commonly called "liver spots." Seborrheic keratoses are described as crusty brown "stuck on" patches, while xanthelasma appear as yellowish, waxy deposits on upper eyelids.

   Reference: p. 1442

   Descriptors:
   1. 51 2. 05 3. Comprehension
   4. IV–4 5. Nursing Process 6. Moderate

9. When the nurse assesses the patient with vitiligo, he or she anticipates finding
   A. nail beds dusky.
   B. ruddy blue face, oral mucosa, and conjunctiva.
   C. bronzed appearance.
   *D. patchy, milky white spots.

   Rationale: With cyanosis, nail beds are dusky. With polycythemia, the nurse notes ruddy blue face, oral mucosa, and conjunctiva. A bronzed appearance, or "external tan," is associated with Addison's disease. Vitiligo is a condition characterized by destruction of the melanocytes in circumscribed areas of skin and appears in light or dark as patchy, milky white spots, often symmetric bilaterally.

   Reference: p. 1444

   Descriptors:
   1. 51 2. 03 3. Application
   4. IV–4 5. Nursing Process 6. Moderate

10. When the patient shows the nurse skin areas that are circumscribed, elevated, palpable masses containing serous fluid, the nurse recognizes that the patient is demonstrating
   A. macules.
   B. papules.
   *C. vessicles.
   D. pustules.

   Rationale: A macule is a flat, nonpalpable skin color change, while a papule is an elevated, solid, palpable mass. A vessicle is a circumscribed, elevated, palpable mass containing serous fluid, while a pustule is a pus-filled vessicle.

   Reference: pp. 1446–1447

   Descriptors:
   1. 51 2. 03 3. Knowledge
   4. IV–1 5. Nursing Process 6. Easy

11. When the nurse reviews the physician's report and physical exam and notes that the patient demonstrates multiple abdominal cicatrix, he or she observes the abdominal area for
   A. ulcerations.
   B. scales.
   *C. scars.
   D. lichenification.

   Rationale: A cicatrix is a skin mark left after healing of a wound or lesion and represents replacement by connective tissue of the injured tissue. Young scars are red or purple, while mature scars are white or glistening.

   Reference: pp. 1446–1447

   Descriptors:
   1. 51 2. 03 3. Application
   4. IV–1 5. Nursing Process 6. Moderate

12. When the nurse observes the patient's nail beds and notes transverse depressions, he or she records the observation as
   A. clubbing of the nails.
   B. paronychia.
   *C. Beau's lines.
   D. spoon nails.

   Rationale: Transverse depressions known as Beau's lines in the nails may reflect retarded growth of the nail matrix secondary to severe illness or, more commonly, local trauma.

   Reference: p. 1449

   Descriptors:
   1. 51 2. 07 3. Application
   4. IV–1 5. Nursing Process 6. Moderate

13. In which of the following types of diagnostic testing is a scalpel blade moistened with oil used to obtain tissue samples?
   A. Skin biopsy.
   B. Patch testing.
   *C. Skin scrapings.
   D. Tzank smear.

   Rationale: Skin scraping samples are obtained from fungal lesions with a scalpel blade moistened with oil so that the scraped skin adheres to the blade. The scraped material is transferred to a glass slide covered with a cover slip, and examined microscopically.

Reference: p. 1450

Descriptors:
1. 51 2. 08 3. Comprehension
4. IV–1 5. Nursing Process 6. Moderate

14. In which of the following types of diagnostic testing are secretions from a suspected lesion applied to a glass slide, stained, and examined?
   A. Skin biopsy.
   B. Patch testing.
   C. Skin scrapings.
   *D. Tzank smear.

Rationale: The Tzank smear is used to examine cells from blistering skin conditions, such as varicella and pemphigus.

Reference: p. 1450

Descriptors:
1. 51 2. 08 3. Comprehension
4. IV–1 5. Nursing Process 6. Easy

15. Which of the following types of diagnostic testing is used to differentiate epidermal from dermal lesions?
   A. Skin biopsy.
   B. Patch testing.
   C. Skin scrapings.
   *D. Wood's light testing.

Rationale: Wood's light produces ultraviolet rays, not harmful to skin or eyes, that differentiate epidermal from dermal lesions and hypopigmented and hyperpigmented lesions from normal skin.

Reference: p. 1450

Descriptors:
1. 51 2. 08 3. Comprehension
4. IV–1 5. Nursing Process 6. Moderate

CHAPTER 52
Management of Patients with Dermatologic Problems

1. The nurse follows which of the following guidelines in providing skin care and protection in bathing a patient with skin problems?
   A. Lather well with antibacterial soap.
   B. Use the friction of a towel rub to stimulate the skin.
   *C. Use pledgets saturated with oil to help loosen crusts.
   D. Use deodorant soaps in the axilla and groin areas.

Rationale: The essence of skin care and protection in bathing a patient with skin problems is as follows: Use a mild, lipid-free soap or soap substitute, rinse the area completely, and blot the area dry with a soft cloth. Avoid deodorant soaps. Pledgets saturated with oil, sterile saline, or another prescribed solution will help loosen crusts, remove exudates, or free an adherent dry dressing.

Reference: p. 1453

Descriptors:
1. 52 2. 01 3. Application
4. IV–1 5. Nursing Process 6. Difficult

2. With the goal of reversing the inflammatory process, the nurse applies which of the following general rules to skin that is acutely inflamed (hot, red, and swollen) and oozing? Apply
   A. ointment.
   *B. wet dressings.
   C. paste.
   D. cream.

Rationale: As a rule, if the skin is acutely inflamed and oozing, it is best to apply wet dressings and soothing lotions.

Reference: p. 1454

Descriptors:
1. 52 2. 01 3. Application
4. IV–1 5. Nursing Process 6. Moderate

3. With the goal of reversing the inflammatory process, the nurse applies which of the following to skin that is dry and scaly? Apply
   A. lotion.
   B. baby oil.
   C. wet dressing.
   *D. ointments.

Rationale: As a rule, in chronic conditions in which the skin surface is dry and scaly, water-soluble emulsions, creams, ointments, and pastes are used.

Reference: p. 1453

Descriptors:
1. 52 2. 01 3. Application
4. IV–1 5. Nursing Process 6. Moderate

4. In order to support the natural wound-healing process, the general rule regarding dressing changes is that
   A. all dressings should be changed daily.
   B. all dressings should be changed every 8 hours.
   *C. all chronic wounds should be left covered for 48 to 72 hours absent infection or heavy discharge.
   D. all acute wounds should be left uncovered.

Rationale: It is now thought that the natural wound-healing process should be disrupted as little as possible. Unless the wound is infected or has heavy discharge, it is common to leave chronic wounds covered for 48 to 72 hours and acute wounds for 24 hours.

Reference: p. 1454

Descriptors:
1. 52 2. 01 3. Application
4. IV–4 5. Nursing Process 6. Moderate

5. In terms of topical pharmacotherapy, the nurse recognizes that gels are
 A. lotions with oil added to prevent crusting.
 *B. semisolid emulsions that become liquid when applied to the skin or scalp.
 C. mixtures of powders and ointments.
 D. mixtures of powders and water.

Rationale: Gels are semisolid emulsions that can become liquid when applied to the skin or scalp. They are not visible after application, greaseless, and nonstaining.

Reference: p. 1457

Descriptors:
1. 52 2. 02 3. Comprehension
4. IV–1 5. Nursing Process 6. Moderate

6. Because skin irritation and itching can interfere with normal sleep, the nurse teaches the patient with a pruritic skin disorder to
 A. take naps when itching is less severe.
 B. take a warm bath at bedtime.
 C. exercise prior to bedtime.
 *D. use a bedtime routine to ease the transition from wakefulness to sleep.

Rationale: Measures to promote sleep include keeping a regular schedule for sleeping, going to bed at the same time and getting up at the same time, using a bedtime routine, and exercising regularly. In general, cool baths are recommended for pruritic skin.

Reference: p. 1462

Descriptors:
1. 52 2. 03 3. Application
4. IV–1 5. Teaching/Learning 6. Moderate

7. Acne vulgaris is characterized by the appearance of which of the following lesions?
 A. Furuncle.
 B. Carbuncle.
 *C. Comedone.
 D. Chelitis.

Rationale: Acne vulgaris is characterized by comedones (primary acne lesions), both closed comedones (whiteheads) and open comedones (blackheads), as well as papules, pustules, nodules, and cysts.

Reference: p. 1465

Descriptors:
1. 52 2. 03 3. Comprehension
4. IV–4 5. Nursing Process 6. Easy

8. Of the following skin problems, the most common fungal skin infection is
 A. impetigo.
 B. shingles.
 C. folliculitis.
 *D. tinea corporis.

Rationale: The most common fungal skin infection is tinea (called ringworm because of its characteristic appearance, like a round ring or tunnel under the skin). Tinea infections affect the head, body, groin, feet, and nails.

Reference: p. 1470

Descriptors:
1. 52 2. 03 3. Comprehension
4. IV–4 5. Nursing Process 6. Moderate

9. The nurse teaches the mother of a young child diagnosed with impetigo which of the following general guidelines?
 A. Mild soap should be used to clean the skin.
 *B. Towels that come into contact with the infected areas will infect others who then touch the towels.
 C. Topical antibiotic should be applied directly to crusted areas.
 D. Topical antibiotic should be applied once daily after bathing.

Rationale: Skin with impetigo lesions should be cleaned with an antiseptic solution to reduce bacterial content in the infected area and prevent spread. Crusts should be removed prior to topical antibiotic application, which must occur several times daily for a week. Impetigo is contagious and may spread to other parts of the patient's skin or to other members of the family who touch the patient or use towels or combs that are soiled with the exudate of the lesions.

Reference: pp. 1467–1468

Descriptors:
1. 52 2. 03
3. Application/Analysis 4. IV–3
5. Teaching/Learning 6. Difficult

10. The nurse teaches the mother of a young child diagnosed with impetigo which of the following general guidelines?
 A. Mild soap should be used to clean the skin.
 B. Impetigo is not contagious.
 *C. Crusted areas must be soaked or washed with soap solution to remove the central site of bacterial growth prior to application of topical antibiotic.
 D. Topical antibiotic should be applied once daily after bathing.

Rationale: Skin with impetigo lesions should be cleaned with an antiseptic solution to reduce bacterial content in the infected area and prevent spread. Crusts should be removed prior to topical antibiotic application, which must occur several times daily for a week. Impetigo is contagious and may spread to other parts of the patient's skin or to other members of the family who touch the patient or use towels or combs that are soiled with the exudate of the lesions.

Reference: pp. 1467–1468

Descriptors:
1. 52 2. 03
3. Application/Analysis 4. IV–3
5. Teaching/Learning 6. Moderate

11. Which of the following general guidelines should the nurse incorporate into health education for school-age children regarding pediculosis capitis?
 A. The disorder is a sign of uncleanliness.
 B. The condition spreads slowly.
 *C. Do not share combs, brushes, or hats.
 D. One thorough shampoo will kill the organisms.

Rationale: Head lice is not a sign of uncleanliness. The condition spreads rapidly, so treatment must be started immediately. Students should be warned not to share combs, brushes, or hats. Lindane (Kwell) should be used for 2 or 3 shampoos as part of therapy to prevent reinfestation.

Reference: pp. 1472–1473

Descriptors:
1. 52 2. 03 3. Application
4. IV–3 5. Teaching/Learning 6. Easy

12. Which of the following general guidelines should the nurse incorporate into health education for parents of school-age children regarding pediculosis capitis?
 A. Combs and brushes must be thrown away.
 *B. All articles, clothing, towels, and bedding in contact with the pediculi must be washed in hot water or dry cleaned.
 C. The infected child must undergo medication treatment.
 D. The organisms may be easily removed from hair shafts by combing.

Rationale: Combs and brushes may be disinfected with the prescribed shampoo. All materials potentially containing the organism must be washed in hot water or dry cleaned. All family members must be treated. The organisms are extremely difficult to remove and may have to be picked off with fingernails, one by one.

Reference: pp. 1472–1473

Descriptors:
1. 52 2. 03 3. Application
4. IV–3 5. Teaching/Learning 6. Moderate

13. The nurse teaches the patient with psoriasis that the most important principle of treatment is
 A. to follow dietary guidelines closely.
 B. to take frequent tar baths.
 *C. to remove scales gently.
 D. that psoriatic areas on the face should be treated with high-potency topical steroids.

Rationale: Genetic makeup and environmental stimuli are believed to play a role in development of psoriasis. Tar baths, an old form of treatment, are rarely used. The most important principles of psoriasis treatment is gentle removal of scales. In general, high-potency topical corticosteroids should not be used on the face and intertriginous areas.

Reference: p. 1476

Descriptors:
1. 52 2. 02 3. Application
4. IV–1 5. Teaching/Learning 6. Moderate

14. Which of the following benign tumors of the skin are caused by human papillomavirus?
 A. Actinic keratoses.
 B. Angiomas.
 *C. Verrucae.
 D. Pigmented nevi.

Rationale: Verrucae (warts) are common benign skin tumors caused by infection with the human papillomavirus, which belongs to the DNA virus group.

Reference: p. 1485

Descriptors:
1. 52 2. 05 3. Knowledge
4. IV–1 5. Nursing Process 6. Easy

15. Which of the following skin tumors represents the most common type of skin cancer?
 A. Dermatofibroma.
 *B. Basal cell carcinoma.
 C. Squamous cell carcinoma.
 D. Melanoma.

Rationale: The most common type of skin cancer is basal cell carcinoma, followed by squamous cell carcinoma. Malignant melanoma is the third most common type of skin cancer.

Reference: p. 1486

Descriptors:
1. 52 2. 05 3. Comprehension
4. IV–1 5. Nursing Process 6. Moderate

16. When the nurse teaches the patient about skin cancer, he or she uses the ABCDs of moles to emphasize which of the following guidelines?
 A. The lesion appears balanced on both sides.
 B. The border of the lesion is round.
 *C. Shades of blue within a single lesion should be reported immediately to the physician.
 D. A lesion larger than 6 mm is likely to be malignant.

Rationale: ABCDs of moles include asymmetry, irregular border, and diameter exceeding 6 mm *in combination* with another sign is significant. Colors that may indicate malignancy if found together within a single lesion are shades of red, white, and blue; shades of blue are ominous.

Reference: p. 1490

Descriptors:
1. 52 2. 05 3. Application
4. IV–3 5. Teaching/Learning 6. Moderate

17. Which type of Kaposi's sarcoma (KS) is characterized as an aggressive tumor that involves multiple body organs?
   A. Classic KS.
   B. African KS.
   *C. AIDS-related KS.
   D. KS associated with immunosuppressant therapy.

Rationale: AIDS-related KS is an aggressive tumor that involves multiple body organs. Classic KS is chronic, African KS may be chronic or progress to lymphadenopathic forms, and KS associated with immunosuppressant therapy is characterized by local skin lesions and disseminated visceral and mucocutaneous diseases.

Reference: p. 1491

Descriptors:
1. 52 2. 07 3. Comprehension
4. IV–1 5. Nursing Process 6. Difficult

18. A nurse recognizes that, in order for a skin graft to survive, which of the following conditions must be met?
   *A. The recipient site must have an adequate blood supply.
   B. The graft must have air space above its bed.
   C. The graft must remain mobile at the recipient site.
   D. Infection of the recipient cite must be controlled.

Rationale: In order for a graft to survive the recipient site must have an adequate blood supply so that normal physiologic function can resume; the graft must be in close contact with its bed; the graft must be firmly fixed so that it remains in place on the recipient site; and the area must be free of infection.

Reference: pp. 1492–1493

Descriptors:
1. 52 2. 08 3. Analysis
4. IV–3 5. Nursing Process 6. Moderate

19. The nurse teaches the patient who has undergone skin grafting which of the following general guidelines regarding donor-site care after healing?
   A. Do not use skin cream on the area.
   B. Apply cold compresses to the area.
   *C. Showering is permitted.
   D. Expose the area to sunlight to promote healing.

Rationale: A membrane dressing is transparent and permits the patient to shower. After healing, the patient is instructed to keep the donor site soft and pliable with cream. Extremes in temperature, external trauma, and sunlight are to be avoided both for donor sites and grafted areas because these areas are sensitive, especially to thermal injuries.

Reference: pp. 1494–1495

Descriptors:
1. 52 2. 08 3. Application
4. IV–3 5. Teaching/Learning 6. Moderate

20. A nurse teaches the patient undergoing which of the following types of facial surgery that cold compresses are usually applied over the treatment area for approximately 6 hours to minimize edema, exudate, and loss of capillary permeability?
   A. Chemical face peeling.
   B. Dermabrasion.
   *C. Argon laser.
   D. Carbon dioxide laser.

Rationale: Cold compresses are used after argon laser treatment. A mask of waterproof adhesive is applied post chemical face peel, while a sterile dressing is applied post dermabrasion. A wound created by carbon dioxide laser is covered with ointment and a nonadhesive dressing.

Reference: pp. 1498–1499

Descriptors:
1. 52 2. 08 3. Analysis
4. IV–1 5. Nursing Process 6. Difficult

CHAPTER 53
Management of Patients with Burn Injury

1. Which of the following terms refers to a graft derived from one part of a patient's body and used on another part of that same patient's body?
   A. Allograft.
   B. Homograft.
   C. Heterograft.
   *D. Autograft.

Rationale: Autografts of full-thickness and pedicle flaps are commonly used for reconstructive surgery, months or years after the initial injury.

Reference: p. 1502

Descriptors:
1. 53 2. 05 3. Knowledge
4. IV–1 5. Nursing Process 6. Easy

2. When the emergency nurse learns that the patient suffered injury from a flash flame, the nurse anticipates which depth of burn?
   *A. Deep partial thickness.
   B. Superficial partial thickness.
   C. Full thickness.
   D. Superficial.

Rationale: A deep partial thickness burn is similar to a second-degree burn and is associated with scalds and flash flames.

Reference: p. 1503

Descriptors:
1. 53 2. 02 3. Comprehension
4. IV–1 5. Nursing Process 6. Moderate

3. Regarding emergency procedures at the burn scene, the nurse teaches which of the following guidelines?
A. Apply ice directly to a burn area.
*B. Never wrap burn victims in ice.
C. Never apply water to a chemical burn.
D. Maintain cold dressings on a burn site at all times.

Rationale: Wrapping burn victims in ice may worsen the tissue damage and lead to hypothermia in patients with large burns.

Reference: p. 1508

Descriptors:
1. 53 2. 03 3. Application
4. IV–3 5. Nursing Process 6. Moderate

4. The first dressing change for an autografted area is performed
A. within 12 hours after surgery.
B. within 24 hours after surgery.
*C. as soon as foul odor or purulent drainage is noted.
D. as soon as sanguineous drainage is noted.

Rationale: A foul odor or purulent infection may indicate infection and should be reported to the surgeon immediately. The first dressing change is usually performed by the surgeon 3 to 5 days after surgery, or earlier in the event of purulent drainage or a foul odor.

Reference: p. 1519

Descriptors:
1. 52 2. 05 3. Comprehension
4. IV–3 5. Nursing Process 6. Moderate

5. Which of the following observations in the patient who has undergone allograft for treatment of burn site must be reported to the physician immediately?
A. Pain at the allograft donor site.
B. Sanguineous drainage at the allograft donor site.
C. Decreased pain at the allograft recipient site.
*D. Crackles in the lungs.

Rationale: Pain at the allograft donor site is anticipated since the nerve endings have been stimulated. Sanguineous drainage at the allograft donor site is anticipated since upper layers of tissue have been replaced. Decreased pain at the recipient site is anticipated since the wound has been protected by the graft. Crackles in the lungs may indicate a fluid buildup indicative of congestive heart failure and pulmonary edema.

Reference: pp. 1512–1515

Descriptors:
1. 53 2. 06 3. Application
4. IV–3 5. Nursing Process 6. Difficult

6. A major burn injury exceeds what percentage of body surface area (BSA)?
A. 10%.
B. 150%.
C. 20%.
*D. 25%.

Rationale: Burns that do not exceed 25% of the total BSA produce a primarily local response, whereas burns that exceed 20% BSA may produce both a local and a systemic response, which is considered a major burn injury.

Reference: p. 1504

Descriptors:
1. 53 2. 01 3. Knowledge
4. IV–1 5. Nursing Process 6. Easy

7. According to the American Burn Association, a second-degree burn of 15 to 25% total body surface area in adults would be classified as which type of burn?
A. Subclinical.
B. Minor.
*C. Moderate.
D. Major.

Rationale: Moderate, uncomplicated burn injury classification uses the following criteria: second-degree burns of 15–25% TBSA in adults or 10–20% in children; third-degree burns of < 10% TBSA not involving special care areas; excludes electrical injury, inhalation injury, concurrent trauma, all poor-risk patients (i.e., extremes of age, intercurrent disease).

Reference: p. 1509

Descriptors:
1. 53 2. 01 3. Analysis
4. IV–1 5. Nursing Process 6. Moderate

8. When the Emergency Department nurse is informed that a public utilities worker injured by electrical current in en route, the nurse informs the staff that the patient's damage will be treated as a
A. subclinical burn injury.
B. minor burn injury.
C. moderate burn injury.
*D. major burn injury.

Rationale: All inhalation electrical injuries are categorized as major burn injuries.

Reference: p. 1509

Descriptors:
1. 53 2. 01 3. Analysis
4. IV–1 5. Nursing Process 6. Moderate

9. A nurse monitors the burn patient's serum values for which of the following fluid and electrolyte disturbances that would be anticipated during the emergent/resuscitative phase of burn injury?
   A. Sodium excess.
   B. Decreased hematocrit.
   *C. Potassium excess.
   D. Base-bicarbonate excess.

Rationale: Anticipated fluid and electrolyte changes that occur during the emergent/resuscitative phase of burn injury include potassium excess, sodium deficit, base-bicarbonate deficit, and elevated hematocrit.

Reference: p. 1510

Descriptors:
1. 53 2. 04 3. Application
4. IV–3 5. Nursing Process 6. Moderate

10. During which of the following time periods does the nurse monitor the aged burn patient very carefully for symptoms and signs of congestive heart failure?
   A. Within the first 4 hours after burn injury.
   B. Beginning 6 to 8 hours after burn injury.
   C. Within 24 hours after burn injury.
   *D. Beginning 48 to 72 hours after burn injury.

Rationale: As capillaries regain integrity, at 48 or more postburn hours, fluid moves from the interstitial to the intravascular compartment and diuresis begins. If cardiac or renal function is inadequate, for instance in the elderly patient, fluid overload occurs and congestive heart failure may result.

Reference: p. 1511

Descriptors:
1. 53 2. 06 3. Application
4. IV–3 5. Nursing Process 6. Moderate

11. The nurse monitors the burn patient's serum values for which of the following fluid and electrolyte disturbances that would be anticipated during the acute phase of burn injury?
   A. Decreased urinary output.
   B. Potassium excess.
   C. Increased hematocrit.
   *D. Sodium deficit.

Rationale: Anticipated fluid and electrolyte changes that occur during the acute phase of burn injury include potassium deficit, sodium deficit, increased urinary output, and decreased hematocrit.

Reference: p. 1515

Descriptors:
1. 53 2. 04 3. Application
4. IV–3 5. Nursing Process 6. Moderate

12. A nurse teaches the parents of a school-age burn victim that the wound is in a dynamic state for which of the following time periods after the burn occurs?
   A. 30 days.
   B. 6 months.
   C. 12 months.
   *D. 1.5 to 2 years.

Rationale: The wound is in a dynamic state for 1.5 to 2 years after the burn occurs. If appropriate measures are instituted during this active period, the scar tissue loses its redness and softens.

Reference: p. 1529

Descriptors:
1. 53 2. 07 3. Application
4. IV–1 5. Teaching/Learning 6. Moderate

13. The nurse teaches the mother of the patient with a burn injury which of the following guidelines regarding prescribed pain medication and dressing changes? Pain medication should be administered
   A. 2 hours before dressing changes.
   *B. 30 minutes before dressing changes.
   C. at the beginning of a dressing change.
   D. as soon as the dressing change is completed.

Rationale: Prescribed pain medication should be administered 30 minutes prior to a painful dressing change to initiate its effects prior to the onset of the painful procedure, with peak activity occurring during and after the dressing change.

Reference: p. 1532

Descriptors:
1. 53 2. 06 3. Application
4. IV–1 5. Teaching/Learning 6. Moderate

14. According to the Rule of Nines, a patient who experiences burns on his anterior and posterior legs would demonstrate what percentage of body burn?
   A. 9%.
   B. 18%.
   C. 27%.
   *D. 36%.

Rationale: Each leg, anterior and posterior, would require multiplying 4 times 9% yielding a 36% total surface area of burn.

Reference: p. 1504

Descriptors:
1. 53 2. 01 3. Application
4. IV–1 5. Nursing Process 6. Difficult

15. The primary cause of nausea and vomiting after a major burn injury is
   A. fluid shift.
   B. medications.
   *C. paralytic ileus.
   D. emotional upset.

Rationale: Nausea and vomiting typically occur after a major burn injury due to paralytic ileus caused by the physiological trauma.

Reference: p. 1508

Descriptors:
1. 53 2. 03 3. Comprehension
4. IV–3 5. Nursing Process 6. Moderate

UNIT 13 SENSORINEURAL FUNCTION

CHAPTER 54 Assessment and Management of Patients with Eye and Vision Disorders

1. Which of the following abbreviations refer to the LEFT eye?
   A. OU.
   *B. OS.
   C. OD.
   D. OTC.

   Rationale: The abbreviation, OU, refers to oculus uterque (both eyes; each eye). The abbreviation OS refers to oculus sinister (left eye), while OD refers to oculus dexter (right eye). The abbreviation, OTC, refers to "over-the-counter" or nonprescription drugs, in general.

   Reference: p. 1540

   Descriptors:
   1. 54 2. 01 3. Knowledge
   4. IV–1 5. Nursing Process 6. Easy

2. Of the following eye structures, which has the function of producing clear aqueous humor?
   *A. Ciliary body.
   B. Anterior chamber.
   C. Conjunctiva.
   D. Posterior chamber

   Rationale: The ciliary body produces aqueous humor, which occupies the anterior chamber and nourishes the cornea.

   Reference: p. 1541

   Descriptors:
   1. 54 2. 01 3. Knowledge
   4. IV–1 5. Nursing Process 6. Easy

3. The eye structure that covers the sclera is termed the
   A. limbus.
   *B. palpebral conjunctiva.
   C. uvea.
   D. fornix.

   Rationale: The conjunctiva provides a barrier to the external environment and nourishes the eye, with the bulbar conjunctiva covering the sclera and the palpebral conjunctiva lining the inner surface of the upper and lower eyelids. The fornix is the junction of the two portions of conjunctiva, palpebral and bulbar.

   Reference: p. 1540

   Descriptors:
   1. 54 2. 01 3. Knowledge
   4. IV–1 5. Nursing Process 6. Easy

4. When the patient asks the nurse what it means when the optometrist tells her that her vision is 20/200, the nurse responds that the patient is able to see
   A. at 200 feet what a person with 20/20 vision sees at 200 feet.
   *B. at 20 feet what a person with 20/20 vision sees at 200 feet.
   C. at 200 feet what a person with 20/20 vision sees at 20 feet.
   D. at 20 feet what a person with 20/20 vision sees at 20 feet.

   Rationale: The fraction 20/20, the standard of normal vision, means that the person can see the letters on the line designed as 20/20 from a distance of 20 feet away. A person whose vision is 20/200 can see an object from 20 feet away that a person whose vision is 20/20 can see from 200 feet away.

   Reference: p. 1543

   Descriptors:
   1. 54 2. 02 3. Analysis
   4. IV–1 5. Nursing Process 6. Difficult

5. The nurse would use which of the following terms to describe the patient's drooping eyelid?
   A. Hyphema.
   B. Chemosis.
   *C. Ptosis.
   D. Strabismus.

   Rationale: Ptosis is the term used to describe a drooping eyelid. Hyphema refers to blood in the anterior chamber. Chemosis refers to edema of the conjunctiva. Strabismus refers to a condition in which there is deviation from perfect ocular alignment.

   Reference: p. 1540

   Descriptors:
   1. 54 2. 02 3. Comprehension
   4. IV–1 5. Nursing Process 6. Moderate

6. Intraocular pressure (IOP) is measured by which of the following methods?
   A. Indirect ophthalmoscopy.
   B. Slit lamp examination.
   C. Ultrasonography.
   *D. Tonometry.

Rationale: Tonometry is used to measure IOP by determining the force necessary to indent or flatten a small anterior area of the globe of the eye.

Reference: p. 1545

Descriptors:
1. 54 2. 02 3. Knowledge
4. IV–1 5. Nursing Process 6. Moderate

7. Which of the following terms refers to the refractive error in which the cornea demonstrates an irregular curve?
   A. Emmetropia.
   B. Myopia.
   *C. Astigmatism.
   D. Hyperopia

Rationale: Emmetropia is the term used to refer to individuals for whom the visual image focuses precisely on the macula. Myopia refers to individuals in whom the distant visual image focuses short of the retina, and hyperopia refers to individuals in whom the distant visual image focuses beyond the retina. Astigmatism refers to an irregularity in the curve of the cornea that may result in a decreased acuity of both distance and near vision.

Reference: p. 1546

Descriptors:
1. 54 2. 02 3. Analysis
4. IV–1 5. Nursing Process 6. Moderate

8. When the patient explains to the nurse that she is experiencing transient blurring of vision, halos around lights, temporal headaches, and ocular pain, the nurse recognizes the combination of symptoms as characteristic of
   A. chronic open-angle glaucoma.
   B. normal tension glaucoma.
   *C. subacute angle-closure glaucoma.
   D. acute angle-closure glaucoma.

Rationale: Subacute angle-closure glaucoma is demonstrated by transient blurring of vision, halos around light, temporal headache and or ocular pain; the pupil may also be semi-dilated.

Reference: p. 1551

Descriptors:
1. 54 2. 03 3. Analysis
4. IV–1 5. Nursing Process 6. Difficult

9. Of the following medications used in managing glaucoma, which increases aqueous fluid outflow?
   A. Beta blockers.
   B. Carbonic anhydrase inhibitors.
   *C. Cholinergics.
   D. Alpha-adrenergic agonists.

Rationale: Cholinergics increase aqueous fluid outflow by contracting the ciliary muscle, causing miosis. Beta blockers, carbonic anhydrase inhibitors, and alpha-adrenergic agonists decrease aqueous humor production.

Reference: p. 1553

Descriptors:
1. 54 2. 04 3. Comprehension
4. IV–2 5. Nursing Process 6. Difficult

10. Of the following medications used in managing glaucoma, which increases uveoscleral outflow?
   A. Beta blockers.
   B. Carbonic anhydrase inhibitors.
   *C. Prostaglandins.
   D. Alpha-adrenergic agonists.

Rationale: Prostaglandins are used to treat glaucoma by increasing uveoscleral outflow. Beta blockers, carbonic anhydrase inhibitors, and alpha-adrenergic agonists decrease aqueous humor production.

Reference: p. 1553

Descriptors:
1. 54 2. 04 3. Comprehension
4. IV–2 5. Nursing Process 6. Difficult

11. Legal blindness is defined as
   A. best corrected visual acuity of 20/70 to 20/200.
   B. best corrected visual acuity of 20/400 to no light perception.
   C. absences of light perception.
   *D. best corrected visual acuity does not exceed 20/200 in the better eye.

Rationale: Legal blindness is a condition of impaired vision in which an individual has a BCVA that does not exceed 20/200 in the better eye, or whose widest visual field diameter is 20 degrees or less. This definition does not equate with functional ability, nor does it classify the degrees of impairment.

Reference: p. 1546

Descriptors:
1. 54 2. 05 3. Comprehension
4. IV–1 5. Nursing Process 6. Moderate

12. A nurse teaches the patient who has undergone cataract extraction with intraocular lens implant to report which of the following signs or symptoms to the ophthalmologist immediately?
   A. Blurring of vision.
   B. Slight morning discharge.
   C. A scratchy feeling.
   *D. Pain.

Rationale: Postoperatively, the patient who has undergone cataract extraction with intraocular lens implant should report new floaters in vision, flashing lights, decrease in vision, pain, or increase in redness to the ophthalmologist. Slight morning discharge and a scratchy feeling can be expected for a few days. Blurring of vision may be experienced for several days to weeks.

Reference: p. 1557

Descriptors:
1. 54 2. 09 3. Application
4. IV–3 5. Teaching/Learning 6. Difficult

13. Which of the following terms refers to acute suppurative infection of the eyelids caused by Staphylococcus aureus?
*A. Hordeolum.
B. Chalazion.
C. Blepharitis.
D. Bacterial keratitis.

Rationale: Hordeolum (sty) is an acute suppurative infection of the glands of the eyelids caused by S. aureus. The lid is red and edematous with a small collection of pus in the form of an abscess.

Reference: p. 1565

Descriptors:
1. 54 2. 03 3. Comprehension
4. IV–3 5. Nursing Process 6. Moderate

14. Which of the following drugs results in miosis?
A. Atropine.
*B. Pilocarpine.
C. Timolol.
D. Acetazolamide.

Rationale: Atropine is a mydriatic agent. Pilocarpine is a miotic. Timolol is a beta blocker. Acetazolamide is a carbonic anyhydrase inhibitor.

Reference: p. 1552

Descriptors:
1. 54 2. 04 3. Comprehension
4. IV–2 5. Nursing Process 6. Moderate

15. Which of the following drugs result in mydriasis?
*A. Atropine.
B. Pilocarpine.
C. Timolol.
D. Acetazolamide.

Rationale: Atropine is a mydriatic agent. Pilocarpine is a miotic. Timolol is a beta blocker. Acetazolamide is a carbonic anyhydrase inhibitor.

Reference: pp. 1552, 1573–1574

Descriptors:
1. 54 2. 04 3. Comprehension
4. IV–2 5. Nursing Process 6. Moderate

CHAPTER 55
Assessment and Management of Patients with Hearing and Balance Disorders

1. The healthy tympanic membrane appears
A. pink.
B. red.
*C. gray.
D. white.

Rationale: The healthy tympanic membrane appears pearly gray and is positioned obliquely at the base of the ear canal.

Reference: p. 1582

Descriptors:
1. 55 2. 01 3. Knowledge
4. IV–1 5. Nursing Process 6. Easy

2. Which of the following terms refers to altered sensation of orientation in space?
A. Vertigo.
B. Tinnitus.
C. Nystagmus.
*D. Dizziness.

Rationale: Vertigo is illusion of movement where the individual or the surroundings are sensed as moving. Tinnitus refers to a subjective perception of sound with internal origin. Nystagmus refers to involuntary rhythmic eye movement. Dizziness is the term used to refer to altered sensation of orientation in space. Dizziness may be associated with inner ear disturbances.

Reference: p. 1579

Descriptors:
1. 55 2. 01 3. Knowledge
4. IV–1 5. Nursing Process 6. Moderate

3. Of the following terms, which describes a condition characterized by abnormal spongy bone formation around the stapes?
*A. Otosclerosis.
B. Middle ear effusion.
C. Chronic otitis media.
D. Otitis externa.

Rationale: Otosclerosis refers to abnormal spongy-bone formation and is more common in females and frequently hereditary. A middle ear effusion is denoted by fluid in the middle ear without evidence of infection. Chronic otitis media is defined as repeated episodes of acute otitis media causing irreversible tissue damage and persistent tympanic membrane perforation. Otitis externa refers to inflammation of the external auditory canal.

Reference: p. 1579

Descriptors:
1. 55 2. 01 3. Knowledge
4. IV–1 5. Nursing Process 6. Easy

4. Ossiculoplasty is defined as
A. surgical repair of the ear drum.
*B. surgical reconstruction of the middle ear bones.
C. incision into the tympanic membrane.
D. incision into the ear drum.

Rationale: Surgical repair of the ear drum is termed tympanoplasty. Ossiculoplasty refers to surgical reconstruction of the middle ear bones and is performed to restore hearing. Tympanotomy or myringotomy is the term used to refer to incision into the tympanic membrane.

Reference: p. 1579

Descriptors:
1. 55 2. 05 3 Comprehension
4. IV–1 5. Nursing Process 6. Moderate

5. Which of the following terms refers to surgical repair of the tympanic membrane?
   A. Tympanotomy.
   B. Myringotomy.
   C. Ossiculoplasty.
   *D. Tympanoplasty.

Rationale: A tympanotomy is an incision into the tympanic membrane. A myringotomy is an incision into the tympanic membrane. An ossiculoplasty is a surgical reconstruction of the middle ear bones to restore hearing. Tympanoplasty is surgery to repair a scarred eardrum.

Reference: p. 1579

Descriptors:
1. 55 2. 05 3. Comprehension
4. IV–1 5. Nursing Process 6. Moderate

6. Of the following tests, which uses a tuning fork between two positions to assess hearing?
   A. Whisper.
   B. Watch Tick.
   *C. Rinne.
   D. Weber.

Rationale: The whisper test involves covering the untested ear and whispering from a distance of 2 or 3 feet from the unoccluded ear, and the ability of the patient to repeat what was whispered. The watch tick test relies on the ability of the patient to perceive the high-pitched sound made a watch held at the patient's auricle. In the Rinne test, the examiner shifts the stem of a vibrating tuning fork between two positions to test air conduction of sound and bone conduction of sound. The Weber test uses bone conduction to test lateralization of sound.

Reference: p. 1583

Descriptors:
1. 55 2. 01 3. Comprehension
4. IV–1 5. Nursing Process 6. Moderate

7. When assessing the patient, which of the following conditions of the inner ear does the nurse anticipate normal hearing?
   A. Meniere's disease.
   B. Labyrinthitis.
   C. Endolymphatic hydrops.
   *D. Vestibular neuronitis.

Rationale: Meniere's disease is associated with progressive sensorineural hearing loss. Labyrinthitis is associated with varying decreases of hearing loss. Endolymphatic hydrops refers to a dilation in the endolymphatic space associated with Meniere's disease. Vestibular neuronitis is a disorder of the vestibular nerve characterized by severe vertigo with normal hearing.

Reference: p. 1596

Descriptors:
1. 55 2. 01 3. Application
4. IV–1 5. Nursing Process 6. Difficult

8. Of the following terms, which refers to the progressive hearing loss associated with aging?
   A. Exostoses.
   B. Otalgia.
   C. Sensoroineural hearing loss.
   *D. Presbycusis.

Rationale: Exostoses refers to small, hard, bony protrusions in the lower posterior bony portion of the ear canal. Otalgia refers to a sensation of fullness or pain in the ear. Sensorineural hearing loss is loss of hearing related to damage of the end organ for hearing and/or cranial nerve VIII. Presbycusis is the term used to refer to the progressive hearing loss associated with aging. Both middle and inner ear age-related changes result in hearing loss.

Reference: p. 1579

Descriptors:
1. 55 2. 01 3. Comprehension
4. IV–1 5. Nursing Process 6. Moderate

9. The nurse closely monitors the patient receiving which of the following categories of medications known to cause ototoxicity?
   A. Non-steroidal anti-inflammatory drugs (NSAIDs).
   *B. Aminoglycoside antibiotics.
   C. Opiates.
   D. Tricyclic antidepressants.

Rationale: Intravenous medications, especially the aminoglycosides (amikacin, gentamycin, tobramycin) are the most common cause of ototoxicity by adversely affecting the cochlea, vestibular apparatus, and cranial nerve VIII.

Reference: p. 1600

Descriptors:
1. 55 2. 07 3. Application
4. IV–2 5. Nursing Process 6. Difficult

10. When the nurse reviews diagnostic testing results and finds that the patient's hearing loss in decibels is 12, the nurse interprets the finding to mean that the patient should demonstrate
   *A. Normal hearing.
   B. Slight hearing loss.
   C. Mild hearing loss.
   D. Moderate hearing loss.

Rationale: Severity of hearing loss in decibels is as follows: 0–15 = normal hearing; >15–25 = slight; >25–40 = mild; >40–55 = moderate; >55–70 = moderate to severe; >70–90 = severe; >90 profound.

Reference: p. 1584

Descriptors:
1. 55 2. 02 3. Application
4. IV–1 5. Nursing Process 6. Moderate

11. When the patient demonstrates which of the following manifestations, the nurse is alert to the potential that patient may be have hearing impairment and loss?
*A. Suspiciousness.
B. Speaking in very soft tones.
C. Asks frequently for statements to be repeated.
D. Hyperresponsive to questions.

Rationale: The hearing-impaired person, who often hears only part of what is being said, may suspect that others are talking about him or her. Suspicion results. The individual with hearing loss generally speaks both in loudness and pronunciation, is reluctant to ask for repeated statements and pretends to hear, and is socially withdrawn.

Reference: p. 1587

Descriptors:
1. 55 2. 02 3. Application
4. IV–4 5. Nursing Process 6. Difficult

12. The nurse assesses the patient diagnosed with acute otitis externa for which of the following typical clinical features?
A. Fever.
B. Rhinitis.
*C. Aural tenderness.
D. Upper respiratory infection.

Rationale: Clinical features of otitis externa include persistent otalgia that may awaken the patient at night and absence of systemic symptoms.

Reference: p. 1590

Descriptors:
1. 55 2. 04 3. Application
4. IV–1 5. Nursing Process 6. Easy

13. The nurse assesses the patient diagnosed with acute otitis media for which of the following typical clinical features?
*A. Fever.
B. Edema of the external auditory canal.
C. Aural tenderness.
D. Ear pain awakening patient at night.

Rationale: Clinical features of acute otitis media include fever, upper respiratory infection, rhinitis, and bulging tympanic membrane. When the membrane ruptures, otorrhea occurs and ear pain is absent.

Reference: p. 1590

Descriptors:
1. 55 2. 04 3. Application
4. IV–1 5. Nursing Process 6. Easy

14. When the nurse notes that the patient who is wearing hearing aids in both ears exhibits whistling noise, it indicates that the
A. batteries must be replaced.
*B. aids are improperly worn.
C. volume is turned off.
D. tubing is disconnected from the aid.

Rationale: Whistling noise noted from hearing aids generally indicates that the aids are improperly made, improperly worn, or worn out.

Reference: p. 1602

Descriptors:
1. 55 2. 07 3. Application
4. IV–1 5. Nursing Process 6. Difficult

15. When the nurse reviews diagnostic testing results and finds that the patient's hearing loss in decibels is 40, the nurse interprets the finding to mean that the patient should demonstrate
A. normal hearing.
B. slight hearing loss.
C. mild hearing loss.
*D. moderate hearing loss.

Rationale: Severity of hearing loss in decibels is as follows: 0–15 = normal hearing; >15–25 = slight; >25–40 = mild; >40–55 = moderate; >55–70 = moderate to severe; >70–90 = severe; >90 profound.

Reference: p. 1584

Descriptors:
1. 55 2. 02 3. Application
4. IV–1 5. Nursing Process 6. Moderate

16. The nurse closely monitors the patient receiving which of the following categories of medications known to cause ototoxicity?
*A. Salicylates.
B. Penicillins.
C. Opiates.
D. Tricyclic antidepressants.

Rationale: At high doses, aspirin toxicity can produce tinnitus.

Reference: p. 1600

Descriptors:
1. 55 2. 07 3. Application
4. IV–2 5. Nursing Process 6. Difficult

UNIT 14 NEUROLOGIC FUNCTION

CHAPTER 56
Assessment of Neurologic Function

1. Which of the following terms refers to the inability to recognize objects through a particular sensory system?
   A. Dementia.
   B. Ataxia.
   C. Aphasia.
   *D. Agnosia.

   Rationale: Agnosia is the term used to refer to the inability to recognize objects through a particular sensory system. Agnosia may be visual, auditory, or tactile.

   Reference: p. 1608

   Descriptors:
   1. 56 2. 03 3. Knowledge
   4. IV–1 5. Nursing Process 6. Easy

2. Of the following neurotransmitters, which demonstrates inhibitory action, helps control mood and sleep, and inhibits pain pathways?
   *A. Serotonin.
   B. Enkephalin.
   C. Norepinephrine.
   D. Acetylcholine.

   Rationale: Serotonin is the neurotransmitter that demonstrates inhibitory actions, helps control mood and sleep, and inhibits pain pathways. The sources of serotonin are the brain stem, hypothalamus, and dorsal horn of the spinal cord.

   Reference: p. 1609

   Descriptors:
   1. 54 2. 02 3. Comprehension
   4. IV–1 5. Nursing Process 6. Moderate

3. Which of the following terms is used to describe the fibrous connective tissue that covers the brain and spinal cord?
   A. Dura mater.
   B. Arachnoid.
   *C. Meninges.
   D. Pia mater.

   Rationale: The meninges is the term used to describe the fibrous connective tissue that covers the brain and spinal cord. The meninges has three layers, the dura mater, arachnoid, and pia mater.

   Reference: pp. 1611–1612

   Descriptors:
   1. 56 2. 03 3. Knowledge
   4. IV–1 5. Nursing Process 6. Easy

4. Upper motor neuron lesions cause
   A. decreased muscle tone.
   B. flaccid paralysis.
   *C. no muscle atrophy.
   D. absent or decreased reflexes.

   Rationale: Upper motor neuron lesions do not cause muscle atrophy but do cause loss of voluntary control.

   Reference: p. 1619

   Descriptors:
   1. 56 2. 01 3. Comprehension
   4. IV–1 5. Nursing Process 6. Moderate

5. Lower motor neuron lesions cause
   A. increased muscle tone.
   B. no muscle atrophy.
   C. hyperactive and abnormal reflexes.
   *D. flaccid muscle paralysis.

   Rationale: Lower motor neuron lesions cause flaccid muscle paralysis, muscle atrophy, decreased muscle tone, and loss of voluntary control.

   Reference: p. 1619

   Descriptors:
   1. 56 2. 01 3. Comprehension
   4. IV–1 5. Nursing Process 6. Moderate

6. When the nurse observes that the patient has extension and external rotation of the arms and wrists and extension, plantar flexion, and internal rotation of the feet, he or she records that the patient's posturing as
   A. normal.
   B. flaccid.
   *C. decerebrate.
   D. decorticate.

   Rationale: In decerebrate posturing, the result of lesions at the midbrain, the patient has extension and external rotation of the arms and wrists, and extension, plantar flexion, and internal rotation of the feet. Decerebrate posturing is the result of lesions at the midbrain and is more ominous than decorticate posturing.

   Reference: p. 1620

   Descriptors:
   1. 56 2. 03 3. Application
   4. IV–4 5. Nursing Process 6. Moderate

7. When the nurse observes that the patient is demonstrating flexion and internal rotation of the arms and wrists, and extension, internal rotation, and plantar flextion of the feet, the nurse documents that the patient's posturing is
   A. normal.
   B. flaccid.

C. decerebrate.
*D. decorticate.

Rationale: In decorticate posturing, the result of lesions of the internal capsule or cerebral hemispheres, the patient has flexion and internal rotation of the arms and wrists, and extension, internal rotation, and plantar flexion of the feet.

Reference: p. 1620

Descriptors:
1. 56 2. 03 3. Application
4. IV–4 5. Nursing Process 6. Moderate

8. When the nurse notes that the cerebral trauma patient is limp and lacks motor tone, the nurse documents that the patient's posturing is
A. normal.
*B. flaccid.
C. decerebrate.
D. decorticate.

Rationale: Flaccid posturing, usually the result of lower brain stem dysfunction, is manifest as absence of motor function, limpness, and absence of motor tone.

Reference: p. 1620

Descriptors:
1. 56 2. 03 3. Application
4. IV–4 5. Nursing Process 6. Moderate

9. Stimulation of the parasympathetic branch of the autonomic nervous system results in
A. dilated pupils.
B. dilated bronchioles.
*C. increased peristaltic movement.
D. relaxed muscular walls of the urinary bladder.

Rationale: Parasympathetic stimulation results in constricted pupils, constricted bronchioles, increased peristaltic movement, and contracted muscular walls of the urinary bladder.

Reference: p. 1617

Descriptors:
1. 56 2. 02 3. Comprehension
4. IV–1 5. Nursing Process 6. Moderate

10. Stimulation of the sympathetic branch of the autonomic nervous system results in
*A. dilated blood vessels in the heart muscle.
B. constricted bronchioles.
C. decreased secretion of sweat.
D. constricted pupils.

Rationale: Sympathetic nervous system stimulation results in dilated blood vessels in the heart and skeletal muscle, dilated bronchioles, increased secretion of sweat, and dilated pupils.

Reference: p. 1617

Descriptors:
1. 56 2. 02 3. Comprehension
4. IV–1 5. Nursing Process 6. Moderate

11. When the nurse assesses the patient's ankle jerks and determines that they indicate a normal reflex, the nurse grades the observation as
A. 0.
B. 1+.
*C. 2+.
D. 3+.

Rationale: Reflex responses are often graded on a scale of 0 to 4+, where 0 = absent reflex; 1+ = hypoactive reflex; 2+ = normal reflex; 3+ = hyperactive reflex, and 4+ = hyperactive reflex with sustained clonus.

Reference: p. 1623

Descriptors:
1. 56 2. 03 3. Application
4. IV–1 5. Nursing Process 6. Moderate

12. When the nurse strokes the lateral aspect of the sole of the foot of the head injured patient and notes that the toes fan out and draw back, the nurse records which of the following observations?
A. Hyperactive reflex with clonus.
*B. Positive Babinski response.
C. Negative Babinski response.
D. Hypoactive ankle reflex.

Rationale: If the lateral aspect of the sole of the foot of a person with an intact CNS is stroked, the toes contract and are drawn together and the Babinski response is noted as negative. In patients who have CNS disease of the motor system, however, the toes fan out and are drawn back—demonstrating a positive Babinski response.

Reference: p. 1625

Descriptors:
1. 56 2. 03 3. Application
4. IV–4 5. Nursing Process 6. Difficult

13. Regarding neurological assessment, the nurse recalls that which of the following findings demonstrates a normal observation?
A. Negative Babinski response in all patient populations.
*B. Positive Babinskin response in the newborn.
C. Positive Babinksi response in the adult.
D. Positive Babinski response in all patient populations.

Rationale: A positive Babinski response is normal in newborns but represents serious abnormality in adults.

Reference: p. 1625

Descriptors:
1. 56 2. 04 3. Application
4. IV–4 5. Nursing Process 6. Difficult

14. When the aged patient informs the nurse that she is experiencing abdominal pain, the nurse's BEST response is to
A. document the finding.

B. assess the patient's diet for sources of roughage.
C. notify the physician.
*D. complete an in-depth physical assessment and history of the pain.

Rationale: Complaints of pain, such as abdominal discomfort or chest pain, may be more serious in the elderly than the patient's perception might indicate, due to the decreasing reaction to painful stimuli that occurs with age. The nurse's BEST response is to carefully evaluate the patient, including detailed data gathering, assessment, and physical examination.

Reference: p. 1625

Descriptors:
1. 56 2. 04
3. Application/Analysis 4. IV–3
5. Nursing Process 6. Difficult

15. To reduce the incidence of post lumbar puncture headache, the nurse suggests which of the following positions for two hours IMMEDIATELY after the procedure?
*A. Prone.
B. Supine, head of bed flat.
C. Supine, head of bed elevated no more than 15 degrees.
D. Supine, head of bed elevated 45 degrees.

Rationale: The lumbar puncture headache may be avoided if a small-gauge needle is used and if the patient remains prone after the procedure. When a large volume of fluid is removed, the patient is positioned prone for 2 hours, then flat in a side-lying position for 2–3 hours, and then supine and prone for 6 or more hours.

Reference: p. 1631

Descriptors:
1. 56 2. 05 3. Application
4. IV–1 5. Nursing Process 6. Moderate

CHAPTER 57
Management of Patients with Neurologic Dysfunction

1. The Monro-Kellie hypothesis refers to
A. unresponsiveness to the environment.
B. the brain's attempt to restore blood flow by increasing arterial pressure to overcome the increased intracranial pressure.
C. a condition in which the patient is wakeful but devoid of conscious content, without cognitive or affective mental function.
*D. the dynamic equilibrium of cranial contents.

Rationale: The hypothesis states that because of the limited space for expansion within the skull, an increase in any one of the cranial contents (brain tissue, blood, or cerebrospinal fluid) causes a change in the volume of the others.

Reference: p. 1634

Descriptors:
1. 57 2. 02 3. Comprehension
4. IV–1 5. Nursing Process 6. Moderate

2. A patient who demonstrates an *obtunded* level of consciousness
A. has difficulty following commands and may be agitated or irritable.
B. sleeps often and shows slowed speech and thought processes.
*C. sleeps almost constantly but is arousable and can follow simple commands.
D. does not respond to environmental stimuli.

Rationale: The obtunded patient sleeps almost constantly but is arousable and can follow simple commands. An obtunded patient stays awake only with persistent stimulation.

Reference: p. 1635

Descriptors:
1. 57 2. 01 3. Comprehension
4. IV–1 5. Nursing Process 6. Easy

3. An osmotic diuretic, such as Mannitol, is given to the patient with increased intracranial pressure (IICP) in order to
A. control fever.
*B. dehydrate the brain and reduce cerebral edema.
C. control shivering.
D. reduce cellular metabolic demands.

Rationale: Osmotic diuretics draw water across intact membranes, thereby reducing the volume of brain and extracellular fluid.

Reference: p. 1638

Descriptors:
1. 57 2. 03 3. Comprehension
4. IV–2 5. Nursing Process 6. Moderate

4. Which of the following positions are employed to help reduce intracranial pressure (ICP)?
A. Keeping the head flat with use of no pillow.
B. Rotating the neck to the far right with neck support.
*C. Avoiding flexion of the neck with use of a cervical collar.
D. Extreme hip flexion supported by pillows.

Rationale: Proper positioning helps to reduce ICP. The patient's head is kept in neutral position. Use of a cervical collar promotes venous drainage and prevents jugular vein distortion, which will increase ICP. Slight elevation of the head is maintained and extreme rotation of the neck and flexion of the neck are avoided. Extreme hip flexion is also avoided because the position causes an increase in intra-abdominal and intrathoracic pressures, which can increase ICP.

Reference: p. 1639

Descriptors:
1. 57 2. 03 3. Application
4. IV–3 5. Nursing Process 6. Moderate

5. Which of the following insults or abnormalities most commonly causes ischemic stroke?
A. Arteriovenous malformation.
B. Trauma.
C. Intracerebral aneurysm rupture.
*D. Cocaine use.

Rationale: Cocaine is a potent vasoconstrictor and may result in a life-threatening reaction, even with the individual's first unprescribed use of the drug.

Reference: p. 1654

Descriptors:
1. 57 2. 07 3. Knowledge
4. IV–3 5. Nursing Process 6. Easy

6. When the patient is diagnosed as having global aphasia, the nurse recognizes that the patient will be unable to
A. comprehend the spoken word.
B. form words that are understandable.
C. speak at all.
*D. form words that are understandable or comprehend the spoken word.

Rationale: Global aphasia is a combination of expressive and receptive aphasia and presents tremendous challenge to the nurse to effectively communicate with the patient.

Reference: pp. 1653, 1659

Descriptors:
1. 57 2. 06 3. Analysis
4. IV–1 5. Nursing Process 6. Moderate

7. Which of the following terms related to aphasia refers to the inability to perform previously learned purposeful motor acts on a voluntary basis?
A. Agnosia.
B. Agraphia.
*C. Apraxia.
D. Perseveration.

Rationale: Apraxia is the inability to perform previously learned purposeful motor acts on a voluntary basis. Verbal apraxia refers to difficulty in forming and organizing intelligible words although the musculature is intact.

Reference: p. 1659

Descriptors:
1. 57 2. 06 3. Comprehension
4. IV–1 5. Nursing Process 6. Moderate

8. Which of the following terms related to aphasia refers to the failure to recognize familiar objects perceived by the senses?
*A. Agnosia.
B. Agraphia.
C. Apraxia.
D. Perseveration.

Rationale: Agnosia refers to the failure to recognize familiar objects perceived by the senses. Auditory agnosia is failure to recognize significance of sounds.

Reference: p. 1659

Descriptors:
1. 57 2. 06 3. Comprehension
4. IV–1 5. Nursing Process 6. Moderate

9. Which of the following terms related to aphasia refers to difficulty reading?
A. Agnosia.
B. Agraphia.
*C. Alexia.
D. Perseveration.

Rationale: Alexia or dyslexia refers to difficulty in reading. Alexia or dyslexia may occur in the absence of aphasia.

Reference: p. 1659

Descriptors:
1. 57 2. 06 3. Comprehension
4. IV–1 5. Nursing Process 6. Moderate

10. Which of the following observations of the head injured patient must the nurse recognize as a late sign of increased intracranial pressure?
A. Disorientation.
B. Impaired ocular movements.
*C. Projectile vomiting.
D. Headache that is constant.

Rationale: Projectile vomiting may occur with increased pressure on the reflex center in the medulla. Disorientation, impaired ocular movements, and constant headache are early signs of increased intracranial pressure.

Reference: p. 1643

Descriptors:
1. 57 2. 02 3. Application
4. IV–3 5. Nursing Process 6. Moderate

11. When the nurse observes that the post-craniotomy patient is wakeful but devoid of conscious content, without cognitive or affective mental condition, the nurse recognizes that which of the following terms BEST describes the patient? The patient is demonstrating signs of
A. unconsciousness.
B. coma.
C. akinetic mutism.
*D. persistent vegetative state.

Rationale: Persistent vegetative state is a condition in which the patient is described as wakeful but devoid of conscious content, without cognitive or affective mental function. In unconsciousness, the patient is unresponsive to and unaware of environmental stimuli. Coma is a clinical state of unconsciousness in which the patient is unaware of self or the environment for prolonged periods. Akinetic mutism is a state or unresponsiveness to the environment in which the patient makes no movement or sound but sometimes opens the eyes.

Reference: p. 1644

Descriptors:
1. 57 2. 04 3. Application
4. IV–1 5. Nursing Process 6. Difficult

12. When performing endotracheal suctioning of the airway of the unconscious patient, the appropriate technique to be used by the nurse is described as
 A. lubricating the tip of the suction catheter with petrolatum.
 B. applying suction as the catheter enters the airway.
 *C. aspirating the airway as the catheter is withdrawn.
 D. inserting the catheter into the airway until it meets resistance.

Rationale: With the suction off, a whistle-tip catheter is lubricated with a water-soluble lubricant and inserted (avoiding stimulation of carina). Then the suction is turned on while the aspirating catheter is withdrawn with a twisting motion of the thumb and forefinger.

Reference: p. 1646

Descriptors:
1. 57 2. 04 3. Application
4. IV–1 5. Nursing Process 6. Moderate

13. The nurse teaches the family of the patient who has suffered a right hemispheric stroke the patient most likely will demonstrate
 A. aphasia.
 B. paralysis on the right side of the body.
 C. slow, cautious behavior.
 *D. spatial, perceptual deficits.

Rationale: Patients suffering right hemispheric strokes demonstrate paralysis on the left side of the body, left visual field defects, spatial-perceptual deficits, increased distractability, impulsive behavior and poor judgment, and lack of awareness of deficits.

Reference: p. 1654

Descriptors:
1. 57 2. 09 3. Application
4. IV–1 5. Teaching/Learning 6. Moderate

14. The nurse teaches the family of the patient who has suffered a left hemispheric stroke that the patient most likely will demonstrate
 *A. aphasia.
 B. paralysis on the left side of the body.
 C. impulsive behavior and poor judgment.
 D. lack of awareness of deficits.

Rationale: Patients suffering left hemispheric strokes demonstrate paralysis on the right side of the body; right visual field defects; aphasia; altered intellectual ability; and slow, cautious behavior.

Reference: p. 1654

Descriptors:
1. 57 2. 09 3. Application
4. IV–1 5. Teaching/Learning 6. Moderate

15. Which of the following terms is used to describe surgical division of spinal roots to control severe pain associated with metastatic malignancies?
 A. Cordotomy.
 *B. Rhizotomy.
 C. Sympathectomy.
 D. Vagotomy.

Rationale: Rhizotomy, the surgical division of the spinal roots, is also an ablative procedure and is used for controlling the severe chest pain of lung cancer and for pain relief in head and neck malignancies.

Reference: p. 1671

Descriptors:
1. 57 2. 11 3. Comprehension
4. IV–1 5. Nursing Process 6. Easy

CHAPTER 58
Management of Patients with Neurologic Trauma

1. Prior to releasing the patient who has been diagnosed as having a concussion from the Emergency Department, the nurse teaches the family or friends who will be attending the patient to contact the physician or return to the ED if the patient
 A. complains of headache.
 B. complains of generalized weakness.
 C. sleeps for short periods of time.
 *D. vomits.

Rationale: Vomiting is a sign of increasing intracranial pressure and should be reported immediately.

Reference: p. 1676

Descriptors:
1. 58 2. 02 3. Application
4. IV–3 5. Teaching/Learning 6. Easy

2. When the nurse reviews the physician's progress notes for the patient who has sustained a head injury and sees that the physician observed Battle's sign when the patient was in the Emergency Department, the nurse knows that the physician observed
 *A. an area of bruising over the mastoid bone.

B. a blood stain surrounded by a yellowish stain on the head dressing.
C. escape of cerebrospinal fluid (CSF) from the patient's ear.
D. escape of cerebrospinal fluid (CSF) from the patient's nose.

Rationale: Battle's sign is demonstrated by an area of ecchymosis (bruising) seen over the mastoid. Battle's sign may indicate skull fracture.

Reference: p. 1675

Descriptors:
1. 58 2. 01 3. Application
4. IV–4 5. Nursing Process 6. Moderate

3. Which of the following findings in the patient who has sustained a head injury indicate increasing intracranial pressure (ICP)?
A. Increased pulse.
*B. Widening pulse pressure.
C. Decreased respirations.
D. Decreased body temperature.

Rationale: Widening pulse pressure indicates increasing intracranial pressure. Additional signs of increasing ICP include increasing systolic blood pressure, bradycardia, rapid respirations, and rapid rise in body temperature.

Reference: p. 1680

Descriptors:
1. 58 2. 02 3. Application
4. IV–3 5. Nursing Process 6. Moderate

4. Which of the following nursing interventions is appropriate when caring for the awake and oriented head injured patient?
A. Do not elevate the head of the bed.
B. Encourage the patient to cough every 2 hours.
*C. Supply oxygen therapy to keep blood gas values within normal range.
D. Use restraints if the patient becomes agitated.

Rationale: The brain is extremely sensitive to hypoxia, and a neurologic deficit can worsen if the patient is hypoxemic. The goal is to keep blood gas values within normal range to ensure adequate cerebral circulation.

Reference: p. 1682

Descriptors:
1. 58 2. 02 3. Application
4. IV–1 5. Nursing Process 6. Moderate

5. Of the following stimuli, which is known to trigger an episode of autonomic hyperreflexia in the patient who has suffered a spinal cord injury?
A. Diarrhea.
B. Placing the patient in a sitting position.
C. Voiding.
*D. Applying a blanket over the patient.

Rationale: A number of stimuli may trigger this reflex: distended bladder (most common cause), distention or contraction of the visceral organs (especially the bowel—constipation, impaction), or stimulation of the skin (tactile, pain, thermal stimuli, pressure ulcer).

Reference: p. 1694

Descriptors:
1. 58 2. 06 3. Application
4. IV–3 5. Nursing Process 6. Difficult

6. When the nurse applies the Glasgow Coma Scale to the assessment of the head injured patient and determines that the patient has scored a 9, the nurse recognizes that the patient
A. is generally interpreted as comatose.
B. is within normal range, but unstable.
*C. indicates need for emergency attention.
D. has scored as a normal individual.

Rationale: The Glasgow Coma Scale (possible scores range from 3–15) is a tool for assessing a patient's response to stimuli. A score of 10 or less indicates a need for emeregency attention; a score of 7 or less is generally interpreted as coma.

Reference: p. 1682

Descriptors:
1. 58 2. 02 3. Application
4. IV–3 5. Nursing Process 6. Moderate

7. When the head injured patient is agitated from his catheter, intravenous lines, and repeated neurologic checks, the nurse's BEST intervention for preventing injury is to
A. restrain the patient.
B. administer opoids.
C. provide repeated instruction to relax.
*D. wrap the patient's hands in mitts.

Rationale: To protect the patient from self-injury and dislodging of body tubes, the nurse uses padded side rails or wraps the patient's hands in mitts. The nurse should avoid restraints, because straining against them can increase intracranial pressure or cause other injury. Opoids as a means of controlling restless should be avoided because these medications can depress respiration, constrict the pupils, and alter the patient's responsiveness.

Reference: p. 1682

Descriptors:
1. 58 2. 03 3. Application
4. IV–3 5. Nursing Process 6. Difficult

8. The population at risk for spinal cord injury is which of the following?
A. Toddlers.
B. School-age children.
*C. Young males.
D. Aged females.

Rationale: Spinal cord injury occurs predominantly in males, with young men accounting for more than 82% of all such injuries.

Reference: p. 1686

Descriptors:
1. 58 2. 04 3. Knowledge
4. IV–3 5. Nursing Process 6. Easy

9. The nurse assesses the thoracic spinal cord injury patient for which of the following features that would be typical of spinal shock?
A. Hyperactivity of reflexes.
B. Hypertension.
*C. Abrupt onset of fever.
D. Hyperventilation.

Rationale: In spinal shock, the reflexes are absent, blood pressure and heart rate fall, and respiratory failure can occur. Because the patient does not perspire on the paralyzed portions of the body because sympathetic activity is blocked, close observation is required for early detection of an abrupt onset of fever.

Reference: p. 1690

Descriptors:
1. 58 2. 05 3. Application
4. IV–3 5. Nursing Process 6. Moderate

10. When the spinal cord injured patient asks why he must wear thigh-high elastic pressure stockings, the nurse responds that the patient is at risk for development of deep vein thrombosis due to
A. dehydration.
B. transection of the spinal cord.
*C. immobility.
D. effects of medications.

Rationale: Thrombophlebitis is a relatively common complication in patients after spinal cord injury. Immobilization and the associated venous stasis, as well as varying degrees of autonomic disruption, contribute to the high risk and susceptibility for deep vein thrombosis.

Reference: p. 1693

Descriptors:
1. 58 2. 05 3. Application
4. IV–1 5. Nursing Process 6. Difficult

11. When the spinal cord injured patient demonstrates signs and symptoms indicative of autonomic dysreflexia (hyperreflexia), the nurse's BEST intervention is to
A. lower the patient's head.
*B. irrigate the patient's urinary catheter.
C. notify the physician.
D. manually remove a fecal mass.

Rationale: When autonomic hyperreflexia occurs, the patient is placed immediately in a sitting position to lower blood pressure. If a urinary catheter is in place, it should be irrigated to be certain it is patent. If a fecal mass is present, a topic anesthetic is inserted 10 to 15 minutes before the mass is removed, because visceral distention or contraction can cause autonomic dysreflexia.

Reference: p. 1694

Descriptors:
1. 58 2. 06 3. Application
4. IV–4 5. Nursing Process 6. Difficult

12. The nurse teaches the patient who has sustained a spinal cord injury resulting in paraplegia that, to promote skin integrity, the maximum amount of time that the patient should remain in any position is
A. 1 hour.
*B. 2 hours.
C. 3 hours.
D. 4 hours.

Rationale: The person with paraplegia must take responsibility for monitoring his or her skin status. This involves relieving pressure and not remaining in any position for longer than 2 hours, in addition to ensuring that the skin receives meticulous attention and cleansing.

Reference: p. 1696

Descriptors:
1. 58 2. 07 3. Application
4. IV–3 5. Teaching/Learning 6. Easy

13. The nurse teaches the patient with quadriplegia or paraplegia which of the following guidelines related to bladder management?
A. The bladder should be emptied every 8 hours.
B. Fluids should be controlled to about 1 liter per day.
C. Underwear should not be worn.
*D. Cloudy, foul-smelling urine should be reported to the physician immediately.

Rationale: The patient must monitor his or her urine for signs of urinary tract infection: cloudy, foul-smelling urine; fever; chills; or hematuria.

Reference: p. 1697

Descriptors:
1. 58 2. 07 3. Application
4. IV–3 5. Teaching/Learning 6. Easy

14. Which of the following nursing interventions are indicated in the treatment of constipation in the conscious patient at risk for development of increased intracranial pressure?
A. Enema administration.
B. Cathartic administration.
*C. Increased roughage in diet.
D. Increasing fluids to 3000 cc/day.

Rationale: The Valsalva maneuver, which can be produced by straining at defecation, raises ICP and is to be avoided. Stool softeners may be prescribed. If the patient is alert and able to eat, a diet high in fiber may be indicated. Enemas and cathartics are avoided.

Reference: p. 1680

Descriptors:
1. 58 2. 02 3. Application
4. IV–1 5. Nursing Process 6. Moderate

15. When the nurse applies the Glasgow Coma Scale to the assessment of the head injured patient and determines that the patient has scored a 14, the nurse recognizes that the patient
A. is generally interpreted as comatose.
B. is within normal range, but unstable.
C. indicates need for emergency attention.
*D. has scored as a normal individual.

Rationale: The Glasgow Coma Scale (possible scores range from 3–15) is a tool for assessing a patient's response to stimuli. A score of 10 or less indicates a need for emergency attention; a score of 7 or less is generally interpreted as coma.

Reference: p. 1682

Descriptors:
1. 58 2. 02 3. Application
4. IV–3 5. Nursing Process 6. Moderate

CHAPTER 59
Management of Patients with Neurologic Disorders

1. Which of the following terms refers to muscular hypertonicity with increased resistance to stretch?
A. Akathesia.
B. Ataxia.
C. Myclonus.
*D. Spasticity.

Rationale: Spasticity is muscular hypertonicity with increased resistance to stretch. Spasticity is often associated with weakness, increased deep tendon reflexes, and diminished superficial reflexes.

Reference: p. 1701

Descriptors:
1. 59 2. 03 3. Knowledge
4. IV–1 5. Nursing Process 6. Easy

2. Of the following terms, which refers to blindness in the right or left halves of the visual fields of both eyes?
*A. Homonymous hemianopsia.
B. Scotoma.
C. Diplopia.
D. Nystagmus.

Rationale: Homonymous hemianopsia refers to blindness in the right or left halves of the visual field of both eyes. It occurs with occipital lobe tumors.

Reference: p. 1701

Descriptors:
1. 59 2. 03 3. Knowledge
4. IV–1 5. Nursing Process 6. Easy

3. Which of the following terms is used to describe rapid, jerky, involuntary, purposeless movements of the extremities?
A. Bradykinesia.
*B. Chorea.
C. Dyskinesia.
D. Spondylosis.

Rationale: Bradykinesia refers to very slow voluntary movements and speech. Choreaform movements are rapid, jerky, involuntary and may also be observed in the face, such as grimacing. Dyskinesia refers to impaired ability to execute voluntary movements. Spondylosis refers to degenerative arthritis of the cervical or lumbar vertebrae.

Reference: p. 1701

Descriptors:
1. 59 2. 08 3. Knowledge
4. IV–1 5. Nursing Process 6. Moderate

4. Which of the phases of a migraine headache usually lasts less than an hour?
A. Prodrome.
B. Headache.
*C. Aura.
D. Recovery.

Rationale: The prodrome phase occurs hours to days before a migraine headache. The headache phase lasts from 4 to 72 hours. The aura phase occurs in about 20% of patients who have migraines and may be characterized by focal neurological symptoms. During the postheadache phase, patients may sleep for extended periods.

Reference: pp. 1702–1703

Descriptors:
1. 59 2. 02 3. Comprehension
4. IV–1 5. Nursing Process 6. Moderate

5. The most common type of brain neoplasm is the
A. angioma.
B. meningioma.
C. neuroma.
*D. glioma.

Rationale: Angiomas account for approximately 4% of brain tumors. Meningiomas account for 15 to 20% of all brain tumors. Neuromas account for 7% of all brain tumors. Gliomas are the most common brain neoplasms, accounting for about 45% of all brain tumors.

Reference: p. 1705

Descriptors:
1. 59 2. 04 3. Knowledge
4. IV–1 5. Nursing Process 6. Moderate

6. Which of the following diseases is a chronic, degenerative progressive disease of the central ner-

vous system characterized by the occurrence of small patches of demyelination in the brain and spinal cord?
*A. Multiple sclerosis.
B. Parkinson's disease.
C. Huntington's disease.
D. Creutzfeldt-Jakob's disease.

Rationale: Multiple sclerosis is a chronic, degenerative progressive disease of the CNS characterized by the occurrence of small patches of demyelination in the brain and spinal cord. The cause of MS is not known and the disease affects twice as many women as men. Parkinson's disease is associated with decreased levels of dopamine due to destruction of pigmented neuronal cells in the substantia nigra in the basal ganglia of the brain. Huntington's disease is a chronic, progressive, hereditary disease of the nervous system that results in progressive involuntary dancelike movement and dementia. Creutzfeldt-Jakob's disease is a rare, transmissible, progressive fatal disease of the central nervous system characterized by spongiform degeneration of the gray matter of the brain.

Reference: pp. 1718, 1723–1729, 1730, 1731

Descriptors:
1. 59 2. 06, 07, 08 3. Analysis
4. IV–4 5. Nursing Process 6. Difficult

7. Which of the following diseases is associated with decreased levels of dopamine due to destruction of pigmented neuronal cells in the substantia nigra in the basal ganglia of the brain?
A. Multiple sclerosis.
*B. Parkinson's disease.
C. Huntington's disease.
D. Creutzfeldt-Jakob's disease.

Rationale: Multiple sclerosis is a chronic, degenerative progressive disease of the CNS characterized by the occurrence of small patches of demyelination in the brain and spinal cord. The cause of MS is not known and the disease affects twice as many women as men. Parkinson's disease is associated with decreased levels of dopamine due to destruction of pigmented neuronal cells in the substantia nigra in the basal ganglia of the brain. Huntington's disease is a chronic, progressive, hereditary disease of the nervous system that results in progressive involuntary dancelike movement and dementia. Creutzfeldt-Jakob's disease is a rare, transmissible, progressive fatal disease of the central nervous system characterized by spongiform degeneration of the gray matter of the brain.

Reference: pp. 1718, 1723–1729, 1730, 1731

Descriptors:
1. 59 2. 06, 07, 08 3. Analysis
4. IV–4 5. Nursing Process 6. Difficult

8. Which of the following diseases is a chronic, progressive, hereditary disease of the nervous system that results in progressive involuntary dancelike movement and dementia?
A. Multiple sclerosis.
B. Parkinson's disease.
*C. Huntington's disease.
D. Creutzfeldt-Jakob's disease.

Rationale: Multiple sclerosis is a chronic, degenerative progressive disease of the CNS characterized by the occurrence of small patches of demyelination in the brain and spinal cord. The cause of MS is not known and the disease affects twice as many women as men. Parkinson's disease is associated with decreased levels of dopamine due to destruction of pigmented neuronal cells in the substantia nigra in the basal ganglia of the brain. Huntington's disease is a chronic, progressive, hereditary disease of the nervous system that results in progressive involuntary dancelike movement and dementia. Creutzfeldt-Jakob's disease is a rare, transmissible, progressive fatal disease of the central nervous system characterized by spongiform degeneration of the gray matter of the brain.

Reference: pp. 1718, 1723–1729, 1730, 1731

Descriptors:
1. 59 2. 06, 07, 08 3. Analysis
4. IV–4 5. Nursing Process 6. Difficult

9. Which of the following diseases is a rare, transmissible, progressive fatal disease of the central nervous system characterized by spongiform degeneration of the gray matter of the brain?
A. Multiple sclerosis.
B. Parkinson's disease.
C. Huntington's disease.
*D. Creutzfeldt-Jakob's disease.

Rationale: Multiple sclerosis is a chronic, degenerative progressive disease of the CNS characterized by the occurrence of small patches of demyelination in the brain and spinal cord. The cause of MS is not known and the disease affects twice as many women as men. Parkinson's disease is associated with decreased levels of dopamine due to destruction of pigmented neuronal cells in the substantia nigra in the basal ganglia of the brain. Huntington's disease is a chronic, progressive, hereditary disease of the nervous system that results in progressive involuntary dancelike movement and dementia. Creutzfeldt-Jakob's disease is a rare, transmissible, progressive fatal disease of the central nervous system characterized by spongiform degeneration of the gray matter of the brain.

Reference: pp. 1718, 1723–1729, 1730, 1731

Descriptors:
1. 59 2. 06, 07, 08 3. Analysis
4. IV–4 5. Nursing Process 6. Difficult

10. Bell's palsy is a disorder of which cranial nerve?
A. Trigeminal (V).
*B. Facial (VII).

C. Vestibulocochlear (VIII).
D. Vagus (X).

Rationale: Trigeminal neuralgia is a disorder of the trigeminal nerve and causes face pain. Bell's palsy is characterized by facial dysfunction, weakness, and paralysis. Meniere's syndrome is a disorder of the vestibulocochlear nerve. Gullain-Barré syndrome is a disorder of the vagus nerve.

Reference: p. 1753–1754

Descriptors:
1. 59 2. 09 3. Knowledge
4. IV–1 5. Nursing Process 6. Moderate

11. Guillian-Barré syndrome is a disorder of which cranial nerve?
A. Trigeminal (V).
B. Facial (VII).
C. Vestibulocochlear (VIII).
*D. Vagus (X).

Rationale: Trigeminal neuralgia is a disorder of the trigeminal nerve and causes face pain. Bell's palsy is characterized by facial dysfunction, weakness, and paralysis. Meniere's syndrome is a disorder of the vestibulocochlear nerve. Gullain-Barré syndrome is a disorder of the vagus nerve.

Reference: pp. 1753–1754

Descriptors:
1. 59 2. 09 3. Knowledge
4. IV–1 5. Nursing Process 6. Moderate

12. Meniere's syndrome is a disorder of which cranial nerve?
A. Trigeminal (V).
B. Facial (VII).
*C. Vestibulocochlear (VIII).
D. Vagus (X).

Rationale: Trigeminal neuralgia is a disorder of the trigeminal nerve and causes face pain. Bell's palsy is characterized by facial dysfunction, weakness, and paralysis. Meniere's syndrome is a disorder of the vestibulocochlear nerve. Gullain-Barré syndrome is a disorder of the vagus nerve.

Reference: pp. 1753–1754

Descriptors:
1. 59 2. 09 3. Knowledge
4. IV–1 5. Nursing Process 6. Moderate

13. The term *secondary headache* would be applicable to the patient who experiences
*A. headache associated with brain tumor.
B. migraine headache.
C. cluster headache.
D. tension headache.

Rationale: A secondary headache is associated with organic causes, such as a brain tumor or aneurysm.

Reference: p. 1701

Descriptors:
1. 59 2. 01 3. Knowledge
4. IV–1 5. Nursing Process 6. Moderate

14. Abnormal metabolism of which of the following neurotransmitters is believed to play a major role in migraine headaches?
A. Epinephrine.
B. Norepinephrine.
C. Acetylcholine.
*D. Serotonin.

Rationale: Abnormal metabolism of serotonin, a vasoactive neurotransmitter found in platelets and cells of the brain, plays a major role in the development of migraine headache.

Reference: p. 1702

Descriptors:
1. 59 2. 01 3. Knowledge
4. IV–1 5. Nursing Process 6. Moderate

15. Of the following signs and symptoms, which may occur with a migraine headache and refers to a defect in vision?
A. Paresthesia.
*B. Scotoma.
C. Myoclonus.
D. Chorea.

Rationale: Scotoma, blind spots in the field of vision, may occur in one or both eyes.

Reference: pp. 1701–1702

Descriptors:
1. 59 2. 01 3. Knowledge
4. IV–1 5. Nursing Process 6. Moderate

UNIT 15 MUSCULOSKELETAL FUNCTION

CHAPTER 60 Assessment of Musculoskeletal Function

1. Which of the following terms is used to refer to the shaft of long bone?
A. Kyphosis.
*B. Diaphysis.
C. Epiphysis.
D. Scoliosis.

Rationale: Diaphysis refers to the shaft of long bone, while epiphysis refers to the end of long bone. Kyphosis refers to an increase in thoracic curvature of the spine, while scoliosis is a lateral curving of the spine.

Reference: p. 1764

Descriptors:

1. 60 2. 01 3. Knowledge
4. IV–1 5. Nursing Process 6. Easy

2. Which of the following terms is used to refer to a lateral curving of the spine?
   A. Kyphosis.
   B. Diaphysis.
   C. Epiphysis.
   *D. Scoliosis.

Rationale: Diaphysis refers to the shaft of long bone, while epiphysis refers to the end of long bone. Kyphosis refers to an increase in thoracic curvature of the spine, while scoliosis is a lateral curving of the spine.

Reference: p. 1764

Descriptors:

1. 60 2. 01 3. Knowledge
4. IV–1 5. Nursing Process 6. Easy

3. Which of the following terms refers to lattice-like bone structure?
   A. Callus.
   B. Endosteum.
   C. Osteoporosis.
   *D. Trabecula.

Rationale: Trabecula is lattice-like bone structure, while osteoporosis refers to abnormal loss of bone mass and strength. Callus is fibrous tissue that forms at the fracture site, and endosteum is the marrow cavity lining of hollow bone.

Reference: p. 1764

Descriptors:

1. 60 2. 01 3. Knowledge
4. IV–1 5. Nursing Process 6. Easy

4. Which of the following terms refers to fibrous tissue that forms at a fracture site?
   *A. Callus.
   B. Endosteum.
   C. Osteoporosis.
   D. Trabecula.

Rationale: Trabecula is lattice-like bone structure, while osteoporosis refers to abnormal loss of bone mass and strength. Callus is fibrous tissue that forms at the fracture site, and endosteum is the marrow cavity lining of hollow bone.

Reference: p. 1764

Descriptors:

1. 60 2. 01 3. Knowledge
4. IV–1 5. Nursing Process 6. Easy

5. Which of the following terms refers to absence of muscle tone?
   A. Clonus.
   *B. Flaccid.
   C. Fasciculation.
   D. Spastic.

Rationale: Clonus refers to rhythmic contraction of muscle, while flaccid refers to a muscle that is limp, not firm, and demonstrates absence of muscle tone. Fasciculation is an involuntary twitch of muscle fibers, and spastic refers to having greater than normal muscle tone.

Reference: p. 1764

Descriptors:

1. 60 2. 01 3. Knowledge
4. IV–1 5. Nursing Process 6. Easy

6. Which of the following terms refers to having greater than normal muscle tone?
   A. Clonus.
   B. Flaccid.
   C. Fasciculation.
   *D. Spastic.

Rationale: Clonus refers to rhythmic contraction of muscle, while flaccid refers to a muscle that is limp, not firm, and demonstrates absence of muscle tone. Fasciculation is an involuntary twitch of muscle fibers, and spastic refers to having greater than normal muscle tone.

Reference: p. 1764

Descriptors:

1. 60 2. 01 3. Knowledge
4. IV–1 5. Nursing Process 6. Easy

7. Which of the following terms refers to a bone resorption cell?
   A. Osteoblast.
   *B. Osteoclast.
   C. Osteocyte.
   D. Osteon.

Rationale: An osteoblast is a bone-forming cell, while an osteoclast is a bone resorption cell. An osteocyte is a mature bone cell, while as osteon is a microscopic functional bone unit.

Reference: p. 1764

Descriptors:

1. 60 2. 01 3. Knowledge
4. IV–1 5. Nursing Process 6. Easy

8. Which of the following terms refers to a mature bone cell?
   A. Osteoblast.
   B. Osteoclast.
   *C. Osteocyte.
   D. Osteon.

Rationale: An osteoblast is a bone-forming cell, while an osteoclast is a bone resorption cell. An osteocyte is a mature bone cell, while as osteon is a microscopic functional bone unit.

Reference: p. 1764

Descriptors:
1. 60 2. 01 3. Knowledge
4. IV–1 5. Nursing Process 6. Easy

9. Which of the following terms refers MOST PRECISELY to special tissue at ends of bone?
*A. Cartilage.
B. Fascia.
C. Ligament.
D. Tendon.

Rationale: Cartilage is special tissue at ends of bone, while fascia is the fibrous tissue that covers, supports, and separates muscles. Ligaments are fibrous bands connecting bones, while tendons are cords of fibrous tissue connecting muscle to bone.

Descriptors:
1. 60 2. 01 3. Knowledge
4. IV–1 5. Nursing Process 6. Moderate

Reference: p. 1764

10. Which of the following terms refers to fibrous tissue that connects muscle to bone?
A. Cartilage.
B. Fascia.
C. Ligament.
*D. Tendon.

Rationale: Cartilage is special tissue at ends of bone, while fascia is the fibrous tissue that covers, supports, and separates muscles. Ligaments are fibrous bands connecting bones, while tendons are cords of fibrous tissue connecting muscle to bone.

Reference: p. 1764

Descriptors:
1. 60 2. 01 3. Knowledge
4. IV–1 5. Nursing Process 6. Moderate

11. Which phase of fracture healing is characterized by neovascularization?
A. Acute phase, soon after fracture.
*B. Inflammatory phase.
C. Reparative phase.
D. Remodeling phase.

Rationale: Soon after a fracture, an extensive blood clot forms in the subperiosteal and soft tissue. The inflammatory phase follows and is characterized by neovascularization and beginning organization of the blood clot. The reparative phase occurs next, characterized by formation of a callus of cartilage and woven bone near the fracture site. During the last phase, the remodeling phase, the bone cortex is revitalized.

Reference: p. 1766

Descriptors:
1. 60 2. 01 3. Comprehension
4. IV–1 5. Nursing Process 6. Difficult

12. Which phase of fracture healing is characterized by formation of a callus of cartilage?
A. Acute phase, soon after fracture.
B. Inflammatory phase.
*C. Reparative phase.
D. Remodeling phase.

Rationale: Soon after a fracture, an extensive blood clot forms in the subperiosteal and soft tissue. The inflammatory phase follows and is characterized by neovascularization and beginning organization of the blood clot. The reparative phase occurs next, characterized by formation of a callus of cartilage and woven bone near the fracture site. During the last phase, the remodeling phase, the bone cortex is revitalized.

Reference: p. 1766

Descriptors:
1. 60 2. 01 3. Comprehension
4. IV–1 5. Nursing Process 6. Difficult

13. Which type of diarthotic joints allow rotation for activities such as opening a doorknob?
A. Ball-and-Socket.
B. Hinge.
*C. Pivot.
D. Gliding.

Rationale: Ball and socket joints (hip and shoulder) permit full freedom of movement, while hinge joints (elbow and knee) permit bending in one direction. Pivot joints, such as the articulation between the radius and ulna, permit rotation such as that required for turning a doorknob. Gliding joints permit limited movement in all directions and are presented by the joints of the carpal bones in the wrist.

Reference: p. 1768

Descriptors:
1. 60 2. 01 3. Analysis
4. IV–1 5. Nursing Process 6. Moderate

14. Which of the following terms is used to describe muscle contraction that results in moving toward midline?
A. Abduction.
*B. Adduction.
C. Supination.
D. Pronation.

Rationale: Abduction refers to moving away from midline, while adduction refers to moving toward midline. Supination refers to turning upward, while pronation refers to turning downward.

Reference: p. 1770

Descriptors:
1. 60 2. 03 3. Knowledge
4. IV–4 5. Nursing Process 6. Moderate

15. Which of the following terms is used to describe muscle contraction that results turning of the extremity upward?
A. Abduction.
B. Adduction.
*C. Supination.
D. Pronation.

Rationale: Abduction refers to moving away from midline, while adduction refers to moving toward midline. Supination refers to turning upward, while pronation refers to turning downward.

Reference: p. 1770

Descriptors:
1. 60 2. 03 3. Knowledge
4. IV–4 5. Nursing Process 6. Moderate

16. Which of the following diagnostic tests is used to detect metastatic and primary bone tumors, osteomyelitis, certain fractures, and aseptic necrosis?
 A. Computed tomography scan (CT, CAT).
 B. Magnetic resonance imagery (MRI).
 C. Bone densitometry.
 *D. Bone scan.

Rationale: A CT scan is used to show in detail a specific plain of involved bone and can reveal tumors of the soft tissue or injuries to the ligaments or tendons. MRI is used to demonstrate tumors or narrowing of tissue pathways through bone. Bone densitometry is used to estimate bone density. A bone scan is used to detect metastatic disease through use of injected, bone-seeking radioisotope.

Reference: p. 1775

Descriptors:
1. 60 2. 04 3. Knowledge
4. I–1 5. Nursing Process 6. Moderate

17. In which of the following diagnostic tests are needle electrodes inserted into selected muscles?
 A. Arthrocentesis.
 B. Biopsy.
 *C. Electromyography (EMG).
 D. Bone densitometry.

Rationale: Arthrocentesis refers to joint aspiration, while biopsy refers to tissue sampling for analysis. EMG uses needle electrodes to provide information about the electrical potential of muscles and the nerves leading to them. Bone densitometry is used to estimate bone density.

Reference: p. 1776

Descriptors:
1. 60 2. 04 3. Knowledge
4. I–1 5. Nursing Process 6. Moderate

18. An elevation of which of the following blood chemistry values would be indicative of early fracture healing?
 *A. Alkaline phosphatase.
 B. Creatine kinase (CK).
 C. Serum glutamic oxaloacetic transaminase (SGOT).
 D. Aldolase.

Rationale: Alkaline phosphatase is elevated during early fracture healing, while creatinine kinase and SGOT are elevated with muscle damage. Aldolase is elevated in muscle diseases such as muscular dystrophy and skeletal muscle necrosis.

Reference: p. 1776

Descriptors:
1. 60 2. 04 3. Knowledge
4. I–1 5. Nursing Process 6. Difficult

CHAPTER 61 Musculoskeletal Care Modalities

1. Which of the following terms refers to surgical fusion of a joint?
 A. Open reduction with internal fixation (ORIF)
 *B. Arthrodesis
 C. Arthroplasty
 D. Arthrotomy

Rationale: Arthrodesis refers to surgical fusion of a joint.

Reference: p. 1779

Descriptors:
1. 61 2. 07 3. Knowledge
4. IV–1 5. Nursing Process 6. Easy

2. The nurse teaches the patient with a plaster cast which of the following general guidelines?
 A. Apply intermittent heat, as prescribed.
 B. Rest the damp cast on a hard edge until it dries.
 *C. Handle a damp cast with the palms of the hands.
 D. Maintain the casted extremity below heart level.

Rationale: The palms of the hands should be used to prevent denting the cast. Ice may be applied, if ordered, and the casted extremity should be elevated to heart level frequently.

Reference: p. 1779

Descriptors:
1. 61 2. 01 3. Comprehension
4. IV–1 5. Teaching/Learning 6. Moderate

3. Which of the following accurate statements does the nurse provide to the patient who is having a cast removed?
 A. Do not move when the saw is being applied to the cast because it may result in skin abrasion.
 B. Do not be alarmed when the saw cuts through the padding.
 C. You may rub the skin gently after the cast and padding are removed.
 *D. You may apply emollient lotion after the skin is washed and dried.

Rationale: Emollient lotion removes dead skin that has accumulated during immobilization and keeps the skin supple. The cast will not cut skin, and scissors are used to cut the padding. The patient should be taught to avoid rubbing or scratching the skin.

Reference: p. 1784

Descriptors:
1. 61 2. 02 3. Analysis
4. IV–1 5. Teaching/Learning 6. Moderate

4. When the patient who has had a leg cast removed drags his foot when ambulating, the nurse recognizes that the cast has likely injured which of the following nerves?
 A. Femoral.
 B. Popliteal.
 *C. Peroneal.
 D. Sciatic.

Rationale: Injury to the peroneal nerve as a result of pressure is a cause of footdrop (the inability to maintain the foot in a normally flexed position). Consequently, the patient drags the foot when ambulating.

Reference: p. 1780

Descriptors:
1. 61 2. 02 3. Comprehension
4. IV–4 5. Nursing Process 6. Difficult

5. Which of the following actions is MOST appropriate when the patient with a cast on his left lower leg tells the nurse that the pain is unrelenting and increasing, despite use of his PCA (patient-controlled analgesia) pump and a recent injection for pain?
 *A. Notify the surgeon.
 B. Teach the patient guided-imagery techniques.
 C. Make certain that the extremity is elevated above heart level.
 D. Increase the frequency of ice bag changes to every 15 minutes.

Rationale: Unrelenting, uncontrollable pain is a symptom of compartment syndrome. Permanent damage may result; therefore, the surgeon must be notified of the finding and provided the opportunity to examine the patient.

Reference: p. 1783

Descriptors:
1. 61 2. 02 3. Analysis
4. IV–3 5. Nursing Process 6. Difficult

6. Which of the following principles guides the nurse caring for a patient in traction?
 A. Skeletal traction may be discontinued when X-rays are obtained.
 B. Weights are never removed.
 C. Knots in the rope or footplate should rest against the pulley.
 *D. Weights must hang free and not rest on the bed or floor.

Rationale: Weights are used to apply the vector of force necessary to achieve effective traction. If they are allowed to rest on the floor or bed, they will not achieve the vector of force required. Weights may be used intermittently when prescribed by the physician and may be removed if a life-threatening situation occurs.

Reference: p. 1787

Descriptors:
1. 61 2. 03 3. Knowledge
4. IV–1 5. Nursing Process 6. Moderate

7. Of the following types of traction, which is used to treat fractures of the elbow and humerus?
 A. Buck's extension.
 *B. Dunlop's.
 C. Russell's.
 D. Cervical head halter.

Rationale: Dunlop's traction is applied to the upper extremity for supracondylar fractures of the elbow and humerus. Buck's extension and Russell's are used for lower leg fractures. Cervical head halters are used to treat back pain.

Reference: p. 1788

Descriptors:
1. 61 2. 03 3. Knowledge
4. IV–1 5. Nursing Process 6. Difficult

8. To manage skin breakdown in the patient who is treated with traction and wearing foam boots, the nurse removes the foam boots to inspect the skin, ankle, and Achilles tendon every
 *A. shift (three times a day).
 B. 24 hours.
 C. 2 hours.
 D. week.

Rationale: The nurse removes the foam boots three times a day. A second nurse is needed to support the extremity during the inspection and skin care.

Reference: p. 1789

Descriptors:
1. 61 2. 04 3. Application
4. IV–1 5. Nursing Process 6. Moderate

9. How often must the nurse inspect the pin sites of the patient in skeletal traction for signs of inflammation and evidence of infection?
 A. Every 2 hours.
 *B. Every 8 hours.
 C. Every 12 hours.
 D. Every 24 hours.

Rationale: Because of the threat of development of osteomyelitis from the wounds created by pin insertion through the fractured bone for attachment of skeletal traction, the nurse must inspect the pin site at least every 8 hours.

Reference: p. 1790

Descriptors:
1. 61 2. 05 3. Application
4. IV–3 5. Nursing Process 6. Moderate

10. Which of the following observations of the patient in traction, if made by the nurse, may indicate to him or her that the patient has developed deep vein thrombosis (DVT)?
A. Decreased circumference of the calf.
B. Calf pallor.
C. Calf coolness.
*D. Discomfort in the calf when the foot is forcibly dorsiflexed.

Rationale: Signs of DVT include calf tenderness, warmth, redness, or swelling, or a positive Homan's sign (discomfort in the calf when the foot is forcibly dorsiflexed). The nurse promptly reports such findings to the physician for definitive evaluation and therapy.

Reference: p. 1791

Descriptors:
1. 61 2. 05 3. Comprehension
4. IV–3 5. Nursing Process 6. Moderate

11. The nurse teaches the patient which of the following guidelines for avoiding hip dislocation after replacement surgery?
A. Keep the knees together at all times.
*B. Never cross the legs when seated.
C. Bend forward only when seated in a chair.
D. Refrain from positioning a pillow between the legs when sleeping.

Rationale: The affected leg should not cross the center of the body. Crossing the affected leg will result in adduction of the affected hip.

Reference: p. 1794

Descriptors:
1. 61 2. 06 3. Analysis
4. IV–3 5. Teaching/Learning 6. Difficult

12. What is the BEST response of the nurse who observes that the drainage from the patient post total hip replacement measures 400 mL in the first 24 hours?
A. Contact the blood bank to determine availability of blood for transfusion.
B. Notify the surgeon immediately.
C. Monitor the patient for signs of shock.
*D. Record the drainage.

Rationale: Drainage of 200 to 500 mL in the first 24 hours post total hip replacement is expected. By 48 hours postoperatively, the drainage in 8 hours usually decreases to 30 mL or less.

Reference: p. 1795

Descriptors:
1. 61 2. 06 3. Application
4. IV–4 5. Nursing Process 6. Moderate

13. When the patient, post total hip replacement, reports to the nurse that she heard a "popping" sensation in the affected hip, the nurse's FIRST response is to
*A. determine if there is shortening of the affected leg.
B. notify the surgeon immediately.
C. document the description in the patient's own language.
D. adjust the hip pillow.

Rationale: Since the nurse was not present to hear the sound, the nurse FIRST assesses the patient for other signs of hip dislocation, such as shortening of the affected leg, abnormal external or internal rotation of the hip, and restricted ability or inability to move the leg.

Reference: pp. 1794–1795

Descriptors:
1. 61 2. 06 3. Application
4. IV–1 5. Nursing Process 6. Difficult

14. Postoperatively, a patient who has undergone total knee replacement and has his leg placed in a continuous passive motion (CPM) machine asks the nurse what the machine does. The nurse responds that the machine
A. eliminates the need for physical therapy.
B. decreases wound drainage.
*C. promotes healing by increasing circulation.
D. strengthens the leg.

Rationale: A CPM device is used to promote healing by increasing circulation and movement of the knee joint. Physical therapy is needed for strength and range of motion exercises.

Reference: p. 1796

Descriptors:
1. 61 2. 06 3. Application
4. IV–1 5. Teaching/Learning 6. Moderate

15. The nurse teaches the postoperative orthopedic patient who is on bedrest that it is important to eat a well balanced diet with
A. large amounts of milk.
B. limited protein.
C. decreased fiber.
*D. adequate vitamins.

Rationale: A well-balanced diet with adequate protein and vitamins is needed for wound healing. Large amounts of milk should not be given to the orthopedic patient on bedrest, however, because this adds to the calcium pool in the body and requires that more calcium be excreted by the kidneys, which increases the risk for urinary calculi. Increased fiber promotes intestinal functioning.

Reference: p. 1803

Descriptors:
1. 61 2. 07 3. Analysis
4. IV–4 5. Teaching/Learning 6. Difficult

CHAPTER 62
Management of Patients with Musculoskeletal Disorders

1. Which of the following terms refers to dead bone in the abscess cavity?
   A. Involucrum.
   B. Radiculopathy.
   *C. Sequestrum.
   D. Sciatica.

   Rationale: Involucrum refers to new bone growth around sequestrum. Sequestrum is commonly found in bone abscesses caused by osteomyelitis. Radiculopathy and sciatica refer to radiating pain felt "down the leg" by the patient and is associated with nerve root impingement in the lumbar vertebral area.

   Reference: p. 1807

   Descriptors:
   1. 62 2. 08 3. Knowledge
   4. IV–4 5. Nursing Process 6. Moderate

2. When the patient preparing to undergo a myelogram asks the nurse to explain the test, the nurse's BEST response is that it is a diagnostic procedure for low back pain used to
   A. demonstrate fracture, infection, dislocation, osteoarthritis, or scoliosis.
   B. demonstrate displacement of epidural veins.
   C. used to evaluate spinal nerve root disorders.
   *D. used to demonstrate degenerative disks or disk protrusion.

   Rationale: A radiograph (X-ray) of the spine demonstrates fracture, infection, dislocation, osteoarthritis, or scoliosis, while an epidural venogram demonstrates displacement of epidural veins. Electromyogram (EMG) is used to evaluate spinal nerve roots disorders, while a myelogram is used to identify a protruding disk. When a myelogram is performed, a small amount of contrast medium is injected into the intervertebral disk to allow graphic visualization of the disc space.

   Reference: p. 1807

   Descriptors:
   1. 62 2. 02 3. Application
   4. III–1 5. Teaching/Learning 6. Moderate

3. A nurse teaches the patient with low back pain that MOST low back pain is
   *A. self-limiting.
   B. treated by surgery.
   C. caused by osteomyelitis.
   D. treated by bed rest.

   Rationale: Most back pain is self-limiting and resolves within 4 weeks with analgesics, rest, stress reduction, and relaxation. Disk degeneration is a common cause of low back pain. Bed rest is recommended for 2 to 4 days ONLY if pain is severe.

   Reference: p. 1807

   Descriptors:
   1. 62 2. 02 3. Comprehension
   4. IV–4 5. Teaching/Learning 6. Moderate

4. When the nurse raises the leg of the patient with low back pain gently, and if the patient complains of back and leg pain with such movement, the nurse recognizes that the result suggests potential
   A. deep vein thrombosis.
   *B. nerve root involvement.
   C. paresthesia.
   D. conversion reaction.

   Rationale: When the patient demonstrates pain with straight-leg raises, the nurse recognizes that the patient's response suggests nerve root involvement. Paresthesia refers to the sensations that the nurse evaluates with by assessing deep tendon reflexes.

   Reference: p. 1808

   Descriptors:
   1. 62 2. 01 3. Analysis
   4. IV–4 5. Nursing Process 6. Difficult

5. The nurse teaches the patient with low back pain which of the following general guidelines?
   A. Seek employment that will allow sitting most of the time.
   B. Bend over from the waist when picking up articles no more than 10 pounds in weight.
   *C. Shift weight frequently if you are required to stand for long periods of time.
   D. Sleep on your abdomen most of the time.

   Rationale: A patient who is required to stand for long periods should shift weight frequently and should rest one foot on a low stool, which decreases lumbar lordosis. Sleeping on one's side or on one's back with knees flexed is recommended. When lifting, the patient should bend his or her knees and tighten abdominal muscles, keeping the load close to the body while picking it up. The patient should avoid sitting for prolonged periods.

   Reference: p. 1809

   Descriptors:
   1. 62 2. 02 3. Analysis
   4. IV–1 5. Teaching/Learning 6. Difficult

6. When the patient with low back pain asks the nurse what type of exercise would be best for her, the nurse recommends
   A. jogging.
   B. running.
   *C. walking.
   D. step aerobics.

   Rationale: To promote a healthy back, the patient should avoid jumping and jarring activities. Walking outdoors and gradually increasing the distance and pace of the walk is recommended.

   Reference: p. 1810

Descriptors:
1. 62 2. 02 3. Application
4. IV–1 5. Teaching/Learning 6. Moderate

7. Carpal Tunnel Syndrome (CTS) refers to a (an)
*A. entrapment neuropathy of the median nerve.
B. impingement syndrome in the shoulder.
C. slowly progressive contracture of the palmar fascia.
D. collection of gelatinous material near the tendon sheaths and joints.

Rationale: CTS is a median nerve entrapment that occurs at the wrist. It is commonly due to repetitive hand activities but may be associated with arthritis, hypothyroidism, or pregnancy. Dupuytren's deformity is a slowly progressive contracture of the palmar fascia, which causes flexion of the fourth and fifth fingers and frequently the middle fingers, rendering them more or less useless.

Reference: pp. 1811–1812

Descriptors:
1. 62 2. 03 3. Knowledge
4. IV–4 5. Nursing Process 6. Moderate

8. Dupuytren's contracture refers to a (an)
A. entrapment neuropathy of the median nerve.
B. impingement syndrome in the shoulder.
*C. slowly progressive contracture of the palmar fascia.
D. collection of gelatinous material near the tendon sheaths and joints.

Rationale: CTS is a median nerve entrapment that occurs at the wrist. It is commonly due to repetitive hand activities but may be associated with arthritis, hypothyroidism, or pregnancy. Dupuytren's deformity is a slowly progressive contracture of the palmar fascia, which causes flexion of the fourth and fifth fingers and frequently the middle fingers, rendering them more or less useless.

Reference: pp. 1812–1813

Descriptors:
1. 62 2. 03 3. Knowledge
4. IV–4 5. Nursing Process 6. Moderate

9. A nurse teaches the patient who has been diagnosed with tendinitis of the shoulder which of the following guidelines?
A. For the first 24–48 hours of the acute phase of the tendinitis, apply cold to the shoulder.
B. Work to raise the affected arm above shoulder level at least three times daily.
*C. Support the affected arm on pillows while sleeping.
D. Use the joint as much as possible to avoid "frozen" shoulder.

Rationale: Supporting the affected arm on pillows while sleeping will keep the patient from rolling over onto the shoulder. Patients with tendinitis will experience severe pain when rolling onto the affected shoulder while sleeping and be awakened throughout the night.

Reference: p. 1812

Descriptors:
1. 62 2. 03 3. Analysis
4. IV–1 5. Teaching/Learning 6. Moderate

10. The nurse teaches the patient who is being discharged after hand surgery to report which of the following signs or symptoms, if experienced in the affected fingers, to the physician promptly?
A. Warmth.
B. Swelling.
*C. Paresthesia.
D. Pain.

Rationale: Pain and swelling are anticipated abnormal findings after hand surgery, and warmth in the fingers indicates positive circulatory status. The patient should be taught to report abnormal findings (e.g., unrelenting pain; paralysis; paresthesia; cool, nonblanching fingers), elevated temperature, and purulent drainage.

Reference: p. 1813

Descriptors:
1. 62 2. 03 3. Analysis
4. IV–4 5. Teaching/Learning 6. Moderate

11. Which of the following terms refers to a condition in which the freed edge of a nail plate penetrates the surrounding skin, either laterally or anteriorly?
*A. Onychocryptosis.
B. Corn.
C. Callus.
D. Hammer toe.

Rationale: Onychocryptosis, ingrown toenail, is a painful condition that is caused by improper self-treatment (nail-clipping technique), external pressure (tight shoes or stockings), internal pressure (deformed toes), trauma, or infection.

Reference: p. 1814

Descriptors:
1. 62 2. 04 3. Knowledge
4. IV–4 5. Nursing Process 6. Moderate

12. When the patient demonstrates a great toe that deviates laterally with osseous enlargement of first metatarsal head, the nurse recognizes that the patient is demonstrating a bunion, or
A. hammer toe.
*B. hallux valgus.
C. pes cavus.
D. morton's neuroma.

Rationale: Hallux valgus (bunion) is a deformity in which the great toe deviates laterally and in which there is a marked prominence of the medial aspect of the first metatarsal-phalangeal joint and exostosis. Hammer toe is a flexion deformity of the interphalageal joint, which may involve several toes, while pes cavus refers to a foot with an abnormally high arch and a fixed equinus deformity of the forefoot. A Morton's neuroma is a swelling of the third (lateral) branch of the median plantar nerve.

Reference: pp. 1814–1815

Descriptors:
1. 62 2. 04 3. Knowledge
4. IV–4 5. Nursing Process 6. Moderate

13. When the patient complains of throbbing, burning pain in the foot that is usually relieved when the patient rests, the nurse recognizes that the patient is MOST LIKELY demonstrating a
A. hammer toe.
B. hallux valgus.
C. pes cavus.
*D. Morton's neuroma.

Rationale: The patient is describing neuropathic pain. A Morton's neuroma is a swelling of the third (lateral) branch of the median plantar nerve. Hallux valgus (bunion) is a deformity in which the great toe deviates laterally and in which there is a marked prominence of the medial aspect of the first metatarsal-phalangeal joint and exostosis. Hammer toe is a flexion deformity of the interphalageal joint, which may involve several toes, while pes cavus refers to a foot with an abnormally high arch and a fixed equinus deformity of the forefoot. A Morton's neuroma is a swelling of the third (lateral) branch of the median plantar nerve.

Reference: p. 1815

Descriptors:
1. 62 2. 04 3. Knowledge
4. IV–4 5. Nursing Process 6. Moderate

14. The nurse teaches the patient who has undergone foot surgery which of the following general guidelines?
*A. Keep the foot elevated at heart level.
B. Change the dressing upon arriving home after surgery and as needed.
C. Refrain from wearing a shoe on the affected foot.
D. Apply weight to the affect foot to tolerance.

Rationale: The patient should not rest the foot below heart level or markedly above heart level. The initial dressing change will be performed by the surgeon. The wound dressing should be covered by special protective shoes. The patient will be prescribed weight-bearing limits, and centrally acting pain medication will affect the patient's perception of pain.

Reference: p. 1816

Descriptors:
1. 62 2. 04 3. Application
4. IV–1 5. Teaching/Learning 6. Difficult

15. Regarding the pathophysiology of osteoporosis, the nurse understands that there is an age-related increase in which of the following hormones that contributes to the development of the disease?
A. Calcitonin.
B. Estrogen.
*C. Parathyroid hormone.
D. Progesterone.

Rationale: Estrogen and calcitonin decrease with age. Parathyroid hormone increases with aging and increases bone resorption. Progesterone is not associated with the disease.

Reference: p. 1817

Descriptors:
1. 62 2. 05 3. Comprehension
4. IV–4 5. Nursing Process 6. Difficult

16. Which of the following groups of white women are at GREATEST RISK for development of osteoporosis?
*A. Small-framed, nonobese.
B. Small-framed, obese.
C. Large-framed, nonobese.
D. Large-framed, obese.

Rationale: Small-framed, nonobese white women are at greatest risk for osteoporosis. African American women, who have a greater bone mass than white women, are less susceptible to osteoporosis.

Reference: p. 1817

Descriptors:
1. 62 2. 05 3. Knowledge
4. IV–4 5. Cultural Awareness 6. Moderate

17. What is the recommended daily intake (in milligrams) of dietary calcium by menopausal and postmenopausal women?
A. 300–500.
B. 800–1000.
*C. 1200–1500.
D. 1800–2000.

Rationale: Menopausal and postmenopausal women are taught to consume a balanced diet with adequate calcium (1200–1500 mg/day). For adolescent and young (nonpregnant and nonlactating) women, 1000–1300 mg/day is recommended.

Reference: p. 1818

Descriptors:
1. 62 2. 05 3. Knowledge
4. II–1 5. Nursing Process 6. Easy

18. Which of the following vitamins is deficient in osteomalacia?
A. A.
B. C.
*C. D.
D. E.

Rationale: The primary defect in osteomalacia is a deficiency of activated vitamin D (calcitriol), which promotes calcium absorption from the gastrointestinal tract and facilitates mineralization of bone.

Reference: p. 1820

Descriptors:
1. 62 2. 06 3. Knowledge
4. II–2 5. Nursing Process 6. Easy

19. When vitamin supplementation is used to treat the patient with osteomalacia, the nurse must stress the importance of monitoring which of the following serum electrolytes?
A. Phosphorus.
*B. Calcium.
C. Magnesium.
D. Chloride.

Rationale: Because high doses of vitamin D are toxic and enhance the risk of hypercalcemia, the importance of monitoring the serum calcium level is stressed. Vitamin D raises the concentration of calcium and phosphorus in the extracellular fluid and thus makes these ions available for mineralization of bone.

Reference: p. 1821

Descriptors:
1. 62 2. 06 3. Comprehension
4. IV–2 5. Nursing Process 6. Moderate

20. When the patient with Paget's disease has been prescribed Calcitonin, the nurse recognizes that the medication is administered
*A. subcutaneously.
B. intramuscularly.
C. intravenously.
D. topically.

Rationale: Calcitonin is administered subcutaneously or by nasal inhalation. The effect of calcitonin therapy is evident in 3 to 6 months.

Reference: p. 1822

Descriptors:
1. 62 2. 07 3. Knowledge
4. IV–2 5. Nursing Process 6. Easy

CHAPTER 63
Management of Patients with Musculoskeletal Trauma

1. Which of the following terms refers to an injury to ligaments and other soft tissue at a joint?
A. Contusion.
B. Strain.
*C. Sprain.
D. Dislocation.

Rationale: A sprain is caused by wrenching or twisting motion. A strain is a "muscle-pull" from overuse, overstretching, or excessive stress, while a contusion is a soft tissue injury caused by blunt force. A dislocation is a condition in which the articular surfaces of the bones forming a joint are no longer in anatomic contact.

Reference: p. 1832

Descriptors:
1. 63 2. 01 3. Knowledge
4. IV–4 5. Nursing Process 6. Easy

2. Which of the following terms refers to soft tissue injury caused by blunt force?
*A. Contusion.
B. Strain.
C. Sprain.
D. Dislocation.

Rationale: A sprain is caused by wrenching or twisting motion. A strain is a "muscle-pull" from overuse, overstretching, or excessive stress, while a contusion is a soft tissue injury caused by blunt force. A dislocation is a condition in which the articular surfaces of the bones forming a joint are no longer in anatomic contact.

Reference: p. 1832

Descriptors:
1. 63 2. 01 3. Knowledge
4. IV–4 5. Nursing Process 6. Easy

3. Which of the following terms refers to a "muscle pull"?
A. Contusion.
*B. Strain.
C. Sprain.
D. Dislocation.

Rationale: A sprain is caused by wrenching or twisting motion. A strain is a "muscle-pull" from overuse, overstretching or excessive stress, while a contusion is a soft tissue injury caused by blunt force. A dislocation is a condition in which the articular surfaces of the bones forming a joint are no longer in anatomic contact.

Reference: p. 1832

Descriptors:
1. 63 2. 01 3. Knowledge
4. IV–4 5. Nursing Process 6. Easy

4. Which of the following terms is used to describe a partial dislocation of the articulating surfaces of a joint?
A. Dislocation.
*B. Subluxation.
C. Sprain.
D. Strain.

Rationale: A sprain is caused by wrenching or twisting motion, while a strain is a "muscle-pull" from overuse, overstretching or excessive stress. A dislocation is a condition in which the articular surfaces of the bones forming a joint are no longer in anatomic contact. A subluxation is a partial dislocation of articulating bone surfaces.

Reference: p. 1832

Descriptors:
1. 63 2. 01 3. Knowledge
4. IV–4 5. Nursing Process 6. Moderate

5. Which of the following terms is used to describe a condition in which the articular surfaces of the bones forming a joint are no longer in anatomic contact.
*A. Dislocation.
B. Subluxation.
C. Sprain.
D. Strain.

Rationale: A sprain is caused by wrenching or twisting motion, while a strain is a "muscle-pull" from overuse, overstretching or excessive stress. A dislocation is a condition in which the articular surfaces of the bones forming a joint are no longer in anatomic contact. A subluxation is a partial dislocation of articulating bone surfaces.

Reference: p. 1832

Descriptors:
1. 63 2. 01 3. Knowledge
4. IV–4 5. Nursing Process 6. Moderate

6. The nurse teaches the patient who has suffered an ankle sprain to
*A. use cold applications to the sprain during the first 24 to 48 hours.
B. expect disability to decrease within first 24 hours of injury.
C. expect pain to decrease within 3 hours after injury.
D. begin progressive passive and active range of motion exercises immediately.

Rationale: Cold applications are believed to produce vasoconstriction and reduce edema. The disability and pain are anticipated to increase during the first 2 to 3 hours after injury. Progressive passive and active exercises may being in 2 to 5 days, according to MD recommendation.

Reference: p. 1832

Descriptors:
1. 63 2. 02 3. Application
4. IV–1 5. Teaching/Learning 6. Moderate

7. Which of the following types of injuries are associated with repeated bone trauma from activities such as jogging, gymnastics, and aerobics?
A. Dislocations.
B. Colles' fractures of the wrist.
C. Metatarsal fractures.
*D. Stress fractures of the tibia.

Rationale: Dislocations are seen with throwing and lifting sports, while Colles' fractures are seen frequently with skaters and bikers. Metatarsal fractures are common in ballet and track and field athletes. Stress fractures are associated with jogging, gymnastics, and aerobics and also with basketball.

Reference: p. 1833

Descriptors:
1. 63 2. 02 3. Analysis
4. IV–4 5. Nursing Process 6. Moderate

8. The nurse anticipates which of the following problems as an early complication of a fracture?
A. Avascular necrosis of bone.
*B. Compartment syndrome.
C. Reflex sympathetic dystrophy.
D. Heterotrophic ossification.

Rationale: Early complications include shock, fat embolism, compartment syndrome, thromboembolism, DIC, and infection. Delayed complications include delayed union and nonunion, avascular necrosis of bone, reaction to external fixation devices, RSD, and heterotrophic ossification.

Reference: pp. 1837–1838

Descriptors:
1. 63 2. 06 3. Analysis
4. I–1 5. Nursing Process 6. Moderate

9. When the patient who has sustained a lower leg fracture and had a cast applied 4 hours earlier complains of deep, throbbing, unrelenting pain that is not controlled by opioids, the nurse's BEST response is to
A. maintain ice packs to the cast at the site of fracture.
B. increase the elevation of the leg.
*C. contact the orthopedic surgeon.
D. review medications for nonopioid analgesics available for administration.

Rationale: Compartment syndrome is manifested by the symptoms described. Permanent function can be lost if the problem continues for more than 6 hours. Therefore, the orthopedic surgeon must be contacted immediately.

Reference: pp. 1837–1838

Descriptors:
1. 63 2. 06 3. Application
4. IV–3 5. Nursing Process 6. Moderate

10. When the family of the young adult patient with a fractured femur informs the nurse that the patient is getting a fever and sometimes confused, the nurse most appropriately assesses the patient for which of the following fracture complications?
A. Compartment syndrome.
*B. Fat emboli syndrome.
C. Deep vein thrombosis.
D. Overmedication with opioids.

Rationale: Fat emboli syndrome is associated with long bone fractures and presenting features include hypoxia, tachypnea, tachycardia, pyrexia, and mental status changes.

Reference: p. 1837

Descriptors:
1. 63 2. 06 3. Analysis
4. IV–3 5. Nursing Process 6. Moderate

11. The nurse evaluates his or her patient teaching as effective when the patient with a closed leg fracture preparing for discharge identifies which of the following signs or symptoms that must be reported to the physician promptly?
   A. Need for pain medication every 4 hours.
   B. Decrease in pain by elevation of the leg on two pillows.
   C. Callouses developing on palms of hands from crutch use.
   *D. Cool, pale toes.

Rationale: Complications to report promptly to the physician include uncontrolled swelling and pain; cool, pale fingers or toes; paresthesia; paralysis; signs of systemic infection; signs of DVT; problems with the mobilization device.

Reference: p. 1841

Descriptors:
1. 63 2. 05 3. Comprehension
4. II–2 5. Teaching/Learning 6. Moderate

12. Which of the following expected outcomes for the elderly patient with a fractured hip would indicate to the nurse that nursing interventions to prevent neurovascular compromise have been successful?
   A. Affected extremity is pale and cool.
   B. Pain on passive flexion of the foot.
   C. Decreased sensation on sole of foot.
   *D. Moderate swelling of the affected extremity.

Rationale: Pale and cool extremity indicates decreased tissue perfusion, which may indicate neurovascular compromise. Pain on passive stretch of foot indicates nerve ischemia. Decreased sensation on sole of foot indicates tibial nerve dysfunction. Moderate swelling is to be expected but the tissue should not be palpably tense.

Reference: p. 1854

Descriptors:
1. 63 2. 08 3. Analysis
4. IV–4 5. Nursing Process 6. Difficult

13. Which of the following nursing diagnoses would be most appropriate for the patient who complains to the nurse that she continues to have pain in the leg that has been amputated?
   A. Pain related to amputation.
   *B. Sensory/perceptual alteration: phantom limb pain related to amputation.
   C. Coping, ineffective (individual) related to failure to accept loss of body part.
   D. Grieving related to loss of body part.

Rationale: The issue of phantom pain must be addressed, and the sensory/perceptual alteration provides the framework for identifying nursing interventions.

Reference: p. 1860

Descriptors:
1. 63 2. 10 3. Comprehension
4. IV–4 5. Nursing Process 6. Moderate

14. Which of the following terms describes a fracture that has several bone fragments?
   A. Greenstick.
   B. Complete.
   C. Open.
   *D. Comminuted.

Rationale: Greenstick fractures are incomplete, while complete fractures demonstrate a break across the entire cross-section of bone. An open fracture is one in which the skin or mucous membrane wound extends to the fractured bone.

Reference: p. 1835

Descriptors:
1. 63 2. 03 3. Knowledge
4. I–2 5. Nursing Process 6. Easy

15. When the nurse reviews the physician's progress note for the patient with an fracture and finds that it has been described as Grade III, the nurse recognizes that the wound is
   A. clean and less than 2 cm long.
   B. larger than 2 cm without extensive soft tissue damage.
   *C. highly contaminated and has extensive soft tissue damage.
   D. the least severe type of bone injury.

Rationale: Grade III open fractures are the most severe, highly contaminated with extensive soft tissue damage.

Reference: p. 1835

Descriptors:
1. 63 2. 04 3. Comprehension
4. IV–4 5. Nursing Process 6. Moderate

UNIT 16
OTHER ACUTE PROBLEMS

CHAPTER 64
Management of Patients with Infectious Diseases

1. Which of the following terms refers to microorganisms being present in a host without symptoms to the host?
   A. Infection.
   B. Bacteremia.

C. Fungemia.
*D. Colonization.

Rationale: Infection refers to a condition in which the host interacts physiologically and immunologically with a microorganism. Bacteremia refers to bacteria in the blood, while fungemia refers to a bloodstream infection caused by fungal microorganisms. Colonization is the term used to refer to presence of microorganisms in a host without host interference or interaction.

Reference: p. 1870

Descriptors:
1. 64 2. 01 3. Comprehension
4. IV–4 5. Nursing Process 6. Moderate

2. Which of the following terms refers to microorganisms being present in a host with the host interacting both physiologically and immunologically?
*A. Infection.
B. Bacteremia.
C. Fungemia.
D. Colonization.

Rationale: Infection refers to a condition in which the host interacts physiologically and immunologically with a microorganism. Bacteremia refers to bacteria in the blood, while fungemia refers to a bloodstream infection caused by fungal microorganisms. Colonization is the term used to refer to presence of microorganisms in a host without host interference or interaction.

Reference: p. 1870

Descriptors:
1. 64 2. 01 3. Comprehension
4. IV–4 5. Nursing Process 6. Moderate

3. Which of the following microorganisms is easily transmitted from patient to patient on the hands of health care workers?
A. Mycobacterium tuberculosis.
B. Clostridium tetani.
*C. Staphylococcus aureus.
D. Human immunodeficiency virus.

Rationale: Tuberculosis is almost always transmitted by the airborne route, and tetanus usually results from exposure to dirt. HIV is a weak virus that does not live long outside the body. Staph microorganisms are ubiquitous and easily transmitted by health care workers who fail to conduct routine handwashing between patients.

Reference: p. 1870

1. 64 2. 05 3. Comprehension
4. II–2 5. Nursing Process 6. Moderate

4. Of the following microbiologic reports, which describes the organism's antimicrobial susceptibility?
A. Smear.
B. Stain.
C. Culture.
*D. Sensitivity.

Rationale: The smear and stain provide information regarding the mix of cells present at the site at the time of specimen collection. Culture refines the information regarding the organisms, and sensitivity identifies the organism's antimicrobial susceptibility.

Reference: p. 1873

Descriptors:
1. 64 2. 02 3. Knowledge
4. I–02 5. Nursing Process 6. Easy

5. Of the following microbiologic reports, which provides information regarding the mix of cells present at the site at the time of specimen collection?
*A. Smear.
B. Drug susceptibility.
C. Culture.
D. Sensitivity.

Rationale: The smear and stain provide information regarding the mix of cells present at the site at the time of specimen collection. Culture refines the information regarding the organisms, and sensitivity identifies the organism's antimicrobial susceptibility.

Reference: p. 1873

Descriptors:
1. 64 2. 02 3. Knowledge
4. I–02 5. Nursing Process 6. Easy

6. In order to demonstrate immunity to measles, mumps, and rubella, a person is required to provide which of the following forms of evidence?
A. Having been born before 1945.
B. Documented administration of one dose of vaccine.
C. Written report by mother of nurse describing childhood infection with the diseases.
*D. Laboratory evidence of immunity.

Rationale: All people who work in health care should demonstrate evidence of immunity to measles, mumps, and rubella by one of the following: (1) having been born before 1957, (2) documented administration of 2 doses of vaccine, (3) laboratory evidence of immunity, or (4) documentation of physician-diagnosed measles or mumps.

Reference: p. 1875

Descriptors:
1. 64 2. 04 3. Knowledge
4. I–2 5. Nursing Process 6. Easy

7. The Centers for Disease Control and Prevention (CDC) are primarily responsible for
*A. reporting and tracking disease outbreaks and environmental hazards.
B. educating the public.
C. reducing the public's risk exposure.
D. treating infected individuals.

Rationale: The CDC's goals are to provide scientific recommendations regarding disease prevention and control in order to reduce disease. The Occupational Safety and Health Administration's goal is to reduce the public's risk exposure.

Reference: pp. 1873–1874

Descriptors:
1. 64 2. 03 3. Comprehension
4. I–2 5. Nursing Process 6. Moderate

8. The goal of the Occupational Safety and Health Administration is to
 A. report and track disease outbreaks and environmental hazards.
 B. educate the public.
 *C. reduce the public's risk exposure.
 D. treat infected individuals.

Rationale: The CDC's goals are to provide scientific recommendations regarding disease prevention and control in order to reduce disease. The Occupational Safety and Health Administration's goal is to reduce the public's risk exposure.

Reference: p. 1874

Descriptors:
1. 64 2. 03 3. Comprehension
4. I–2 5. Nursing Process 6. Moderate

9. The patient who has been diagnosed with shingles asks for the name of the childhood disease that is caused by the same microorganism as shingles. The nurse responds that the disease is
 A. measles.
 B. rubella.
 C. smallpox.
 *D. chickenpox.

Rationale: Varicella zoster is the causative viral agent of chickenpox and herpes zoster, shingles.

Reference: p. 1876

Descriptors:
1. 64 2. 09 3. Knowledge
4. IV–4 5. Nursing Process 6. Moderate

10. Which of the following statements regarding infection caused by Methicillin-resistant Staphylococcus aureus (MRSA) is accurate?
 A. MRSA is more virulent than other strains of staphylococci.
 *B. MRSA acquired in the hospital may persist as normal flora in the patient in the future.
 C. Only identified MRSA-infected patients are colonized.
 D. Only identified MRSA-infected patients transmit MRSA.

Rationale: There is no evidence that MRSA is more virulent than other strains of staph, and MRSA acquired in the hospital is known to persist as normal flora. The nurse must assume that every patient contact offers the possibility of MRSA exposure, and colonization by MRSA is seldom recognized. Persons who are colonized serve as reservoirs and may transmit the microorganism.

Reference: p. 1877

Descriptors:
1. 64 2. 01 3. Analysis
4. I–2 5. Nursing Process 6. Difficult

11. Of the following statements, which presents a general guideline regarding handwashing?
 A. Handwashing calls for at least 30 seconds of vigorous scrubbing.
 B. Special attention should be paid to the palm of each hand.
 *C. There is high bacterial burden between fingers.
 D. Antimicrobial soap must always be used.

Rationale: Effective handwashing calls for at least 10 seconds of vigorous scrubbing with special attention to the area around nail beds and between fingers where there is high bacterial burden. Antimicrobial handwashing agents should be used in the intensive care unit and when the patient is known to be colonized with antibiotic-resistant bacteria.

Reference: p. 1878

Descriptors:
1. 64 2. 09 3. Knowledge
4. I–2 5. Nursing process 6. Easy

12. Droplet precautions must be used when caring for the patient demonstrating
 A. measles.
 *B. streptococcus (Group A) infection (ex. pharyngitis).
 C. clostridium difficile infection.
 D. herpes simplex viral infection.

Rationale: Airborne precautions are indicated for patients with measles, while contact precautions are indicated for patients with C. difficile and herpes simplex. Standard precautions apply to all forms of infection.

Reference: p. 1880

Descriptors:
1. 64 2. 09 3. Analysis
4. I–2 5. Nursing Process 6. Difficult

13. The nurse teaches which of the following patients the importance of antibiotic prophylaxis for events and procedures that may introduce the risk of endocarditis? The patient who has
 A. undergone coronary artery bypass.
 B. had a below-knee amputation.
 *C. undergone aortic valve replacement.
 D. had resection of a lobe of the lung.

Rationale: Patients with valvular disease, congenital heart disease, intracardiac prostheses, and previous endocarditis should be taught the value of antibiotic proplylaxis for events and procedures that may introduce risk of endocarditis.

Reference: p. 1897

Descriptors:
1. 64 2. 09 3. Comprehension
4. II–2 5. Teaching/Learning 6. Moderate

14. Which of the following signs or symptoms, if demonstrated by the patient with recognized infection, may indicate onset of septic shock?
 A. Bradycardia.
 B. Subnormal temperature.
 *C. Hypoxemia.
 D. Polyuria.

Rationale: Signs of septic shock include fever, tachycardia (>90 beats/minute), tachypnea (> 20 respirations/minute), change of mental status, hypoxemia, elevated lactate levels, and urine output less than 30 cc/hour.

Reference: p. 1896

Descriptors:
1. 64 2. 09 3. Analysis
4. II–2 5. Nursing Process 6. Moderate

15. Which of the following statements used in promoting disease reduction through influenza vaccination programs is accurate?
 A. Once a person is immunized with an influenza vaccine, repeat immunization is unnecessary.
 *B. Although less effective in the elderly, influenza vaccine decreases the severity of the illness in those who do get infected.
 C. The vaccine is not recommended for individuals with chronic pulmonary disease.
 D. The vaccine is not effective in preventing pneumonia and hospitalization in those who become infected.

Rationale: Each year a new vaccine is available; therefore, annual vaccination is recommended. It is recommended for those with chronic pulmonary or cardiovascular disease, diabetes, immunosuppression, or renal dysfunction. The vaccine is 50 to 70% effective in preventing pneumonia and hospitalization of those who get infected with the disease.

Reference: p. 1876

Descriptors:
1. 64 2. 09 3. Comprehension
4. II–2 5. Nursing Process 6. Moderate

CHAPTER 65
Emergency Nursing

1. Which of the following terms is used to describe minor injuries or illnesses requiring first-aid level of management?
 A. Triage.
 *B. Urgent.
 C. Emergent.
 D. Immediate.

Rationale: The term, urgent, is used to denote individuals who require first aid, but not immediate treatment.

Reference: p. 1902

Descriptors:
1. 65 2. 02 3. Knowledge
4. I–1 5. Nursing Process 6. Easy

2. When field triage has occurred and the patient is admitted to the ED with a yellow tag, the ED nurse recognizes that the tag indicates that the patient requires which type of care?
 A. Emergent.
 *B. Immediate.
 C. Urgent.
 D. Psychological support.

Rationale: A yellow tag from field triage indicates the patient has a nonacute, non-lifethreatening injury or illness requiring attention and management without significant delay.

Reference: p. 1902

Descriptors:
1. 65 2. 02 3. Knowledge
4. I–1 5. Nursing Process 6. Easy

3. When the patient arrives at the emergency room and is unconscious, which of the following actions by the nurse is most important regarding obtaining consent to examine and treat?
 A. Ask the physician to sign the consent form.
 B. Contact the nearest relative.
 C. Seek a court order for treatment.
 *D. Document the patient's critical status in his or her medical record.

Rationale: Although the consent to examine and treat is required, if the patient is unconscious and brought to the ED without family or friends, the information is documented and treatment is not delayed.

Reference: pp. 1903–1904

Descriptors:
1. 65 2. 01 3. Analysis 4. I–2
5. Nursing Process/Documentation 6. Difficult

4. When family members arrive at the ED and are informed that the family member has died, the nurse responds with which of the following actions?
 A. Offer to obtain a physician order for sedation.
 B. Volunteer details of the event leading to the death.
 C. Inform the family members that the patient has "passed on."
 *D. Show acceptance of the deceased's body by touching when the family members view the body.

Rationale: Sedation may mask grieving, and the nurse must avoid euphemisms and volunteering unnecessary information (e.g., patient was drinking and driving). When the nurse touches the body, it gives the family "permission" to touch the body and may help the family integrate the loss.

Reference: p. 1904

Descriptors:
1. 65 2. 01 3. Analysis
4. IV–1 5. Caring 6. Difficult

5. Which of the following injuries, if demonstrated by the patient entering the ED, would take HIGHEST priority?
 A. Open leg fracture.
 B. Open head injury.
 *C. Stabbing to the chest.
 D. Traumatic amputation of thumb.

Rationale: Only a few conditions, such as obstructed airway or a sucking chest wound, take precedence over control of hemorrhage. Stabbing to the chest generally results in a sucking chest wound that can result in lung collapse and mediastinal shift causing death.

Reference: p. 1905

Descriptors:
1. 65 2. 02 3. Analysis
4. IV–3 5. Nursing Process 6. Difficult

6. Which of the following signs or symptoms, if observed by the nurse in the patient who has sustained multiple trauma but was admitted awake, alert, and oriented, would most likely indicate internal bleeding?
 A. Complaints of increased pain at wound sites.
 B. Decreased pulse rate.
 C. Increased blood pressure.
 *D. Complaints of thirst.

Rationale: Complaints of thirst accompanied by apprehension may indicate internal bleeding. With shock, the nurse would anticipate that the pulse would increase and the blood pressure would decrease.

Reference: p. 1909

Descriptors:
1. 65 2. 04 3. Comprehension
4. IV–4 5. Nursing Process 6. Moderate

7. Which of the following blood types *must* be infused to treat massive blood loss in the newly admitted female patient of childbearing age?
 A. AB positive.
 B. AB negative.
 C. O positive.
 *D. O negative.

Rationale: Packed red blood cells are infused when there is massive blood loss (O negative is used in women of childbearing age and O positive is used for men and postmenopausal women).

Reference: p. 1905

Descriptors:
1. 65 2. 03 3. Analysis
4. IV–4 5. Nursing Process 6. Moderate

8. For which of the following conscious patients are chest thrusts recommended to manage a foreign body airway obstruction?
 A. Overweight child, 8 years and under.
 B. Elderly adult of normal weight.
 *C. Female demonstrating late stage of pregnancy.
 D. Slender, middle-aged adult.

Rationale: Chest thrusts are used only in the advanced stages of pregnancy or in the markedly obese person who requires intervention for foreign body airway obstruction.

Reference: p. 1906

Descriptors:
1. 65 2. 02 3. Knowledge
4. I–2 5. Nursing Process 6. Moderate

9. Why must the nurse be careful not to cut through or disrupt any tears, holes, bloodstains, or dirt present on the clothing of the patient who has experienced trauma?
 A. The clothing is property of another and must be treated with care.
 B. Such care will facilitate repair and salvage of the clothing.
 *C. The clothing of the trauma victim is potential evidence with legal implications.
 D. Such care will decrease trauma to the family member receiving the clothing.

Rationale: Trauma in any patient (living or dead) has potential legal, or forensic, implications. Clothing itself, as well as patterns of stains, debris, etc., are sources of potential evidence and must be preserved.

Reference: p. 1910

Descriptors:
1. 65 2. 02
3. I–1 4. Application
5. Nursing Process 6. Moderate

10. Which of the following activities does the nurse teach the patient who has experienced frostbite to the extremities?
 A. Prior to rewarming, massage the extremities to restore circulation.
 B. After rewarming, open blebs that form on the skin with gentle pressure.
 *C. After rewarming, actively move the affected digits hourly.
 D. As part of rewarming, apply hot compresses to the tissues.

Rationale: Massage, opening of blebs, and use of hot compresses are contraindicated in the treatment of frostbite. Hourly active motion of the affected digits is encouraged to promote maximal restoration of function and to prevent contractures.

Reference: p. 1915

Descriptors:
1. 65 2. 05 3. IV–4
4. Analysis 5. Nursing Process 6. Difficult

11. Vomiting is INDUCED when the patient has ingested which of the following substances?
*A. A bottle of baby aspirin.
B. Toilet bowl cleaner.
C. Calculator battery.
D. Kerosene.

Rationale: Vomiting is NOT induced with alkaline or acid products (B, C) or petroleum distillates (D). It is induced with supervision in salicylate poisoning.

Reference: pp. 1919–1920

Descriptors:
1. 65 2. 06 3. Comprehension
4. I–2 5. Nursing Process 6. Moderate

12. When the nurse is assisting with gastric lavage of the obtunded patient who has ingested a known poison, he or she
A. places the patient in a left lateral position with the head elevated 30 degrees.
B. instills the antidote and then aspirates gastric contents.
C. informs the conscious patient that an endotracheal tube must be placed prior to lavage.
*D. lubricates the tube with a water-soluble lubricant.

Rationale: The patient's head is lowered 15 degrees, and gastric contents are aspirated and sent for analysis prior to instillation of any substance. The unconscious patient will undergo endotracheal intubation, and oil-based lubricants must not be used.

Reference: pp. 1920–1921

Descriptors:
1. 65 2. 06 3. Analysis
4. IV–1 5. Nursing Process 6. Difficult

13. When the nurse suspects that the aged patient admitted to the ED with areas of skin hemorrhage at various stages of resolution may be a victim of maltreatment, which of the following questions is phrased appropriately?
A. "Who's been hitting you?"
B. "Where did you get these bruises?"
*C. "Has anyone failed to help you take care of yourself when you needed help?"
D. "Do you have a balance problem?"

Rationale: Questions must be open-ended, nonaccusatory, and nonconfrontational. The nurse encourages the patient to confide in him or her and indicates that the nurse is in a position to protect the patient's safety.

Reference: p. 1927

Descriptors:
1. 65 2. 01 3. Application
4. I–2 5. Nursing Process 6. Moderate

14. When the alert patient is admitted to the ED with a severe laceration of the lower leg, the nurse's FIRST action is to
A. lower the limb.
B. apply a tourniquet.
C. establish a patent IV site.
*D. apply a sterile pressure dressing.

Rationale: Most bleeding can be stopped by applying direct pressure over the wound, unless an artery has been severed. Limbs should be elevated, and a tourniquest is used only as a last resort when hemorrhage cannot be controlled any other way.

Reference: p. 1908

Descriptors:
1. 65 2. 02 3. Application
4. I–1 5. Nursing Process 6. Moderate

15. Completion of which of the following activities by the nurse is most critical to the patient who is awake, alert, and oriented but known to have lost a large amount of blood from multiple wounds when admitted to the ED?
A. Providing ventilatory support.
*B. Establishing a patent intravenous access site.
C. Obtaining specimens for arterial blood gas level, blood chemistries, and hemoglobin and hematocrit.
D. Administering pain medication.

Rationale: An awake, alert, and oriented person is not demonstrating respiratory difficulty and appears to be tolerating his or her pain. Restoration of the circulating blood volume is accomplished with rapid fluid and blood replacement as prescribed based upon ABG levels, chemistry studies, and hemoglobin and hematocrit values.

Reference: pp. 1908–1909

Descriptors:
1. 65 2. 04 3. IV–2
4. Synthesis 5. Nursing Process 6. Difficult

16. The ED nurse anticipates administration of which of the following medications to the patient admitted after stepping on a nest of yellow-jacket insects, suffering multiple stings, and demonstrating signs of an anaphylactic reaction?
A. Antivenin.
*B. Epinephrine.
C. Morphine.
D. Benadryl.

Rationale: Aqueous epinephrine (1:1000 dilution) as prescribed is administered to provide rapid relief of hypersensitivity reactions. Antivenin is used for snake bites, and morphine is contraindicated due to respiratory depression effects. While benadryl is antihistaminic in action and effect, it is not used to treat anaphylactic reactions.

Reference: pp. 1917–1918

Descriptors:

1. 65	2. 02	3. Analysis
4. IV–2	5. Nursing Process	6. Moderate

17. The sexual assault nurse examiner performs which of the following activities in the care of the rape victim?
    A. Shaving all pubic hair for laboratory analysis.
    B. Using ample lubricant on the speculum for the pelvic examination.
    *C. Offering antibiotic prophylaxis for exposure to STDs.
    D. Placing each item of clothing in a separate plastic bag.

Rationale: Pubic hair is combined or trimmed for sampling and plastic bags are not used because they retain moisture, which promotes mold and mildew that can destroy evidence. Water is used to lubricate the speculum because chemicals in lubricants may interfere with testing of specimens obtained. Rocepth IM and Vibramycin orally may be prescribed for prophylaxis against gonorrhea, syphyllis, and chlamydia.

Reference: p. 1928

Descriptors:

1. 65	2. 08	3. Analysis
4. I–1	5. Nursing Process	6. Difficult

18. Which of the following interventions is indicated early in the treatment of the overactive patient who has been admitted to the ED after a "bad reaction" to a hallucinogen?
    A. Application of restraints.
    B. Administration of psychotropic medication.
    C. Seeking police protection.
    *D. Telling the patient, "I am here to help you."

Rationale: Approaching the patient with a calm, confident, and firm manner is therapeutic and has a calming effect. Restraints are used as a last resort and as ordered, and police should be nearby if the patient is potentially violent.

Reference: p. 1929

Descriptors:

1. 65	2. 09	3. Application
4. I–2	5. Nursing Process	6. Difficult